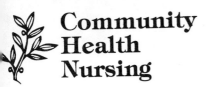

**Community
Health
Nursing**

Community Health Nursing
Patterns and Practice
Second Edition

Sarah Ellen Archer, R.N., Dr.P.H.
University of California,
San Francisco

Ruth P. Fleshman, R.N., Ph.D.
Nursing Dynamics Corporation
Mill Valley, California

Duxbury Press, North Scituate, Massachusetts

Community Health Nursing: Patterns and Practice, 2nd edition, was edited and prepared for composition by *Sylvia Dovner* Interior design was provided by *Dorothy Booth.* The cover was designed by *Elizabeth Rotchford.*

Duxbury Press
A Division of Wadsworth, Inc.

Library of Congress Cataloging in Publication Data
Archer, Sarah Ellen.
  Community health nursing.
  Bibliography: p.
  Includes index.
  1. Community health nursing.   I. Fleshman,
Ruth P., joint author.   II. Title.
RT98.A73   1979   610.73'43   78–12720
ISBN 0-87872-198-3

Printed in the United States of America
2 3 4 5 6 7 8 9 — 83 82 81 80 79

In memoriam
Carol Edgerton Mitchell

Dedication
To our student colleagues:
Past: who helped us realize the need for this book
Present: who helped us by their comments and
support
Future: who we hope will find this useful and who
will help us revise our thinking.

Contributors

Sarah Ellen Archer, R.N., D.P.H.

Associate Professor, Community Health Nursing and Administration,
School of Nursing, University of California, San Francisco
Lecturer, School of Public Health, University of California, Berkeley
Secretary-Treasurer and Community Nurse Practitioner, Nursing
Dynamics Corporation, Mill Valley, California

Teresa A. Bello, R.N., M.S.

Assistant Clinical Professor, Community Health Nursing, School of
Nursing, University of California, San Francisco

Fay Bower, R.N., D.N.S.

Chairperson and Professor, Department of Nursing, San Jose State
University, San Jose, California

Carol Dana Brancich, R.N., M.S.

Formerly Director of Nurses, Santa Cruz County Health Services
Agency, Santa Cruz, California
Vice-President, Nursing Dynamics Corporation, Santa Cruz, California

Suzanne Brodnax, R.N., M.S.

Formerly: Public Health Care Nurse, Home Care Referral Unit, Alameda
County, Health Department, Oakland, California
Graduate Research Nurse, Commune Health Education Project, School of
Nursing, University of California, San Francisco

Ruth P. Fleshman, R.N., Ph.D.
President and Community Nurse Practitioner, Nursing Dynamics Corporation, Mill Valley, California

Margaret J. Jacobson, R.N., Ph.D.
Professor and Associate Dean for Curriculum, School of Applied Arts and Sciences, San Jose State University, San Jose, California

Carol Ann Lockhart, R.N., M.S.
Chief, Office of Local Health Services, Arizona Department of Health Services, Phoenix, Arizona
Adjunct Assistant Professor, Health Services Administration, College of Business, Arizona State University, Tempe, Arizona

Carol Edgerton Mitchell, R.N., M.N.
Assistant Professor, Community Mental Health Nursing, School of Nursing, University of California, San Francisco (deceased, July 1978)

Jean Moorhead, R.N., M.S.
Formerly Nursing Consultant/Legislative Representative, California Nurses' Association
Assemblywoman, California 5th District

Dorothy S. Oda, R.N., D.N.S.
Assistant Professor, Community Health and School Nursing, and Project Director, Nurse Specialist in School Health Program, School of Nursing, University of California, San Francisco
Member, Board of Trustees, Nursing Dynamics Corporation, Mill Valley, California

Patricia Porter, R.N., M.S.
Director, Home Care Program, O'Connor Hospital, San Jose, California
Member, Board of Trustees, and Community Nurse Practitioner, Nursing Dynamics Corporation, Santa Cruz, California

Ruth Ann Terry, R.N., M.P.H.
Assistant Clinical Professor, Community Health Nursing School of Nursing, University of California, San Francisco

Contents

Preface

Feedback from our colleagues about the first edition of this book made it clear that they would like several major topics added to make this a more all-purpose text. However, we have had to realize, like nursing as a whole, that we cannot be all things to all people unless we go far beyond the limits of one volume. Nonetheless, we have acted on some of this feedback. For example, we have added a whole new section covering family theories and their application in community health nursing. We have also expanded other portions with chapters on discharge planning, quality assurance, and legislation. Even though each of these topics is worth an entire book itself, we have included them here briefly because we believe community nurses need to be just as aware of these aspects of our work as we are of the more traditional elements.

Every chapter from the first edition has been substantially rewritten both to bring it up to date and to refine our particular viewpoints. Because we continue to be actively practicing community health nurses, our areas of interest change with the years. Our times change too and the ways we practice must reflect these changes. Thus, although vast sums of money are still concentrated on institutional services, some groups are becoming aware of the limitations of an illness focus. Of course, that approach has always been able to produce more than enough work for all the health professionals around. It does not seem likely, however, that we could ever stem the tide of disease by waiting to treat it. Now we are beginning to realize that if we are ever to develop an emphasis on health instead, we must be concerned with preventing disease and enhancing the healthful qualities of life for our population. We are also becoming aware that health and illness are much more than just microorganisms and medicines. The health of any population depends directly on the quality and quantity of food available, housing, transportation, the quality of the social and physical environment—in fact, all of the elements that make up the essentials of daily life. It soon begins to look as if everything is hooked to everything else, and health is far too big to be left to the professionals.

If it sounds like a very big order, you can see why we believe that no single book can handle it all. A field like community health, constantly shifting, expanding, experimenting, and changing, doesn't hold still long enough to be written down. For that reason we have picked only a few of the pertinent theories, a selection from the fields of information, and put these together with examples of how nurses actually work with them. By using specific settings and real clients, we suggest ways these theories and information bits can be transferred to other situations. This is planned to illustrate the usefulness of learning generalized theories precisely because they *can* be transferred. The deluge of facts we deal with daily will, discouragingly enough, be obsolete before you can turn around. Thus it is more important, then, to learn the processes involved in getting up-to-date facts, in applying the most recent technology, in evaluating the effectiveness of the most current therapies.

With this in mind, we have asked a number of colleagues to share their own special areas drawn from real experiences. Although we agree about the underlying principles, how we put them into operation varies with the style and circumstances of each individual. We hope you will notice the thread of the basic concepts through the various experiences we all report. In the end you should be able then to get a feel for both the complexities of this field of nursing and the unifying ideas that make us all colleagues in a very exciting enterprise.

ACKNOWLEDGMENTS

We thank the following people for their help:

H. Ross Archer for his counsel and information on Health Insurance.

Mary Heatherman and Margaret Hoff of the Learning Information Resources Center, School of Nursing, University of California, San Francisco, for their assistance in revising the Yellow Pages.

Our colleagues who contributed in their areas of expertise.

Our many colleagues whose feedback has helped us in the revisions and expansions of the second edition.

Introduction

In a field as bursting with innovation as community health, practitioners seldom have the time to formalize the organizing beliefs, experiences, and principles that direct their activities. Many academicians skilled at theorizing have never developed comparable levels of ability in the practitioner's field. Our desire to teach is thoroughly grounded in real-world work experience, which is essential in a book such as this. Because the ground we cover is too extensive for any single writer, we have engaged in collaborative work with several colleagues with various special experiences in the community. This approach is especially appro priate since community health itself is nearly always a teamwork business and the better for it. So too with this book.

None of us pretends to being balanced, objective, or even restrained about our topics. Each of us has worked at it in the community and is thoroughly partial to the work we have done. Like any group of individuals, we do not necessarily share each other's enthusiasms. Although we are not all equally expert in all areas, we try to speak only to our own strong suits, with an end result of covering a wide range of nursing activities with an enthusiasm that seldom shines through most writing about nursing. Thus we hope to stir a similar response in our readers.

There is a real conflict between trying to share our feelings about our work and the way texts are traditionally written. Proper academic style often seems to us to be synonymous with dull, so we have deliberately chosen to violate a number of the proprieties that govern such writing. We know this offends a few, but feedback from students all over the country has suggested that the audience we want to talk to hears what we are saying. Because community nursing is made up of many different kinds of workers with varieties of ways of working, we have tried to keep each writer's style intact. Some might have preferred the whole to speak with a single tone, but that's not the nature of the enterprise. Not only have we kept a difference in writing style, we deliberately drew on a number of people with widely differing backgrounds to illustrate the differences within our common field. However, we have also all worked together so that our shared perspective has been worked out face to face.

While first developing this book our work group had several meetings to thrash out some of the minor problems of style. How to refer to nurses? We know there are a growing number of men in the field, and in this era of awareness of all kinds of chauvinisms, we hoped we could avoid offending them. We tried various avoidance devices like "the nurse does this and then the nurse . . ." or "he/she," or "in nursing, one does this" and so on. But these were painful to the ear and we finally gave up the fight. Nursing is, after all, still a predominantly women's occupation and in spite of all our men friends in the field, we chose to refer to our colleagues as "she" in many of the examples we present in this book.

There is also the whole notion of pronouns. Really proper academic writings avoid any sense of the personal, even at the expense of using very stilted circumlocutions. However, we decided to let each writer decide for herself what felt most comfortable. For the most part, if any one of us means that "I did this" we use "I"; if it was more than one we use "we." There are a lot of "we's" in this text, but that seems properly reflective of the ease we community nurses feel in working in team situations. Nowhere is the word used in the editorial or imperial sense. Even the editors—this section's "we"—actually worked jointly on the portions of the book labeled with either or both of our names. Finally, we all also use the term to refer to ourselves as part of that larger group with whom we hope you also will identify yourself—community health nurses.

In the planning stages of this book, we kept receiving interesting suggestions that we felt reflected a general underestimation of the ability of students to deal with complex material. Since we intended it for undergraduate as well as graduate nurses, we were urged not to make it too far beyond our readers, too hard to understand. Since we had all been frequent and sometimes recent students, we have all been mightily offended by nursing writing that condescended to its readers to the point that we simply turned it off. For that reason we have tried to avoid talking down to you, using neither super-simple terms that save you from thinking nor the specialized jargon that insiders often use to keep ideas suitably obscure for outsiders. We also tried out several chapters on baccalaureate students in our area, made changes as they suggested, and found they had no complaints about our incomprehensibility. In the years since this book first came out we have received varieties of positive feedback from students and none seemed troubled by our level of discussion. We presume that if there are words or concepts you don't know, you'll look them up or ask some community health faculty.

We do hope that you won't be lulled, however, by the conversational nature of some of the material. High-flown gobbledegook does not necessarily imply heavy-duty content nor does a casual writing style mean the material is trivial. Many issues in community health can be revealed by pondering some of the simpler phrases we all tend to take for granted. All you need to do as an example is consider awhile each of the words in the phrase, "health care system."

OTHER WORD GAMES

We have generally tried to avoid using the term "patient" and instead refer to "client" or "consumer." For us, "patient" has come to imply a superior-inferior exchange—a game of one-up, one-down. "Client" or "consumer" on the other hand suggests a more nearly equal position, a collaborative relationship. Included in this is the realization that a client is one who pays for, has bought our services and is not accepting charity. This is consonant with increased consumer participation in the health care delivery system. There are times when "patient" is used but we have tried to limit it to when a client has moved into that relation with some other care provider and especially when one-down is implied.

Articles and whole books have been devoted to attempts to define, describe, and quantify health, wellness, and other synonyms. Rather than engage in that pursuit, we have defined in chapters 1 and 2 an operational term, Optimum Level of Functioning (OLOF). Even when we use the word "health" we still deal with it in terms of our definition of OLOF. But acronyms become boring and "health" is used here as a synonym for OLOF.

On the other hand we are trying to suggest a clear difference when we use the terms "medical care" and "health care." The former refers to the services rendered by a physician or physicians in aggregate. Health care is the total package of services which includes but is not limited to medical care.

Although some writers do not choose to make such a distinction, we have defined a difference between public health and community health. For us, public health refers to a practice limited to official health agencies—local, county, state, and national. They join other generalized health workers operating in nonofficial (that is, nongovernmental) agencies, in nonhealth agencies or even independently in a wide variety of community settings. For this broader category we retain the term "community health." The specifics of the definition are left to the context.

Many formal presentations of nursing theory proceed with dignity from concept to various kinds of application. As knowledge proliferates, theories become dominant and the experiential bases are lost or omitted for lack of space. Some people are apparently very comfortable functioning with this deductive style of learning and can easily move from the abstract to the concrete. We go in the opposite direction: with the inductive style that utilizes a number of specific events from which principles and concepts can be derived. Committed to a foundation in real experiences, we have inserted many incidents and events as examples to serve as concrete definitions of the abstract ideas we are presenting. Thus we ground our theory in the observed data from which we derived it. These slices of reality will also provide opportunities for you to derive other kinds of theories, since we can't hope to treat any incident in an exhaustive fashion. Both the deductive and inductive are useful methods. We hope our fellow travellers will learn to move comfortably in both directions to the enrichment of their nursing practice and the benefit of their clients.

Our inductive frame of reference has led us to try to maximize the applicability of our materials in situations that we have faced and our readers will too. Thus we have minimized the references and citations within our presentations. As it is, every chapter could be expanded into a book of its own. So each chapter is really an introduction to the topics discussed and is intended to be a stimulus for further study rather than an exhaustive treatment. The bibliographies that appear at the end of each chapter are planned to reflect the materials we talk about and can be used for more intensive study.

Community nursing is, if nothing else, eclectic and will borrow any theory that helps explain observable phenomena. By keeping citations to a minimum, we know we risk offending the academic purist who demands endless footnotes. Those persons interested in tracing the development of the theories our observations have confirmed can look forward to absorbing lifetime careers in the library. Those who are concerned, as we are, with using theory can go a long way without knowing the name of its originator.

Even before the onset of nursing's version of future shock, we who worked in the community knew that what we learned in school was never enough. The scientific and social information explosion of the last decade has made it even more urgent that nurses establish a lifelong pattern of learning. Some of this comes from continuing education, workshops, books, and journals. Equally important is the learning that occurs through experience. To aid you in sifting through the mountain of material produced each year, we include one chapter as a guide. The experience we leave to you.

THE SHAPE OF THINGS TO COME

Each of the five parts in this book begins with a brief rundown of the chapters it contains. Part I begins with general introductory materials: definitions, the overall perspective, and our conceptual framework for community health nursing. In Part II we present a whole new set of material on families as clients that was not included in our first edition. This addition was the result of direct feedback from many of the first edition's readers. It isn't possible to find any single theory to apply to such complex situations as we encounter with our most common client in the community: the family. For that reason we present several theories that have their own strong and weak points as far as application goes. However, a theoretical understanding of families is never enough, and Part II goes on to provide examples of health counseling situations and the care of the sick at home in the context of family. Part III takes up some of the tools of particular interest to community nursing. Like so many other nursing techniques, these are neither invented by us nor are they our monopolies. But, by showing examples of how we use them, we expect to give you a better notion of their particular applicability to community health nursing practice. Some of the fascinating complexities of nursing roles described by nurses actually involved in these areas are presented in Part IV. Then in the last section we wind up a few loose ends, bits and pieces that were too interesting (to us) to be left out but too short to be expanded into full chapters. Some are dilemmas—situations with at least two unsatisfactory solutions—and a few are warnings of some unexpected hazards out here in the community. In general, however, we expect you will realize that we are not only committed to work in the community, we actually enjoy it!

PART I

Community Health Nursing Concepts and Processes

EDITORS' INTRODUCTION

We begin this book with selected concepts and processes we have found particularly applicable in community health nursing. Most theories that work in the real world have been developed by the practitioners only after long contact with that world. Thus, our choices represent our various work experiences that have led us to a comfortable conceptual framework. This inductive process for developing workable theories fits our general approach to community health nursing, and our desire in this section is to provide a guide for ourselves and others in approaching nursing practice with intuitive, pragmatic, and theoretical strengths. This approach is one way of becoming socialized into thinking like community health nurses—that is, of seeing the world through nurse-colored glasses.

Chapter 1: An Introduction to Community Health Nursing
Ruth Fleshman and Margaret Jacobson start us off with an overview of our conceptual framework. They provide a number of crucial concepts, definitions, and special terms that are derived from the general field of nursing, from community nursing, and from our other parent field, public health. The terms they discuss are used throughout the rest of the book in a variety of contexts by our other writers. By spelling out a number of roles community nurses may be called upon to play,

1

the authors also give us an idea of the wide range of activities we community nurses have open to us.

Chapter 2:   Selected Concepts for Community Health Nurses
Sarah Ellen Archer discusses a number of concepts that are pivotal to community health nursing practice. Communities are our clients, and to dispell any notion that a community is merely a geographic place, she describes a number of kinds of communities as well as examples of community health nurses' activities in them. Optimum level of functioning (OLOF) is our conceptualization of health. OLOF comes from a holistic perspective and emphasizes peoples' abilities, not their disabilities. To measure OLOF of communities or individual clients, community health nurses need a grasp of the sources of health indicator data and some of the uses to which these data can be put. Some examples are presented in this chapter, which concludes with a brief discussion of holism and a plea for community health nurses to look at the whole client.

Chapter 3:   Selected Processes for Community Health Nurses
Sarah Ellen Archer discusses the concept of exchange as a fundamental part of all human interrelationships. Systems theory is introduced and discussed in terms of family analysis. Planning, a process essential for change, is elaborated upon and examples for community health nurses are given.

1. An Introduction to Community Health Nursing

Ruth P. Fleshman
Margaret J. Jacobson

COMMUNITY HEALTH NURSING: WHAT IT IS

As a student in any program in nursing you are beset with numerous definitions of nursing and its many facets. In considering only a few of them, you become aware of how hard it is to get nurses, let alone outsiders, to agree on what nursing is. The same is true for community health nursing, since definitions depend on the frame of reference of those trying to do the defining. We feel the following statement is one upon which many of us can generally agree. *Community nursing is a learned practice with the ultimate goal of contributing, as individuals and in collaboration with others, to the promotion of the client's optimum level of functioning* (OLOF) *through teaching and the delivery of care.* This definition draws from the philosophy of Winslow's classic description of public health:

> Public health is the science and the art of preventing disease, prolonging life, and promoting physical and mental health and efficiency through organized community efforts toward a sanitary environment; the control of community infections; the education of the individual in principles of personal hygiene; the organization of medical and nursing service for the early diagnosis and treatment of disease; and the development of the social machinery which will ensure to every individual in the community a standard of living adequate for the maintenance of health [Winslow 1952:30].

3

Since the time Winslow wrote this description, there have been many changes in our field. The ways we practice have become so diverse that we can no longer describe it by listing the things we do; nor are the titles by which we are called a particularly helpful way of creating categories. We will later describe a number of types of community health nurse activities and the roles we can all play.

You will note that we use the term *community health,* while Winslow uses *public health.* For many people, the latter term means the activities of those who work for governmental bodies, at all levels, in the delivery of health care to various populations. However, too many nongovernmental groups are involved in the same kind of work from the same perspective to not be seen in much the same way. For this reason, we use the term *community health* as an umbrella under which we all, government workers and otherwise, pursue our professional goals.

CHALLENGES FOR COMMUNITY HEALTH

To help clients toward their optimal levels of functioning, community health nurses are concerned with three levels of prevention.

Primary prevention deals with health promotion and specific protection against diseases. Teaching expectant mothers about nutrition and how to care for themselves and their infants are examples of health promotion. Specific protection activities include immunizing elderly and high-risk individuals against influenza each fall.

Secondary prevention focuses on early diagnosis and prompt intervention in disease processes. Examining our own and teaching our women clients to examine their own breasts in a systematic search for early stages of breast cancer is an example of secondary prevention. The earlier a diagnosis can be made, the greater is the likelihood of successful, life-saving treatment. Most primary care services are aimed at secondary prevention.

Tertiary prevention uses rehabilitation activities to prevent further complications and to restore as much as possible in the way of optimal functioning. For example, physical fitness and stress management training after heart attacks can help victims regain their abilities to function and decrease the probability of subsequent heart attacks. Crisis intervention involving counseling after a disaster is another example, as is discussed in chapter 5.

Winslow's concern with a sanitary environment is as pertinent today as ever, although the actual environmental hazards may have shifted from microorganisms, at least in industrial societies. Contemporary hazards include pollution of air, water, food, and land from human, industrial, and agricultural activities.

Because of the past successes of health technology, we have become lax about the measures needed to prevent communicable diseases. Illustrative of this laxity is the fact that in some locales fewer than 50 percent of young children entering school have been immunized against the leading communicable disease of childhood. Our great dependence on medical interventions results in a growing number of drug-resistant pathogens.

Variable levels of personal hygiene still contribute to the disease process, and the areas of concern can be suggested by observing how many people leave public rest rooms without washing their hands. For the most part, the major diseases affecting modern society are no longer amenable to simple immunization or other single-faceted solutions. Our health concerns must increasingly be with personal lifestyle changes in such areas as diet, exercise, stress management, and substance abuse. Clearly, peoples' optimal levels of functioning more than ever depend on how they choose to live their lives relative to these factors.

The scope of contemporary health problems and the tools for their solution make it impossible for any one or two health disciplines to render the services needed for a whole community. Although medicine and nursing are still the predominant care disciplines for much of public and community health, we are being joined by many new specialties who bring sophisticated techniques to bear on community needs. More than ever, community health is a multidisciplinary enterprise whose team members need to learn how best to utilize their own talents and those of the others around them to further the ultimate goals of health.

One of the greatest challenges facing the multidisciplinary community health team is the fact that we must take into account the entire range of personal and environmental factors that impinge on the maintenance of health. Many of our clients have passed the level of mere adequacy in their standard of living, and the result is often greater health problems than we had before. For example, too many calories from too rich foods, the use of automobiles instead of bicycles and foot power, and sedentary, high-stress occupations rather than physically taxing jobs are all signs of the affluence that creates hazards to life that were not expected while we still strove toward a higher standard of living.

You may have already noticed that we use the term *client* here and in community nursing practice to indicate not only the individual but in the broader generic sense to refer to a family, a variety of other kinds of groups, or a total community. Implicit in this term is the notion that clients need not be ill; "patients" are ill. Use of the term *patient* carries the connotation of a one-up, one-down relationship between the provider and the consumer of health care, both psychologically as well as literally since a patient can be considered to be a horizontal client. Use of the term *client* suggests a reciprocal relationship to the health care provider—that is, their status is (or should be) more nearly equal, thereby allowing the client to *expect* service, rather than be humbly grateful for it. The shift from the singular individual as the focus of concern to entire groups is often difficult to do. Additionally, considering a family or group as a single client rather than as a group of clients requires taking into account the ways in which it functions as a social entity.

Community health nurses' activities geared toward promoting client OLOF are of three distinctly different kinds of services.

Direct client services are those in which the nurse is a deliverer of care or services to the client, whether individual, family, or larger group. That care may be physical nursing, such as bed baths or injections, or the direct action may take the form of crisis counseling or physical assessment. Alternatively, deliberate nonactions may be the preferred intervention. Examples include supportive nonassistance as a client undergoing rehabilitation therapy struggles to tie his shoe or as a new widow painfully tries to make her own decisions after forty years of marriage.

Semidirect client services are those that enable direct care to take place. For example, your faculty member teaches you how to give direct client services: You provide the direct client service because you work with the client; the faculty person provides semidirect service because she works with you. Another example is the responsibilities of nursing supervisors that ensure sufficient supplies are available for direct client services to be given effectively and efficiently. Semidirect services may also be a part of the work done by a nurse primarily involved in direct client service. For example, calling a meeting of workers from a variety of service agencies working with several members of a client family may be necessary in order to increase the degree of continuity in the services and counseling the family is getting. Nurses working on advisory boards, special task forces, or planning bodies also aid in improving the distribution of health services to groups or total communities. In any case, without adequate semidirect client services, quality direct care cannot be given.

Indirect client services focus on the creation and management of the systems within which consumer-provider exchanges or transactions occur. Thus, the nurse-administrator of a health agency is engaged in indirect client service as is the dean of a school of nursing. Such nurse-administrators facilitate both semidirect and direct client services by establishing a climate within the system that allows these activities to take place. This type of indirect service may entail insuring that a fair share of the total institution budget is allocated to nursing services or redirecting present funds to support newly identified client service areas (see figure 1.1).

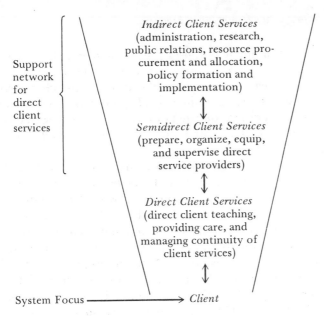

Support
network
for
direct
client
services

Indirect Client Services
(administration, research,
public relations, resource procurement and allocation,
policy formation and
implementation)

↕

Semidirect Client Services
(prepare, organize, equip,
and supervise direct
service providers)

↕

Direct Client Services
(direct client teaching,
providing care, and
managing continuity of
client services)

↕

System Focus ⟶ Client

(individual, family, group, population, community)

1.1   *Subsystems of Client Service*

Source: Sarah Ellen Archer, "Community Nursing Practitioners: Another Assessment,"
Copyright © 1976, American Journal of Nursing Company. Reproduced with permission
from *Nursing Outlook,* August Vol. 24, No. 8.

THE SYSTEMS PERSPECTIVE

A systems viewpoint will help put our concepts into perspective. In chapter 3 we deal more explicitly with a systems view of health care, but at this point you may need a few basic systems terms to begin to understand our frame of reference.

> A system is an entity comprised of parts which is designed and built by man into an organized whole for the attainment of a specific purpose [Banathy 1968:90].

The three main aspects of any system are purpose, process, and content. The sum of the parts that make up a system are called its *content*. A system's content is organized to accomplish some specific *purpose*. And the operations or functions by which its parts or components work together to accomplish its purpose are called the *process* of the system (Banathy 1968:4). The components of a system are called *subsystems*. These, in turn, may be thought of as systems of their own but on a smaller scale. A useful analogy is that of a box within a larger box within yet a larger box.

Nursing is a subsystem of a larger system, the so-called health care delivery system. As a subsystem of nursing, community health nursing contributes to nursing's ultimate purposes just as nursing adds its inputs to the larger health care delivery system's attainment of its ultimate purposes. Community health nursing has the three major characteristics common to all systems: (1) an ultimate goal, (2) organization—that is, a series of actions or operations directed toward accomplishing that goal— and (3) ongoing adaptability and innovation in a rapidly changing society (Bevis 1973:6–7).

The *ultimate goal* of the community nursing process, whether direct, semidirect, or indirect, and regardless of whether the focus is primary, secondary, or tertiary prevention, is consonant with that of nursing and the health care system: the attainment and maintenance of an optimal level of functioning by whatever client or community is being served. The *organization,* the steps taken to achieve the goal, is centered on the quality of life, the prevention of dysfunctions, and the development and delivery of continuous, pertinent health care service to consumers. The final characteristic essential to the viability of community health nursing is its continuous *ability to adapt* and change. Community nursing must be flexible and innovative in relation to the lifestyle of consumers; otherwise the ultimate goal may not be met and community nursing's reason for being will cease. The basic philosophical stance of community nursing is client centered and concerned with the quality of life.

COMMUNITY NURSING PRACTICE

Community nursing is done in a variety of settings ranging from agricultural workers' camps to the ambulatory clinics of major hospitals through whatever agency or facility finances such services. Community nursing may also be carried out on an independent basis when the community nurse engages in an individual contractual type of practice. Community nursing is collaborative, interrelated, and on occasion overlapping with other health disciplines—that is, roles may become blurred depending on the situation. In a medical center the roles of nurses, physicians, and social workers may be well circumscribed, but where there is no social worker, few physicians, and long distances between population centers, the community nurse's roles are often greatly expanded.

The functions of community nursing practice are independent, interdependent, and dependent according to the role, setting, and the laws pertaining to that practice. For example, different states have a variety of laws regulating the practice of the certified nurse-midwife. Some states limit the midwife to *dependent practice* by vesting authority entirely in the obstetrician. Other states, and some European countries such as Great Britain, permit *interdependent practice* through laws establishing the purview of midwives to include normal pregnancy and delivery with pathology referred for a physician's care. A few states permit *independent practice* either by refusing to enact restricting laws or by delegating to physicians only certain activities, such as the prescription of drugs or the breaking and entering of the skin.

Throughout this book the terms *community health nurse* or *community nurse* are used to mean a nurse practicing in a wide variety of community-based services and consumer advocate areas and in a variety of roles, at times including independent practice. The public health nurse in an official agency—that is, a governmental agency—practices community health nursing, but community nursing is certainly not confined to public health nursing agencies.

Traditional texts separate community health agencies into official, voluntary, and proprietary. These divisions have little effect on nursing practice and are based on the various structures of the institutions within which nursing practice takes place. *Official agencies* are those established within government hierarchies, controlled by legislation, and funded and staffed by employees or contractors of the applicable jurisdiction. Thus, we have city, county, state, and federal health agencies. *Voluntary agencies* are private groups of many varieties, organized as charitable, educational, or welfare service organizations. Examples of these are such national or worldwide organizations as the Red Cross or the American Heart Association. The term *voluntary* also refers to church-affiliated services or free-standing community services, such as the Visiting Nurses Associations, and community hospitals. Another major subdivision is based on the agency's financial purpose. Many voluntary agencies are also legally designated as nonprofit corporations. Those designed to make profit for their owners are referred to as *proprietary agencies*. Many nursing homes and some hospitals fall into the proprietary category. Being designated nonprofit does not, however, mean that an agency has to lose money; just that whatever money is left over after salaries and other expenses cannot be used to enrich any individual or group in the position of owner of the organization.

Several new categories of health agencies have begun to emerge but still have not taken on enough form to match the foregoing groupings. One is the notion of alternative agencies, such as free clinics, minority-group community services, experimental combinations of orthodox and unorthodox health approaches geared to the needs of a specific population or community (see chapter 16). Another movement is developing from consumer-initiated programs for self-help. These may involve professionals as consultants, but the ability and right of clients to learn how to care for themselves is stressed.

Community agencies and hospitals are all parts of the larger health care system that is supported by a major portion of the national economy (see chapter 2). Although the greatest resources are available for acute care, individual clients may spend only a minute fraction of their lives in such episodes. Far more time and effort are spent trying to avoid either the episodic event (through primary prevention) or a recurrence of it (through tertiary prevention). When communicable diseases were the major killers, short and dramatic public health interventions were effective; sanitation and mass immunization could reduce or even eliminate significant acute diseases. Now, however, the health care consumer can no longer be a passive client in preventing disease. Only through knowledge and changed lifestyle can the incidence of chronic diseases be reduced (see chapter 9).

Community nursing is primarily involved with nonacute events, the prevention of acute events, and the interrelation and continuity of care as clients move between episodic and distributive events (National Commission 1970). Such continuity leads to an awareness that consumers of medical and nursing care are not different people inside and outside of hospitals. For this reason, community nursing may also be practiced within hospital walls (see chapter 19).

SOME ROLES OF COMMUNITY NURSES

Since community health nurses function in a variety of roles, the skills needed to function should be a part of the educational preparation for nursing practice. Some important examples of these skills are communication, teaching and learning, interpersonal relationships, problem solving, and decision making. Neither facts nor process are enough in themselves. Learning how to learn and to continue learning is a skill in itself that does not become dated as do facts and some concepts. Continuously updating the content of nursing is necessary since our scientific base is expanding as explosively as every other field of knowledge.

Defining community nursing is no longer possible by describing particular jobs. We do, however, find a number of recurrent roles that we community nurses are playing wherever we work. The interpretation of possible roles depends to a great extent on the system within which these roles must be enacted. The same role looks very different when carried out in a free clinic and when in an urban medical center. We find *all* of the roles being done in different places but seldom all together. Often systems impose severe restraints on a nurse's ability to use the full range of nursing skills, and nurses are always wise to test the atmosphere before assuming some of the more controversial functions of a given role. The roles we feel are especially important for community nursing are described in the following sections.

ADVOCATE

An advocate is any person who speaks for and on behalf of some other person or group. Attorneys are advocates for their clients and speak to support their legal cases by arguing for their innocence or the extenuating circumstances that led to the clients' present position. The community nurse can be a client-advocate in at least two ways: by assisting clients to obtain what they are entitled to from the system, and by trying to make the system more responsive to client needs, either in particular cases or in general. Client-advocacy can range from calling the welfare department before referring a family in an effort to pave the way for the members to testifying in court on behalf of a client. You may hear *advocate* and *ombudsman* used interchangeably, but the terms are not synonymous. An advocate speaks in favor of something, while the ombudsman is a mediator and intentionally does not take sides. For example, in family counseling we may at times assume the role of ombudsman among family members, in conflicts such as those centering around changes in values between generations. As in most mediator situations, this role involves a great deal of interpretation to the people on both sides of the issue. As an advocate, we would be concerned with explaining the views of a particular client to others.

COLLABORATOR AND TEAM MEMBER

Although we often operate on a one-to-one basis with clients, we are seldom isolated in our practice. Both within our employing agencies and the health care system, we work with others: nurses, physicians, social workers, receptionists, psychologists, nutritionists, community aides, clients, and so on. Collaboration implies a collegial relationship with other nurses, health discipline members, and clients. Inherent in collaboration is the belief that each person has a unique contribution to make and should participate equally in decision making. Collaboration thrives in settings where communication is open and participants hold a mutual respect for one another. As a client-advocate the nurse may have to ensure that clients have an opportunity to collaborate in decisions that affect them.

COMMUNITY ORGANIZER

The effectiveness of group action to create change has been well documented in recent years. Such groups do not spring full grown from the neighborhoods but are often focused by one or a few energetic organizers into issues that concern the whole group. Such gatherings can, of course, be used by people with their own special interests, but they can also reflect a need to restore the power balance more equitably between service providers and recipients. Many people may question the propriety of nurses working in this area, but since development of health services is a legitimate nursing concern, utilizing nursing skills to help community groups develop their own health-related organization is, by extension, quite proper. This role may be seen as a step beyond advocacy: Nurse-organizers are trying to move communities to learn to speak for themselves. Importantly, a nurse involved here must be careful to promote a client-centered process—that is, to enable the consumers to express their own wants, not those they think are expected by the providers. This type of activity may be very uncomfortable since we are, after all, brainwashed about health care delivery to some extent by our own professional background. The experience can be rewarding, though, to see groups emerge and become able to make their voices heard in the agencies that determine how health care is delivered. It is also rewarding to be a part of that process as a facilitator, a role characterized by being temporary, to be ended when the group is self-sustaining.

CONSULTANT

Due to our expertise and information, we community nurses are often consultants to clients and to other people. Working in collaboration with the physician, we give observations of and information about a client and receive specialized information about the physician's therapy program. Other consultative exchanges occur with schoolteachers, legislators, probation officers, or anyone else who maintains a helping relationship with our clients. Although many community nurses take a generalist approach to their work, others develop special expertise in some particular aspect of what they do. Some expand into clinical specialization in such areas as contraception, genetic counseling, or chronic illness management. Some become known for special skill with certain nursing tools, such as interviewing, data analysis, teaching strategies, or crisis counseling. The forte of other nurses may be expansion into the basic knowledge underlying nursing practice, such as minority group ethnology, nutrition, and growth and development. All of these provide the basis for expertise and consultation.

COORDINATOR AND FACILITATOR

Often the community nurse is the member of the health care team who makes care accessible and effectively coordinates the services available to the client. Without some coordination the client may receive a duplication of services from different agencies and still have some essential needs unmet. One ambulatory clinic client who needed to limit her activities once said, "Everyone I talk with asks me if I have stairs to climb where I live. Each time I answer yes, but no one has told me what I can do about it." A social worker, a sanitarian, a schoolteacher, and a community worker may all see a client in the home, but the community nurse may well be the one who coordinates their efforts, sets up lines of communication and collaboration, and assists the client in making decisions and in planning for such things as following through on a positive tuberculin test, getting necessary immunizations for the family, and seeing a physician.

DELIVERER OF SERVICES

There is some confusion and disagreement about what is and what is not appropriate for a nurse to deliver in the way of direct services to clients. As a beginning student you may think that you are not doing nursing unless you do something for or to the client, such as change a dressing, give an injection, or take a temperature or a blood pressure reading. It is important to you to be able to "do something" in order to feel like a nurse, but as we have noted, what you do may be direct, semidirect, or indirect nursing care. A combination of all three kinds of service is the more usual and desirable situation. In reality, a visible direct service may often be the act that gives credibility to the semidirect and indirect services that are an important and essential part of nursing. Conant's study of home visits gives some examples of client responses to nurse visits and points up the need for credibility and the impact of "doing something" that can be identified as nursing (1965:119). We often fail to acknowledge our indirect nursing services, and thus we often reinforce the fallacy that nursing is not nursing unless something is done directly to or for the client. Actually community nursing is what we do ourselves and through other people to help the clients do something for themselves.

EDUCATOR

The community nurse must be able to teach many kinds of people many kinds of things, even though the education need not be schooling in a formal sense. In order to teach, we must have something to teach—that is, we must have the information or know where to get it in order to pass it on. Obviously we must keep this information active and updated. To teach successfully, it follows that we should know some essential things about the learner and the teaching-learning process. The aim of learning is to change behavior, but such alterations are not always immediate or observable. In community nursing we rarely get immediate feedback from the learner's behavior, yet the teaching that we do may be of great value as it is probably the only primary prevention for a number of chronic illnesses. Sometimes changes in vital statistics in the community will indicate some effects of our teaching, although we must be aware that many other variables are operating in the situation.

The establishment of objectives and the ability to measure how well the objectives are met are essential to the teaching-learning process. Simply telling someone a bit of information can't be considered teaching, particularly if there is no evidence that the client has learned or met the objective of the teaching. An important part of the teaching-learning process is that the community nurse and client share some objectives.

EVALUATOR

Deciding what health service is needed and seeing that it is delivered is, for many health workers, the most challenging part of their job. Equally crucial, though, is that the impact of the particular service be evaluated somehow. We are beginning to see what happens when such evaluation is left undone: In many communities, public health nursing jobs are being downgraded or eliminated because we have never documented how what we do makes any difference to anyone. Just as our service to clients needs to be assessed, so do we need to develop means to evaluate the performance of ourselves and other health workers. Such appraisals are often very threatening, as all of us who have suffered through unhappy student ratings well know! But the development of usable standards of practice as well as criteria for various levels of competence is most appropriately done by the people actually working in the field. On an even larger scale, important considerations are whether the entire system is actually achieving its purpose, meeting its ultimate goals, and how efficiently its process is moving in those directions. Many of us are convinced that some systems devote more resources to maintaining the system than to the supposed output, and we're sure you can think of some examples not too far away! As nurses in community settings, we have special awareness of the impact of health agencies on the lives of clients, which may thus place us in a position to evaluate that impact with particular acuity.

INFORMATION-GATHERER, RESEARCHER

Data gathering may be a step in the process of nursing diagnosis, research, or decision making. It is also a role of its own that requires a continually questioning approach to whatever field is being examined. We prefer to think of data gathering as systematic curiosity about what's really going on in community health. Better health care interventions are based on organized information, which must be sought from a wide variety of sources by the nurse who is developing a care plan, working with clients to reach their own care decisions, or trying to demonstrate to the agency administrator that a new service is needed. Innovative programs are most in need of a solid data base since these are most likely to be resisted by administrators and others who control the needed resources. Skill in collecting information must be practiced and should become a regular nursing tool that we have many chances to use in our work as community health nurses.

Manager

The solo practitioner is no longer the most effective means for delivering health care to a community. However, putting many health workers together does not guarantee a better delivery system. An effective team evolves only with time and a good deal of facilitative work. If one does emerge, generally in any but an authoritarian model, it still needs a designated manager who will create the conditions under which the other team members will be able to carry out their specialized tasks, but without letting them forget the overall task of the team. Surprisingly, many such managers turn out to be social workers or nurses. Not everyone wants to do that kind of work nor is everyone suited to do it. But we have many experiences as nurses that prepare us for that particular role. We have been characterized as having the widest appreciation of the client's lifestyle and being most concerned with the client's day-by-day life. Further as health professionals, we also understand the special views and language used by our other colleagues in this field. Thus, with some abilities to organize and mediate, we may find ourselves the best suited to coordinate and manage the performance of a disparate group of health professionals to achieve a unified task of care. The manager role differs from the coordinator-facilitator role, which focuses on care the client receives, often from uncoordinated providers, in that the nurse-manager works with providers so they present a balanced program of care.

Referrer

Making referrals of clients to other services has become nearly stereotypical of the public health nurse. Nonetheless, this activity has a great deal of importance because we must work with many different kinds of clients with wide varieties of concerns related more or less directly to health. Thus, we are often confronted with matters of importance that are beyond or outside the scope of our own professional skills. Knowledge of the resources available to deal with such a spectrum of problems is one hallmark of an experienced community health nurse. Elsewhere we mention that one attribute of a professional is to know when and where to begin looking for help. Often clients are so hemmed in by crises that they cannot step back far enough to see how anyone else could help, let alone to look among the many community services for one that would fit their special circumstances. Community nurses must often take on this task, by turning first to their immediate colleagues or going directly to community agencies to facilitate the use of their services by clients. It is not enough, of course, to simply write down a phone number for the client; a referral is not properly complete until the client is actually linked to the service provider who is able and willing to deal with the presenting issue. Thus follow-through contacting is essential to be sure that yet another client has not fallen into some interagency crack.

RESEARCH AND COMMUNITY NURSING

"Although there has been a great deal of rhetoric about the need for nursing research, the amount of research actually carried out by nurses has been minimal when compared with other applied sciences" (Jacox 1974:382). Community nursing is noted for its limited amount of research in the development of theoretical bases for action. Much of our nursing practice is still done on a prescribed and ritualistic basis. Some things are done in certain ways because students have modeled themselves after teachers or because a time-honored policy or a procedure exists for the action. However, many challenging problems are encountered each day by the nurse in active practice, and many of these lend themselves to systematic study.

For many years nurse educators held the notion that research in nursing was a prerogative of graduate education, and this notion may account for how few nurses become interested in research. It may also have produced the idea that research is something imposed from outside on practice and teaching. Fortunately, more and more baccalaureate nursing programs are developing the research component as a continuous strand throughout the undergraduate program. Hopefully, as a consequence, graduates may view research as an integral part of practice and as a guide to practice.

Broadly speaking, there are two main approaches to conducting research: the experimental and the nonexperimental designs (Abdellah and Levine 1965:45–65). These might be viewed as two entirely separate and dichotomous methods, but in fact, they are best considered as points on a continuum.

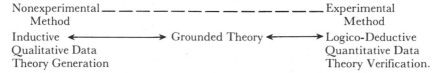

In the purest sense, experimental research, at one end of the continuum, derives its data under controlled conditions; the data are predominantly quantitative and subject to statistical inference with tests of
probability. Experimental research begins with a theory, or hypothesis. It
sharply limits the number of factors being observed and keeps uniform all
but the particular element being tested. This method is best suited to
simple phenomena and rigorously controlled environments, such as lab-
oratories. The experimenter is expected to maintain an objective role in
the research. There are explicit rules in quantitative analysis applicable
to such items as sampling, reliability, validity, frequency distributions,
hypothesis construction, and the presentation of evidence. In fact, there
are classic or true experimental designs (Campbell and Stanley 1963:13).

Nonexperimental research, at the other end of the continuum, is
appropriate in situations that cannot be controlled; the person conducting the research is frequently a participant in the phenomenon being
observed. Instead of a precise design, as in experimental research, the observation takes place in the reality situation where the events occur—that
is, artificial comparisons are not introduced. The data derived are usually
qualitative and descriptive. There are also explicit, but flexible, guides in
qualitative analysis depending upon the researcher's goal—such as
developing hypotheses for provisional testing or for theory development
by using a constant comparative method of analysis (Glaser and Strauss
1968:101–15).

The purpose of this comparison of the experimental method and quantitative analysis with the nonexperimental method and qualitative analysis is primarily to emphasize that the two methods need not be mutually
exclusive. Glaser and Strauss hold that there is no fundamental clash between the purposes and capacities of qualitative and quantitative analysis
methods (Glaser and Strauss 1968:17). Qualitative data can be quan-
tified and quantitative data can be qualified. To perceive the two approaches as related on a continuum is helpful to the novice researcher
who often may think that only studies that use statistical measurements
may be considered research.

Qualitative data available to us hold a great potential for the development of grounded theory, which is theory based on and derived from the
reality of the setting and context in which the events occur. Grounded
theory is placed in the midpoint of the continuum because in using the

constant comparative method of analysis, it evolves from an inductive method to arrive at a tentative theory that can then be tested deductively in some form of the experimental research design. This test, in turn, serves as further data to modify or advance the original theory (Glaser and Strauss 1968). The actual methods used to gather data depend on the kind of research questions being asked and the environment in which the research must be carried out.

Families, communities, and other groups do not lend themselves neatly, conveniently, or ethically to controlled research. The protection of human rights and the choices of individuals and groups may indeed create dissonance between the role of the nurse as a client-advocate and the role of the nurse in the testing of theory by experimental methods. Field methods of research that yield qualitative data are more compatible with the roles and functions of the community nurse (Schatzman and Strauss 1973). A more detailed discussion of field methods appears in chapter 8.

SUMMARY

This chapter introduces our conceptual framework for community nursing. It is largely devoted to presenting definitions and examples of the pivotal ideas that will be developed further in subsequent chapters. These include optimum level of functioning (OLOF); primary, secondary, and tertiary prevention; direct, semidirect, and indirect service; individuals, families, groups, and communities as clients; systems theory; community health agencies; and various community nurse roles, such as advocate, collaborator and team member, community organizer, consultant, coordinator and facilitator, deliverer of services, educator, evaluator, information-gatherer or researcher, manager, and referrer. We end with brief comments on perspectives on research that may make it more useful for community nurses. We have set community health nursing in a very broad context and discussed some of the roles community nurses may assume in promoting clients' optimum levels of functioning.

REFERENCES

ABDELLAH, FAY G., and LEVINE, EUGENE. *Better Patient Care Through Nursing Research*. New York: Macmillan Co., 1965.

ARCHER, SARAH ELLEN. "Community Nurse Practitioners: Another Assessment." *Nursing Outlook* 24 (August 1976): 499–503.

BANATHY, BELA H. *Instructional Systems*. Belmont, Calif.: Fearon Publishers, 1968.

BEVIS, EM O. *Curriculum Building in Nursing: A Process.* St. Louis: C. V. Mosby Co., 1973.

BYERLY, ELIZABETH L. "The Nurse Researcher as a Participant Observer in a Nursing Setting." *Nursing Research* 18, no. 3 (1969):230–36.

CAMPBELL, DONALD T., and STANLEY, JULIAN C. *Experimental and Quasi-Experimental Designs for Research.* Chicago: Rand McNally and Co., 1963.

CLARK, DUNCAN W., and MACMAHON, BRIAN, eds. *Preventive Medicine.* Boston: Little, Brown and Co., 1967.

CONANT, LUCY. "Give and Take in Home Visits." *American Journal of Nursing* 65 (July 1965):119.

COULTER, PEARL PARVIA. *The Nurse in the Public Health Program.* New York: G. P. Putnam's Sons, 1954.

DICKOFF, JAMES, et al. "Theory in a Practice Discipline," Part II of "Practice Oriented Research." *Nursing Research* 17, no. 6 (1968):545–54.

FREEMAN, RUTH B. *Community Health Nursing Practice,* 4th ed. Philadelphia: W. B. Saunders Co., 1970.

GEORKE, LENOV S., and STEBBINS, ERNEST L. *Mustard's Introduction to Public Health,* 5th ed. New York: Macmillan Co., 1968.

GILBERT, RUTH. *The Public Health Nurse and Her Patient.* Cambridge, Mass.: Harvard University Press, 1955.

GLASER, BARNEY G., and STRAUSS, ANSELM L. *The Discovery of Grounded Theory: Strategies for Qualitative Research.* Chicago: Aldine Publishing Co., 1968.

——*Awareness of Dying.* Chicago: Aldine Publishing Co., 1965.

HALL, JOANNE E., and WEAVER, BARBARA R., *Distributive Nursing Practice: A Systems Approach to Community Health.* Philadelphia: J. B. Lippincott Co., 1977.

HANLON, JOHN J. *Principles of Public Health Administration,* 5th ed. St. Louis: C. V. Mosby Co., 1969.

HILLEBOE, HERMAN, and GRANVILLE, W. LARIMORE, eds. *Preventive Medicine,* 2nd ed. Philadelphia: W. B. Saunders Co., 1965.

JACOBSON, MARGARET J. "Qualitative Data as a Potential Source of Theory in Nursing." *Image* 4 (1969):10–14.

JACOX, ADA. "Nursing Research and the Clinician." *Nursing Outlook* 22 (1974):382–85.

KALINS, ETHEL L. *Textbook of Public Health Nursing.* St. Louis: C. V. Mosby Co., 1967.

LEAHY, KATHLEEN M., COLILI, M. MARGUERITE, and JONES, MARY C. *Community Health Nursing,* 2nd ed. New York: McGraw-Hill Book Co., 1971.

LEAVELL, HUGH R., and CLARK, R. GURNEY. *Preventive Medicine for the Doctor in His Community: An Epidemiologic Approach,* 3rd ed. New York: McGraw-Hill Book Co., 1965.

MAHONEY, ROBERT F. *Emergency and Disaster Nursing.* London: Collier-Macmillan Ltd., 1969.

NATIONAL COMMISSION FOR THE STUDY OF NURSING AND NURSING EDUCATION, Jerome P. Lysaught, director. *An Abstract for Action.* New York: McGraw-Hill Book Co., 1970

OLESON, VIRGINIA L., and WHITAKER, ELVI W. *The Silent Dialogue.* San Francisco: Jossey-Bass, 1968.

OSBORNE, OLIVER H. "Anthropology and Nursing: Some Common Traditions and Interests." *Nursing Research* 18 (1969):251–55.

SARTWELL, PHILLIP E., ed. *Maxcey-Rosenau Preventive Medicine and Public Health,* 10th ed. New York: Appleton-Century-Crofts, 1973.

SCHATZMAN, LEONARD and STRAUSS, ANSELM L. *Field Research, Strategies for a*

Natural Sociology. Englewood Cliffs, N.J.: Prentice-Hall, 1973.

SMOLENSKY, JACK, and HOAR, FRANKLIN B. *Principles of Community Health,* 3rd ed. Philadelphia: W. B. Saunders Co., 1972.

WENSLEY, EDITH. *Nursing Service Without Walls: A Call to Action to All Communities Coast to Coast.* New York: National League for Nursing, 1963.

WILLIAMS, CAROLYN. "Community Health Nursing—What Is It?" *Nursing Outlook* 25 (April 1977):250–54.

WINSLOW, C. E. A. *Man and Epidemics.* Princeton, N.J.: Princeton University Press, 1952.

2. Selected Concepts for Community Health Nurses

Sarah Ellen Archer

INTRODUCTION

In this chapter we discuss some of the concepts basic to community nursing. You probably know about some of them; others may be less familiar, especially in the context used here. The purpose is to show the use to which we can put these concepts in working with our clients: individuals, families, groups, and communities.

There are many types of *communities*. The typology we present has proven useful for us in analyzing different kinds of communities to learn more about their structures and functions. Although most of us end up working in communities that are defined by agency, census, or legal criteria, these don't define the actual community that we must serve to be effective. Needs go beyond census tract or city limit boundaries, and we must be concerned with the larger area even though we may focus much of our attention on the community to which we are assigned.

Community health nurses must view the community as a client and so learn to work with communities as effectively as we do with individuals and families. This goal requires that we learn to assess communities and that we become actively involved in a variety of community activities. This involvement will not only help us increase our knowledge of the communities we serve but also provide us with opportunities to be more visible in the communities. Since many of our community activities must

21

be undertaken as volunteers, we also discuss some of the benefits of volunteerism in this chapter.

Others have spent many pages defining and redefining health. Rather than do that all again, we have decided to focus primarily on peoples' and systems' abilities to function as our indicator of health. Thus, from our viewpoint, community health nurses' basic goal is to promote clients' attainment and maintenance of their *optimum level of functioning* (OLOF). We believe that this goal should be the purpose of the entire health care delivery system as well. To help clients reach their OLOF we must consider the personal, social, biological, and environmental forces that impinge upon and therefore influence their abilities to function. Thus in this chapter we illustrate some of these factors to encourage community health nurses to look beyond the health care delivery system for influences on OLOF.

Later in the chapter, the many levels of functioning that exist are shown on a *continuum of function*. A number of positive and negative functional indicators ranging from OLOF to dysfunction are placed on the continuum. To assess the individual's or a population's location at any given time on the continuum of function, a variety of *health indicators* have been developed. These are measurements of many kinds of variables that are thought to describe the health status of the population. They include morbidity and mortality data, environmental and social characteristics, provider records, census data, and interview surveys of samples of the population. Data from all these health indicators, taken together as well as used separately, provide health workers with information about the client populations with whom they work and are useful in identifying high-risk groups and geographic areas. A number of sources of health indicator data are identified.

The chapter concludes with a brief discussion of the concept of *holism*. A holistic approach to the care of people is currently a very prevalent theme. Community health nurses have long dealt with whole clients in their own environment. As is shown in the discussion of the factors impinging on peoples' attainment and maintenance of OLOF, we must consider social, economic, political, environmental, behavioral, hereditary, and health care system influences on our clients if we are to help them promote their levels of functioning. We emphasize the environmental influences on people in order to expand the factors generally of concern in most holistic approaches. We feel this expansion is essential and is consonant with our systems approach to clients discussed in chapter 3.

COMMUNITY

There are almost as many definitions of community as there are people trying to define it. The purpose of this section is to present and discuss a typology of definitions so that each of us can develop or decide upon those that are meaningful and helpful to us. Definitions of types of communities can be divided into three general groups: emotional, structural, and functional. The three groups, as well as the individual types of community described in each one, are neither discrete nor mutually exclusive. In short, all the definitions tend to run together, which often results in people simply refusing to attempt to define community at all, even to the point of saying that community does not exist. We believe that community does exist in many forms, and we present some of them here.

EMOTIONAL COMMUNITIES

Emotional communities are elusive of definition. They center around a sense or feeling of community.

Belonging Communities.   This type of community may be viewed as a place where you belong; a place where you have "roots." Keyes states that ambivalence permeates the quest for this kind of community:

> To me, community   real community—is the place where I'm known, where I'm safe to be known for better or worse, on many levels. But it's so powerful to be unknown, to be anonymous, even if it's lonely. Am I willing to trade in my freedom to come and go unobserved for some 'sense of community'?
>
> We hate mass society and its institutions, hate the feeling of not being known anywhere—but it's power, a power we'd give up very reluctantly [Keyes 1973:14].

He attributes our lack of community to our fondness for three things: mobility, privacy, and convenience (Keyes 1973:15).

Americans' mobility is well known and redocumented by every new census. Mobility has contributed to the development of the nuclear family as young people move away from their relatives because of jobs, or adventure, or just "because." Children grow up without knowing their grandparents. People get old and have no family close by to care for them. Mobility is a mixed blessing.

Community has been defined as the opposite of privacy (Chermayeff and Tzonis 1971:28). This view seems reasonable since, as Keyes mentioned, being unknown is inherent in privacy. Toffler speaks of the value of anonymity and disposable relationships (1970:95–123). Certain analysts consider the increase in burglaries and street crime directly related to lack of a feeling of community—that is, where neighbors don't want to know each other and can be counted on *not* to get involved or even notice when things aren't going as usual in the neighborhood. This lack of feeling is a kind of quest for privacy.

Many convenience factors in our homes have reduced our opportunities to communicate with each other. Doom-crying authors have long talked about the deterioration of the American family; television is one modern scapegoat. Although it brings many new things to us, we sit alone and silent to receive its offerings. Another example is the combination of the desire for privacy and convenience that is among the reasons for the failure of many efforts to organize car pools. For many, driving is the only time they have to be alone, and they're not about to give it up without a struggle, regardless of the soaring price of energy.

Community nurses who have the opportunity to work where people are known and relate closely to each other have many allies when families and individual people need help. If the mother in one family is ill, another mother can be counted on to help out. In communities where these kinds of personal relations among neighborhood residents do not exist, the nurse and the client must find other resources for help, often at great expense, *if* any can be found at all.

Special Interest Communities.   These communities are bound together by a common set of interests or needs that make members alike in at least the area of their special interest (Blum 1974:501). For example, nurses tend to identify, at least to a point, with other nurses insofar as we share common experiences. This identification goes beyond the scope of professional organizations, although these structural communities may reap some benefits from the emotional community that exists among those sharing a common profession. Special interest communities may come and go with the rise and fall of issues. Mothers may become a special interest community until a stop light is placed at an intersection where their children must cross a busy street. When the cause is removed the community may dissolve, at least temporarily. Animal owners, sports fans, and foreign car owners are illustrations of special interest communities.

Special interest groups offer ready-made opportunities for our use for the benefit of our clients. Mothers who will work together to get a stop light can be encouraged to undertake other kinds of activities, and the community nurse can help spark and encourage them. Special interest groups can also be formed if a sufficiently important issue is raised or even if a relatively trivial cause is sufficiently well publicized.

STRUCTURAL COMMUNITIES

Structural communities involve time and space relationships among people. These communities are physical ones such as towns and cities. Obviously, many functional communities develop in these structural ones where people live and work.

Aggregates.   Probably the most general structural definition of a community is any aggregate of people, regardless of why they are gathered. In this definition stress is on "togetherness" for its own sake. Almost any conceivable group, from a nation to a casual crowd, can fit under this classification. An advantage of this kind of definition for community nurses is that they can relate to any cluster of people as a client-community. In nursing, "community" has often been applied to all that space *outside* "the hospital," which has been the *inside*. Thus, the realization that at least in this one sense the hospital can be a community can free us from an artificial division. In my own classes, I use this context in teaching community organization and stress that a hospital unit or the hospital as a whole is a perfectly appropriate community to try to organize.

Special Risk Groups or Aggregates.   Williams defines aggregates in another way. She uses the term to refer to groups of persons who have one or more personal or environmental characteristics in common. Her examples include groups of people with hypertension whose risk of stroke or coronary heart disease is greater than those people whose blood pressure is within normal limits. Black men are a higher risk group for hypertension than are the other aggregates in the population (1977:251). People who live in areas of high environmental risk such as near nuclear waste disposal sites, refineries, chemical plants, and other environmental hazards are high-risk aggregates from radiation and other types of environmental pollution. Smokers, alcohol, and other drug abusers are self-induced high-risk aggregates within the population. Community nurses may work specifically with any one or several of these kinds of high-risk groups as their community.

Face to Face Communities.   This type of community is, the "primary" community of groups such as families, neighborhoods, parishes, and other closely knit, relatively small groups (Blum 1974:498). In face-to-face communities news travels fast and everyone knows everybody else's business. These are the communities about which Keyes was so ambivalent and the kind of community about which Ross observed, ". . . the social structure of a community constitutes a whole, and . . . change in any one part of the structure reacts on all other parts" (1967:111).

Such communities can be found in rural areas and in the "ethnic" communities of eastern cities where people of European descent have lived for a period of time. Because of the closeness and commonalities of the people in the community, help and care are often freely exchanged. The community nurse's job of finding caretakers and other kinds of assistance for clients (see chapter 7) is easier than in other types of communities.

Communities of Problem Ecology.   The boundaries of these communities encompass the geographical areas affected by ecological problems (Blum 1974:500). Epidemiologists have long realized that ecological problems ignore geopolitical boundaries; the Great Plagues of the Middle Ages were an early and bitter lesson to this effect. The ecological problem of urban and industrial pollution of an inland river can be an example of this kind of problem-defined community. All the people, municipalities, and industries located in its drainage basin must act in concert if the waterway is to be cleaned up.

Another example of a community of problem ecology is the social climate or environment in which we, particularly in the United States, live. Toffler describes the effects on people of the exponential changes that are taking place in this society (1970). Inabilities to cope with the techno-logical and social changes are thought to be reflected in the increasing rates of drug and alcohol abuse, violence, suicides, and other symptoms of alienation. All these problems are highly pertinent for community nurses working with clients in today's society since we are seeing increasing numbers of people with these kinds of needs.

Geopolitical Communities. These communities are units of political jurisdiction and have definite legal, geographic boundaries; examples are cities, towns, states, and nations. They are the seat of regularized political and legal power and are often the site to which client-centered advocacy actions must be directed. The fact that problems and needs, as well as potential solutions, often spread over many political jurisdictions means that cooperation and coordination must be sought. Thus, tradeoffs, terri-torial conflicts, and inadequate programs often arise. Some of these phe-nomena are discussed in chapter 11 on politics and economics.

Organizations. These kinds of communities include health departments, hospitals, churches, labor unions, and other bureaucracies. These institu-tions have a structure that binds members together. They have power, in varying degrees, to regulate the activities their members undertake. The fact that organizations have boundaries or jurisdictional limits is manifest in the recognition that some client needs can be met more appropriately by other organizations than the one for which the community nurse works. This recognition can make a gross difference, such as sending a sick child to the hospital or to another physician because the well baby clinic does not serve sick children. More subtly, it may mean referring a client who cannot afford private health services to a governmental agency or free clinic rather than to a private care facility.

Community of Solution. This community was defined by the National Commission on Community Health Services as a community with "boun-daries within which a problem can be defined, dealt with, and solved" (1966:2). The Commission also talked about "environmental problem-sheds" and "health services marketing areas" as well as the interdependence of communities on each other for the solution of health and environmental problems (1966:4). Communities of solution transcend geopolitical areas in their effort to define an area large enough to provide the solutions for problems.

Community nurses can make excellent use of the idea of community of solution when searching for resources to help clients meet their needs. Because communities of solution extend beyond geopolitical limits, the nurse should be sure to inquire about agency eligibility requirements for people from other jurisdictions, since some agencies confine their services to their own locale. Town A has a special education program and town B does not. You're the community nurse in town B and you have a family with a child who needs to be in the special education class in town A. The community of solution for this problem includes both towns A and B. Before referring the family to the special class in town A, you had best make sure that they will accept the referral from another jurisdiction. Of course the family can probably find out for themselves, but part of your responsibility in making referrals is to be sure that the referrals are appropriate and therefore will be accepted. In other words, the nurse needs to be sure that the special education program in town A is part of the realistic community of solution for the client who needs to be enrolled there, even though he or she lives in town B.

FUNCTIONAL COMMUNITIES

Definitions of functional community have a common baseline in the belief by the local people involved that ". . . community is whatever sense of the local common good citizens can be helped to achieve" (Hayes 1962:153). Functional definitions are predicated on the assumption that community is an achievement rather than the result of mere geographic placement. Functional communities are not fixed; they change as a result of experience and in accordance with alterations in problems that catch people's attention (Biddle and Biddle 1965:77).

Communities of Identifiable Need.   These communities are based on a common problem such as might be had by migrant workers or women wishing to have abortions (Blum 1974:499). This type is much like the communities of special interest and problem ecology already cited. Municipalities or institutions can join together in communities to meet shared needs; an example is the Association of Bay Area Governments in the San Francisco Area or the consortia being developed by institutions of higher education to help them stretch their resources through programs of sharing with other schools.

Community nurses often work with communities of identifiable need in such positions as state health department staff assigned to direct, semi-direct, or indirect activities focusing on such a community. Programs such as abortion counseling, computerizing migrant children's school records and all migrant persons' health records for easy transmission to other locations, and arranging for special education classes for handi-capped children are all community nursing activities related to com-munities of identifiable needs.

Critical Mass Communities. This functional community is much like Blum's community of resources (1974:503–04) in which there are suf-ficient resources—money, personnel, consumers, influence with other communities and jurisdictions, and material—or whatever else is needed to do something about a problem, need, or situation. "Critical mass" in general usage means sufficient resources to support a program or service; for example, the number of people needed in an area to provide economic support for and sufficient utilization of a facility. In higher education the term is used to denote the presence within the institution of sufficient numbers and specializations of faculty to attract research funds, excep-tional graduate students, and other well-qualified faculty. Thus the con-stituents and numbers of persons or resources vary with the situation. Six people may be the critical mass community to deal with a particular need, provided they are the right people.

Since the critical mass community is identified here as a functional one, it is not bound to a set of geographical boundaries, however they are defined, as is the community of solution discussed before. The basis for a critical mass community may be geographic, such as the areas that must be considered in trying to solve the pollution problems of our inland lakes and rivers. However, the critical mass community for these problems must also include Washington, D.C., where the power and the capital are located to bring plans for cleanup to at least partial fruition. The critical mass community, then, must be an amalgam of whatever kinds of communities—functional, emotional, structural—are needed to deal with the problem at hand. Hopefully, critical mass communities could be put together to deal only with specific issues and then dissolved. Such tem-porary goal-directed organizations, or *adhocracies*, could free their compo-nents to create new configurations to deal with other problems.

A conference of all of the agency representatives who are working with a client can be a critical mass community function. Often the community nurse arranges these meetings. Their outcomes may vary from plans to continue activities with a client as they have been, to institute new activi-ties, or to discontinue some if the agencies decide services are no longer needed. Quite frequently this kind of meeting points up the fact that other agencies and services are needed by the client. This decision is based on the realization that the present group cannot meet its objectives; therefore, the group is not a critical mass community. For example, a patient is about to leave the hospital following a stroke; the nurse in charge of discharge planning calls together the community nurse, the physical therapist, the social worker, and the other personnel directly involved with the patient to discuss plans for home care. Soon after the meeting begins, the community nurse points out that the group really cannot plan unless the client, the spouse, or whoever will be giving care at home is involved in the discussions. Thus, the group present comes to the realization that it is not a critical mass community for this situation. By adding the client's spouse to the planning group, the community nurse is striving to create a critical mass community that can function to help the client's family cope with its needs.

We community nurses need to be aware of the many kinds of communities that exist and in which we work. This discussion can serve as a baseline for your initial community nursing experience. As you experience these kinds of communities and read further about the changes in our society, doubtless you will begin to identify and define your own classification of communities.

COMMUNITY NURSES' INVOLVEMENT IN COMMUNITY ACTIVITIES

Nurses, particularly community health nurses, must become increasingly involved in the variety of community activities that influence peoples' health and their abilities to function optimally. This kind of participation requires that we view the entire community—regardless of what kind it is—as our client. We must learn to relate to groups of people and organizations with the same ease and effectiveness that we have developed in dealing with individuals and families. Thus we must know our communities as well as we do the individuals within them. There are many techniques for community assessment and organization that you may find useful (Altshuler 1970; Bello 1975; Cox 1974; Kahn 1970; Kent 1972; Kramer 1975; Milio 1970; OM Collective 1971; Ross 1967; Ruybal, Bauwens, and Falsa 1975).

As community health nurses, we bring a unique perspective to all kinds of community organizations. There's very little that goes on in communities that doesn't influence someone's ability to cope. We are generally the group of health care professionals that has the most ongoing contacts with people in their own territory. We are able, therefore, to make observations and ask questions as well as be told things that our clients are less likely to discuss with other professionals in other settings. Because of our preparation in nursing in general and community nursing in particular, we have a whole set of tools and skills not only for assessing what we see and hear, but also for using these data to help influence change. Community nurses can serve as a vital link in the communication network between all kinds of community agencies and our clients since we can have a foot in both camps. We can do so by encouraging clients to come to meetings and speak their piece or, if that doesn't work, at least make sure that our clients have information about what is going on. We should be able to speak both our clients' and our colleagues' languages and thus play an interpreter role. I have found the consumer members of boards and committees are often less intimidated in talking to nurses than they are with other disciplines represented. With participation in community planning for health also come opportunities to be client advocates, a legitimate and essential role for community nurses.

CONDITIONING AS WOMEN

For all of us, much of the decision to participate in community activities has to do with our conditioning as women that influences the way we view work. Men are raised from infancy with the idea that they will work to support themselves and probably several other people as well. Women are more ambiguous about work and about how long they will work. Although this pattern is undergoing some change, it is still the norm rather than the exception. Our ambiguity underlies and influences much of what we do with regard to our professional development and whether we view nursing as a career rather than a series of jobs. Hennig and Jardim (1977) have observed that most women make career decisions ten years later than men do for a variety of reasons: ambiguity about work itself, assumptions that they will marry and devote their time to family responsibilities, or that their income would always be supplementary and, therefore, less important. Women also tend to be more passive than are men in seizing, much less creating, career opportunities. We tend to wait to be chosen rather than to assertively go after what we want and believe is our due. We also tend to see each job or position as an end in itself rather than a means to a subsequent position or professional attainment. For nursing to evolve as a profession and for us to take our appropriate and responsible place in the array of health care providers, nursing itself and the women in nursing must become more assertive and career oriented.

VOLUNTEERISM

Another real problem in working in community activities is that much of such involvement must be on our own time and is without pay. Most community and professional organizations at best reimburse their officers and board members only for their actual expenses. Many faculty members in schools of nursing participate in community activities as a requirement of their positions. A growing number of service agencies are also seeing the value of having their nurses involved in community activities. However, this community involvement is still too often seen more as a responsibility for nurses at the higher administrative or academic levels than for all of us. Thus in most instances all of the time devoted to community work must be our own time. Opinions of the value or cost of volunteerism run the gamut from outright exploitation to invaluable growth experiences. For example, I am hard pressed to figure out where I have learned the most—in academic preparation, paid work experience, or as a volunteer. All three kinds of experiences have contributed immensely to my personal and professional development. Naturally, one must be able to afford the time involved in volunteer work, both from an hours and a money stand point.

Being a volunteer also calls up ideas of doing trivial chores or simply getting in the staff's way. As anyone knows who has participated in a well-organized and-maintained volunteer program, these problems need not occur. My experience both as a volunteer and as a staff person working with volunteers confirms my belief that volunteers enable services to be given that otherwise would never occur—like the whole free clinic movement. Also volunteers can do things in and to the system in which they function that paid staff wouldn't dare attempt. Volunteers can't be fired by an irate administrator. Volunteers, therefore, have a whole different set of vested interests and opportunities than do staff people.

Volunteers can gain a good deal of power by using their social position and occupational stature to add prestige to their volunteer activities. I learned this as a youngster watching my parents, both of whom are hopelessly addicted volunteers in all sorts of community organizations. Before one is permitted to have a voice in what happens in a group, as noted before, one must pay one's dues. Nurses who pay their dues to organizations, however they can do so, earn the right to contribute to the information that goes into decision making and to be listened to when making suggestions about directions an agency might take. Nurses following this pattern will also have access to information about the community's power structure and be able to develop linkages that can be helpful in efforts to bring about change.

Much progress has been made in the last few years in nurses' involvement as paid staff and as volunteers in community planning and development activities. We've come a long way, but we still have considerable distance to go. We are the numerically largest group of health care providers but our scope of influence does not reflect our numbers. Many still lack skills and incentives to become involved in community activities at all, much less those related to promoting and maintaining the ability of people and communities to function optimally. Clearly, involvement in the community is not for the community health nurse who wants an 8-to-5 job with weekends off. As we illustrate in our description of the community nurses' activities in Pomo County (see chapter 14), legitimation of our role in community activities is far more time consuming. We must be ready to speak out or act as a community health nurse whenever and wherever the opportunity or need arises. No matter where our professional or personal interests lie, there are community groups who need and would welcome our participation.

PERSONAL VALUES OF VOLUNTEERING

More personally valuable spillovers from involvement as a volunteer include opportunities to explore fields of possible interest, resumé building, and job creation. Using voluntary participation as a means to learn more about an area or field in which you think you may be interested is one way to gain this information without having to make the same kind of commitment as is involved if you sought employment in the field. For example, many people have learned about working with older people from volunteering at senior centers or visiting home-bound people through their church or other groups. This kind of experience can lead to the pursuit of a career in gerontology. Others may explore their interests in children and young people by volunteering in day care, girl or boy scouting, and athletic programs. Still others can learn about the needs of people with cancer or heart disease by working through their local chapter of the American Cancer Society or Heart Association. Most communities of any size abound with these kinds of opportunities if we only look for them. Rural areas may have more limited formal resources and therefore even greater needs for our volunteer services.

Resumé building is an essential activity for us all. When you initiate a job application, are invited to apply for a position, or seek admission to an educational program, your resumé must be the selling tool to people you often do not know by describing clearly your experience and skills. Therefore, your resumé must put your best foot forward. Inclusion of a description of your volunteer work, particularly if you have been an officer or chaired a committee, can be a valuable addition to your resumé. If nothing else it tells prospective employers or admissions' committees that you have an interest in your community that extends beyond the requirements of your job. Documentation of volunteer work can also serve at least as a partial substitute for paid work experience. For example, many of the women whose applications for graduate school I have seen have been able to document activities in community health nursing by showing that they worked as volunteers for the Red Cross in setting up and running blood bank programs, or for the Cancer Society as volunteers in "Reach for Recovery" programs and "Ostomy Clubs," or for the local hospice in supporting and caring for a family whose member is dying at home. The list can go on and on. In addition, people with whom you have worked as a volunteer can be an excellent source of letters of reference.

Finally, jobs can often be obtained and even created as a result of volunteer activities. For example, several of the nurses in Pomo County were able to create jobs for themselves as a result of demonstrating the need for their services, the demand for those services in the community, and organizing others to help them put the needed pressure on the power structure to create the jobs and allocate sufficient money. The Pomo health center we describe is still functioning four years later with two full-time family nurse-practitioners (see chapter 14). Many of our other graduate students have helped the positions they now hold to evolve through their field work as students, basically a volunteer activity, and their work as volunteers in the same or related agencies. For example, the present codirectors of a senior day services program helped write the grant proposal that Nursing Dynamics Corporation submitted to create the day services program (Archer and Fleshman, forthcoming, and Part V, Postscripts and Cautionary Tales). Their original job-sharing position was less than 50 percent time each. Through their own efforts, supported by the corporation, they have increased the revenues for the program to the point where they are now both 75 percent time. All of this came about through their becoming known in a community as graduate students doing field work and volunteering with other agencies. The process takes time and patience, but it's paid off for them. It can pay off for you, too.

We realize that many readers may have difficulty seeing themselves as consultants, volunteers, and advocates because their own life experiences and circumstances have not yet brought them to the point where they feel confident enough or see sufficient need to embark on such activities. I come from a middle-class background where I had many role models for these kinds of activities. Perhaps I made a career decision earlier than many women do and so have had more time to learn how to participate in community activities. I am a fairly high energy person—although I must admit that I am having to slow down at least a little, lately. I am in an academic setting where I am expected to be active in public service as part of my job responsibilities. As a community health nurse, the community, its people and its organizations, are my clinical area of practice, and so to remain a competent clinical practitioner in my own eyes as well as those of my colleagues and students, I must continue to work in a variety of kinds of communities. My career goals and all of these circumstances have combined to influence my choice of activities. Each of you has your own set of goals and circumstances. Each of you will develop your own patterns of response to them. We hope that many of you will become involved in community activities both for the personal and professional rewards inherent, but also for the contributions you have to make to others.

OPTIMUM LEVEL OF FUNCTIONING (OLOF)

We have chosen to use the term *optimum level of functioning* or OLOF as our definition of health. OLOF is the best *possible* functioning, taking all things into account. It is a goal toward which we strive, but like all absolutes, is probably impossible to achieve since we live in a world where absolutes are more easily defined than attained. Most other definitions of health share the same ideal, goal-like characteristic.

The point we wish to emphasize in our selection of OLOF is that an individual's *abilities*, not disabilities, should be the focal point of consideration. This emphasis is analogous to "high-level wellness" (Dunn 1961). Few of us are without some so-called disability: the need for glasses, allergies, emotional hangups, and as we grow older, chronic noninfectious conditions. The important thing is not whether we have such conditions, but rather, what we do with or about them. In assessing the degree to which people have attained OLOF, we must consider many kinds of data including so-called "subjective" data on how individuals feel and perceive their own status. These perceptions will change since we live in an everchanging environment and must constantly adapt to personal and environmental alterations (see figure 2.1).

OLOF as we have defined it here is consonant with Terris' suggested revision of the WHO definition of health:

> Health is a state of physical, mental and social well-being and ability to function, and not merely the absence of illness or infirmity [Terris 1975:1038].

As we shall see later in the chapter, OLOF comes from a holistic perspective in dealing with whole client environment. This holistic point of view is illustrated in figure 2.1.

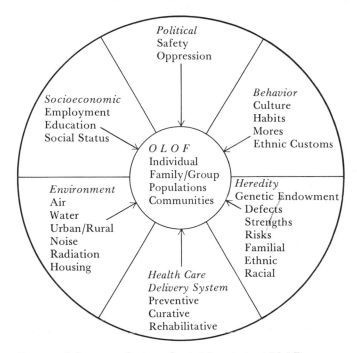

2.1   *Ecosystem Influences on Optimum Level of Functioning (OLOF)*

Each individual has a unique OLOF that he or she strives to attain and maintain. The paraplegic who, as a result of rehabilitation and modification of his environment, is able to be independent, hold down a job, and enjoy life *by his own evaluation* is functioning at his OLOF. His abilities outweigh his disabilities, and in his own eyes he is able to be a productive person.

In figure 2.1, which is modified from Blum (1974:3), we show some of the ecosystem influences acting on and therefore influencing our OLOF. We will briefly discuss each of these influences beginning at the top of the figure and proceeding clockwise.

Political Influences.   These influences have a great effect on the social climate in which we live (see chapter 11). Political jurisdictions have the power and authority to regulate much of our surroundings. The two variables listed in figure 2.1 are safety and oppression. Crime and lack of safety rank among our highest concerns. For example, the decision to expend police department resources in pursuit of victimless crimes while violent crimes increase is a political one. Many minority groups suffer from oppression, institutionalized racism and sexism, differential treatment by law-enforcement officers and school counselors. All of these are political influences having profoundly negative effects on both the oppressed and the oppressors (see chapter 20).

Behavioral Influences.　Habits such as smoking, lack of exercise, and substance abuse adversely affect our OLOF. Culture and ethnic heritage shape much of our lifestyle, including what we eat, and many of our attitudes about those around us, health care, and child-rearing practices.

Hereditary Influences.　Boundaries of abilities and potentials set by heredity are often less modifiable than other influences. Knowledge is increasing about genetics and the possible interventions to prevent or at least minimize their effects. Genetic counseling is more available now, but is still inadequate to meet the population's needs (Jolly 1972).

Health Care Delivery System Influences.　The health care delivery system really plays a relatively minor role in the array of influences on OLOF. It is a disease-oriented system far more than a health- or OLOF-oriented one. The rise of health maintenance organizations and the shift in health insurance coverage to help pay for preventive care may alter this focus. Much more emphasis is needed on primary, secondary, and tertiary prevention measures by health professionals such as community nurses who are concerned with OLOF and not illness (Leavell and Clark 1965). Many of these interventions will have to occur outside as well as inside the health care delivery system as we now define it.

Environmental Influences.　When I first studied environmental health, we had a cliché: "The solution to pollution is dilution." The ecology movement a few years later made clear that there was no longer enough air or water or earth to dilute our wastes. We are a polluting species, and our lack of concern until recently with our environment has caused many irreversible changes. Builders seem determined to cover the entire earth with concrete. Our health is also being affected. Air pollution is linked with lung cancer and emphysema. Chemical water-borne poisonings are an increasing threat to wildlife and man. Environmental influences have begun to produce adverse responses and interfere with our ability to attain and maintain OLOF.

Socioeconomic Influences.　A colleague of ours who has long worked with migrant workers is fond of pointing out that her clients' problems could be solved very well and easily: Give them enough money to live on. Given decent and consistent wages, they could care for their own educational, medical, social, and environmental needs. There are many points of view on this matter, but she may very well be right in terms of her own clients. Most complex problems, however, are not generally amenable to single-approach solutions.

Together, the influences on OLOF shown in figure 2.1 make up our ecosphere. Realization that promoting OLOF must include consideration of the effects of all of these influences on our clients means that we must take a much broader view of our responsibilities. Again the focus on primary, secondary, and tertiary prevention forces us to consider *all* these other influences since that's where these preventive activities must take place. That's the major reason for the inclusion in this book of chapters on research, epidemiology, health education, politics and economics, health insurance, and the variety of settings in which community nurses apply these skills and knowledge.

We should also take a long look at the health care delivery system's components closest to us. We've got to become committed to shifting the system's concern to a more client-centered one. A place to start is rethinking many of the procedures we follow. Such changes are not easy nor can they be implemented without considerable resistance from colleagues and employing agencies. However, if we are committed to meeting client needs, we must think more in terms of fitting our schedules to clients' convenience rather than our own. Most people work during the day, Monday through Friday; so do most nurses in health departments. Many nurses pick community health because of the 8-to-5 schedule with weekends off. The system is not here to take care of nurses' needs, but rather to serve clients' needs. We are in for some interesting information when clients' voices become more dominant in evaluations of services received. If we really want to be where things are happening or could be helped to happen, we're going to have to go to meetings and gatherings at 7:30 A.M. and 8 P.M. and on weekends. This example is only one of many possible. We need to look around at our own system and see what other alterations we can and should make to facilitate our helping clients attain and maintain their OLOF.

CONTINUUM OF FUNCTION

The use of *function* as our measure of health status provides the opportunity to look at factors that positively influence function as well as those that negatively affect it. This view of ability to function is illustrated in figure 2.2, the Continuum of Function. The continuum is conceptualized as a seesaw that is balanced at a neutral point of functioning at the center. This neutral point of functioning, as the name implies, is neither positive nor negative, good nor bad. Instead it is the fulcrum upon which we seesaw back and forth between our optimum level of functioning and dysfunction.

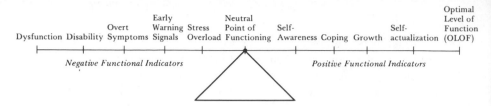

2.2   *Continuum of Function*

Traditionally most of our so-called health indicators, as we shall see later in this chapter, have dealt with disease, disability, and death. They look at the prevalence and causes of these deviations from health or ability to function as surrogate measures for assessing health. This perspective can lead us to tell people, "Well, we can't find anything wrong with you so you can consider yourself healthy." We submit that there must be more to health then the mere absence of disease, particularly since, as we noted earlier, few of us are without some sort of disease or disability.

Thus, the continuum of function can be useful since it requires that we look at both positive and negative functional factors as indicators. The positive indicators are those with which we as community nurses are particularly concerned in helping clients attain and maintain their optimum level of functioning. In short, our efforts should be to help clients tip their continuum of function toward the positive side. The first step is *self-awareness*, which we can facilitate by helping clients see where they are and understand what's happening to them. Until we are aware, we cannot begin to cope. *Coping*, which is the ability to deal constructively with what is happening, is the second phase. We can work effectively with clients in this phase by providing support, by listening, by helping them find and utilize resources, and finally, by assisting them to define and explore alternatives. Growth involves change, while coping involves dealing with the status quo.

Most often *growth* means change in oneself or one's attitudes toward a situation, since changing oneself is often easier than actually altering the situation itself. This process begins in the coping stage when a client starts to look for new avenues or alternatives rather than stay where he or she is. Often the community nurse is the first to know about this change in attitude and desire for a change. We can help clients evaluate alternatives and then make their own changes, or we can steer them to appropriate agencies where they can get assistance. *Self-actualization*, the next phase on the continuum, means that the clients have attained their level of aspiration or achievement and are successful in their own eyes. It is but a short jump from this point to attainment of OLOF.

Community nurses can help varieties of clients move through these positive steps toward OLOF in many ways. We can teach the new mother to become increasingly comfortable in caring for her infant until the point at which she feels secure and confident in her abilities. We can work with school-age children who are having trouble with their studies because of problems at home until they can at least cope more effectively with the situation while we or other agency people help the family work through their difficulties. We can support and push when the young quadraplegic starts to slip into depression and feelings of uselessness and use self-awareness as a steppingstone to coping rather than as the prelude to stress overload. We can reassure and reinforce as we work with the older woman who has had a mastectomy or stroke and who now wants to return to her independent status. These are all positive activities to help people toward their OLOF. Some will attain it; others will not. Almost all can be helped to be more aware and to cope better; many can grow toward self-actualization. More than we know can attain OLOF. We won't know how many until we change our own attitudes to ones of promoting function rather than preventing dysfunction. This notion closely parallels our emphasis on primary prevention in chapter 9

HEALTH INDICATORS

As noted earlier in this chapter what are traditionally called *health indicators* are indeed for the most part measures of disease and disability. The trend now is to develop positive measurements of health status although these are slow in coming and accompanied with much debate (Davies 1975; Goldsmith 1973; Terris 1975; Belloc and Breslow 1972). For the purposes of our discussion here, we will review some of the kinds of health indicator data with which community health nurses need to be familiar. (See the glossary at the end of chapter 9 on epidemiology for a number of epidemiologic terms and the appendix to that chapter for formulas for computing rates used in vital statistics.)

Because health, however it is defined, cannot be readily measured directly, a wide variety of sources of information are considered in order to derive indirect measurements or indicators of the health status of populations. The basic assumption is that if these indicators are themselves optimal, then the health status of the people to whom these indicators apply will probably be good. Thus, if the incidence of infectious diseases is low in a population, we may assume that their health is likely to be better than if the rate is high. Infant mortality, which is higher in the United States than in fourteen other countries (*Social Indicators 1976*), is an indicator that is used frequently to compare health statuses of different populations. Its value is that it infers information about many health-related variables such as the health status of childbearing-age women, the quality of medical care, sanitation, and access to medical and prenatal care. The relationship of these kinds of indicators is relatively easy to see. It is not so easy to make the connection, perhaps, but health is also likely to be better where most or all of the people have indoor toilets that work, more years of education, and are not living in crowded housing conditions.

The study of health indicators and the making of inferences from them about the health status of a population is dependent on a sound base of data about factors affecting that population. One of the earliest recorded instances of the specific use of data to look at the health status was in the early 1600s in England where John Graunt began to summarize the numbers of deaths that occurred each week in London. His data source was the London Bill of Mortality, a forerunner of our modern death certificate. By 1728, Bills of Mortality had been expanded to include the sex and age of the person as well as their cause of death. In 1837 William Farr analyzed information from a number of sources in terms of deaths, sickness rates, and days of sickness for individuals and groups. This work was the beginning of the use of morbidity as well as mortality data as a basis for estimating the health status of the people. Massachusetts produced the first statewide mortality data tabulation in 1857. Birth and death registration became nationwide in the United States in 1933. Thus, many of our people who must prove age eligibility for Social Security must use family *Bible* records, school entry and baptismal certificates, and affidavits from relatives to establish their date of birth, since they never had a birth certificate. Interview surveys of the population to determine the prevalence of various conditions date back at least to the Irish census of 1851. In 1880 the U.S. federal census included some questions whose answers were obtained through household canvassing. These data enabled the Census Bureau to describe morbidity for fourteen million people by age and geographic location. Social and economic interests in the late nineteenth and early twentieth centuries led the U.S. Department of Labor in 1893 to survey workers in major eastern cities about their illnesses during the preceding twelve months. Private firms like Metropolitan Life Insurance Company also did surveys to determine the seasonable distributions of illnesses. A number of small-scale health surveys continued through the Second World War (Katz et al. 1973).

By the late 1940s the reality of the major impact chronic diseases were having on the population became increasingly apparent. In 1949 the Commission on Chronic Illness was established to find ways to solve the problems of chronic illnesses and to serve the chronically ill. Methods developed toward these ends included multiphasic screening, medical examinations, and interview surveys. In 1956 passage of the National Health Survey Act gave rise to the National Center for Health Statistics whose charge is to develop and use methods to obtain current data on illness, disability, and other related phenomena (Katz et al. 1973). All of these approaches to the gathering of information indicating the health status of the population are in current use. We shall consider some of them specifically.

Census Data.   Census data provide a great deal of information especially about urbanized populations in what are called Standard Metropolitan Statistical Areas (SMSA)—that is, communities whose population exceeds 50,000. Many of these data can be used to assess health status and health needs in the population they describe. For example, census data are given by census tracts, which are geographic areas within the SMSA defined on the basis of approximately equal numbers of people residing within the census tract. Thus, census tracts can vary greatly in geographic size. In SMSAs, the urban area is divided into census tracts each of which has several city blocks in it, while the large, sparsely populated rural area of the county is divided into a few very large census tracts. Your area, if you live in an SMSA, is divided in a similar manner.

Data available on census tracts include breakdowns of the population by a number of characteristics: age, sex, ethnic background, marital status, educational level, type of occupation, and income. Environmental information includes condition of housing, population density (numbers of people per dwelling), means of transportation to work, and much more. Taken together, these census data can help us identify potentially high-risk groups of people. For example, families with small children, low incomes, and limited education, crowded into substandard dwellings should have their situations explored by community health nurses. They can be suspected to have some of these kinds of risks and needs: The people may have inadequate information about what services are available in their community and how to use them; if the housing is old, the small children may run a risk of lead poisoning from peeling paint as well as many other kinds of environmental hazards; the people living under these circumstances are more prone to a variety of infectious conditions, including tuberculosis, than are people living in other environments; and infant mortality and general morbidity are likely to be higher for these groups, especially if they are ethnic people of color, than they are for the total population. To be sure, census data cannot provide conclusive information about these and other risk factors facing groups in the population, but they can be of great help in identifying population groups and areas where priorities for investigation should be directed.

Most city and state libraries as well as those at colleges and universities have copies of census data for their area. Planning departments of Health Systems Agencies are other courses for these materials. We suggest that you locate the census data for your locale and take time to read through them. I was amazed the first time I did this how much information is contained there and to how many uses it can be put.

Vital Statistics. Vital data are another source of health indicator information. Each state has its own forms for birth certificates, death certificates, marriage licenses, and procedures for filing for divorce and separation. These forms must be filled out completely and filed with the state or other geopolitical jurisdiction. Data on causes of death are collected from death certificates, which must clearly specify what brought about the person's death as certified by the attending physician or coroner. Causes of death must conform to the nomenclature for disease entities and conditions in the current International Classification of Diseases. A few recent examples of vital data are as follows: Between 1953 and 1974 the annual number of divorces increased by 150 percent (from 390,000 to 977,000 annually); between 1945 and 1975 life expectancy for men in the United States increased from 63.6 years to 68.7 years and for women from 67.9 years to 76.5 years; and infant mortality dropped from 24.7 infants per 1,000 live births in 1965 to 16.7 infants per 1,000 live births in 1974. Compilation of vital data is a worldwide phenomenon that enables comparisons between countries to be made. Thus, statistics people tell us that the United States ranked seventeenth in terms of longevity for males and seventh for females internationally in 1975. This information means that men in sixteen and women in six other countries live longer than do men and women here. We also ranked fifteenth in infant mortality (Social Indicators 1976). These rankings, assuming that the data on which they are based in other countries are comparable to ours (and the World Health Organization strives to see that this is the case), raise questions about our general quality of life here in terms of the health or ability to function, or whatever definition one wishes to use, of our population.

Reportable Diseases. The incidence of occurrence of certain infectious diseases must be reported to health authorities with varying degrees of haste. For example, Class 1 diseases require universal reporting under International Health Regulations. These diseases include cholera, plague, smallpox, yellow fever, louse-borne typhus fever and relapsing fever, paralytic poliomyelitis, influenza, and malaria (Benenson 1975:xxiv). Because of their potential for epidemic spread, these diseases must be reported by telephone or telegraph so that swift measures can be instituted on the scale necessary to protect the population.

Class 2 diseases must also be reported whenever and wherever they occur. Diseases like typhoid fever and diphtheria are reportable by phone or telegraph. Others such as brucellosis and leprosy are reportable weekly by mail (Benenson 1975:xxiv). Again this mandatory reporting is to enable health officials to take appropriate action. Local jurisdictions may add other diseases to the list of mandatory reportable diseases and specify the manner in which reporting is to be done. The requirement to report extends to all practitioners who may have opportunity to see people with any of the Class 2 diseases. Private physicians, clinics, hospitals, and other practitioners are generally supplied with detailed instructions on what to report and how to report it. Many health departments have printed postcards that the practitioner merely fills out and drops in the mail. The case study at the beginning of chapter 9 describes a typical reporting procedure. As community health nurses, we must be aware of the diseases that are reportable in our area and be sure that reporting is carried out promptly. This task may involve reminding other practitioners that a report is required and monitoring the procedure or filing the report ourselves. Again the point of reporting the required information is to permit health department personnel to make the necessary decisions to prevent or control the spread of these diseases among susceptible people.

Record Review as a Source of Health Indicator Data.   Data for reports of morbidity, disability, facility utilization, days lost from work or school, numbers and types of insurance claims filed, incidence of infectious diseases, and many more indicators of the population's health status are compiled by governmental and private agencies for a variety of purposes. Statistical data are being collected from all kinds of facilities, individual and groups of providers, third-party payers, and other sources of medical care to form the bases of these reports. Health Systems Agencies and other planning and regulatory bodies are also busily compiling data on health and social indicators in their communities as a basis for drafting legislation, plans, regulations, standards, budgets, and a number of other documents that require a data base. Never before has there been such emphasis on developing data bases for planning and evaluation of programs that can influence peoples' health. Rather than dwell on endless tables of current morbidity and lost-time data that are quickly out of date unless one is doing longitudinal studies, we concentrate here on some of the major sources of reported information and give a few samples of the types of reports issued.

The government, as might be expected, is a tremendous compiler and supplier of endless reports. The National Center for Health Statistics (NCHS) publishes a number of series of reports entitled *Vital and Health Statistics*. Among this series is Series 10 *Data from the Health Interview Survey*, which presents tabulations and discussions of data obtained from the National Health Survey. This survey uses a questionnaire to obtain information from a carefully selected sample of the civilian, non-institutionalized population about personal and demographic characteristics, illnesses, impairments, chronic conditions, as well as other health topics. Series 11 *Data from the Health Examination Survey* deals with the results of physical examinations of samples of the population. Series 13 *Data on Health Resources Utilization* lays out the ways in which the population uses various kinds of health manpower and facilities to provide long-term, ambulatory, and acute care as well as family planning services. These series of reports are in most university or medical center libraries or may be obtained free of charge from the Scientific and Technical Information Branch, National Center for Health Statistics, Public Health Service, 5600 Fishers Lane, Rockville, MD 20857.

In addition to these series of reports, the government produces many special reports and other publications both on a regular and a periodic basis. One example is *The Nation's Use of Health Resources*, 1976 edition (DHEW 1977). This report presents information compiled from the NCHS sources, all involved governmental agencies, and such non-governmental sources as the American Hospital Association, the Professional Activity Study, the Center for Health Administration Studies at the University of Chicago, and others into one comprehensive report on our utilization of ambulatory, inpatient short-term, inpatient long-term, and home care. The Center for Disease Control publishes *Morbidity and Mortality Weekly Data*, in which outbreaks of specific infectious diseases are discussed and the tabulation of the number of cases of specified, notifiable diseases reported for the week is given by state. Departments of the federal government other than Health, Education and Welfare also prepare reports dealing with health and social indicators. The Department of Commerce's annual *Social Indicators* is an example.

Individual institutions and organizations also prepare special and annual reports, self-studies, and review materials for such examining bodies as the Joint Committee on the Accreditation of Hospitals, the American Public Health Association–National League for Nursing Accreditation Program for Home Health Agencies and Community Nursing Services, and others. Some of these reports are available to the public for examination. They contain much information about utilization, personnel, and costs of running the various programs reviewed. As Health Systems Agencies (HSAs) become more organized and ready to function, they will be assembling data from their health services area on all kinds of health indicators. Thus HSAs can be viewed as something of a clearinghouse and reservoir for health-related data in a locale. Contact your local HSA and ask what kinds of health indicator data it has on file.

Insurance companies are another source of health and social indicator information. Metropolitan Life Insurance Company, for example, has published its *Statistical Bulletin* for almost sixty years. Some of these reports are based on data from the National Center for Health Statistics, but many are from the company's experience with its own employees as well as people it insures. Other insurance companies publish similar reports. The Health Insurance Institute annually publishes its *Source Book of Health Insurance*, which provides detailed information about types, amounts, and utilization of health insurance by people insured by its member companies. See chapter 12 for some of the kinds of information it contains.

USING HEALTH INDICATOR DATA TO MOTIVATE LIFESTYLE CHANGES

In chapter 9, we talk at length about the need for people to be taught how to reduce their own risk factors as means to prevent the development of chronic noninfectious diseases and conditions. Many of these changes require alterations in the person's lifestyle. A potentially effective means for facilitating the needed changes is through tools such as the Health Risk Profile (*Interhealth* 1976) and the Health Hazard Appraisal (Robbins and Hall 1974) Note that we use *potentially* to describe the effectiveness of these instruments since they are relatively new and we need longitudinal studies to ascertain just how effective they are. The questions in table 2.1 are illustrative of those asked on the Health Risk Profile. The questions selected for presentation here are some of those that deal with personal behavior and environmental influences.

In essence what is done in using the health appraisal or profile instruments is that the person is asked a number of questions such as those in table 2.1. The answers to the questions are combined with results of laboratory tests and in some instances physical examinations. The combined data are used to determine what the person's current risks are and

TABLE 2.1 *Selected Questions from* Interhealth's *Health Risk Profile*

Do you now smoke?	____ No	____ Yes
If yes, mark all correct answers:		
I smoke:	____ Cigarettes – 2 or more packs per day.	
	____ Cigarettes – 1½ packs per day.	
	____ Cigarettes – 1 pack per day.	
	____ Cigarettes — ½ pack per day.	
	____ Cigarettes – less than ½ pack per day.	
	____ Cigars or pipe – 5 or more per day (combined total).	
	____ Cigars or pipe – less than 5 per day (combined total).	

TABLE 2.1 *(Continued)*

Did you smoke, but no longer do?   ____ No   ____ Yes

    If yes,

        How long ago did you stop?   ____ years ago

        If less than one year: ____ months ago

        If you did smoke, mark all correct answers:

        I smoked: ____ Cigarettes – 2 or more packs per day.

                              ____ Cigarettes – 1 ½ packs per day.

                              ____ Cigarettes – 1 pack per day.

                              ____ Cigarettes – ½ pack per day.

                              ____ Cigarettes – less than ½ pack per day.

                              ____ Cigars or pipe – 5 or more per day (combined total).

                              ____ Cigars or pipe – less than 5 per day (combined total).

How many total miles per year do you travel in a car or motor vehicle as a driver or passenger?   _____ miles per year

    To help you in estimating the number of miles you drive or ride, the national averages for the following categories of driving are listed below:

        Driving to and from work – 8000 miles per year.

        Driving to and from shopping and other personal business – 4000 miles per year.

        Driving to and from school and church – 1000 miles per year.

        Driving to and from pleasure, recreation and miscellaneous – 5000 miles per year.

How many of these miles are on a freeway, expressway, toll road or other similar limited access highway?

    ____ Most (75% or more)   ____ Some (25–74%)   ____ Little (0–24%)

When in a motor vehicle (car), do you wear a seat belt or shoulder harness?
____ No   ____ Yes

    If yes, mark when you wear it:

    ____ Less than 10% of the time.

    ____ 10–24% of the time.

    ____ 25–74% of the time.

    ____ 75% or more of the time.

TABLE 2.1 (*Continued*)

Mark any of these that you do:

_____ Fly a private plane

_____ Sky dive

_____ Skin dive – scuba dive

_____ Drive a racing car, dune buggy, snowmobile, or motorcycle in *dirt* (off the road)

_____ Drive a motorcycle on the street

Mark any of the medicines you are now taking

_____ Mood elevators (pills of depression)

_____ Pep or diet pills (like dexadrine)

_____ Tranquilizers, sedatives, nerve or sleeping pills (Miltown, Librium, Phenobarbital, Nembutal, Seconal, etc.)

_____ Pain pills (Demerol, codeine, morphine, etc.)

_____ Antihistamines or allergy pills

Do you now drink any alcoholic beverages (beer, wine, whiskey, gin, vodka, etc.)?   _____ No   _____ Yes

   If yes, mark the one correct answer:

   I drink: _____ 2 or less drinks per week.

                   _____ 3 to 6 drinks per week.

                   _____ 7 to 14 drinks per week.

                   _____ 15 to 24 drinks per week.

                   _____ 25 to 40 drinks per week.

                   _____ More than 40 drinks per week.

Did you formerly drink any alcoholic beverages (beer, wine, whiskey, gin, vodka, etc.) and no longer do?   _____ No   _____ Yes

   If yes, mark the one correct answer:

   I drank: _____ 2 or less drinks per week.

                   _____ 3 to 6 drinks per week.

                   _____ 7 to 14 drinks per week.

                   _____ 15 to 24 drinks per week.

                   _____ 25 to 40 drinks per week.

                   _____ More than 40 drinks per week.

Have you ever been told you had liver disease due to drinking?   _____ No   _____ Yes

Source: Reprinted with permission from *Interhealth*, Inc., 2970 Fifth Avenue, San Diego, CA 92103.

to project future risks of developing life-threatening diseases or conditions. The risks are calculated on the basis of known probabilities, like those insurance companies use, and are given in terms of years of life left for the individual. Concrete suggestions are made to help the person zero in on the kinds of lifestyle and environmental changes that need to be made to increase the number of years the individual can expect to live. Table 2.2 shows part of a model client printout based on the Health Risk Profile data. At the top of the table are the factors from the subject's Health Risk Profile responses that if adopted, offer the greatest risk reduction. The combined years the person can add to her life expectancy by considering these factors is at the upper right of the table. Thus, if the subject stops smoking, she can increase her life expectancy over what it is now by 2.7 years. The printout then continues with listings of the ten leading risks for this person based on her age, sex, and health indicator data. If the subject were to follow the specific suggestions given in this printout, she could, potentially, reduce her risks by a total of 43 percent!

TABLE 2.2 *Example of a Health Risk Profile Printout*

STAYWELL PROGRAM   DATE: 12-22-77   ID   000018108   F

- -

CURR B.P. 144/080 PREV B.P. NOT GIVEN CURR CHOL. 200 MG % PREV CHOL. NOT GIVEN
HT. 67 IN. WT. 166 LBS. CURR TRIG. 231 MG % PREV TRIG. NOT GIVEN

- -

AVERAGE TEN YEAR RISK OF DEATH PER 100,000   6,489 YOUR PRESENT AGE   51
YOUR CURRENT TEN YEAR RISK OF DEATH PER 100,000   8,893 YOUR CURRENT RISK AGE   55
YOUR ACHIEVABLE TEN YEAR RISK OF DEATH PER 100,000   4,994 YOUR ACHIEVABLE AGE   48

- -

AN AVG. WOMAN YOUR AGE HAS 6,489 CHANCES OF DYING PER 100,000 IN THE NEXT 10 YRS.
YOUR RISKS ARE 37% GREATER THAN THE AVERAGE.
YOU COULD REDUCE YOUR RISKS BY 43%

- -

NOTE   SOME DATA SUGGESTS THE FOLLOWING DISEASES WHICH MAY SIGNIFICANTLY INCREASE RISK.
        TUBERCULOSIS
NOTE   THIS PROFILE DOES NOT INCLUDE ANY RISK FOR THE FOLLOWING DISEASE(S) DUE TO THE
        REMOVAL OF THE ORGAN FOR NON-CANCEROUS REASONS
        CANCER OF THE CERVIX
        CANCER OF THE UTERUS

- -

FACTORS THAT MAY OFFER THE   COMBINED ACHIEVABLE BENEFIT
GREATEST REDUCTION IN RISK   WITH CHANGE OF THESE FACTORS
        NOT SMOKING . . . . 2.7 YRS
        NOT DRINKING . . . . 1.1 YRS
        EXERCISE PROGRAM . . . . .9 YRS

TABLE 2.2 (*Continued*)

FACTORS THAT MAY OFFER THE GREATEST REDUCTION IN RISK	COMBINED ACHIEVABLE BENEFIT WITH CHANGE OF THESE FACTORS
WEIGHT REDUCTION	.4 YRS
BLOOD PRESSURE REDUCTION	.3 YRS
CHOLESTEROL REDUCTION	.1 YRS
OTHER	1.5 YRS
TOTAL REDUCTION IN RISK	7.0 YRS

- -

YOUR RISKS IN DESCENDING IMPORTANCE. #1 IS HIGHEST.
A RISK FACTOR OF 1.0 IS AVERAGE. A RISK FACTOR LESS THAN 1.0 CARRIES LESS THAN AVERAGE RISK. A RISK FACTOR ABOVE 1.0 CARRIES GREATER THAN AVERAGE RISK.

- -

#1 ARTERIOSCLEROTIC HEART DISEASE   (HEART ATTACK)
AVERAGE RISK   1,260☆ ☆ ☆ ☆ ☆ ☆ ☆ ☆ ☆
YOUR CURRENT RISK   3,276☆ (2.6 X AVG)
YOUR ACHIEVABLE RISK   743☆ ☆ ☆ ☆ ☆   (.6 X AVG)

CONTRIBUTING FACTORS	RISK FACTOR	RISK REDUCING FACTORS	RISK FACTOR
B.P. (CURR)—144/080	.8	B.P. 120/80 OR LESS	.6
CHOL (CURR)—200MG%	.7	CHOLESTEROL 180 OR LESS	.6
DIABETES—NO	1.0		1.0
EXERCISE—SEDENTARY	1.4	SUPERVISED EXERCISE	1.0
FH ASHD NO EARLY DEATHS ..	.9		.9
SMOKER—1 PACK/DAY	1.9	NOT SMOKING	.9
WEIGHT—166 LBS.	1.2	WEIGHT—134 LBS. OR LESS	1.0
NO HX. OF ABNORMAL ECG	1.0		1.0
TRIG.—(CUR)—231MG%	1.8	TRIGLYCERIDES – 151 MG%	1.0

EXCESSIVE STRESS MAY INCREASE RISK. EXACT RISK FACTOR NOT YET AVAILABLE.

- -

#2 LUNG CANCER
AVERAGE RISK   386☆ ☆ ☆ ☆ ☆ ☆ ☆ ☆ ☆
YOUR CURRENT RISK   772☆ ☆ ☆ ☆ ☆ ☆ ☆ ☆ ☆ ☆ ☆ ☆ ☆ ☆ ☆ ☆ ☆ ☆ (2.0 X AVG)
YOUR ACHIEVABLE RISK   618☆ ☆ ☆ ☆ ☆ ☆ ☆ ☆ ☆ ☆ ☆ ☆ ☆ ☆ (1.6 X AVG)

CONTRIBUTING FACTORS	RISK FACTOR	RISK REDUCING FACTORS	RISK FACTOR
SMOKER—1 PACK/DAY	2.0	NOT SMOKING	1.6
		REMAIN STOPPED 5 YEARS	.6

- -

#3 CIRRHOSIS OF LIVER
AVERAGE RISK   284☆ ☆ ☆ ☆ ☆ ☆ ☆ ☆ ☆
YOUR CURRENT RISK   710☆ ☆ ☆ ☆ ☆ ☆ ☆ ☆ ☆ ☆ ☆ ☆ ☆ ☆ ☆ ☆ ☆ ☆ (2.5 X AVG)
YOUR ACHIEVABLE RISK   57☆ ☆   (.2 X AVG)

CONTRIBUTING FACTORS	RISK FACTOR	RISK REDUCING FACTORS	RISK FACTOR
ALCOHOL—25–40 DRINKS/WK	2.5	NOT DRINKING	.2
LIVER FUNCTION	1.0		1.0

TABLE 2.2 *(Continued)*

#4 BREAST CANCER
    AVERAGE RISK   684☆ ☆ ☆ ☆ ☆ ☆ ☆ ☆ ☆ ☆
    YOUR CURRENT RISK   479☆ ☆ ☆ ☆ ☆ ☆ ☆   (.7 X AVG)
    YOUR ACHIEVABLE RISK   342☆ ☆ ☆ ☆ ☆   (.5 X AVG)

CONTRIBUTING FACTORS	RISK FACTOR	RISK REDUCING FACTORS	RISK FACTOR
CURRENT FACTOR	.7	ACHIEVABLE FACTOR	.5
FAMILY HISTORY—NO			
MONTHLY SELF-EXAM—YES			
YEARLY MD EXAM—YES			
YEARLY MAMMOGRAPHY—NO		YEARLY MAMMOGRAPHY	

- -

#5 STROKE
    AVERAGE RISK   422☆ ☆ ☆ ☆ ☆ ☆ ☆ ☆ ☆ ☆
    YOUR CURRENT RISK   405☆ ☆ ☆ ☆ ☆ ☆ ☆ ☆ ☆ ☆   (1.0 X AVG)
    YOUR ACHIEVABLE RISK   177☆ ☆ ☆ ☆   (.4 X AVG)

CONTRIBUTING FACTORS	RISK FACTOR	RISK REDUCING FACTORS	RISK FACTOR
B.P. (CURR)—144/080	.8	B.P. 120/80 OR LESS	.6
CHOL (CURR)—200MG%	.7		.7
DIABETES—NO	1.0		1.0
SMOKER—1 PACK/DAY	1.4	NOT SMOKING	1.0
NO HX. OF ABNORMAL ECG	1.0		1.0

- -

#6 CANCER OF INTESTINES AND RECTUM
    AVERAGE RISK   277☆ ☆ ☆ ☆ ☆ ☆ ☆ ☆ ☆ ☆
    YOUR CURRENT RISK   277☆ ☆ ☆ ☆ ☆ ☆ ☆ ☆ ☆ ☆   (AVERAGE)
    YOUR ACHIEVABLE RISK   83☆ ☆ ☆   (.3 X AVG)

CONTRIBUTING FACTORS	RISK FACTOR	RISK REDUCING FACTORS	RISK FACTOR
INTESTINAL POLYP—NO	1.0		1.0
RECTAL BLEEDING—NO	1.0		1.0
ULC. COLITIS—NO	1.0		1.0
ANNUAL SIGMOID.—NO	1.0	ANNUAL IN FUTURE	.3

- -

#7 CANCER OF OVARIES   NO FACTORS FOR THIS CAUSE OF DEATH
    AVERAGE RISK   227☆ ☆ ☆ ☆ ☆ ☆ ☆ ☆ ☆ ☆
    YOUR CURRENT RISK   227☆ ☆ ☆ ☆ ☆ ☆ ☆ ☆ ☆ ☆   (AVERAGE)
    YOUR ACHIEVABLE RISK   227☆ ☆ ☆ ☆ ☆ ☆ ☆ ☆ ☆ ☆   (AVERAGE)

- -

#8 SUICIDE
    AVERAGE RISK   131☆ ☆ ☆ ☆ ☆ ☆ ☆ ☆ ☆ ☆
    YOUR CURRENT RISK   131☆ ☆ ☆ ☆ ☆ ☆ ☆ ☆ ☆ ☆   (AVERAGE)
    YOUR ACHIEVABLE RISK   131☆ ☆ ☆ ☆ ☆ ☆ ☆ ☆ ☆ ☆   (AVERAGE)

TABLE 2.2 *(Continued)*

CONTRIBUTING FACTORS	RISK FACTOR	RISK REDUCING FACTORS	RISK FACTOR
NO DEPRESSION	1.0		1.0
FH SUICIDE—NO	1.0		1.0
ALCOHOL—25-40 DRINKS/WK	1.0		1.0

- -

#9 CHRONIC RHEUMATIC HEART DISEASE

AVERAGE RISK	111☆ ☆ ☆ ☆ ☆ ☆ ☆ ☆ ☆		
YOUR CURRENT RISK	11☆		(.1 X AVG)
YOUR ACHIEVABLE RISK	11☆		(.1 X AVG)

CONTRIBUTING FACTORS	RISK FACTOR	RISK REDUCING FACTORS	RISK FACTOR
NO HX. RHEUMATIC FEVER			
NO HX. HEART MURMUR	.1		.1

- -

#10 CANCER OF CERVIX

AVERAGE RISK	103☆ ☆ ☆ ☆ ☆ ☆ ☆ ☆ ☆		
YOUR CURRENT RISK	0		(.0 X AVG)
YOUR ACHIEVABLE RISK	0		(.0 X AVG)

CONTRIBUTING FACTORS	RISK FACTOR	RISK REDUCING FACTORS	RISK FACTOR
☆ ☆ ☆ ☆ ORGAN REMOVED	.0		.0

- -

OTHER: ALL OTHER CAUSES OF DEATH (APPROX 1000) WHOSE TOTAL RISK IS 2,604

- -

THIS APPRAISAL IS BASED ON POSSIBLE 10 YEAR RISK USING DATA BELIEVED TO BE VALID. PRE-EXISTING DISEASE MAY TOTALLY INVALIDATE THE RESULT. THE RISK REDUCING MEASURES HOWEVER ARE ONLY GUIDELINES FOR THE INDIVIDUAL AND SHOULD BE UNDERTAKEN ONLY WITH THE SUPERVISION OF A PHYSICIAN. THE 1974 GELLER TABLES ARE UTILIZED IN THE COMPUTATIONS. RISK FACTORS ARE CONSTANTLY APPRAISED AND UPDATED AS DATA WARRANTS.

Source: Reprinted with permission from *Interhealth*, Inc., 2970 Fifth Avenue, San Diego, CA 92103.

The value of these kinds of individual health indicator data being available to the person is that he or she can see specifically, insofar as our present knowledge permits any of us to see, what personal risks are being run, how "bad" these risks are, and what can be done to reduce these risks. The health education and health promotion activities that community health nurses could help clients with if these kinds of data were available to each one, are tremendous. Of course, obtaining these kinds of data is the easiest part of changing risks, but they are a start. Because they are personal and based on the individual client's own history, tests, and responses, their potential for motivating lifestyle change is greater than if they were impersonal. These kinds of data in the hands of the people upon whose own lives the data are based has a much more potentially persuasive effect than the general warning printed on the cigarette pack or birth control pill label. Clients need help and support over time to make changes—as any of us who ever tried to lose weight know too well. This is where community health nurses can work with individuals or groups to make and maintain the needed changes. Groups are particularly valuable in these situations since this format enables people to be aware that others share their risks and facilitates clients' developing their own support systems.

The use of these kinds of health appraisal and motivational techniques are increasing. Explore your own community for the kinds being used there. A friend who uses the Health Hazard Appraisal in his health education practice says the results do not have their greatest impact on the client the first time, or even the second time, they are seen by the client. But when clients keep getting the same message about the life-shortening effect of things they keep on choosing to do, they finally get very serious about changing their lifestyles. High-awareness times seem to be particularly associated with client's entry into a new decade in their age. Thus, a thirty-year-old woman may become much more concerned than she was at twenty-nine. A particularly valuable learning experience is to have one of these health appraisals done on your own risks. See how you react.

HOLISM

When Ruth Fleshman and I began our independent practice working with older people at a local senior center in 1974, we publicized our work in terms of health counseling and blood pressure monitoring. Interestingly enough, blood pressure monitoring was what people heard and came to us for. We were amazed and amused at the number of clients who came in, sat down, and immediately rolled up one sleeve, only to be surprised by a lengthy interview about their lifestyle, their health history, and their abilities to cope with stress and loss—all before we did anything about their blood pressure. We carefully explained to each one our belief in the importance of understanding something about the whole person before dealing with any specific health concern. Admittedly, "whole person" is a concept that realistically cannot be grasped in even repeated interviews, but at least we have opened up the idea that we are interested in much more than blood pressure. Recently a long-time client was overheard telling a new one what to expect on her first visit. It went something like this: "They ask you to talk about what you do for exercise, where you go for fun, where you live and can you get transportation to places, what medicines you take and why, do you examine your own breasts for lumps, did you have flu shots—all kinds of things." That isn't all we talk with them about, but it's a good start.

As noted earlier in this chapter, OLOF comes from a holistic perspective that looks at the whole client. If we really are to try to consider the whole client—and that's easier to talk about than to do—we must look at psychosocial, physical, and environmental influences. Most holistic approaches place heavy emphasis on the psychological. As Lee notes:

> It's unfortunate that because of medicine's focus on technology and the delivery of specialized care we have let marginal practitioners preempt the word holistic when these practitioners neglect the organic, biological, and often the social aspects of health and deal almost exclusively with psychological factors [Lee 1978:20].

One of our big concerns in the area of holism is that many, including Lee, pay little attention to environmental factors that very heavily influence many of us, particularly the very young and the very old. All of the influencing factors in the OLOF ecosystem model shown in figure 2.1 must be considered. Ornstein has captured something of what we mean when he says:

> To many, it [holism] means only freaky things, so we end up with just another fragmented approach to health instead of a holistic one. Holistic is an attitude. The term should not be used to describe a system of treatment or an institute, but an understanding of the whole situation [Ornstein 1978:20].

The importance of adopting a holistic attitude toward clients is increasingly vital as more information becomes available about the effects of lifestyle, stress, environmental pollutants, social repression, and loneliness on our abilities to function. As community health nurses, along with nurses in general, we have always taken pride in ourselves for looking at the whole client. However, we may have talked about this approach to clients more than we have practiced it. In a world where everything, especially medical and health care, is becoming increasingly superspecialized and compartmentalized, clients' needs for someone to put it and them all together has never been so great. Community health nurses can do much to meet this need if we truly look at the whole client.

SUMMARY

Five basic concepts are discussed in this chapter. Community is presented as a typology of kinds of communities: emotional communities, structural communities, and functional communities. Selected characteristics of each of these kinds of communities are given. The discussion of community nurses' involvement in community activities stresses the community health nurse's unique contributions to community activities and the benefits that can be accrued from this kind of participation.

OLOF, which stands for optimum level of functioning, is offered as a holistic definition of health that emphasizes peoples' abilities rather than their disabilities. An ecosystem model is developed to show political, behavioral, hereditary, health care delivery system, environmental, and socioeconomic influences on OLOF. The Continuum of Function places peoples' abilities to function on a continuum between OLOF and dysfunction.

Health indicators are those data that give indications about the health status of a population or an individual person. Often these indicators are of illness or disability such as days of work lost or utilization of health resources. Many sources of health indicator data useful to community health nurses exist and are discussed. Individual health indicator data generated by the use of health hazard appraisals and health risk profiles are suggested as very valuable tools for community health nurses to use in working with clients to help them change their lifestyles to promote their own OLOF and reduce their risks.

Holism is equated with the ecosystem perspective of OLOF found in figure 2.1. Many of the current popular definitions fall short of looking at the total client, either by overemphasizing psychological factors or ignoring environmental influences. Note is taken that holism is an attitude not a thing. A plea is made in this world of increasing specialization and fragmentation for community health nurses, at least, to adopt a holistic attitude toward clients.

REFERENCES

ALTSHULER, ALAN A. *Community Control*. New York: Pegasus, 1970.

ARCHER, SARAH ELLEN, and FLESHMAN, RUTH P. "Doing Our Own Thing: Community Health Nurses in Independent Practice." *Journal of Nursing Administration*, forthcoming.

BELLO, TERESA A. "Community Health Nurses and Community Organizations." in S.E. Archer and R.P. Fleshman, eds. *Community Health Nursing: Patterns and Practice*, 1st ed. North Scituate, Mass.: Duxbury Press, 1975, pp. 386–405.

BELLOC, NEDRA B., and BRESLOW, LESTER. "Relationship of Physical Health Status and Health Practices." *Preventive Medicine* 1 (1972):409–21.

BENENSON, ABRAM S., ed. *Control of Communicable Diseases in Man*, 12th ed. Washington, D.C.: American Public Health Association, 1975.

BLUM, HENRIK L. *Health Planning*. New York: Human Sciences Press, 1974.

CARDUS, DAVID, and THRALL, ROBERT M. "Overview: Health and the Planning of Health Care Systems." *Preventive Medicine* 6 (1977): 134–42.

CHERMAYEFF, SERGE, and TZONIS, ALEXANDER. *Shape of Community: Realization of Human Potential.* Baltimore, Md.: Penguin Books, 1971.

COX, FRED. *Strategies of Community Organization.* Itasca, Ill.: F.E. Peacock, Publishers, 1974.

DAVIES, DEAN F. "Progress Toward the Assessment of Health Status." *Preventive Medicine* 4 (1975):282–95.

DUNN, H.L. *High Level Wellness.* Arlington, Va.: R.W. Beatty, Ltd., 1961.

GOLDSMITH, SETH B. "A Reevaluation of Health Status Indicators." *Health Services Reports* 88 (1973):937–41.

HAYES, WAYLAND J. "The Problem of Community Intelligence." *International Review of Community Development,* no. 10, 1962.

HEALTH INSURANCE INSTITUTE. *Source Book of Health Insurance Data, 1976–1977.* New York: Health Insurance Institute, 1977.

Health Risk Profile. San Diego, Calif: Interhealth, 1976.

HENNIG, MARGARET, and JARDIM, ANNE. *The Managerial Woman.* New York: Anchor Press, 1977.

International Classification of Diseases, 8th ed. Geneva: World Health Organization, 1965.

JOLLY, ELIZABETH. *The Invisible Chain: Diseases Passed on by Inheritance.* Chicago: Nelson Hall, 1972.

KAHN, SI. *How People Get Power: Organizing Oppressed Communities for Action.* New York: McGraw-Hill Book Co., 1970.

KATZ, SIDNEY, et al. "Measuring the Health Status of Populations." In *Health Status Indexes: Proceedings of a Conference Conducted by Health Services Research,* ed. Robert L. Berg. Chicago: Hospital Research and Educational Trust, 1973, pp. 39–59.

KENT, JAMES. *Descriptive Approach to Community Organization* (videotape). Denver: Foundation for Urban and Neighborhood Development, 1972.

KEYES, RALPH. *We, the Lonely People: Searching for Community.* New York: Harper & Row, 1973.

KRAMER, RALPH M., and SPECHT, HARRY, eds. *Readings in Community Organization Practice.* Englewood Cliffs, N.J.: Prentice-Hall, 1975.

LEAVELL, HUGH R., and CLARK, R. GURNEY. Preventive Medicine for the Doctor in His Community: An Epidemiological Approach, 3rd. ed. New York: McGraw-Hill Book Co., 1965.

LEE, PHILLIP R. "What the Experts Say." *San Francisco Chronicle,* January 19, 1978, p. 20.

LYNCH, JAMES J. *The Broken Heart: The Medical Consequences of Loneliness.* New York: Basic Books, 1977.

MILIO, NANCY. *9226 Kercheval: The Storefront that Did Not Burn.* Ann Arbor: University of Michigan Press, 1970.

Morbidity and Mortality Weekly Report. Atlanta: U.S. Department of Health, Education and Welfare, Public Health Service, Center for Disease Control, published weekly.

NATIONAL COMMISSION ON COMMUNITY HEALTH SERVICES. *Health Is a Community Affair.* Cambridge, Mass.: Harvard University Press, 1966.

NISBET, ROBERT A. *The Quest for Community.* New York: Oxford University Press, 1953.

OM COLLECTIVE. *The Organizer's Manual.* New York: Bantam Books, 1971.

ORNSTEIN, ROBERT. "What the Experts Say." *San Francisco Chronicle,* January 19, 1978, p. 20.

Robbins, Lewis C., and Hall, Jack H. *How to Practice Prospective Medicine.* Indianapolis: Methodist Hospital of Indiana, 1970.

Ross, Murray G. *Community Organization: Theory, Principles and Practice,* 2nd ed. New York: Harper & Row, 1967.

Statistical Bulletin. New York: Metropolitan Life Insurance Company, published monthly.

Ruybal, S.E., Bauwens, E., and Falsa, M.J. "Community Assessment: An Epidemiological Approach." *Nursing Outlook* 23 (1975):2154–70.

Terris, Milton. "Approaches to an Epidemiology of Health." *American Journal of Public Health* 65 (October 1975):1037–45.

The Nation's Use of Health Resources, 1976 ed. Washington, D.C.: U.S. Department of Health, Education and Welfare, DHEW Publication No. (HRA) 77–1240, Public Health Service, Health Resources Administration, National Center for Health Statistics, 1977.

Toffler, Alvin. *Future Shock.* New York: Random House, 1970.

U.S. Department of Commerce. *Social Indicators 1976.* Washington, D.C.: U.S. Government Printing Office, 1977.

U.S. Public Health Service. *Forward Plan for Health, 1977–1981.* Washington, D.C.: Department of Health, Education and Welfare, DHEW Publication Number (OS) 76–50024, U.S. Government Printing Office, 1975.

Vital and Health Statistics. Washington, D.C.: U.S. Department of Health, Education and Welfare, Public Health Service, Health Resources Administration, National Center for Health Statistics, several series, published periodically.

Warren, Donald I., and Warren, Rachelle B. "Six Kinds of Neighborhoods." *Psychology Today* 9 (June 1975):74–80.

Ward, Barbara, and Dubos, Rene. Only One Earth: The Care and Maintenance of a Small Planet. New York: W. W. Norton & Co., 1972.

"What High Level of Wellness Means." *Canadian Journal of Public Health* 50 (1959):447–57.

Williams, Carolyn. "Community Health Nursing: What Is It?" *Nursing Outlook* 25 (April 1977):250–54.

3. Selected Community Health Processes

Sarah Ellen Archer

INTRODUCTION

This chapter discusses a few community health processes that are useful to us in community health nursing. They are placed here in the beginning of the book because they are needed before we proceed to look at community nursing's relationship to the family in great detail in Part II. Later in the book, other key community health processes—research, epidemiology, health education, politics and economics, health insurance, and quality control—are topics of specific chapters. The basic processes discussed here will be revisited in these chapters as well as in others that describe specific kinds of community health nurses' roles. The three processes introduced in this chapter can be viewed as fundamental components in our conceptual framework of community health nursing.

Exchanges are basic building blocks for interactions and relationships. We see community nurse-client relationships as exchanges between peers, which is consonant with our emphasis on the informed and participating client in client-centered community nursing. We do not see our clients in the traditional one-down role characteristic of Western medicine. We seek throughout this book to help our colleagues develop a frame of reference that will facilitate working productively and at a mutually satisfying level of exchange with clients who are active and in-

57

formed participants in decision making. We believe that this is the most effective way to facilitate clients' attaining and maintaining their optimum level of functioning (OLOF).

Systems theory enables us to take a holistic view of our clients and their environments, whether the client is an individual, a family, a group, or a community. It is a handy method for understanding interactions between clients and their environments and for seeing the value of considering outcomes and consequences of actions. As Donovan sings it, "everything's a part of everything, anyway." That's why we think it's important to use the holistic approach upon which systems theory is based. A glossary of systems terms and their definitions is included at the end of the chapter.

Planning is basically a process of bringing about change. In our conception of planning, clients are essential participants in the development, implementation, and evaluation of plans that affect them. The cyclic planning process we discuss relies heavily on feedback and considerations of consequences. The cyclic nature of planning is stressed by proposing that evaluation, the final step in any planning cycle, is the initial assessment or first step of the next cycle. In this way we seek to promote continuity and coordination in what could otherwise be a disjointed series of occurrences. This continuity will reduce the chance that clients will fall through the cracks between the planning cycles and get lost.

EXCHANGE

You smile at a guy and he smiles back; that's an exchange. You and he have engaged in a basic unit of social relation. Actions have reciprocals or reactions they produce. Your smile signalled him that your intentions were friendly and, generally, unless there is some specific reason not to do so, he will respond appropriately by smiling back. The transaction was thus completed smoothly. If, in response to your smile, he had turned and fled or made menacing motions toward you, your probable response would have been surprise and bewilderment, since these reactions to a smile would have been inappropriate and therefore unexpected. Another common form of exchange involves material goods and is the basis for trade. Thus you go to the store and obtain a dozen eggs in exchange for paying the stated price. In chapter 11, tradeoffs and games, both political exchanges, are discussed. Thus exchanges can involve both material and nonmaterial goods.

Figure 3.1 shows a model of an exchange relationship. In the model, the community nurse is circle A and the client is circle B; the two circles

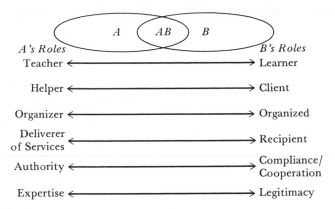

A's Roles   B's Roles

Teacher ←————————————————→ Learner

Helper ←————————————————→ Client

Organizer ←————————————————→ Organized

Deliverer
of Services ←————————————————→ Recipient

Authority ←————————————————→ Compliance/
Cooperation

Expertise ←————————————————→ Legitimacy

3.1   *Complimentary Exchange and Interdependent Relationships*

are partially overlapping to indicate that the community nurse and the client are interdependent. The two-way arrows between the selected roles listed for the community nurse and the client symbolize that the roles are complementary and reciprocal. For example, to be a teacher one must have a learner, and to be a learner one must have someone or something from which to learn.

Eisenstadt has described some basic aspects of exchanges (1965: 32–35) that can be applied to community nursing: There are some material and nonmaterial things that are nonexchangeable and what these are must be learned. For example, adherents of Jehovah's Witness religion will not under any circumstances consent to blood transfusions. Diet counseling is made much more complicated by food habits that are an integral part of the client's culture or lifestyle and so are extremely resistant to exchange for other food habits. These two examples, respectively, illustrate absolute and relatively firm nonexchangeable or nonnegotiable patterns of behavior.

Much emphasis in the epidemiology chapter (9) is placed on health education (chapter 10) to help clients change their lifestyles to promote their OLOF as well as to prevent or forestall the development of chronic noninfectious diseases and conditions. This process requires client behavior changes, even though, as noted, some are nonexchangeable while others are more amenable to alteration. The nonnegotiable ones should be identified first, for once these are identified, areas of bargaining can be set up. For example, militant smokers who refuse to stop smoking even though they have elevated blood pressure and complain occasionally of shortness of breath will not stop no matter how persistent our admonitions or persuasive our arguments. If we continue to nag at them, we are likely to lose whatever influence we may have with them in this and other areas of health behavior where change may be possible. Recognizing this fact, we would be well advised to work with these clients to reduce the amount they smoke, to change to one of the lower "tar" and nicotine brands, to concentrate on not inhaling, and to build an exercise and fitness program that can counteract some of the adverse effects of smoking. Through this kind of an exchange in which both nurse and client participants compromise, the clients' risk from smoking will be reduced. We will have approached our objective of persuading clients to stop smoking without losing our rapport with them or jeopardizing our chances of successful subsequent exchanges with them. Both the clients' responsibility for themselves and our legitimacy as helping people are furthered in this kind of a relationship. Besides, very often when smokers become hooked on some form of moderate to strenuous exercise, they will quit smoking because it interferes with their new enjoyable activity. Under these circumstances, the smokers stop smoking because they *want* to do so and exchange smoking for more rewarding activities. This exchange is a positive experience and a self-induced change. Behavior changes under these circumstances are likely to be long-lasting.

The media of exchange vary with the types of people or institutions involved. In a barter economy, exchange media are generally in kind; thus lettuce is traded for eggs. Services such as medical care may be paid for with commodities such as chickens or clients' labor rather than money.

Developing various frameworks, organizations, and norms for exchange insures relatively smooth functioning. People who must receive blood transfusions are dependent on blood donors. Except in rare instances—war, disaster, and the movies—direct transfusions (exchanges) between the blood donor and the blood recipient do not take place. Instead, institutions, most notably blood banks and hospitals, play a middleman function in the exchange. The presence of these middleman institutions insures that the right amount or the right type of blood is available at the right time, thus making for a much smoother transaction than would be the case if the right number of blood donors had to be found at the exact moment the blood recipient needed them. Community nurses serve a similar middle person function in our role of coordinator of services to be sure that the client and the service are brought together at the appropriate time and that each knows enough about the other to be able to make the exchange a successful one.

The point in introducing the concept of exchange is that it is fundamental in our relationships with clients and colleagues. The nurse-client relationship is built on exchanges of such reciprocals as expertise and legitimacy, teaching and learning, delivery of services and receipt of services. Likewise our collegial relationships with members of other health care disciplines are exchanges. We get information from the physician or hospital about a client; we use that information in our exchanges with the client, and we feed back information to the physician or hospital about these exchanges. Thus, exchanges come in cycles, with each leading to the next one. Bearing in mind that no sound social relationship is based on one-way transactions, we should periodically stop and take stock of the state of our exchanges with our clients and colleagues. Viewing our relationships with clients in the context of an exchange model can help us consider clients as equals rather than as patients. As we have previously suggested, the latter term implies a one-down or inferior role to that of the helping person. Although this nurse-patient, doctor-nurse, one-up and one-down relationship is traditional, we believe it is inappropriate to our emphasis on client-centered care—that is, planning *with* rather than *for* clients and helping clients attain and maintain what in *their* definition, not *ours,* is their optimal level of functioning. For these reasons, exchange is an appropriate component in our conceptual framework of community nursing.

SYSTEMS THEORY

In chapter 1, we introduced systems theory as an aid to analyzing and understanding how the component parts of organizations work together to help the system attain its predefined goals. A system is basically a set of interacting and interdependent parts. Branden and Herban (1976:6) classify all systems into three types.

1. Physical or mechanical systems such as solar system or the internal combustion engine;
2. Biologic systems such as those that comprise plants and animals;
3. Human and social systems such as families, communities, and political parties.

The following illustration using a biologic system will serve to help us understand some of the fundamental functions of a system and set the stage for our consideration of more complex social systems. The glossary of systems terms at the end of the chapter gives the meanings of the italicized words in this discussion.

Most systems such as our digestive system are composed of components, in this case mouth, esophagus, stomach, and intestines. These individual parts can be considered to be *subsystems* of the digestive system. In turn, the digestive system is a *subsystem* of the person along with cardio-vascular, genito-urinary, nervous system, and others. Each system is a subsystem of another, larger system. Our digestive system is an *open system* that obtains its *inputs* of food and fluids from the environment. The *outputs* of the digestive system go to other *subsystems* in the body and out into the environment in the forms of energy and waste products. *Subsystems* within a larger system are interrelated to and interdependent upon one another; affect one and the others will also be affected, to some degree at least. The digestive process, which converts *inputs* of food and fluids into *outputs,* in systems jargon is called *throughput.*

Feedback can and does occur at any point within our digestive system. It can also come from other *subsystems* within the larger system and from the environment. The value of *feedback* is that if its messages are heeded, *cybernation* can occur—that is, the system can correct itself to be more efficient or more effective or both. A few examples of these concepts may help. Some people have an immediate and unpleasant reaction to spiced foods. This *feedback* may influence the digestive system only, and so the treatment may be to deal with the immediate symptoms and not to eat spicy food again. The *input* of too much alcohol for the digestive system to handle can result in effects on other *subsystems* within the person or on the person's entire system, such as in the case of a hangover. This *feedback* should enable the person to think clearly about not having so much alcohol again. Environmental *feedback* can occur as a result of unpleasant conduct at a party or as a result of an accident caused by driving while under the influence of alcohol. All these kinds and sources of *feedback* can help the person in charge of the system alter his or her behavior on the basis of the messages received from these sources inside and outside the system. Failure to *cybernate* the system can result in many *consequences* with an ever widening *ripple effect.* This simple example demonstrates the basic principles of systems theory. We go on now to a more complex social system, the family. In chapter 11 systems theory is used to describe the functioning of a community, a still more intricate social system.

The systems approach is consonant with the comments in chapter 2 on taking a holistic approach to clients whether they be individuals, families, groups, communities, organizations, or whatever. All of these clients are made up of many interacting and interdependent parts or subsystems. All interact with each other and with their greater environment. To ignore or underestimate the importance of any of these interactions is to diminish our ability to work with the whole client.

FAMILY: A MODEL OF AN OPEN SYSTEM

The family unit as an example of an open system is illustrated in figure 3.2. In this model the family is shown as an entity in an environment or ecosystem with which it interacts—that is, from which it derives its inputs and to which it gives its outputs. This interaction with its environment is the characteristic that makes the family an open system. Our family model is composed of four subsystems: two adults, A and B, and two children, c and d.

The family's environment is made up of the geographic, social, educational, economic, religious, political, ecological, ethnic, and interest communities surrounding it and of which it is a part or subsystem. Inputs into this family system include such obvious things as income, influence of jobs and schools, and goods and services that the family uses. More subtle but equally important inputs from the environment include feelings of acceptance or discrimination based at least in part on the family's actions or outputs as well as on the prevailing attitudes in the environment toward "those" kinds of families. An example of such environmental attitudes toward different kinds of family constellations is the city ordinance in one community that prohibits any more than four people not related by blood, adoption, or marriage from living in the same dwelling. Other communities have similar laws (*Time,* April 15, 1974:104).

The internal workings of the family system are extremely important. Each member, A, B, c, and d, is a subsystem of the family system. Since all of these subsystems are interrelated and interdependent, what happens to any one member affects all of the others, although often to varying degrees. Loss or incapacitation of any one member profoundly affects all other members. Therefore, should something happen to A, the breadwinner, we can predict that the emotional, financial, and social support for the other family members will decrease and that the stresses on them will increase. A's incapacity will decrease the family's income, cause changes in the dependence/independence balance within the family, and generally increase the stress on the total family. The community nurse's most important function in working with family systems at times of crisis may be to help with the provision of support for the other members. Conceptualizing the family as a system composed of interacting and interdependent subsystems makes this need for support for the other family members a predictable one. The community nurse's functions of bringing the family together with resources in its community is a recognition that the family itself is a subsystem of the environment in which it lives. As such, family and environment not only exchange goods and services but also are interdependent. Should the family lose its income to the point that it must seek public assistance funds in order to survive, its social/economic environment will have to bear that cost.

Family systems have goals and objectives that they strive to attain. Progress toward these goals may be interrupted by internal or external crises. Unless some catastrophe occurs to alter them, most families continue on their way toward some kinds of goals. These may include saving money for a down payment on a house in the suburbs or country, pushing children to get good grades so they can go on to college, planning for next

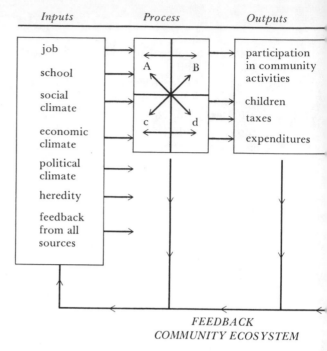

Inputs	Process	Outputs

Inputs	Outputs
job	participation in community activities
school	
social climate	children
economic climate	taxes
political climate	expenditures
heredity	
feedback from all sources	

FEEDBACK
COMMUNITY ECOSYSTEM

3.2   *The Family as an Open System Model*

year's vacation, a new TV or car, or trying to figure out how to apply for food stamps. To work effectively and efficiently with families as community nurses, we must know our clients' goals. We may be the appropriate persons to facilitate the achievement of some of these goals.

Banathy points out:

> . . . the key criterion by which the effectiveness or adequacy of the performance of a system can be evaluated is how closely the output of the system satisfies the purpose for which it exists [Banathy 1968:13].

Thus, if the family's outputs meet its own objectives or reasons for being, then we may say that the family system's activities have been successful. As community nurses, we can have input into family's decision-making processes based on our rapport with them and their recognition of our desire to help them as well as our expertise to do so. We must remember, however, that we are part of the family's environment, not part of the family system. As such, we must respect the family's goals and wishes and help them cope with the outcomes and consequences whether or not we agree with their decisions. At all times we must remember that the family is responsible for itself and its decisions. Our responsibility is to provide the family or individual member with information about alternative actions and their consequences. In the final analysis, the family, not the nurse, makes the decisions. Feedback from these decisions may motivate the family to make changes or to continue as they are going.

Primary Consequences	Secondary Consequences
positive acceptance	mental and physical disruptions
rejection	bankruptcy or social status
financial difficulties	consequences to infinity ∞
respect	success failure

FEEDBACK

The family system also interacts with its environment in terms of its outputs. These outputs include participation in community activities, the way the family maintains its home and grounds or apartment—in short, the actions that family members undertake. For most families the ultimate output is children, who eventually leave the family and go out into the environment. Feedback results from all these outputs from the family system. The family will soon hear about the activities of any one of its members whom the environment judges noteworthy. This feedback may come in the form of praise and commendation for particularly valuable community service or equally vigorous censure and criticism for behavior of which the community disapproves. In between are the vast number of actions that go unnoticed, which often signifies that everything is OK. In some circumstances no news is good news.

Outputs generate consequence and the ripple effects or geometric results of these effects go on and on. Families may be entangled in networks of circumstances, both positive and negative, as a consequence of some of the family's outputs. Persons who for reasons of conscience could not participate in the Vietnam conflict involved themselves and their families in a series of consequences, the full impact of which will take years to understand and more years to subside. The feedback to these young people and their families for their actions and the consequences of those actions is far greater than many had anticipated. Usually, consequences of actions tend to be more far-reaching than expected. For this reason, time and effort should be spent trying to understand and anticipate the probable consequences of the outcomes of actions before actions are taken. Such considerations may not alter the family's actions but may at least prepare the system for some of the probable results—both positive and negative. Community nurses working with families can play a valuable role assisting clients to consider the consequences of their actions. We can do this by asking such questions as, "If you do this, what do you think will happen immediately, next month, next year, or a couple of years from now?" Such questions may help the family focus on the immediate feedback and long-range consequences.

Another, larger-scale example of the consequences to a system's eco-system or environment occurring as a result of the system's outputs may help in understanding their importance. A hospital (system), due to demands for higher salaries and increasing costs of material and supplies (inputs), may decide to increase its rates to clients (outputs). The results of increased hospital charges (consequences) may include increased insurance claims, which in turn will cause an increase in insurance premiums. Some will be unable to pay the higher premiums and will drop their insurance. Clients with no insurance may ignore subsequent illness as long as possible. When they do seek care, they will have to pay the expenses as best they can from their own pocket. The part of the costs they cannot pay and for which the health care facility is not reimbursed from other sources is passed on to other clients and their insurance companies. The ripple effect then starts the whole cycle over again.

ANALYZING A FAMILY SYSTEM

Families have a history and a future as well as the present point at which we see them. In assessing family systems the community nurse must consider the family's passage through time and stages. The child-bearing family is expanding; families with older children are contracting. Families may be at the peak of their earning power, they may be poor, they may be just beginning, they may be retired. To understand and therefore be able to work with clients, the community nurse must have some appreciation of where they came from and where they're going as well as where they are now (Goode 1963; Haley 1971; Kay 1972; Skolnick 1971; see also Part II).

Churchman suggests five basic considerations for analyzing any system (1968:33–34). Under each one we suggest questions you may want to use in assessing family systems.

Performance Considerations.   Here we are concerned with how well and in what ways the family functions. As with all systems, the final evaluation must be made in terms of the extent to which the system attains its preset goals.

What are the family's goals now, in several years? Have these changed? Why? Are they clear enough to be measured?

Who makes decisions? Does the family work together in arriving at what it wants to do or is one member dominant? As community nurses, our input will be more likely to have an effect if we work with the member(s) who make the final choices than if we try to work through other members. Thus the community nurse may have to arrange to meet with the family in the evening or on weekends when the decisionmaker(s) can be present.

What things will the family system knowingly sacrifice to obtain others? What are their priorities? Often we become concerned about the way families use their resources, usually because we think they "ought to" do something else. Just because we think good nutrition and dental care are essential doesn't mean our clients must think so too. If we know where the family is cutting corners to save money or for whatever reason, we may be able to help with budgeting suggestions, low cost food ideas, and referrals to community resources. Even if we can't help, we can explain some probable consequences of their actions. Parents are often unwilling to spend money having children's baby teeth maintained or restored and often say "they're going to fall out anyway." We can help them understand that the probability of sound permanent teeth is increased by caring for deciduous teeth.

Environmental Considerations.   Every system functions in an environment that affects it, but which it does not control.

What are the constraints or givens in the family's environment? Family income is inadequate to support the family and so its working members are looking for additional jobs. The fact that so far none can be found is an environmental constraint. The nurse may be able to assist by suggesting ways to stretch the family's present income. Sometimes environmental constraints can be alleviated; other times they must be accepted and families encouraged to devote their energies to things they can affect.

What are the environmental conditions over which the family has no control, but which are subject to at least some degree of nursing intervention? Often we know more about how other systems in the family's environment function. Because of our professional status and agency connections, we often have a kind of access to these systems that clients simply do not have. We may be able to help a family get through the red tape at the welfare department, particularly if we know someone in the department. Often we can help families deal with environmental forces by preparing them in advance for the kinds of procedural obstacles they will face.

Resource Considerations.   In this part of the analysis we are concerned with helping our clients make the most of what they have.

What are the family's resources? Consideration should be given not only to material resources but also to the abilities and strengths, as well as the liabilities of each member. Many of these considerations are discussed in chapter 6 on nursing care in the home. Helping the family understand the extent of its health insurance coverage is another way community nurses can help families make the most of their resources (health insurance is discussed in chapter 12).

What alternative resources can be mobilized for and used by the family? In times of crisis, assistance from the environment may be forthcoming. At the death or birth of a family member, friends and relatives often support the family. These crisis resources are usually short term. For families with long-term needs such as chronic illness and disability, help is harder to find. The resources listed in chapter 15 provide a starting point for looking at community resources. Chapter 6 again can be of assistance.

Financial crises are common for us all. Clients often seek to borrow money to meet special and ongoing obligations. Many persons are unaware of the differences between bank and loan company interest rates, even with the Truth in Lending Law. We need to remember that families often make less than sound decisions in crisis situations. In their haste to get funds they may turn to quick money sources that charge exorbitant interest rates. Clients' credit ratings may be poor, thereby making them ineligible for regular bank loans. Many people are so intimidated by orthodox lending agencies that they prefer doing business with the friendly neighborhood usurer. We may be able to help them understand what they're getting into if we at least ask about their plans.

Who in the family decides how and when resources are to be used? We must work with the decisionmakers, as noted before, since planning that does not involve those who actually decide on family resource allocations is bound to be less than successful. Most community nurses work for agencies whose hours of service coincide with normal Monday-through-Friday working hours; most other people are also at work. Nurses are not realistic, especially in times of diminished resources and increased need for them, to expect working members of the family to risk a day's pay to leave work to participate in a planning meeting. Better that we should rearrange the meeting by changing our own schedules.

Subsystem Considerations.   Here we are concerned with who the family subsystems are and how they function.

Who are the components of the family? The family is a functional unit or system. This concept makes possible consideration of a single individual as a family and as fulfilling alone many or all of the tasks that are part of family life. All the people who have the same last name or live under the same roof are not necessarily functional members of the family system. For example, the mother of three children has remarried recently; the new stepfather takes no part in family decisions, activities, or discipline. His standard answer is "go ask your mother." There is little sharing of such functions as emotional support for and socialization of the children. In working with this family, the community nurse must understand how each person does or does not function in the system and how each's part affects the other members and the system as a whole.

How do the components of the family system interact? The community nurse is in an excellent position to assess ways family members interact. As outsiders, our vested interests are different from those of the family as a unit and of its members, and so our perspective in most situations is different from theirs. The community nurse needs to have a thorough knowledge of family dynamics (Ackerman 1966; Delora 1972; Hadden and Borgatta 1969; Otto 1970; Satir 1967). Families often play games, some of which may be detrimental to some members (Berne 1964; see also Part II).

Helping family members see how their behaviors may interfere with other member's optimal level of functioning often enables them to consider making adjustments. For example, while doing a developmental assessment of a child, the nurse has many opportunities to talk with parents about ways of reinforcing some behaviors and extinguishing others. We may counsel them on techniques of behavior modification (Loomis and Horsley 1974; Reese 1966). In this type of situation our role is that of ombudsman since our interest is in helping the family improve its level of functioning and does not include "taking sides" with either the children or their parents.

Management Considerations.   Here the question is how can the management or running of the family be improved? Having done the first four steps in the analysis, we are ready to suggest ways that the family may be able to increase its efficiency and effectiveness as a system. Sharing our observations with the family can add to the information input they use in deciding whether to modify their functioning.

PLANNING

Client-Centered Planning

No one should be more interested and involved in the planning process than the people on the receiving end. This is true whether we are planning for mass transit or health care delivery. However, much planning takes place without the knowledge of, much less the participation of, the people affected. Unless the situation is one in which the "planned for" people have little choice but to accept what is in store for them, noncompliance is quite possible by those who are told what is going to happen to them. We believe that people should have the opportunity to participate in decisions that affect them. Helping the people who will be most affected actually to become involved in the planning process often involves both salespersonship and considerable education. The end results are worth the time and energy required.

In our view, planning is a cooperative process. Clients or consumers should be actively involved in deliberations and decisions, selection of alternatives, and evaluations of the outcomes and consequences. This stance is clearly stated in Public Law 89–749 "Comprehensive Health Planning and Public Health Service Amendments of 1966" and repeated in P.L. 93–641 "The National Health Planning and Resources Development Act of 1974" and its extensions. The implementation of community representation on planning councils has always been easier to talk about than achieve. In the past, attempts to "represent" community residents have recruited the successful business executive or the social leader with time for volunteer work. People with vested interests in what the group was constituted to do also were eager to be involved.

Efforts have been made to seek out representatives from other segments of the population to serve on planning councils and committees. In addition, wider input from the total clientele can be obtained through public hearings and referenda on crucial issues. Even more important is the control by consumers of the implementation and evaluation of the plans that are made.

Underlying many planning efforts is a desire to involve people in activities that bring about change. Ross defines three factors or scales (see figure 3.3) for consideration in working with people in change-related activities (1967:27–39).

Time Scale.   The time scale is a continuum between a tight time schedule

3.3   *Influences on Client Participation*

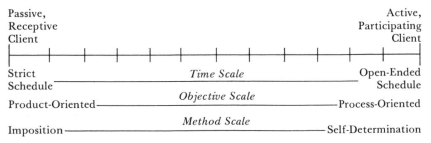

to open-ended or sufficient time. Strict time limits are appropriate in emergency situations or when other actions must take place in sequence following completion of the one at hand. In other situations people can take as much time as they need to question and discuss before reaching a decision on a course of action. For example, discharge planning, to be effective, must be completed before the client goes home and so has a strict time limit. Since elective surgery, on the other hand, can be scheduled when convenient, the planning involved is less time oriented. Since time is often a variable resource, most planning situations fall somewhere toward the middle of the time scale, especially if any action is ever to be taken.

Objective Scale.   Product orientation is at one end of this scale and process orientation is at the other. Product focus means we're concerned with a specific outcome, while process focus deals with learning to do the thing. A meeting dealing with business items will proceed with a different style and pace than will a meeting set up to teach group members parliamentary procedure or group process. In the former case, the objective is task oriented since it focuses on getting through the agenda. The latter is concerned with providing participants with an experience they can use in other circumstances.

Method Scale.   There is fairly general consensus that people involved in making a decision are more likely to carry it out than are people on whom a decision is imposed. A common reaction to attempts at imposition is passive agreement as long as the authority is present, followed by prompt contrary action when the oppressor leaves. A child told not to eat cookies before dinner obeys as long as mother is there; the minute her back is turned he makes a beeline for the jar.

As with all continua, many positions exist between each of the extremes and most activities cluster toward the center. If we are concerned about assisting clients to attain and maintain their OLOF, our activities are more likely to facilitate this outcome if they cluster toward the right side—that is, the client participation side—of the scale.

An example of these scales and the various roles played by providers of health care services and their consumers is found in the proverb: Give a man a fish and you satisfy his hunger for one day; teach him to fish and you satisfy his hunger forever. Generally, giving something to clients is a lot quicker than teaching them to do it for themselves. Thus, the choice of action in this example can be determined according to the time and objective scales. If, further, we decide they should have fish and not poultry, we impose our decision on them. These activities that cluster on the lefthand side of the continuum place health care providers in a more active role and consumers in a recipient or passive role. This position carries a rather high probability that the consumers will not be able to do things for themselves and will remain dependent on the providers to meet their needs. Teaching the man to fish, once he has decided that he really wants to learn, and permitting him to learn at his own speed illustrates activities at the right side of the continuum. A benefit is that one successful learning experience can be modified and transferred to other situations. Given the breadth of influences on people's OLOF already discussed, providers cannot always be present to "do for" clients and so clients must not only be encouraged but assisted to take more responsibility for themselves. That is the rationale underlying our commitment to helping clients become as self-sufficient and independent as possible.

We are also convinced that increased client involvement is vital throughout the health care delivery system. One risk, however, of consumer participation, especially at the beginning, is a devaluation of the professionals' contributions. The value of professionalism lies precisely in the area of special knowledge. When it is needed, the consumer has the right to insist that the professional do the job but not run the whole enterprise. Nowhere is consumer involvement and participation more important than in the planning process.

Regretfully, a note of caution must be added here: Not all practitioners, including nurses, administrators, or agencies agree on anything, much less the value of client participation in planning. My own experience also leads me to believe that not all of us agree on the value of planning, either. The one-up and one-down attitudes that persist in our health care system and social structures make meaningful collaboration between professionals and clients and among professionals difficult if not almost impossible. There is evidence that many kinds of collaboration are becoming more prevalent, if not yet universal. If professionals and clients alike can become committed to the overriding goal of promoting the highest level of functioning for all, ways can be found to work together and to provide needed services in an equitable and dignified manner.

PLANNING PROCESS

The planning process outlined in this section is deceptive, for on paper each step appears as a clear-cut unit, separate from other steps. In reality things don't work like that. We find that none of the steps is discrete, all overlap, and there is much moving back and forth among them. As we discuss and illustrate each step, this overlapping will become more obvious. In real practice, planning is not a linear activity beginning at point A and moving on a straight line through all the other points until we reach the end. Rather, planning is like a system in which each step is a subsystem in itself. The interdependence and interrelatedness of subsystems should prepare us to expect that any step of the process will be subject to change as a result of feedback from the activities in any other step. As frustrating as it may seem, planning, like most other processes, requires that we do many steps or elements simultaneously. In many instances feedback may make clear that we must go back to a previous step in the process and change what we have decided before proceeding with the next step. If we do not build in feedback mechanisms all along the way or if we choose to ignore the input this early warning system sends back to us, we are very likely to make serious mistakes. Almost without exception, a process is more easily corrected than is a completed product. Nevertheless, to have some order in the presentation of the steps of the planning process, they do have to be presented in linear fashion. But don't be fooled that that's the way the process actually works, whether you're planning a dinner party or developing a Health Systems Agency plan. Lots of later steps depend on other steps being carried out first, while many steps must be done simultaneously. Planning is not a simple matter.

The nursing or helping process has been variously defined but usually includes these elements: assessment, planning, implementation, and evaluation (see chapter 13). The planning process, as we use the term, includes all of these components. The steps of the planning process, listed in the order in which we will discuss them, are as follows:

1. Formation of precursor or overriding goals;
2. Initial assessment;
3. Initial formation of objectives and evaluation criteria;
4. Assessment of past trends, present realities, and desired futures;
5. Choice and ordering of needs and priorities;
6. Evaluation of alternative courses of action and their probable consequences;
7. Redefinition of objectives, evaluation criteria, and priorities;
8. Plan formation;
9. Implementation;
10. Evaluation of outcomes in terms of predefined criteria;
11. Redefinition of objectives, evaluation criteria, and priorities;
12. Assessment of past trends, present realities, and desired futures.

The planning is done in cycles, and steps 11 and 12 of the process in planning cycle A are the initial steps in planning cycle B (see figure 3.4). Thus, planning is a continuous process. We should bear in mind that the steps are subsystems and so influence and are influenced by all the other steps or subsystems as we consider each of the steps of the planning processes.

Formation of Precursor or Overriding Goals.   Precursor goals are those goals or values that exert influence on all of our activities. I have already indicated my own very strong belief in the need for and value of client-centered planning. We are more conscious of some precursor beliefs and values than of others. For example, values such as "health care is a right for everybody, not a privilege for the wealthy" and "all people are equally valuable regardless of their age, sex, ethnic background, kind or amount of ability or disability, or any other factor" are based on very different beliefs than are comparable values such as "health care is a commodity that must be bought" and "some groups of people are more valuable to society and so should have first access to limited services." These two sets of precursor values give rise to very different objectives, priorities, and evaluation criteria. All too often agencies and individuals go merrily off on their way without having looked at their values and defined the overriding goals they want to accomplish by the action being planned.

Whenever conflicting value sets are at work in the same ecosystem, there are bound to be disagreements, which is precisely the situation in the health care delivery system in the United States. Conflicts in values and beliefs are inevitable and desirable. If we all thought alike, life would be very dull and little change would take place. However, some meeting ground can be found on which action to meet client needs can take place if the protagonists on the various sides of the arguments can agree that meeting client needs is more important than having their own way on issues (Bondurant 1958).

We need to understand our own value system since it influences the way we look at everything. We have personal values and professional ones. The process of becoming a nurse is one of socialization into a fairly uniform set of values. We, therefore, view the world through "nurse-colored" glasses. There may be discrepancies between our personal and professional goals. We may, for example, hold a personal belief in the absolute equality of value among human beings. However, if we work with kidney dialysis clients, we learn that the limited numbers who may be accommodated by existent facilities have been selected according to some relative value scale. Those of "lesser" value are not accepted for dialysis maintenance or transplant and hence are likely to die sooner than those who are accepted. This conflict can create unbearable internal tensions that we must find some means to resolve.

We must also be aware that there are differences between what we as persons believe and what we actually do. Interpretations of our actions differ depending on the values of those doing the interpreting. Your mother probably views your activities in a far different perspective than does your immediate supervisor.

The organizations with which we work also have goals based on values. One way of testing for a system's real goals is to look for the goals for which the system will knowingly sacrifice other goals. The agency's budget is a good place to begin assessing for real goals. We have long advised our colleagues to read an organization's stated goals and objectives and then examine the organization's budget. If the two disagree, believe the budget. The way a system allocates its resources is the "proof of the pudding" in terms of its real goals. Obviously, then, one of the quickest ways to become a change agent is to gain control of the budget-making process, a goal that draws some nurses into administration.

Precursor or overriding goals, then, are those guides and belief systems that color what we do and how we view the world. We need to be conscious of our goals and, in so doing, modify them as the need arises. Goals are more general and all inclusive than are objectives, which we will discuss shortly.

Initial Assessment.   This step initiates each subsequent cycle in the planning process. As noted, precursor goals are general and fairly static so that we proceed within the broad framework they provide. In this initial assessment, we determine that all is not what we and others thought it was or want it to be. Therefore, change is needed. Information gathering at this point may be relatively unfocused. We have a suspicion or feeling that there is something in one of our families that needs further study, or we may be apprised of the need through referral from another agency. For example, a referral comes from the hospital that a member of one of our client families is ready for discharge and will need care at home. Initial assessment would involve contacting the client's family, seeing the home, talking with the client and family, discussing the client's conditions and care with the discharge planner and other nursing staff at the hospital, exchanging information with the physician, and in general sizing up the situation. These data together with our goals and beliefs about "good client care" combine to give us our basic objectives for beginning to plan with the client, family, and others involved to help in the OLOF process (see chapters 6, 7, and 19).

Initial Formation of Objectives and Evaluation Criteria.   The relationship of goals, objectives, and evaluation criteria can be visualized as an open umbrella. Goals are the top or covering of the umbrella. The objectives are the supports or ribs that give the goals or covering of the umbrella its shape. The ribs come together to form the handle; this handle represents the criteria by which we evaluate the degree of success we have in achieving the plan's objectives.

The goal in planning with the family whose member is about to be discharged from the hospital is to promote and preserve the family's OLOF. This goal is too general to be measured in a specific situation; thus the objectives come into use. Objectives are specific and measurable statements of what we plan to do (Mager 1967). They describe how we will go about attaining our goals. Our objectives with the client family are to rearrange the home so that the ill member gets needed rest, has enough privacy, and yet does not become isolated from the family. These objectives may involve switching bedrooms so that the client is nearer the bathroom, arranging for wheelchair rental so that the client can move about, and placing railings and other aids in the bathroom to enable the client to move about in there.

The evaluation criteria are set up to determine to what extent we did what we set out to do. Did we rearrange the home, get the wheelchair, modify the bathroom? These questions can be answered objectively. Subjective criteria must also be considered. Did our interventions and modifications help the client cope with the situation? The client is the only one who can really evaluate this kind of subjective criterion, and our getting this kind of evaluation is essential. Our interventions may be technically quite correct and adequate from an objective point of view, but they may be inadequate from the client's point of view. We must have both professional and client evaluations so that we can change both our objectives and the ways in which we evaluate their achievement.

Assessment.   We shall talk at length about assessment since it is a basis for evaluating alternatives, forming plans, and evaluating their outcomes (Blum 1974:160–217). Assessment involves examining past trends, present realities, and desired futures. Assessment is illustrated in table 3.1. On a personal level, assessment takes place in our considerations of what we have done, what we are doing, and what we want to do. Somewhere along the line each of us picked nursing as a career. Many factors influenced our decision. Some of these were the realities of our present situation, such as an opportunity to enter a school of nursing, inability to do other things, and so forth. For many of us past experiences with nurses or as a patient also influenced our thinking. Perception of the kinds of future we want and the probabilities of attaining it also figured into our decision. The same process takes place in all assessments.

Our assessment model is placed on a time continuum from past to future. We will apply this model to a family assessment. First we look at the family's past, which includes the individual members' histories as well as the experiences of the family as a unit. In some instances we may

TABLE 3.1 *The Assessment Step in the Planning Process*

Past Trends + Reality of What "Is" + Future Mapping = Assessment		
Trends	*Reality of What "Is"*	*Future Mapping*
Experience of individuals, groups, communities	Indicators	Normative approach
	"Problems"	—"should be" perspective
—long enough period of time to show changes which have occurred	Needs and desires	—planning *from* a desired future
	—observations	
—small enough time intervals so as not to miss changes nor misread patterns or possible cause/effect relationships	—statistics and other data sources	Explorative approach
		—"could be" perspective
	—exchange of data with other agencies/ personnel	—planning *for* desired futures by considering alternative means
	—individuals' statements	
	—validations with persons involved	

Past	*Present*	*Future*

TIME SCALE

need to consider only the length of time the family has been together; in others we need a longer time frame. Deciding what is an adequate length of past history to consider must be tailored to fit each situation. Intervals must be both long and short enough to allow us to see changes. In a family in which one member suffers from allergies, we must know the parents' childhood allergy histories as well as *their* parents' histories. Many allergies are hereditary but tend to "skip a generation." We must also be concerned with the intervals at which the allergy occurs, such as spring only, after certain foods, around animals, or all the time. These data give us valuable clues to the kind of allergy the person may have; from this we can begin to advise the family about what to do.

Assessment of the present seeks to answer the question, "What's really going on here now?" The field method of data gathering offers ideal tools for this phase of our assessment (Schatzman and Strauss 1973). Community nurses generally make first contact with individuals and families as a result of a referral or request for a specific kind of service. Validation and additional information may be sought from the referring agency both before and after contact with the client. Regular feedback to the referring agency is an essential component of continuity of care for our clients; maintaining this continuity is largely our responsibility. We must also seek validation from the client. Nothing is more embarrassing than making an antepartal visit following a referral only to learn, after you've announced your reason for calling, that the client is not now nor does she intend to become pregnant. One way to find out what's really going on is to ask clients how they define their problem or need: "Are you really having problems with your diet? The doctor says you are. What do you think?" Such questions can help clients express what they think about their diet or whatever and also gives us a point at which to begin.

In assessing the present situation, we seek to obtain relevant information from many sources. Data gathering can be carried to ridiculous extremes so that all our time is spent assessing, thereby leaving none for implementation. We can't ever get *all* the relevant information and so must be selective and constantly alert for additional information that may appear at a later time.

In *future mapping* (Blum 1974:186–208), we first consider a *normative,* "should be" statement based on our values and beliefs. These normative ideas make up the utopian scenario or picture in our heads of how the future should look. Examples of other people's utopias include *Walden Two* (Skinner 1960; see also More 1973 and Huxley 1958). Many of our desired futures are expressed in negative terms. "There should not be so much pollution, traffic congestion, and noise in urban areas." Utopias aren't realistic and so can't come into being. However, our desired normative future based on values does rule out some possibilities as unacceptable and leaves many for further exploration. These are the options that the *explorative* approach takes into consideration in weighing alternatives for attaining a future as close to the normative one as possible. Go back to our selection of nursing as a career: For most of us, other fields were at least worth considering before we made a decision. Among the reasons they were rejected was that they did not enable us to approach our utopia. The combination of a normative desired future and selection of the alternative most likely to get us nearest to this goal combine to determine our "shall be" future, which we then go about bringing into reality.

The more people you involve in the assessment process the more input will be obtained about the present and about desired and undesired futures. This breadth of opinion is essential for sound planning. Continued attention to this kind of information throughout the process enables planners to adjust and correct their course on the basis of feedback and new data. Thus assessment is an ongoing process.

Choice and Ordering of Needs and Priorities.   Needs rapidly become apparent as we study and analyze the data generated in the assessment step. We prefer the term "needs" to "problems" and define *needs* as discrepancies between what *is,* as determined in the assessment step, and what *ought to be* as defined by the combination of the normative and explorative conceptions of a desired future. Finding ways to deal with these discrepancies—that is, to bring the present state of affairs closer to the ideal one—is what planning is all about.

There is always more to do than can possibly be done. Before we rank needs in the order of their relative importance, we must go through a sorting or triage process. The triage process helps us select those areas where our potential for intervention is greatest. The triage process is based on the economic principle of opportunity costs, which simply means that resources that are spent for one kind of commodity or activity cannot be spent for any others (see chapter 11). The triage process that we recommend is based on a hierarchy of needs and should follow such guidelines as these: Some needs are impossible to do anything about. We must recognize this reality and direct our efforts to other needs where change can be brought about. It's stupid to beat our heads against a wall at the expense of other things we could affect but will not have the energy left to do so. Many policies in any agency we work for will prove too restrictive and interfere with what we feel are our responsibilities to our clients. An attempt to change policies is relatively fruitless for individual nurses, especially at a staff level. Groups of nurses can and are having a great impact on change in many agencies and institutions. Remember the principle of strength in numbers. We can often influence the guidelines by which policies are interpreted and so be able to work productively with clients within the stated policies of the agency.

Some needs will resolve themselves, given time, without any interventions at all. We should recognize these and leave them to their own resolution: "An untreated cold lasts two weeks; a treated one, a fortnight." Reasonably healthy people have ample resources for dealing with the usual range of stress. To insist on intervening is poor allocation of energies and may actually create problems that did not previously exist. Many penicillin allergies are due to the use of antibiotics in illnesses not susceptible to them or in amounts inadequate for therapy.

Some needs require more resources, for example, time, money, personnel, than we can reasonably spend on them. Trying to meet these needs must, therefore, be done at the expense of other activities. Often the activities that are foregone are those in which our productivity potential is greatest. A clear illustration of choices based on available resources is found in triage as it is done in disaster nursing. Under disaster conditions resources are allocated in exactly the opposite manner than in the rest of the health care delivery system. In disaster we initially sort casualties into three groups. The first group are only minimally injured and so will manage with or without treatment; we do not treat these people at all.

The second group are those who are so severely injured that even with expert and extensive treatment our chances of saving them are minimal. We make these people comfortable and leave them in the care of the clergy or whoever else can stay with them. The third group are those people who are injured in such a way or to such an extent that treatment will have significant effects. These are the people on whom we expend our supplies and energies. The decisions are hard ones to make, but they are reality decisions.

Some needs require actions by other persons or agencies over whom neither we nor our clients have any or sufficient control. Until such time as enough power can be gained to mobilize these other resources, using our energies on them may be relatively futile. Federal or state budget priorities may, for example, veer away from providing funds to support mental health services. Although long-range action needs to be taken on government policymakers to pressure them into reassessing their priorities, the present needs of mental health clients can't wait for that. Support may possibly be gotten faster from local funding sources that are often responsive to local demand.

Some needs are beyond the scope of our expertise. If the expertise required is something we should know, then we had better get it; if not, we should seek others who have it. We can use both consultation and referral. For example, as community nurses, performing tracheotomies is not within our purview but it is our responsibility to recognize when someone is moving toward a need for one, and we must make an urgent type of referral to make that need known. On the other hand, colostomy care is within our scope of responsibilities; if we don't know how to do it, then we had better learn.

Some needs can be met by anyone on the scene and therefore don't require the intervention of the community nurse. However, we may want to meet some of these needs as a means of increasing our credibility with clients. Taking a client to the grocery store, we may be told, is not an appropriate activity for a community nurse. If we use this activity as an opportunity to assess what foods the client actually buys, we are in an excellent position to counsel on nutrition. If the cereal chosen is one of the nonfortified varieties, we can point out the nutritional value of that cereal relative to fortified brands by comparing the box descriptions of nutritional values. This process can also alert the client to the importance of reading all labels. The decision whether to buy the fortified cereal rather than the other one is still the client's, but our teaching may have some influence on purchasing and therefore on nutritional patterns. One corollary to this premise is that certain things need to be done and if no one else is on the scene, the community nurse is humanly obligated to do them. In one case a regular home visit had been cancelled by the home care client and the visiting nurse only glanced down the street as she drove past. When she saw the client sitting on the sidewalk, clutching her freshly broken arm, the nurse turned back, placed the ambulance call, and waited with the client until it took her away before going on to the day's scheduled house calls.

Some needs can be more effectively and efficiently met by community nurses than by anyone else. These are the needs we must identify and on which we should concentrate our efforts. Often, treatments are taught to clients in the hospital and must be modified for implementation when the client goes home. A woman, convalescing from a heart attack, has been told to do no lifting or reaching when she goes home. These instructions necessitate a number of changes in the home that we can help the family understand and implement. The most frequently used kitchen items should be put on the lower shelves within easy reach. Should other items, out of reach of the client, be needed then other members of the family will have to get them down or a very sturdy stepladder will be necessary.

In most of the examples cited under these triage guidelines, some alternative courses of action and their consequences have been considered. The examples illustrate again that the steps of the planning process are not separate and discrete entities but are interrelated and interdependent. The triage process can help reduce our frustrations. Community nurses have long faced the expectation that we can and will do everything. Apparently this expectation is an interpretation of our statement that we are generalists. We have all heard the statement, "Let nursing do it." This attitude of our colleagues has been perpetuated largely by our willingness to take on almost anything that came along. The predictable result has not only been overload but also diminished quality of services in the areas where we, as community nurses, can be most effective. We must define the parameters of our expertise and learn that to say "I cannot do that" is part of professional responsibility and not an admission of failure.

Once needs that can be effectively and efficiently met are identified, they must be ordered or ranked according to their magnitude and importance to the client. There is often a disjuncture between how the professional views client needs and what clients *want* in dealing with their lives. Only by ranking priorities from the client's viewpoint can plans for action have any hope of success. Thus selecting needs and ordering priorities are based not only on the clients' needs but also on the providers' abilities to meet these needs.

Evaluation of Alternative Courses of Action and their Consequences. There is almost always more than one way to deal with the needs that are assigned the highest priority in the preceding step. In this part of the planning process we consider not only the immediate outcomes of our actions but also the long-range consequences. In the proverb cited earlier, the immediate outcomes of giving the man the fish and teaching him to fish are basically the same: The man eats. However, the long-range consequences of the two actions are very different. In the first instance the immediate need is met but the person remains dependent on the giver. In the second situation the person gains the potential for meeting his own needs through fishing as well as increased independence and growing pride with his ability to care for himself.

This analogy can be transferred to our work with clients. If we provide care and services *for* people, we meet their needs but they remain dependent on us for subsequent care. If, in providing this care, we teach the individual or family to give some or all of the same care, we move the client toward independence and we help family members contribute to the disabled member's recovery. Thus the consequences of client-teaching can reduce feelings of helplessness and frustration as well as assure that necessary care is given. Obviously this transfer of responsibility from nurse to client must be done at the client's pace rather than the nurse's. If our desired future for clients is that they return to or attain their OLOF following disability, then we must consider this aim in weighing the consequences of our actions. Clients' independence is the primary priority under which all other activities and alternatives are ranked. Chapter 11 presents a section on decision making that can be of use in evaluating the relative consequences of courses of action.

There are examples of consequences that should be avoided as well as those to be sought out. A client has been exposed to rubella during her first trimester of pregnancy. Tests reveal that she has no immunity to rubella. We must talk with her and the father about the risk of the infant being deformed and introduce the alternative of abortion. The parents must have opportunities to talk about the consequences of any decision they make in terms of the child, other children, and their own feelings. Our responsibility is to make the probable consequences of the possible alternatives as clear to the parents as we can. We cannot make their decision for them. Our professional judgement may lead us to advocate one particular decision. That advocacy, however, should not create guilt for clients who choose another alternative nor should it lead us to withdraw from the client's support system. This latter often appears as though we were punishing them for not making what we think is the right choice. Clients have the ultimate authority and responsibility for the outcomes of their own decision making.

There are courses of action whose direct outcomes and consequences are less than ideal but are far better than what clients now have. We have faced this kind of decision in the development of the so-called alternative medical care system that includes free clinics. Much criticism has been leveled at the free clinics as being less than "first-class medicine." Perhaps this is true, whatever first-class medicine is. However, the consequences of the development of free clinics include the facts that they provide medical care in an acceptable and accessible way to clients who are unable or unwilling to seek care from other sources. The same kinds of arguments have been directed at the use of nurse-practioners in unserved and underserved areas. In terms of consequences, the point worth making is that the free clinic and the nurse-practitioner, regardless of their special virtues, are better than no care at all, which was the situation before their arrival.

Part of evaluating possible courses of action includes comparing them with norms, standards, or protocols (see chapter 13). In this process we consider our alternatives in light of already developed and tested ways to deal with similar situations. For example, if a protocol or standard already exists planning the care of a newborn infant through well child conferences for his or first year, we would be well advised to begin with this predefined and tested alternative. To be sure, some modifications may be appropriate for the individual child or family situation, but the basic plan is already there for us to use. The use of standardized plans not only helps us to provide care, but also frees us from having to invent a plan of care for every single client. Finally, standards or protocols are based on what the agency expects us to do and are upon what the agency is evaluated.

Redefinition of Objectives, Evaluation Criteria, and Priorities.   This step is the last one before we form the plan. We are wise to stop and take one last look to be as sure as possible that we have not forgotten anything. If no new data are available to change things and the planning group is satisfied with the priority ordering and consideration of alternatives, then the next step is formation of the actual plan.

Plan Formation.   Plans take many forms. Care plans are the result of client assessment and all the other steps thus far in the process. The plan lays out what we're going to do, who's going to do it, and when it's to be completed. This accountability mechanism is very important since it enables us to follow the plan's implementation and enables the actors to know exactly what is expected of them. A final review of the plan with everyone involved before implementation begins is advisable to answer questions and catch missed items. Program Evaluation Review Technique (PERT) is a method for plan formation and control that some of us have found valuable (Archer 1974).

Plan Implementation.   In this step we actually do something—the something that we have planned so far. Often people and agencies become so engrossed in earlier steps of the planning process that they lose sight of the ultimate purpose: to initiate carefully planned action whose results move toward attaining the plan's objectives for a more desirable future.

Implementation must take place before the assessment data on which the plan is partially based are out of date.

Careful observation must continue during the implementation step so that unforeseen and undesirable outcomes can be detected and dealt with by altering the plan as necessary. As noted, we can never know all we need to know. Thus we begin with our antennae out to gather new information, which is another reminder that feedback never ceases to be an essential source of data.

Evaluation of Outcomes in Terms of Predefined Evaluation Criteria. Although evaluation has been built into every step of the process so far through both constant assessment and feedback, this step is a full-dress evaluation. One of the greatest problems in evaluating many programs' outcomes is the paucity of measurable objectives. The evaluation criteria we will use are the ones we developed in step three of this process. We now apply these criteria to the outcomes of our plan's implementation to judge its effectiveness.

The first question—"Did we do what we said we would?"—is a fairly objective kind of analysis. In an earlier example our purpose was to assist an incapacitated member of a family to socialize with the family and still have a convenient place for rest and privacy. This goal involved modifications of the home that were planned with the client and family and included moving bedroom furnishings and obtaining a wheelchair, as well as considerable family teaching. Evaluation criteria derived from these objectives include both objective and subjective ones. Objective measures are often easier to use, since they deal with observable facts. Either we got the wheelchair or we didn't; we modified the sleeping facilities or we didn't. This part of the evaluation involves basically yes or no answers.

Evaluation of the more subjective kinds of outcomes must be done by the persons directly involved—the clients. Only they can tell us whether and to what extent the alterations which we jointly planned were successful from their point of view. It is not enough for community nurses to have *delivered* good care and sound interventions. Our clients must judge whether they *received* services they found acceptable and useful, which is not to imply that clients should judge procedures from a technical point of reference; that's our job. However, they are the only ones who can evaluate the results of our services in terms of how what we did made them feel—physically and emotionally. If we want to plan and deliver effective as well as efficient services to clients, they must have equal participation in the planning process, and they must also have the final word in evaluation of the results.

If the outcomes of the plan failed to meet or only partially met our clients' and our own objectives, then we must reexamine the entire planning process to locate the points at which feedback failed to alert us to needed changes. We may have misinterpreted data from the assessment step and so made faulty decisions. We may not have considered all the possible alternatives or we may have neglected glaring consequences of some we did consider. If these points of error can be found, we must determine why we didn't pick up on the information and make alterations. If no such feedback failures can be found, then we must examine the whole planning cycle to see where we could have built in feedback but did not. This kind of evaluation of the entire planning process can turn failures into valuable learning experiences since we can transfer what we learned in this cycle to the next one to avoid repeating the same mistakes.

Even if evaluation proves that our outcomes met our objectives for this planning cycle, we would do well to reexamine the whole process to find areas where our effectiveness and efficiency could be increased. Also, successful outcomes may be the result of luck more than sound planning technique. Since we will need to repeat the planning process in many situations, we must be as sure as possible that our methods are sound. Sound methods can be transferred to a variety of situations; luck can't be. We've reached the end of planning cycle A and have begun planning cycle B with the evaluation/assessment step just completed. This relationship of the planning cycles is shown in figure 3.4. The point of intersection is the evaluation step. Cycle A ends and cycle B continues with the redefinition of objectives, criteria for evaluation, and priorities (Arnold 1969:13). In this way the planning cycles are linked together in series rather than being separate and isolated projects. This continuity means that clients are less likely to fall through the holes in the system and be lost than is the case with many separate projects. In the long run these continuous planning cycles are all moving in a more or less orderly

3.4   *Overlapping of Assessment and Evaluation Steps to Provide Continuity among Planning Cycles*

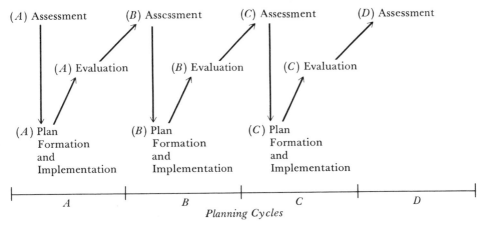

process toward attaining the overriding or precursor goals which initiated step one of cycle A.

SUMMARY

Selected concepts that are basic for the practice of community nursing are presented in this chapter. The concept of exchange is introduced as the basis for relationships between community nurse and client. Nurse-client transactions are seen as peer exchange rather than a one-up and one-down relationship. The description of systems theory uses a family as an example of an open system. Methods of analyzing a system are given, and systems terms appear in the glossary that follows.

Planning is an essential element at all levels of community nursing. To be effective and efficient, the planning process must involve all those who will be affected by decisions, plans, and their outcomes. For this reason some strategies are presented for making planning client centered. Planning is seen as a rational process that does not follow a linear progression, but rather as a system with many feedback loops enabling constant adjustment while the process is underway. The ultimate purpose of planning is to select and implement actions that will bring about changes geared to attain a desired future based on overriding goals and values.

GLOSSARY OF SYSTEMS THEORY TERMS

All special fields have their own particular language. This glossary contains some of the most common terms used in systems theory. Knowing them will make reading about the theory easier and help you to be able to apply it.

Adaptation   The adjustments that systems make to enable them to survive in their environment and carry out their tasks.

Black Box   An operations research term for the system's internal workings that transform inputs into outputs and that are concerned with system maintenance (see Throughput).

Boundaries   The parameters or limits of the system that help the system to maintain its integrity and therefore survive. An open system's boundaries permit exchanges with its environment; a closed system's boundaries do not. A primary management task in open systems is boundary maintenance.

Centralization   Usually one subsystem within a system that plays a dominant part in the operation of the whole system. Changes in the subsystem where this dominant function is centralized are reflected and amplified throughout the system.

Closed System   A system that functions without interacting with its ecosystem and therefore must depend on recycling internal resources to be able to survive. These systems are subject to the second law of thermodynamics, entropy, which predicts an eventual running down as nonrenewable resources are consumed and therefore no longer available for use.

Consequences   The results of the outputs of the system. Outputs' effects on the environment and on the system via feedback loops are geometric rather than arithmetic—that is, each output has results that in turn have more results or consequences. These consequences go on to infinity. Planners must be concerned with consequences as far as they can be predicted. Computer simulation is a useful aid in considering and planning for the possible long-range consequences of systems' activities.

Control   Constant monitoring (cybernation) of whether and to what extent plans are being carried out and the system is functioning properly. Planning to change plans as feedback indicates change is warranted is a critical aspect of control in systems theory. Control is not a coercive term as applied to systems management.

Cybernation   A term derived from the Greek word for steersman that means guiding or correcting the system's course. Cybernation is a constant monitoring of what is actually going on in the system as a basis for making alterations or adaptations in order to keep the system moving toward its predefined goals.

Differentiation   The effect of the tendency of systems to move toward specializing and dividing the labor among the subsystems—that is, each subsystem's functions become clearly differentiated from those of other subsystems. Bureaucratic systems with their specialized departments and divisions are an example of differentiation.

Environment   The ecosystem in which the system functions. Open systems depend on their environment as a source for their inputs and as a market for their outputs. There are many factors in a system's environment that affect the system, but over which the system has no control; the environment, therefore, imposes a number of givens on the system.

Equifinality   The sense of purposefulness with which the system adjusts itself in order to achieve its goals and remain adapted to its environment so that it can survive. A young system may use many paths and means to reach its objectives; its approach may be quite pragmatic. As more regulatory mechanisms, such as rules and policies, are developed, the need for equifinality decreases. Regularized procedures, or hardening of the categories, reduces the need for constant monitoring to be sure that the system is proceeding as planned; there is no other way that the system can operate.

Feedback   The portion of the system's outputs that returns to the system as an input and brings with it information from the environment and other subsystems in the environment about the effects, quality, and consequences of the system's outputs as well as suggestions for changes and new outputs. Feedback may also occur internally as subsystems receive reactions from other subsystems about their work. Feedback occurs naturally in most situations; however, this natural phenomenon can be improved by planning feedback loops that constantly supply the system with information about its performance.

Input   Resources that come into the system from its environment and are used to maintain the system and to produce outputs.

Open System   A living system that engages in exchange relationships with its environment. In these exchanges, the system obtains inputs and produces outputs as well as retains some resources to assure its own survival.

Optimization   Modifying and adapting a system to enable it to concentrate its efforts on one particular kind of activity to achieve the best possible outputs. The principle of opportunity costs—that is, resources used for one purpose cannot be used for other purposes also—is operational here and means that optimizing one subsystem can only be done at the expense of other subsystems since some of the resources they would have received went instead to the subsystem being optimized. In systems jargon then, optimizing one subsystem results in suboptimizing all of the rest.

Outputs   The products that an open system releases into its environment.

Progressive Segregation   The phenomenon in which subsystems move toward independence and unrelatedness. Progressive segregation takes two forms. The first is decay or degeneration in which the system falls apart. The second type is characterized by subsystem growth and increasing independence as its functions become increasingly differentiated. This second type of progressive segregation occurs in creative and evolutionary processes.

Progressive Systemization   The drawing together of parts of a system and strengthening of existing relationships, which is the opposite of progressive segregation.

Ripple Effect   The continuation of consequences as a result of a system's outputs, as illustrated in figure 3.2. It derives its name from the effect noted when one drops an object into a calm pool: The ripples go on until the entire pool may be filled. The consequences of outputs from a system can have a ripple effect far beyond and different from those the planners may have intended or envisioned.

Steady State   A dynamic equilibrium rather than a static homeostasis. Through continuous actions and reactions the system maintains a constantly changing but stable relationship with the environment.

Subsystems   The component parts or units of a system that together make up the system. The subsystems are interrelated and interdependent so that a change in one subsystem spills over and affects all of the others.

System Maintenance   The system's seeking to survive, when all else fails, by using inputs for this purpose rather than for conversion into outputs. Under normal circumstances as well as those of stress, the system uses some of the resources available to it to maintain its operations.

Throughput   The process that takes place inside the system by which inputs are converted into outputs (see Black Box).

REFERENCES

ARCHER, SARAH E. "PERT: A Tool for Nurse Administrators." *Journal of Nursing Administration* 4 (September–October 1974):26–32.

ARNOLD, MARY F. "Evaluation: A Feedback Model." In *Health Planning 1969,* ed. Henrik L. Blum. Berkeley: University of California, School of Public Health, 1969.

BACHRACH, L. "Developing Objectives in Community Mental Health Planning." *American Journal of Public Health* 64 (1974):1162–63.

BAUM, M., BERGWALL, D., and REEVES, P. "Planning Health Care Delivery Systems." *American Journal of Public Health* 65 (1975):272–75.

BERNE, ERIC. *Games People Play.* New York: Ballantine Books, 1964.

BIDDLE, WILLIAM W., and BIDDLE, LAURIDE J. *The Community Development Process: The Rediscovery of Local Initiative.* New York: Holt, Rinehart and Winston, 1965.

BLUM, HENRIK L., et al. *Notes on Comprehensive Health Planning.* Berkeley: University of California, 1969.

BLUM, HENRIK L. *Health Planning.* New York: Human Sciences Press, 1974.

BONDURANT, JOAN. *Conquest of Violence.* Princeton, N.J.: Princeton University Press, 1958.

BRADEN, CARRIE J., and HERBAN, NANCY L. *Community Health: A Systems Approach.* New York: Appleton-Century-Crofts, 1976.

BRODBECK, MAY. "Logic and Scientific Method in Research on Teaching." In N.L. Gage, ed., *Handbook on Research on Teaching.* Chicago:Rand McNally & Co., 1963.

BRUHN, JOHN G. "Planning for Social Change: Dilemmas for Health Planning." *American Journal of Public Health* 63 (July 1973):602–05.

BUCKLEY, WALTER. *Sociology and Modern Systems Theory.* Englewood Cliffs, N.J.: Prentice-Hall, 1967.

CATANESE, ANTHONY J. *Planners and Local Politicians: Impossible Dreams.* Beverly Hills, Calif.: Sage Publications, 1974.

CHERMAYEFF, SERGE, and TZONIS, ALEXANDER. *Shape of Community: Realization of Human Potential.* Baltimore, Md.: Penguin Books, 1971.

CHURCHMAN, C. WEST. *The Systems Approach.* New York: Dell Publishing Co., 1968.

COWAN, PETER, et al. *The Future of Planning.* Beverly Hills, Calif.: Sage Publications, 1973.

EISENSTADT, S. N. *Essays on Cooperative Institutions.* New York: John Wiley and Sons, 1965.

EMERY, F. E., ed. Systems Thinking. Selected Readings. Baltimore, Md.: Penguin Books, 1969.

ETZIONI, AMITAI. *The "Semi-professions" and Their Organization.* New York: Free Press, 1969.

FULLER, R. BUCKMINSTER. *Operating Manual for Spaceship Earth.* Carbondale: Southern Illinois University Press, 1969.

GAGE, N. L., ed. *Handbook of Research on Teaching.* Chicago: Rand McNally & Co., 1963.

GOFFMAN, ERVING. *The Presentation of Self in Everyday Life.* New York: Doubleday and Co., 1959.

HAYMAN, HERBERT H. *Health Planning: A Systematic Approach.* Germantown, Md.: Aspen Systems Corporation, 1975.

LEAVELL, HUGH R., and CLARK, R. GURNEY. *Preventive Medicine for the Doctor in His Community: An Epidemiologic Approach,* 3rd ed. New York: McGraw-Hill Book Co., 1965.

LINDBLOM, CHARLES E. "The Science of Muddling Through." *Public Administration Review* 19 (1959):79–88.

LOOMIS, MAXINE E., and HORSLEY, JO ANNE. *Interpersonal Change: A Behavioral Approach to Nursing Practice.* New York: McGraw-Hill Book Co., 1974.

McDONALD, FREDERICK J. *Educational Psychology,* 2nd ed. Belmont, Calif.: Wadsworth Publishing Co., 1965.

MAGER, ROBERT F. Preparing Instructional Objectives. Belmont, Calif: Fearon Publications, 1967.

MANKIN, DOUGLAS C., and GLUECK, WILLIAM F. "STRATEGIC PLANNING." *Hospital and Health Services Administration* 22 (Spring 1977): 6–22.

MORE, SIR THOMAS. *Utopia.* New York: E.P. Dutton Co., 1973.

ORWELL, GEORGE. *1984.* New York: Harcourt, Brace and Co., 1949.

OTTO, HERBERT C., ed. *The Family in Search of a Future: Alternate Models for Moderns.* New York: Appleton-Century-Crofts, 1970.

PIERCE, LILLIAN M. "Usefulness of a Systems Approach for Problem Conceptualization and Investigation." *Nursing Research* 21 (1972):509–12.

REESE, ELLEN P. *The Analysis of Human Operant Behavior.* Dubuque, Ia.: Wm. C. Brown Co., 1966.

ROEMER, RUTH, KRAMER, CHARLES, and FRINK, JEANNE E. *Planning Urban Health Services: From Jungle to System.* New York: Springer Publishing Co., 1975.

ROSS, MURRAY G. *Community Organization: Theory, Principles, and Practice,* 2nd ed. New York: Harper & Row, 1967.

SCHATZMAN, LEONARD, and STRAUSS, ANSELM L. *Field Research: Strategies for a Natural Sociology.* Englewood Cliffs, N.J.: Prentice-Hall, 1973.

SKINNER, B. F. *Walden Two.* New York: Macmillan Co., 1960.

SOMERS, ANNE R., and SOMERS, HERMAN M. *Health and Health Care: Policies in Perspective.* Germantown, Md.: Aspen Systems Corporation, 1977.

SUTHERLAND, J. *A General Systems Philosophy for the Social and Behavioral Sciences.* New York: Braziller, 1973.

VON BERTALANFFY, L. *General Systems Theory.* New York: Braziller, 1968.

PART II

Community Health Nurses Working with Families

EDITORS' INTRODUCTION

One of the fundamental points made in basic nursing education is to consider individual patients/clients/consumers and devise nursing care plans to fit their individual needs. To move from that point of view of community health nursing to one that approaches its clients at other levels is very often difficult to do. Elsewhere we talk about nursing specialization linked to population groups and to places.
The idea of dealing with groups as intensively and distinctively as we deal with individual people is very hard to grasp. However, one major theme of community health practice is its relation to families. For that reason we present an entire section on the topic.

Chapter 4: Family Theories: Frameworks for Nursing Practice
Fay Bower and Margaret Jacobson present a very fast, very packed run-through of three major viewpoints for considering families: the structural-functional (mainly from anthropology), the developmental (mainly from psychology), and the interactional (mainly from sociology). There is no way any one theory can completely describe something as complex and evolutionary as the American family, but this chapter is an attempt to bring these three theoretical frameworks together in one place to see how each may contribute toward better understanding the client.

To be even more helpful, the authors suggest some of the limitations to each theory as well as the strong points to reinforce the need for care in applying any one.

Chapter 5:   *Crisis Intervention*

Carol Edgerton Mitchell describes a major method for managing the problems so often presented by the families we are visiting. Although there are exceptions, we generally are not involved with families unless they are in some form or another of crisis—often involving issues of illness, life development, or problems with some larger system. Using some examples, this chapter introduces the major themes and processes of the tool of crisis intervention.

Chapter 6:   *Working with Families in Community Health*

Ruth Ann Terry and Teresa Bello exemplify some of the theoretical points in the previous chapters with a series of case studies. Our intent is that this chapter be the basis for creative discussions of elements both of the various theoretical frameworks and the crisis techniques. Since writing down all of the action that occurs in a home visit isn't possible, even as much information as is given in this chapter is, of course, only a small part of the entire event. We suggest that after picking out areas that illustrate the theories mentioned, you try to think what further kinds of information you would have looked for or what other questions you would have wanted to ask if you were trying to use one particular theory in assessing these families.

Chapter 7:   *Family-Focused Community Health Nursing Services in the Home*

In the final chapter in this section, Carol Lockhart uses an extended case example to illustrate how an experienced nurse utilizes a wide range of skills to promote the functioning not only of the individual client but of the family as a whole. In demonstrating nursing services at home, this chapter specifically deals with communication, mutuality of goal setting, and joint contracting for truly client-centered care, a format for rating a family's repertoire of coping resources, and the position of community nursing in the spectrum of care delivery.

4. Family Theories: Frameworks for Nursing Practice

Fay L. Bower
Margaret J. Jacobson

INTRODUCTION

Traditionally community health nursing practice has focused on aggregates of people—that is, on groups of people who have common concerns, problems, or characteristics. Sometimes that group is at high risk of developing a health problem; for instance, persons with hypertension who are high risk for developing a stroke. The group may be people of certain age groups, such as children and older persons who have less ability to deal with certain conditions, or it may be a group that has similar goals and functions, such as the family. This last group, the family, is discussed in this chapter. Specifically, various theoretical and conceptual approaches or frameworks for analyzing and working with the family are presented. Although each approach is presented in its entirety before another is discussed, the reader is cautioned to remember three things: the frameworks presented are in no way inclusive of all the possible approaches; no one approach is endorsed by the authors over another; and in practice, more than one approach may be used. For example, a group of sociologists working in research, teaching, and family counseling were found to employ multiple frameworks (Hays 1977).

Even though it is theoretically possible for a society to exist without family units, every known society has some form of family structure, and with few exceptions the basic social unit is the nuclear family (Brown

93

1963:31–33; see also Bell and Vogel 1968:2). Although most academicians accept the universality of the nuclear family, they continue to debate whether that family has the four requisite functions of socialization, economic cooperation, reproduction, and sexual relations (Murdock 1949:1–11); two irreducible functions, the primary socialization of children and the stabilization of adult personalities (Parsons and Bales 1955:308), or but one universal function, the nurturant socialization of children (Reiss 1965:443–53).

Likewise, there is variance in the literature and among the disciplines regarding the structure of the family. Typically the nuclear family has consisted of a father, mother, and children, with the extended family being all persons related to the primary unit (Shusky 1972). In many parts of the world this kind of composition is still prevalent, but in the United States (U.S. Department of Labor 1976) and in some European countries there is a trend toward childless families and other arrangements of persons who identify themselves as family.

Definitions of family really depend on the frame of reference of the definer. For example, some definitions are dependent on affinal (married) and consanguinal (blood kinship) relationships excluding any fictive arrangements (unrelated persons living together). Other definitions would include fictive arrangements as invented forms of family. Thus, we could say that all marriages are families, but not all families are married (Eschleman 1974:87).

As community health nurses, we need to be aware of and understand the varied definitions of family since our approach will be influenced by the choice of definition. For instance, genetic counseling services will be offered according to the relationships within the family to the person with the gene under consideration. Other services will be determined by certain legal structures that make one family member responsible for the action of another, such as with minor children. In addition, the community health nurse can interact more appropriately when the behavior of clients is understood within the context of their own social unit.

Social anthropologists and family sociologists have posed five or more conceptual or theoretical frameworks for the study of family. The terms *conceptual* and *theoretical* are not to be interpreted as synonomous, but are used together here because the literature uses both. We prefer *conceptual* when discussing the family, but at the same time want to acknowledge the terminology used by others. Broderick (1971:141) and Hays (1977:59–65) have identified three such frameworks that have remained viable and distinguishable from one another over the past decade and that provide frame of reference useful to the community health nurse who is working with families in the delivery of health care services. These three frameworks are structural-functional, developmental, and interactional.

THE STRUCTURAL-FUNCTIONAL APPROACH

The structural-functional approach has its roots in social anthropology, predominantly in the writings of Radcliffe-Brown (1952) and Malinowski (1945) who emphasized the interrelatedness and interdependence of all aspects of society and its subcultures. Structural-functional theory is essentially concerned with the identification, description, and explanation of the arrangement of the parts of a system (structure), with the interrelatedness of those parts (functions), and of how those parts interact with other components of the system (Bell and Vogel 1968:1–34).

CONCEPTS DEFINED

In order to understand the use of the structural-functional framework, several concepts are defined:

Society is a social system that survives its original members, replaces them through biological reproduction, and is relatively self-sufficient (Winch 1963:8).

Social system is a system seen as two or more interdependent units that are at the same time actors and social objects to each other. The properties of social systems are differentiation, organization, boundary maintenance, and equilibrium tendency (McIntyre 1966:53–73).

Equilibrium is an internal state of regularity, or balance, of a system relative to its environment (Parsons 1961:338).

Role is an organized part of an actor's behavior that constitutes and defines his or her participation in an interactive process. Roles involve a set of complementary expectations concerning the actors' own actions and those of others with whom they interact (Parsons and Shils 1954:23).

Role differentiation is the distribution of persons among the various positions and activities distinguished in the structure and hence the differential arrangement of the members of the structure (Levy 1949:8).

Structure is the arrangement of the roles of which a social system is composed. Structure can, then, be divided into relational and unit categories. In this view, the most significant unit of social structure is not the person but the role (Parsons and Shils 1954:23).

Function is the contribution that an activity or role makes to the whole—that is, the consequence of the activity for the system.

Position is a location in a social structure that is associated with a set of social norms (Bates 1956:314).

From a structural-functional point of view the family is a social system with members that have specific roles and functions. Each family member is a part of the family unit and how that member acts will affect how others will behave and how the total unit will relate to other families and groups of people. An analogy has been made to the human system in that the anatomy and physiology of the human organism are inextricably related—that is, the structure of a part influences its function and conversely the functions influence the structure.

The structure and function of the family can be analyzed in three ways. One can look at the relationship of the family to broader social systems, the internal relationships within the family, and the reciprocal relationship between family and personality (McIntyre 1966:55). What is learned by the community health nurse as a result of an analysis in these three ways can provide challenging opportunities for the testing of the structural-functional approach with families and can add to the value of the framework as a basis for nursing action.

Relationship of the Family to Broader Units.   One major emphasis concerning the relationship between the family and the broader social system has been on the role the family plays in the socialization of the family members for society. A family inevitably lives in a broader social context of other individuals, families, and social groups. The family members, whether related or not, must learn certain roles and behaviors for living and interacting outside the family. Certain norms, values, and behaviors must be learned by family members if they are to live harmoniously with their neighbors, be successful in their jobs, or be influential in how the community in which they live is governed or changed. Parsons and Bales (1955:26–31) claim only the family can adequately carry out these socialization responsibilities. Others have not agreed (Spiro 1960; Levy 1955; Fallers 1959). Nevertheless, Parsons and Bales single out socialization and the stabilization of the adult personalities as the two major functions of the family for society.

Internal Relationships within the Family.   Much of the emphasis in studies on the internal relationships within the family has been on the division of labor between the members of the family and on the functions of the division of labor for the maintenance of the family. The work of Parsons, Bales, Shater, and Zelditch (1955) on "expressive" and "instrumental" role differentiation has been to explain and predict this division of labor. According to Zelditch (1955:313), "expressive roles are primarily the integrative or solidifying activities that bring emotional satisfaction to the family members." The wife-mother usually specializes in these activities as she is the integrative force within the home. "Instrumental" roles are primarily activities that occur external to the family but that also include satisfactory goal attainment of the family. The husband-father in his breadwinner role tends to specialize in instrumental activities.

In a practical sense, designating such roles for males and females has implications for how the community health nurse relates with family members. For instance, assigning the expressive role to a woman involved in women's liberation or to a divorced, working mother would be inappropriate. Because of their values and lifestyles, these women behave in more inclusive ways and incorporate characteristics from both categories into their roles. In addition, many men's groups consider it stifling to the development of their own emotional balance to force them into a stereotyped role as instrumental worker. However, when the nurse is working with a family that accepts and practices rigid male-female behaviors, such as the "macho" father and the "homemaker" mother, such labeling is appropriate as it explains why they get along and what could be expected if one or the other decided to make a change in role behavior.

The assignment of the expressive role to the female has received much criticism, particularly from women. Women's liberation groups, consciousness-raising groups, and women in general have strong feelings about the submissiveness of the concept and of the stereotyping of such a conceptualization. Many are concerned about the impact such a framework might have on perpetuating such stereotypes in the socialization of female children.

Eschleman (1974:46) believes such a categorization is arbitrary and cautions against the mutual exclusiveness of the framework, thereby suggesting the impossibility of clearly splitting the expressive and instrumental functions. This view is substantiated by a U.S. Department of Labor survey indicating that the mythical typical American family with a breadwinner husband, a homemaker wife, and two children now only comprises 7 percent of the nation's families.

On the other hand, men who choose to become nurses can give evidence that this dichotomous view of expressive and instrumental functions remains in force in that nursing has traditionally been described as a feminine occupation that utilizes expressive behaviors "best" performed by women. Additionally, relatively few women have become engineers or physicians, which are more traditionally men's jobs with predominantly instrumental aspects.

The ways that roles may be enacted are, within narrow limits, fixed and standarized. Rules or expectations for behavior associated with the role govern the way the individual will function (Parsons and Shils 1954). Cultural norms—the result of values and attitudes ascribed by society— act as a guide for conduct of the occupant of the role. These same values and attitudes assign status, and the rights and privileges that constitute the status of the role must be assumed by the occupant of the role if overt expression of the role is to be fully realized.

Much of the guilt working mothers feel could be due to their acceptance of the ascribed values and attitudes of the traditional mother role. The same can be said about the depression and poor self-image of the aged who have been removed from the work force and who believe they possess low-status positions. Another example includes middle-aged men who due to cardiac problems must alter their ways of living and find that not being the "breadwinner" creates feelings of second-class citizenry.

The community health nurse has many opportunities where counseling and teaching clients about how to cope with changing roles and the feelings generated by these changes are paramount to their health. Assessing the family structure and functions and knowing when the use of a structural-functional framework is beneficial is essential if the nurse is to be effective.

Reciprocal Relationships between Family and Personality.   The third way to approach the family in using the structural-functional framework is to look at the personality of the individual family member and its reciprocal relationship to the family as a whole. As Ackerman states:

> Clearly the configuration of family determines the forms of behavior that are required in the roles of husband and wife, father, mother, and child. Mothering and fathering, and the role of the child, acquire specific meaning only within a defined family structure [Ackerman 1958].

Thus the family molds the kinds of persons it needs in order to carry out its functions. The work of Virginia Satir (1972) exemplifies this concept by suggesting the family keeps its psychotic member in the "sick" role in order to keep the family structure intact and functional. By scapegoating all that happens onto the psychotic member, the family never has to look at its behavior or do anything to change it. The same phenomenon could explain the "cardiac cripple syndrome." The family's insistence on coddling the "sick" member reinforces their expectations that the person "needs" dependent waiting on. In a reciprocal fashion, the sick person's acceptance validates their assumptions, thereby setting the stage for continued dependency on other family members. This interplay is hard to change, particularly if the family needs this kind of arrangement for their functional adaptation to the cardiac problem.

Several factors affect this reciprocal relationship and its impact on personality development. The integration and solidarity of the family are a potent influence on personality development in that too much or too little may have negative effects. For instance, solidarity during infancy may be very effective, yet inhibitive when the child tries to form emotional ties outside the family when he or she is older.

The locus of authority and coordination in the family also affects the personality development of family members. This aspect is best illustrated by parents who act out their own conflicts by implicitly assigning the parental role to the child. The child not only does not get direction, limit setting, or support but must provide them for the parent and at a time when skill for such behaviors is not yet learned. In families where the authority is clearly parental and the children are given appropriately increasing responsibility, the end result is quite different than one would expect from the earlier example.

Another facet to the family-personality reciprocal relationship is the part it plays in developing individuals capable of functioning in society. Children not only learn how to be "wives and mommies" or "husbands and daddies," but how to be managers, salesmen, politicians, nurses, and any number of other roles. However, if the family members are to develop personalities that equip them to cope with the outside world, the assignment of tasks must be appropriate to the capabilities and motivations of each. Community health nurses are aware of the problems a school child has when family expectations go beyond the achievement potential of the child, both physically and intellectually.

The process of value integration is also a family-personality interchange that affects the way the individual member will function in society. The internalization of values derived from the family goes on unconsciously as the children learn their roles. There is considerable continuity from generation to generation, even though values are tested and some modification occurs through the influence of peer groups and situational factors. Much of how adults behave in their jobs and in social relationships outside of the home is influenced by the values they have learned from the family.

BASIC ASSUMPTIONS

Several basic assumptions can be extracted from the structural-functional framework and can guide study and work with families. As community health nurses, we might use the following list of assumptions to screen the appropriateness of the framework for the families we are working with.

1. The family is a social system with functional requirements comparable to those of larger systems (Bell and Vogel 1968:19).

2. The family as a social system is composed of interdependent subsystems (Hill and Hansen 1960).

3. The family system tends to homeostasis (equilibrium) (Hill and Hansen 1960).

4. The family is also a small group possessing certain generic characteristics common in all small groups (Parsons 1961; Zelditch 1955).

5. In every society, one or more basic functions are fulfilled by the family (Bell and Vogel 1968:8; Winch 1963:31).

6. Families perform individual-serving functions as well as society-serving functions (Winch 1963:20).

ADVANTAGES AND DISADVANTAGES OF THE
STRUCTURAL-FUNCTIONAL FRAMEWORK

Although there has been much research concerning the family, relatively few of these studies have used a structural-functional approach. Despite this paucity of use, the framework has had a greater impact on research than its use would indicate. Regardless of the theoretical orientation of the investigator, there are generally many references to the functions of the family. A major part of many family studies is detailed attention to each family member's functions or roles.

In practice the impact of the structural-functional approach has been more difficult to trace (McIntyre 1966). Students may see this impact most clearly in the references that nearly every textbook on the family makes to the functions of families in society. But for psychologists, nurses, social workers, and particularly for those involved with marriage counseling, the influence has been more indirect. Counselors often place emphasis on the client as part of a family system to help the individual deal with his or her role in relation to the other roles in the family, but this emphasis on structural-functionalism is not often directly explored. Kargman (1957) claims that counselors ought to make structural-functionalism explicit since he believes it is an excellent way of orienting the client to the problem situation.

Critics of structural-functionalism suggest the framework tends to promote maintenance of a traditional definition of family because of its focus on social equilibrium. It does follow that authors who make the greatest use of the framework do find a positive social function for the typical contemporary urban middle-class nuclear family with conventional roles based on sex (Parsons and Bales 1955). More recently Goode has pointed out how the modern emerging family has a potential for a new kind of functionalism:

> . . . I see in it and in the industrial system that accompanies it the hope of greater freedom . . . . For me, then, the major and sufficing justification for the newly emerging family patterns is that they offer people at least the potentialities of greater fulfillment [Goode 1963:380].

Another criticism is that the structural-functional approach is teleological—that is, it defines the family's functions and by doing so, creates the functions. Writers using the structural-functional framework have at times seemed to assume that an explanation of the family's functions is also an explanation of the family's origin. Furthermore, many writers point to different functions for the same item.

Thus the functional approach presents a number of logical difficulties. It can be so deceptively simple and sensible that we might easily assume that more has been proved than really has. Nevertheless, as a way of explaining the family and its behavior, the structural-functional approach has been very useful.

DEVELOPMENTAL APPROACHES

A developmental study of the human life cycle makes clear the stages individuals go through as they mature. This same approach has also been applied to families as entities. The developmental framework transcends the boundaries of several approaches by joining the social system approach with the closely related structural-functional concepts and the social-psychological idea that family members are also individuals. The developmental framework is indebted to the rural sociologists for the life-cycle concept; the psychologists, the demographers, and human development specialists for the concept of developmental needs and tasks; the social anthropologists and sociologists for structural-functional concepts; and the symbolic interactionists for the concepts of interacting personalities within the family (Rowe 1966; Hill and Hansen 1960; Hill and Rodgers 1964).

Drawing on Erikson's eight stages of man, Havighurst (1956) formalized the term "developmental tasks" for each stage of family life from birth to old age. Duvall (1957) was the first person to put together all these various concepts into a textbook entitled *Family Development*. Later Rodgers (1962) incorporated role theory with Duvall's developmental tasks and devised what he termed family life-cycle categories.

The developmental framework utilizes the family life-cycle concept as a descriptive tool to compare the structure and functions of the family in different stages of development. The major focus is on the process of change in internal family development with the dimension of time as central. According to the developmental approach, the family is viewed as a semiclosed system engaged in interactive behavior within the system. Since the family is not entirely independent of the larger social system or wholly dependent, it is considered a semiclosed system. As a small-group system that is interrelated, changes do not occur in one part of the system without a series of resultant changes in other parts.

Concepts Central to Developmental Approaches

A number of concepts that comprise the developmental approach are defined below as a basis for the succeeding discussion.

Development is a process that occurs in an organism or a living structure over an extension of time (Harris 1957:10). The successful development of the family is contingent upon the satisfactory accomplishments of biological requirements, cultural imperatives, and personal aspirations and values (Hill 1951).

Family is a unit of interacting personalities (Burgess 1926:3–9). The number of interacting processes can be separately named and described, but they are difficult to dissociate (Duvall and Hill 1948).

Position is location of family members in the family structure; for example, husband-father, wife-mother, son-brother, daughter-sister (Hill and Rodgers 1964).

Role is the dynamic part of a position defined by the norm of the culture (Hill and Rodgers 1964).

Positional career is the longitudinal history of an individual family position composed of ever-changing clusters of roles.

Role sequence is the longitudinal character of a single role (Rodgers 1962:44).

Norm is a behavioral expectation commonly shared by family members.

Family career is the longitudinal expression of the role complex of the family structure as it develops (Rodgers 1962:44).

Developmental tasks comprise a set of norms (role expectations) arising at a particular point in the career of a position in a social system, which if incorporated by the occupant of the position as a role or part of a role cluster, brings about integration and temporary equilibrium in the system (Rodgers 1962:55). The importance of this concept for family development is the realization that developmental tasks are faced by family members who are simultaneously at different stages of their own development.

Family developmental tasks are growth responsibilities that arise at a certain stage in the life of a family, successful achievement of which leads to satisfaction and success with later tasks, while failure leads to unhappiness in the family (Duvall 1962:45). The nine developmental tasks of the family throughout the life span as proposed by Duvall (1958) are:

1. An independent home,
2. Satisfactory ways of getting and spending money,

3. Mutually acceptable patterns in the division of labor,
4. Continuity of mutually satisfying sex relationships,
5. Open system of intellectual and emotional communication,
6. Workable relationships with relatives,
7. Ways of interacting with associate and community organizations,
8. Competency in bearing and rearing children,
9. A workable philosophy of life.

Family life cycle represents critical transitional phases of the life span of a family. The demarcation of one phase to the next is determined by the amount of transition that is required in the family by a particular event. Numerous attempts have been made to delineate the phases of the family life cycle, but in general there have been two broad divisions: expansion and contraction. Table 4.1 traces the trends in definitions of the stages of the family life cycle since 1931.

The developmental framework encompasses the internal dynamic processes in the life cycle of the nuclear family of procreation and is viewed as a semiclosed system that is neither entirely dependent on nor

TABLE 4.1 *Delineations of Stages in the Family Life Cycle*

Family cycle stage	Sorokin, Zimmerman, and Gilpin (1931)	National Conference on Family Life (1948)	Duvall (1957, p. 8)	Feldman* (1961, p. 6)	Rodgers (1962, pp. 64–65)
I	Starting married couple	Couple without children	Couple without children	Early marriage (childless)	Childless couple
II	Couple with one or more children	Oldest child less than 30 months	Oldest child less than 30 months	Oldest child an infant	All children less than 36 months
III		Oldest child from 2½ to 5	Oldest child from 2½ to 6	Oldest child at preschool age	Preschool family with (a) oldest 3–6 and youngest under 3; (b) all children 3–6
IV		Oldest child from 5 to 12	Oldest child from 6 to 13	All children school age	School-age family with (a) infants, (b) preschoolers, (c) all children 6–13
V		Oldest child from 13 to 19	Oldest child from 13 to 20	Oldest child a teenager, all others in school	Teenage family with (a) infants, (b) preschoolers, (c) school-agers, (d) all children 13–20

TABLE 4.1 *(Continued)*

Family cycle stage	Sorokin, Zimmerman, and Gilpin (1931)	National Conference on Family Life (1948)	Duvall (1957, p. 8)	Feldman* (1961, p. 6)	Rodgers (1962, pp. 64–65)
VI	(III) One or more self-supporting children	When first child leaves till last is gone	When first child leaves till last is gone	One or more children at home and one or more out of the home	Young adult family with (a) infants, (b) preschoolers, (c) schoolagers, (d) teenagers, (e) all children over 20
VII	(IV) Couple getting old with all children out	Later years	Empty nest to retirement	All children out of home	Launching family with (a) infants, (b) preschoolers, (c) schoolagers, (d) teenagers, (e) youngest child over 20
VIII				Elderly couple	When all children have been launched until retirement
IX			Retirement to death of one or both spouses		Retirement until death of one spouse
X					Death of first spouse to death of the survivor

*Feldman enumerates Stages IX, X, and XI to classify childless families to correspond to families with children in the stages of childbearing, childrearing, empty nest, and old age (Stages II to VIII).

Source: George P. Rowe, "The Developmental Conceptual Framework to the Study of the Family," in Ivan F. Nye and Felix M. Bernardo, eds., *Emerging Conceptual Frameworks in Family Analysis* (New York: Macmillan Company, 1966).

independent of any other social system. Thus, the family as a unit is influenced by the social system and in turn influences the social milieu. Each family member occupies a position in the family that is characterized by roles related reciprocally to at least one role of the other family member positions. Likewise, each position contains roles that are reciprocally related to roles outside of the family. For example, the father of the family reciprocally relates to the mother and the children as part of the family system, while he also holds an occupational role that is reciprocally related to some other role(s) in his job situation.

The family as an interacting and interrelated group of people is such that if there is change in one position or role, there is also change in the roles or positions of the others. For instance, if the mother decides to abandon "mothering behaviors," someone else will need to assume the "mothering" functions. To a great extent, the family members' roles and positions are defined by the wider culture in which the family system functions. This fact is most recently evident in the way that the women's liberation movement has changed the roles of many women who have sought "out of the home" job satisfaction. Finally, the family system changes through time due to changes in age composition, in membership, and in the functions and status of the family.

Stages or categories of the family life cycle have been delineated on the basis of the transitions and adjustments required by particular situations. Thus the newly formed family, usually a new couple, must evolve styles of interaction and sharing they did not use before. The birth of a child drastically alters the interactions, the family configuration, and even the in-family work to be done. Each stage of the family cycle is related to the previous one and has implications for future stages as the family matures.

Family development is inherently related to the degree that each position and the family role complex complete their individual and family developmental tasks respectively. Biological requirements, cultural imperatives, and personal values and aspirations are the bases of these tasks and role expectations. Achievement of family developmental tasks at each family life-cycle stage is interrelated with the accomplishment of each individual developmental task simultaneously by each family position. This sequential linking of the family role complexes over the cycle of the family life is identified as the family developmental career.

Basic Assumptions about Developmental Approaches

Several basic assumptions must be accepted if the developmental framework is to be used either as a basis for studying families or for working with them.

1. The family is defined as a nuclear unit—that is, a family of procreation from the wedding until the death of the surviving spouse. In most cases the family has children, either by birth or adoption.

2. Families and individual members change and develop in different ways although they both are stimulated by forces from within and from the social milieu (Hill and Hansen 1960).

3. Specific individual and family developmental tasks must be completed before other tasks currently being attempted can be mastered. These tasks are goal directed rather than specific jobs to be done. Also, they are "not looked upon as an all-or-none proposition. Seldom in the family cycle are all its members 'caught up' with themselves and with what is required of them" (Kenkel 1960).

4. The emphasis is on individual members and how each functions within the family. Although the family system as a whole is important, it

is dependent on the behavior of its members (Hill and Hansen 1960).

5. Each individual family and each individual family member is unique in its complex of age-role expectations in reciprocity (Hill and Rodgers 1964). Families vary widely as to the number of positions, age composition, and occupational status of the breadwinner(s). For example, a husband and wife in their late thirties who were married when young would be married long enough to be in the teenage stage of the life cycle (if they had children) while a man of forty who marries a young woman may not reach the teenage stage until he is in his sixties.

6. Human conduct is best seen as the function of the preceding as well as the current social milieu (Hill and Hansen 1960).

ADVANTAGES AND DISADVANTAGES OF DEVELOPMENTAL APPROACHES

The developmental framework has been used widely by researchers and practitioners to study child-rearing practices (Duvall 1946), and it has been found effective in the study of *internal* family change. However, due to the time-consuming and costly aspects of investigating a particular group of families through their entire life history, the use of the developmental framework has been limited. Several alternatives have been suggested. Stott (1951; 1954) doubts the possibility of inferring process and change by looking concurrently at the average differences between families in different stages of the life cycle. Cross-sectional studies of different ages are rightly criticized for their inability to take account of the different history each age group has lived through. The method of retrospective history taking raises the question of validity, since memory is a questionable basis for establishing consistent data. Recent attempts to capture family change by means of segmented longitudinal panels has been encouraging (Rowe 1966). These have studied controlled groups of families at similar stages over relatively short periods of time. In addition, Rowe suggests:

Families could be pinpointed and sampled prior to entering critical transition stages in the family life cycle and then restudied at six-month intervals or so up to two or more years until they are established in a new developmental stage. This could be particularly profitable in the early stages when the time period from one stage to the next is usually not so long [Rowe 1966].

Conclusion: The developmental framework is an attempt to transcend the boundaries of several approaches through incorporation of a number of compatible concepts from other frameworks into one unique schema (Hill and Hansen 1960). As the framework is presently developing, an individual set of basic assumptions is emerging but these, as will be shown, are very similar to those of the interactional school. Whether the framework is variant or an extension of interactional analysis will be determined only as more research is completed.

Community health nurses have found the developmental approach very practical for making family assessments. However, the framework is in actuality culturally bound to the white middle-class American culture, since the research has centered on the traditional American family of father, mother, and children. Additionally, it is strongly child centered with much less emphasis on the individuality of the adults in the family or on the childless family. The fact that fluctuations in birth rates and improvements in survival rates have had an effect on the composition and thus the life-cycle stages of the family should be kept in mind by nurses when utilizing the developmental framework while working with families. For example, the increasing postponement of marriage on the part of women; more single-parent families as a result of premarital childbearing, separations, and divorce; reduction in the size of the average family resulting in shorter periods of family building; more reliable contraceptive measures and a much longer "empty nest" period during which husbands and wives associate together without their children (Glick 1977:5–12) make the developmental framework "out of sync" for most families that the community health nurse encounters.

INTERACTIONAL APPROACH

The interactional framework is a way of viewing the personal relationships of the members of a family. The family is conceived as a unity of interacting personalities (Burgess 1926). It is a living, growing, and changing thing that is made up of persons. Burgess uses the term *unity* rather than *unit* to distinguish between the view of the family as a collection of interacting people and a unity of interacting persons (1926:3–7). From an interactional point of view, the family need not be based on legal or contractual agreements.

Within the family each member occupies a position or positions to which a number of roles are assigned. The individual holds a role(s) that has norms or role expectations because he or she has the attitudes and behaviors to fit the role. The responses of the others in the family serve to reinforce or to challenge the individual's role behaviors. In other words, people define their role expectations in a given situation in terms of reference groups and by their conception of what the role demands. A basic interactional assumption is that all family behaviors stem from individual members' playing their various roles. The group can thus be studied directly by looking at their overt interactions (Hill and Hansen 1960).

The unique and differentiating characteristics of the interactional approach is that it is based on the actions of the family resulting from communication processes (Schvaneveldt 1966). The primary focus is not on external or environmental factors but on the action of the family members. However, the interactional approach can be used for analyzing the relationship between the larger system and the family system. The processes of interaction within the family can be related to the social structure of society, but little attempt is made to view the overall institutional or cross-cultural relationship of family structure and function.

History of the Framework.   Many writers have contributed to the development of the interactional framework. Stryker (1964) indicates the origin of the framework goes back to Hegel with contributions by Baldwin, Dewey, Cooley, and Mead coming later. Waller, Burgess, Hill, and Foote as well as others have conducted research using the interactional framework. Additionally, Simmel, Weber, and Sorokin wrote much concerning the concept of *interaction in society* (Schvaneveldt 1966), but Ernest W. Burgess first suggested that the family be perceived within an interactional framework.

Through time the framework has had a variety of names. Some writers have referred to the framework as *action theory,* while those from psychology have called it *role theory.* To some it is known as the *Chicago Tradition,* since early contributors to the framework came from the University of Chicago. Kirkpatrick (1955) referred to it as the *role-process approach.* The term *interactional* has been used in the most recent writings.

Concepts Defined

Concepts of the interactional family framework are often those of other frameworks, but are predominantly credited to the social psychology school of interactionalism. Since not all of the interactional concepts are applicable to family study, the ones presented here are only those directly useful for studying and working with families.

Interaction is a whole set of processes that takes place between people. Interaction means the social behaviors involved when two or more persons communicate with each other and hence modify each other's behaviors.

Communication is the exchange of meaningful symbols so that "concensus is developed, sustained, or broken" (Shibutani 1961:141).

Symbolic environment is the learned meanings and values that are placed on a situation and are defined before the individual acts. Only humans are assumed to have a symbolic environment.

Act is the purposive behavior that begins as an impulse requiring some adjustment to appropriate objects in the external world (Stryker 1959:113).

Status is a position one maintains in groups because of the way in which one is evaluated as a person. *Personal status* is usually associated with primary groups and rests upon intimate interaction processes. *Social status* refers to relative rank in the community and is determined by norms that govern one's social class (Schvaneveldt 1966).

Position is the pattern of consistent behavior of a single actor. The pattern of consistent behavior refers to clusters of values and interpretations that guide an individual's behavior in a specific social setting.

Role taking is the selective perception of the actions of others and imagining how one looks from another person's viewpoint (Mead 1934).

Role playing is organization of conduct in accordance with group norms by responding to the responses of another in a consistent pattern of behavior.

Role making is the creation and modification of existing roles (Turner 1962).

Group is any number of human beings in reciprocal communication. It is not a mere collection of individuals but a *set* in which relationships are involved.

Primary group is one that has a high degree of intimacy and extensive communication.

Family, according to Burgess (1926), is a unity of interacting personalities. It does not consist or exist on a purely legal or contractual basis, and it lives as long as the interaction is taking place.

Task behavior is the interaction directed toward the completion of group or individual tasks.

Adaptation is the process of adjusting to new or different conditions— that is, the process of acquiring fitness to live in a given environment.

These concepts combine to form a distinctive framework for both the study of and work with families. The term interaction is the key to the approach as it means human beings *interpret and define* each other's actions instead of merely *reacting* to them. For example, the husband does not merely react to the wife's actions but also to the meaning that both persons attach to the actions.

The major distinguishing aspect of this approach is that of communication. Family members act and react by use of symbols. The symbols are interpreted by family members and interaction takes place by determining the meaning of one another's actions. As Burgess (1953) states, interaction does not describe a state, it describes a process.

Role taking is a central process in the interactional approach since a role cannot exist without some counterrole toward which it is oriented.

Interaction is always a dynamic process of continually testing the concept one has of the role of the other. As Turner points out:

> In the socialization of the children in a family and also continuously in family interaction, the product of the testing process is stabilization or the modification of one's own role [Turner 1962:2].

At least three distinctive characteristics of the interactional framework warrant attention here. First, social life in the family is assumed to be in process rather than in equilibrium. This emphasis distinguishes the approach from structural-functional theory. It also differs from psychoanalytical theory in that it does not focus on or give thought to unconscious processes in family interaction. Second, the objects of social interaction, whether human or not, are interpreted by the individual family member and are given special meaning. These social objects are never viewed as just physical stimuli but as the definition of the situation. This aspect of the framework distinguishes it from behavioral theories. Third, the interactional approach focuses on naturalistic phenomena. Thus the methodology for study and practice is observational rather than experimental. Participant observation, interviews, and questionnaires as techniques for study allow the practitioner to get *inside* the family group. This approach is particularly useful to nurses not only because it provides a practical way to study the family, but also because it allows for the isolation of and working through of difficulties of the family members with the nurse as they are happening.

BASIC ASSUMPTIONS

Basic assumptions of the interactional approach have developed over time. Mead (1934) presented the first ones that were refined, organized, and elaborated by Rose (1962), Stryker (1959;1964), and Hill and Hansen (1960). The following assumptions are reflective of this evolution and are based on the work of all those cited so far:

1. People live in a symbolic as well as a physical environment and are stimulated in social situations to act by symbols as well as by physical stimuli (Rose 1962). Symbols are learned through interactions with other people, particularly family members.

2. People communicate with others in order to evoke meanings and values that they intend to evoke (Rose 1962).

3. The process of socialization in which people learn cultural and subcultural values and roles is learned by interacting with other persons.

4. A person is likely to play many roles in the course of a day (Rose 1962).

5. Thinking is a symbolic process based on the values of the thinker. In thinking, people manipulate their own roles by imagining themselves in possible situations.

6. Interactions must be viewed in the context of how the participants define one another (Hess and Handel 1959). Any particular action is formed in the light of the situation in which it occurs.

7. The human being is an actor as well as a reactor. People do not simply respond to stimuli outside of themselves (Stryker 1959).

8. The study of humanity is antireductionistic—that is, human psycho-social behavior cannot be derived from the study of nonhuman forms (Stryker 1959:112).

9. People are the basic autonomous units in the social setting and from their interactions the individual and society are derived (Stryker 1959).

10. The human infant is neither social nor antisocial, but rather asocial, since the child possesses potentialities for social development (Stryker 1959).

11. Social organizations enter into action only to the extent to which they shape social situations.

12. The interaction relationship is more than the sum of the personalities that make it. Additionally, the dynamics of the two units, individual and group, are not interchangeable; the processes appropriate to one unit cannot be imposed upon the other.

ADEQUACIES AND INADEQUACIES OF THE INTERACTIONAL FRAMEWORK

The interactional framework has been widely used for many reasons. Mainly it allows for study of the internal workings of groups such as the family. The greatest merit of the interactional approach is that it furnishes an inclusive framework into which may be fitted all kinds of contributions having to do with the human nature aspects of the family.

The contributions of the framework are manifold; particularly important is the ability to use the framework to teach and understand family dynamics, and its use as a research model for all phases of family functioning. Probably the most important aspect of the framework is that it removes the study of family from the realm of speculation to the field of analysis (Schvaneveldt 1966).

Criticisms of the interactional approach have primarily centered on its failure to recognize the biogenic and psychogenic influences on family behavior. The interactionist would probably believe these influences only set *limits* and that they are not the determining factors in regard to specific family interactions.

Another criticism deals with the concepts and assumptions of the framework. Because of the diversified origin of the framework, there is little agreement among researchers and practitioners concerning the concepts and assumptions. Thus, the original formulations of Mead (1934) and specifically Burgess's work in the family (1926) have been widely used but extended very little.

SUMMARY

This chapter has presented three frameworks for studying family as a basis for working with the family. No attempt has been made to select one framework over another, but rather the concepts, basic assumptions, and advantages and disadvantages of each have been presented. Although only three frameworks have been discussed here, the reader is reminded that other frameworks exist that may offer other approaches and sets of concepts that may deal as effectively, or more so, than the frameworks offered here. The following three chapters attempt to demonstrate how these frameworks can be used to study and work with family dynamics.

REFERENCES

ACKERMAN, NATHAN W. *The Psychodynamics of Family Life*. New York: Basic Books, 1958.

BATES, FREDERICK L. "Position, Role and Status: A Reformulation of Concepts." *Social Forces* 34 (May 1956): 313–21.

BELL, NORMAN, and VOGEL, EZRA F. *A Modern Introduction to the Family*. New York: Free Press of Glencoe, 1968.

BRODERICK, CARLFRED. "Beyond the Five Conceptual Frameworks: A Decade of Development in Family Theory." *Journal of Marriage and the Family* 24 (February 1971): 139–56.

BROWN, INA CORINNE. *Understanding Other Cultures*. Englewood Cliffs, N.J.: Prentice-Hall, 1963.

BURGESS, ERNEST W. *Engagement and Marriage*. Philadelphia: J.B. Lippincott Co., 1953.

———. "The Family as a Unit of Interacting Personalities." *The Family* 7 (March 1926): 3–9.

DUVALL, EVELYN. *Family Development*, 2nd ed. Philadelphia: J.B. Lippincott Co., 1962 (1st ed., 1957).

———. "Implications for Education Through the Family Life Cycle." *Marriage and Family Living* 20 (November 1958): 334–42.

———, and HILL, REUBEN. *Dynamics of Family Interaction*. National Conference on Family Life, Chicago 1948.

———. "Conceptions of Parenthood." *American Journal of Sociology* 52 (March 1946): 193–203.

ESCHLEMAN, J. ROSS. *The Family: An Introduction*. Boston: Allyn and Bacon, 1974.

GLICK, PAUL C. *American Families*. New York: John Wiley & Sons, 1957.

GOODE, WILLIAM J. *World Revolution and Family Patterns*. New York: Free Press of Glencoe, 1963.

HARRIS, DALE B., ed. *The Concept of Development*. Minneapolis: University of Minnesota Press, 1957.

HAVIGHURST, ROBERT J. "Research on the Development Task Concept." *School Review* 64 (May 1956): 215–23.

HAYS, WILLIAM. "Theorists and Theoretical Frameworks Identified by Family Sociologists." *Journal of Marriage and the Family* (February 1977):50–65.

HESS, ROBERT D., and HANDELL, GERALD. *Family Worlds: A Psychological Approach to Family Life*. Chicago: University of Chicago Press, 1959.

HILL, REUBEN, and RODGERS, ROY H. "The Developmental Approach." In H.T. Christensen, ed., *Handbook of Marriage and Family*. Chicago: Rand McNally & Co., 1964.

———, and HANSEN, DONALD A. "The Identification of Conceptual Frameworks Utilized in Family Study." *Marriage and Family Living* 22 (November 1960):279–311.

———. "Interdisciplinary Workshop on Marriage and Family Research." *Marriage and Family Living* 13 (February 1951):13–28.

KARGMAN, MARIE W. "The Clinical Use of Social System Theory in Marriage Counseling." *Marriage and Family Living* 19 (August 1957):263–69.

KENKEL, WILLIAM F. *The Family in Perspective*. New York: Appleton-Century-Croft, 1960.

KIRKPATRICK, CLIFFORD. *The Family: As Process and Institution*. New York: Ronald Press, 1955.

LEVY, MARION J. "Some Questions About Parson's Treatment of the Incest Problem." *British Journal of Sociology* 6 (September 1955):277–85.

———. *The Family Revolution in Modern China*. Cambridge, Mass: Harvard University Press, 1949.

McINTYRE, JENNIE. "The Structure-Functional Approach to Family Study." In F.I. Nye and F.M. Bernardo, eds., *Emerging Conceptual Frameworks in Family Analysis*. New York: Macmillan Co., 1966, pp. 53–73.

MALINOWSKI, BRONISLAW. *The Dynamics of Cultural Change:* New Haven: Yale University Press, 1945

MEAD, GEORGE HERBERT. *Mind, Self and Society*. Chicago: University of Chicago Press, 1934.

MURDOCK, GEORGE P. *Social Structure*. New York: Macmillan Co., 1949, pp. 1–11.

PARSONS, TALCOTT. "An Outline of the Social System." In Talcott Parsons et al., eds., *Theories of Society*. New York: Free Press of Glencoe, 1961.

———, and BALES, ROBERT F. *Family Socialization and Interaction Process*. Glencoe, Ill.: Free Press, 1955.

———, and SHILS, EDWARD A. "Values, Motives, and Systems of Action." In Talcott Parsons and Edward Shils (eds.), *Toward a General Theory of Action*. Cambridge, Mass.: Harvard University Press, 1954.

RADCLIFFE-BROWN, A.R. *Structure and Function in a Primitive Society*. Glencoe, Ill.: Free Press, 1952.

REISS, IRA L. "The Universality of the Family: A Conceptual Analysis." *Journal of Marriage and the Family* 27 (November 1965):443–53.

RODGERS, ROY H. *Improvement in the Construction and Analysis of Family Life Cycle Categories*. Kalamazoo: Western Michigan University, 1962.

ROSE, ARNOLD M. *Human Behaviors and Social Processes: An Interactional Approach*. Boston: Houghton Mifflin Co., 1962.

ROWE, GEORGE P. "The Developmental Conceptual Framework to the Study of the Family." In F.I. Nye and F.M. Bernardo, eds., *Emerging Conceptual Frameworks in Family Analysis*. New York: Macmillan Co., 1966.

SATIR, VIRGINIA. *People-Making*. Palo Alto, Calif.: Science and Behavior Books, 1972.

SCHVANEVELDT, JAY D. "The Interactional Framework in the study of the Family." In F.I. Nye and F.M. Bernardo, eds., *Emerging Conceptual Frameworks in Family Analysis*. New York: Macmillan Co., 1966.

SHIBUTANI, TOMATSU. *Society and Personality: An Interactionist Approach to Social Psychology*. Englewood Cliffs, N.J.: Prentice-Hall, 1961.

SHUSKY, ERNEST L. *Manual for Kinship Analysis,* 2nd ed. New York: Holt, Rinehart and Winston, 1972, pp. 7–17.

SPIRO, MELFORD E. "Is the Family Universal? The Israeli Case." In Norman W. Bell and Ezra F. Vogel, eds., *A Modern Introduction to the Family*. New York: Free Press of Glencoe, 1960.

STOTT, LELAND H. "The Longitudinal Approach to the Study of Family Life." *Journal of Home Economics* 46 (February 1954):79–82.

———. "The Problem of Evaluating Family Success." *Marriage and Family Living* 13 (November 1951):149–53.

STRYKER, SHELTON. "The Interactional and Situational Approaches." In Harold T. Christensens, ed., *Handbook of Marriages and the Family*. Chicago: Rand McNally & Co., 1964.

———. "Symbolic Interaction as an Approach to Family Research." *Marriage and Family Living* 21 (May 1959):111–19.

TURNER, RALPH H. "Role-Taking: Process Versus Conformity." In Arnold M. Rose, *Human Behavior and Social Processes*. Boston: Houghton Mifflin Co., 1962.

WINCH, ROBERT F. *The Modern Family*. New York: Holt, Rinehart and Winston, 1963.

ZELDITCH, M., JR., "Role Differentiation in the Nuclear Family: A Comparative Study." In T. Parsons and R.F. Bales, eds., *A Family Socialization and Interaction Process*. Glencoe, Ill.: Free Press, 1955.

5. Crisis Intervention

Carol Edgerton Mitchell

INTRODUCTION

Crisis Intervention is a problem-solving approach to the major pitfalls of life. "Crisis," as a doom-invoking headline banner or solemnly entoned television pronouncement, has become the representative word for our era. Even as all our words are both individually and culturally unique, "crisis" has a multitude of meanings. Within this chapter, it is defined as a person's sense of acute disruption suffered in response to an overwhelming threat or loss. It is an internal state of stress triggered by perception of an external event, or stressor. This personal disruption, which may be as acute and as overwhelming as a spiking fever, triggers an intense motivation for problem resolution—that is, the acuity of the emotional pain ensures its own brevity—and reorganization at some level will be achieved within four to six weeks. This motivation is what gives the crisis state such an unusual opportunity for positive or negative progression.

Health interruptions often precipitate crisis, and more often than not, a nurse is there. The "unreasonable" patient in the emergency room or the depressed and abruptly withdrawn patient in coronary care; the pregnant adolescent or the "child-abusing" father are examples where a nursing assessment may identify the internal turmoil of crisis. Each case may be a candidate for crisis-generated growth.

HISTORY

Crisis Intervention is a young health therapy. Measured against the traditional models of health care, it is an energetic adolescent with a philosophy of wellness and a unique cognitive approach. Although mentioned almost as often in the health institutions as in the media, the seemingly straightforward crisis therapy model is frequently misinterpreted, for unlike traditional psychotherapy, crisis therapy maintains its problem-solving focus on the client's present and on various cause-effect interactions shaping that present. This approach is an outgrowth of the pioneer community psychiatry work: Erich Lindemann's (1944) study of grief, Edwin Schneidman and Norman Farberow's (1961) and Farberow's (1964) studies of suicide, and Gerald Caplan's (1964) operationalization of primary prevention programs for mental health.

We can identify the contributions of many basic sciences to the final blend of crisis intervention. The approach begins with an assumption that people can be aided through normal stress and normal disruption. Epidemiology is involved since understanding the patterns of both incidence and process is important. Moreover, host, agent, and environmental interactions figure in prevention, as well as diagnosis and treatment, of crisis. Familiarity with physiology of the central and autonomic nervous systems provides recognition of the physical-emotional interrelationships of stress, while knowledge of psychology contributes insight into the dynamics of behavior. Theories of sociology and anthropology extend all these considerations, thereby adding a concern for both social group tendencies and their cultural variations. Crisis theory is holistic. Intervention strives to promote clients' integration as well as their most harmonious adaptation to their environment.

FOUNDATIONS

A few considerations are basic for studying crisis intervention. The universal process of growth and adaptation is reflected, for each of us, in our *maturational drive* (see chapter 17). Responding to myriad intervening variables, this life-long maturational force constantly alters our crisis potential. Ralph Audy has conceptualized four levels of functioning for this adaptive process: ample, threshold, compensated, and with predisposition (Audy 1971). Ample signifies an abundance of health and energy available for optimal adaptation, while *threshold* indicates apparently normal function but depleted reserves. A level of *compensated* function is able to appear healthy only at the cost of considerable energy, while *with predisposition* indicates a potential problem is already present. Each of these levels, in turn, represents a dynamic composite of our physiological, immunological, and psychological-sociological areas of function, and each suggests a varying resiliency against the "slings and arrows" that can precipitate crisis. Only rarely would one have ample health in all areas of function, and the profile of strengths and vulnerabilities in the various areas can be both diagnostic and prognostic.

COPING STRATEGIES

Our interaction patterns, or ways of coping, both reflect and determine our level of effective functioning. Certainly, genetic tendencies are important here. Personality differences are evident in the newborn nursery, and consistent life-long reaction styles individualize us all. Genetic tendencies are the nucleus of personality, and learned coping strategies are its outer evidence. Fragments of the events we have experienced are encoded in our memory banks, and four-star ratings go to those strategies that have succeeded over time. Experience generalizes—that is, the success-failure tone of one event tends to influence our perception of similar events. For example, if a student's first experience with pediatrics proves dismal and the second—approached with misgiving—is disastrous, then a third, fourth, or fifth contact may never occur. Child care may thus be categorized as miserable and avoided like the plague. A whole routine of maneuvers may be designed for avoidance, and even for denial of the avoidance, so that stereotyped expectations and preferred routes of action follow. These develop into our repertoire of coping strategies, or our "tried and true" response patterns that are readily available for use. These strategies include our customary moods (elation, depression, enthusiasm, and the like) as well as our preferred actions (such as attack, avoidance, placation), and these strategies group into our patterns for social interaction.

SUPPORT SYSTEMS

Support systems act as buffers from—or instigators of—environmental threats and influence all levels of adaptive function. These systems can be seen as the connecting web between us and our surroundings, and each can be consistently or occasionally experienced in a positive or negative way. Formal support systems include such institutions as family, health, education, and judicial systems. The informal support systems include community, peer group, social clubs as well as the whole, individually designed "comfort system" we each develop. As the help-hurt experiences with these systems accumulate, our perception of their value will generalize and influence tendencies to link with other support systems. Still another coping strategy is an inclination to link with either the positive or negative potential each system represents. Some people consistently "use the system," some are used by it, and some avoid the known system at all cost. Whether individually health promoting or otherwise, each stance has emerged from experience and is self-perceived as appropriate.

THE PERSON IN CRISIS

Each of us, armed with coping strategies, armored by support systems and motivated toward maturational adaptation, negotiates the environmental hazards that clutter our pathway. Crisis interrupts that progression. The crisis experience is triggered by perception of a provocative "precipitating event" and is compounded by inadequacy in satisfying some essential need. Perception, essential need, and precipitating event merit delineation.

PERCEPTION

Variability in perception shapes the crisis potential of every situation. This interpretation arises from our inherent tendencies, memories of past events, present adaptation level, and confident feelings of worth, or personal value, or self-esteem. The intrusiveness of the event is also interpreted as is one's adequacy-inadequacy in its face. All of these factors in turn determine whether an environmental stressor will be coded as inconsequential or as posing a challenge, a threat, or a loss to one's self-esteem. Maintenance of self-esteem is the core concern. If the present stressful event links with memories of previous failure, it will seem to reinforce feelings of inadequacy and thus threaten this esteem.

An example of this individualized perception can be found in the reaction of two neighborhood women to their partners' illnesses. One woman, long accustomed to comfortable dependency, may see the event as a threat—or loss—to her vulnerable sense of personal worth. She may throw up her hands in despair and cry out, "I can't cope!" Her neighbor, who is equally dependent, but strengthened by a rich repertoire of effective coping strategies, may become energized by her spouse's disruptive illness and face it as a challenge.

This individualized interpretation of the event determines the coping strategies that will be chosen to manage it (figure 5.1). If the event—no matter how grave it appears to the bystander—is processed as inconsequential to the participant's own well-being, the response will be casual, selective inattention. The same event may trigger an anxious alarm-reaction in another person sensitized by earlier difficulty who sees it as a threat to self-esteem. A third person may see the event as a stimulating challenge since successful past experiences have heightened this person's

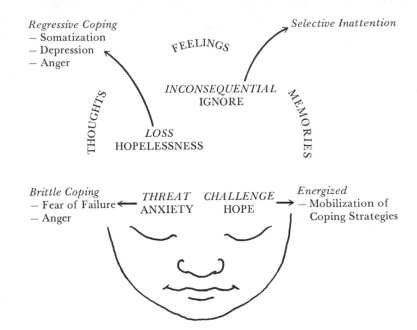

Regressive Coping
— Somatization
— Depression
— Anger

FEELINGS

Selective Inattention

INCONSEQUENTIAL
IGNORE

THOUGHTS

MEMORIES

LOSS
HOPELESSNESS

Brittle Coping
— Fear of Failure
— Anger

THREAT   CHALLENGE
ANXIETY   HOPE

Energized
— Mobilization of
   Coping Strategies

5.1   *Perception of the Event*

hope and esteem, thereby permitting the belief that events bring opportunity rather than disaster. The "identical situation" devastates the fourth individual. Experience has taught this person that life changes mean failure and that challenges will deteriorate into loss. With no confidence in adaptive coping strategies, this person regresses through stress-related illness into a state of passive dependency.

For each of us, the perception of an event is translated into physiological and psycho-social response. As all things interact, this response will magnify or modify the original event and lead to further interpretations and reactions. Individually interpreted events of grave consequence to the concerned individual, are ambiguous at best to the outside observer. Thus, a person may be devastated by the thought of submitting to a "simple" physical exam. Many fears and apprehensions can be linked to an apparently innocent event: whispered allusions overheard as a child, a grandmother's lingering death, detailed description of a celebrity's surgery, fragments that will be individually shaped into a stereotyped response to the stressor.

ESSENTIAL NEEDS

The essential needs we seek to satisfy and defend provide strong motivation for our adaptive efforts. Physiological well-being, as valued and perceived by each person, seems an obvious "essential need." It becomes perplexing in the variety of definitions given to the concept. Innumerable health (or, to our eyes, nonhealth) beliefs are clustered here. A client with no concern for fat-soluble vitamins may swear by the "healthfulness" of a jigger of mineral oil after each meal, while another insists that all the windows be closed at dusk to prevent arthritis. A threat to any one need may precipitate crisis for one individual while it is casually overlooked by another. Only as the need's significance is understood, can the dynamics of the disorganization precipitated by the threat be appreciated.

Self-esteem sums all the essential psycho-social needs. Sexual role mastery is included—as a need to function successfully in culturally appropriate areas of sexuality—as is the satisfaction of dependency-independency needs—the dynamic balance of an assertiveness-passivity equation. Self-esteem itself is the belief in one's intrinsic value. This belief generates energy to defend and augment that value even while it acknowledges the possibility of its own vulnerability. Low self-esteem, on the other hand, invites defeat; its hopelessness depletes energy and discourages linkage with potential support systems. The experience of positive crisis resolution is instrumental in combating poor self-esteem.

PRECIPITATING EVENTS

The stressors that nudge us into personal disorganization are known as precipitating events. There are three categories: maturational, situational, and combined. Through each category of event, our essential needs may be compromised into crisis. *Maturational precipitants* are those self-esteem–threatening events that are inherent in developmental cycles, for our maturational status determines both our own and others' demands for our social performance. Further compounding the maturational complexity are the variations in support systems it brings. The positive support of a preteen's nurturing family may develop into an independency-thwarting negative support system for the adolescent. Then, as the young adult leaves home, the associated loss of customary feedback may threaten self-value, or conversely, it may open avenues for greater self-esteem through a perceived independence appropriate for the new stage of maturational development. When the interacting demands are not well synchronized with maturing abilities, they may seem to threaten esteem and may precipitate crisis.

Situational precipitants are lightning bolts to emotional and physical well-being. These are the specific events that complicate our maturational progression. Weddings, separations, missed appointments, graduations, accidents, and relocations are situational events—whether major or minor—that carry both plain and symbolic messages related to self-esteem.

Combined precipitants are those that occur when a situational event magnifies a particular stage of maturational disruption. The combination may seem devastating, for each aspect seems to amplify the threatening characteristics of the other. A maturational upheaval lowers the level of health function and establishes a susceptibility for further disruption, even as a situational event leaves less energy available for dealing with maturational demands.

PROCESS OF CRISIS CYCLE

We bring our selves to the potential crisis event: our perception of and reaction to the stressor, our experiences, our fears and hopes, our level of functioning, and our strategies for coping. If we are successful in the encounter, our self-esteem is enhanced, our adaptive level moves higher, and there is no crisis. If success eludes us, confidence soon evaporates, anxiety mounts, and rational problem solving deteriorates (figure 5.2). This discomfort of disorganization can produce innovative or regressive coping efforts. They may lead to success and thus bring relief and well-being. If the predicament should worsen, we may choose to redefine success and settle for a more easily negotiated goal.

The fox, frustrated by the inaccessibility of the luscious grapes in Aesop's tale, consoles himself by redefining them as sour. If, however, there are no feasible alternatives, yet "success" remains blocked, disorganization proceeds into defeat. At every stage of the process, the interaction of person and event continues. This dynamically alters the situation as well as its memory and will be instrumental in shaping the situations still to come.

EXPERIENCE OF CRISIS

Somatic complaints are an early indicator of experienced maladaptation. Perhaps the reason is because our culture is more tolerant of physical than of emotional pain, or perhaps because emotional distress wreaks physiological havoc, or perhaps because our organ systems possess symbolic meaning (a broken heart, sick to the stomach, pain in the neck, and such). Somatic complaints may also be the nonspecific physiologic response to some stressor. Whichever the case, perceived loss or threat to a basic need quickly translates into insomnia, gastric disturbance, and musculoskeletal complaints. As the physical discomfort intrudes, less energy is available for general adaptation. Environmental demands, once merely difficult, may appear overwhelming as one's health level

122

5.2   *Process of Crisis Cycle*

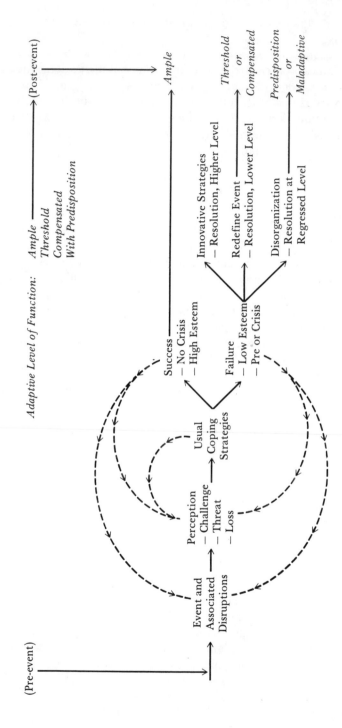

(Pre-event) ──────────────────→ (Post-event)

Adaptive Level of Function:

Ample
Threshold
Compensated
With Predisposition

Event and
Associated
Disruptions

Perception
— Challenge
— Threat
— Loss

Usual
Coping
Strategies

Success
— No Crisis
— High Esteem

Failure
— Low Esteem
— Pre or Crisis

Innovative Strategies
— Resolution, Higher Level

Redefine Event
— Resolution, Lower Level

Disorganization
— Resolution at
   Regressed Level

Ample

*Threshold
or
Compensated*

*Predisposition
or
Maladaptive*

deteriorates from ample to compensated. The distress of personal inadequacy escalates and generalizes. Not only is the original problem area acutely sensitive, but adjacent spheres of function become contaminated by hopelessness and helplessness. The constricted focus of acute anxiety is aggravated by the regressive drawing-in of loss. Anxiety is typically associated with tunnel vision, and perception of loss encourages personal retrenchment. The two reactions tend to amplify each other so that a person experiencing these emotions loses sight of both the intricate causes and their subtle solutions. A simplistic either-or, love-hate, or win-lose view becomes the norm and restricts flexibility; it hinders every phase of problem solving. The experience of crisis is of pain and futility.

OBSERVATION OF CRISIS

As the acuity of crisis escalates, personality disorganization is readily observable. While somatic symptoms may not reach critical levels, significantly, the deterioration in adaptive efforts such as decision making becomes unmistakable. Behavior seems brittle; its rigidity stems from anxiety and a fear of failure that inhibits flexibility. As tension mounts, the desperate person flips from one coping strategy to another. Yet, before one strategy is evaluated, it may be abruptly abandoned and another approach tried. As a response to perceived inadequacy, suggestibility may be high, as well as an apparently ambivalent dependency. Objectively, the crisis state appears as a puzzling personal deterioration.

RESPONSE OF OTHERS

Crisis tends to mobilize concern from others. As the victim's distress becomes more evident, energetic interventions from those in the near environment will increase. They move into the vacuum created by the victim's withdrawal; they offer suggestions, take charge, and wonder at the disorganization. There may be considerable conflict regarding these interventions on the part of both rescuer and rescued, for the status shifts they may suggest imply major changes in power and powerlessness. Surprising solutions can emerge from the disruptions of old norms, for such realignment may encourage innovation and creativity.

Although both formal and informal support systems will generally rally to help the crisis victim, a contrary situation may arise. Crisis can be contagious. Its anxiety and hopelessness can infect a susceptible surrounding group. If the group leader has decompensated and if no alternate leaders are forthcoming, the victim's disruption may spread into a generalized group deterioration. Families with inflexible interaction styles may suffer this "domino" principle should their heads become unable to direct operations. We see the same dynamics in business and professional groups with rigidly centralized leadership.

INTERVENTIONS

Crisis therapy is designed for the acute problems of living. Its interventions are tailored for their resolution. As the situations are acute, so the focus is upon immediacy. Since the problems are those of normal living, the therapy is growth oriented, with emphasis on avoiding dependency and further regression. Since the problems resound within the client's lifestyle, their solutions derive from joint efforts of both client and crisis counselor. A rational problem-solving approach, suggested in all of the above, is the basic intervention style. This cognitive approach emphasizes the natural cause-effect relationship between event and difficulty. It is instrumental in clearing the client's confusion, encouraging hope, and generating a sense of competence.

LEVELS OF INTERVENTION

There are four general categories or levels of crisis intervention. Each successive level incorporates actions taken in the preceding level, thereby adding more complex strategies to the basic interventions.

Environmental manipulation, the most basic type of intervention, includes actions taken generally to enhance the distressed person's physical environment: Meals may be provided, transportation arranged, utilities reconnected. Such impersonal, but pragmatic, assistance encourages a supportive environment that permits the client's physical and emotional reorganization.

General support, the second category of intervention, attends the physical setting with a personally focused, supportive interest. Neighborly concern and helpfulness illustrate this level of intervention.

The generic approach, the third level of intervention, adds an understanding of the usual, or generic, crisis process to the supportiveness of the earlier interventions. At this level, the intervener is familiar with the usual stages of adaptation associated with the major disruptions of life. Grieving for a loss—whether surgical removal of a body part, death of a spouse, or separation due to geographic mobility—is understood as patterned behavior. Manifestations of anxiety and depression are similarly understood. Use of such categorical strategies can promote the client's progression through the cycle of disruption. Generic understanding can also anticipate problem areas and promote primary prevention.

Individually focused intervention, the fourth level, expands the earlier levels with a knowledge of psychodynamics and counseling skills. Primarily used by specially prepared mental health workers, this level incorporates all of the earlier techniques, modifies them to the particular emotional need of each client, and then works with the client and his or her support systems for movement toward crisis resolution.

PROCESS OF INTERVENTION

Just as sequential patterns of behavior exist during the crisis cycle, sequential intervention strategies exist for the third and fourth levels of intervention. The precise ordering of the sequence may vary with the practitioner, place, and client, but the intervention process is organized along an orderly cause-effect relationship that reflects its problem-solving style.

FOUNDATIONAL PHASE

A supportive foundation precedes and facilitates crisis work. Accessibility, both physical and emotional, is essential for this foundation. The best of services are valueless if they are unknown or impossible to reach. Crises erupt with urgency. Availability of resources can change solitary regression into mutual problem solving.

An approach-avoidance conflict seems inherent in the crisis state. While disorganization encourages victims to seek assistance, hopelessness discourages their doing so. A client may also believe his or her perceived worthlessness and inadequacy merit no concern from others. Emotional accessibility can cut through this hopelessness. Rapid rapport facilitates client-practitioner connectedness and also allows renewal of the hope and energy needed for active problem solving. "Tough love," a humanistic concern framed in reality and crisis theory, describes this rapport. It characterizes the first stage of intervention, acknowledges the client's pain, sets a contract for mutual problem solving, and quickly moves client and practitioner to the second stage.

PRELIMINARY PHASE

The practitioner now prepares for the main intervention efforts by assessing the client's level of disruption. Is there a danger to self, to others? What are the indicators of this danger? What are the client's responses to queries in this area? How specific—and realistic—are any threats? Does the mood, or emotional tone, support the client's statements? The practitioner elicits the client's clearly expressed commitment to abstain from destructive actions during the contracted course of intervention. Occasionally there is neither the emotional stability for this kind of agreement nor enough physical organization for self-care. In these instances, a more protective environment must be established. Relatives and friends may be able to provide this support; if not, the health agency will have access to other facilities.

Conversely, the initial assessment may establish that the client is actually in a noncrisis state. Even though coming to a crisis care unit, clients may be cool, calm, casual, and collected. Previous use of the unit may have taught some, especially helpless, passive clients or manipulative ones, that the health agency is a primary coping strategy. When noncrisis seems to be the case, the practitioner can use the joint acknowledgment of the situation for problem solving (rather than the ostensible crisis event) to build more appropriate coping mechanisms or make a referral to more suitable services. Somatic complaints are also considered in the assessment. When their severity or grouping suggests a medical problem, consultation is justified. Too often, real physiological deterioration is discounted as hypochondria.

Ordinarily, initial assessment will determine either a pre- or a crisis condition, suggest a level of distress amenable to the mutuality of crisis intervention's approach, and establish an informal "contract" for the problem area to be worked upon. This contract, or "plan of attack," verbally sketches out expectations of time, effort, and activity. It suggests that resolution of the present distress is forthcoming and conveys the practitioner's belief that the crisis condition, too, will prove to be a cause-effect life problem, a predicament appropriate for a team approach to problem solving.

PROBLEM RECOGNITION PHASE

The global disorganization of the client's perception needs begins to focus. As anxiety and helplessness have generalized from the symbolic event that inspired them, this precipitating event has been masked from painful awareness. The emotional picture presented by crisis has fuzzy outlines, overlapping images, and distorted perception.

Events are seen as wholly "terrible," "overwhelming," "hopeless." Their component parts are undifferentiated; each portion of the event is tarred by the same gloomy brush and through this blurring, are kept inaccessible to individualized attention. The practitioner's task is to clarify, to guide discovery of cause and effect, and to facilitate development of alternate approaches to the central problem.

"Here and now" data pertaining to the central problem area are gathered, their significance considered, and their patterns discussed. Support systems are identified; their potential as well as actual strengths are considered, and their weaknesses weighed. Coping strategies that have been effective for the client are examined. What seems to be interfering with their effectiveness at this time? When was this first evident? What was going on at that moment? What other coping strategies are possible? In what way could they be put into operation?

As the client shares his or her perception of the difficulty, painful memories may surface. Since adaptive energy is now at threshold level, at best, these emotional stressors need to be contained at this time. Their reconsideration when sense of esteem is stronger will be appropriate. Emotional catharsis at this early stage of intervention only fosters additional disorganization.

The mutual detective work now underway is designed to strengthen the client's cognitive control, to foster self-esteem, and to encourage responsibility. Consistent focus on the predicament enables the client to perceive relationships within the event. Actions and reactions resume their meaningfulness, and diffuse anxiety is narrowed to regain its specific—and appropriate—target. As this process occurs, the client's adaptive energy is also focused upon detection of the actual precipitating event.

Identifying the precipitator is now the first order of business. Most presenting complaints are ambiguous and thus conceal the extremely sensitive focal point. Yet, the significance this perceived threat, or loss, holds for the client is the clue to the whole predicament. This precipitator represents an area of self-esteem threatened more by the client's perceived ineffectiveness than by the external event. As the client comprehends the precipitator and the part his or her coping strategies played in its disruption, there is an opportunity for developing more effective ways of coping with this essential life need. Since clients tend to mask any awareness of the precipitating event and its significance, identification is difficult.

A few clues for its detection are helpful. Seven areas yield information for its discovery: themes, mood, forgotten areas, point of decompensation, anniversaries, essential needs compromised, and recency.

Themes in the client's conversation point to significance. For example, a woman, sixty years old, demoralized by her husband's second hospitalization with emphysema, sprinkled her speech with melancholy mention of children moving away from home, death of an aged parent, deterioration of her own health. Her theme of loss and abandonment offered her insight into the deeper significance her husband's hospitalization held for her.

Mood also measures significance. In the example above, the mood in the conversation shifted within a narrow range. Depression was its general tone and became deeper at mention of the hospitalization. General despondence supports a hypothesis of loss; both demoralization and depression suggest a quality of hopelessness.

Content that is "forgotten" or avoided indicates a *forgotten area* of particular sensitivity. A client may forget the events that reinforce a sense of pain or, conversely, may forget areas of hope when immersed in hopelessness. Both provide clues for detection of the precipitator, as well as an illustration of the client's coping strategy. In the example above, the woman was surprised that she had forgotten her husband's hospitalization was expected to be very brief.

The *point of decompensation* is that at which the situation is diagnostic. Whatever aggravated the predicament to such a degree probably held considerable symbolic meaning. The final instigators, or precipitators—a crying child, a worrisome letter, or a derogatory comment—often appear minor in themselves. Through personal symbolism, however, such precipitators may initiate disruption.

Anniversaries tend to dredge up old unresolved pain. We all carry myriad "times of significance"—birthdays, seasons of the year, days of the week—each of which is an individualized time of meaningfulness laden with resurfacing memories and emotions. As with other symbolic events, these times of significance offer a new opportunity to problem solve each time they cycle around. They will continue to resurface until their central issues of self-esteem have somehow been resolved.

Compromised needs are specific areas of threat or loss. Detecting their challenge to one of the essential needs provides another clue for establishing the precipitating event. Need compromise is at the heart of crisis; the specific event serving as vehicle for this threat may be the precipitator.

Recency is the last indicator. A crisis state is acute and limited to about six weeks' duration. Therefore, the event initiating it must be recent. The more strongly integrated an individual's self-concept, the more resistant to disorganization. Such a person may manage to defend against anxiety and hopelessness for two to three weeks of stressful coping before finding either a solution or decompensation. The reverse is equally true: a person at threshold function may become disorganized immediately after perception of the symbolic event. In either case, the precipitating event is of recent origin, and its discovery should emerge from the client's recounting events from the last two to three weeks.

These seven clues help unravel the disorganization of the crisis state. Clients' "ahh haa!" sense of discovery as this identification is shared should confirm the delineation while it also more firmly engages their problem-solving efforts. The detective work erases the magical or global sense of powerlessness clients feel in the face of encompassing stress. The rational, team approach permits a matter-of-fact exploration of what is now seen as "only" a problem of living.

PROBLEM-SOLVING PHASE

After the crisis situation has been delineated and the significance of the precipitating event considered, alternative approaches are sought for problem solution. Mutuality is important here. Interventions that are unilaterally designed by the crisis practitioner seldom maintain "proper fit" in the client's eyes and have small likelihood of compliance. Yet, the client's own interaction skills have already proved ineffective in this area of living; skills and confidence are limited. Through combined resources, the client's reality and ability are extended and guided by the practitioner's experiential and theoretical perspectives. Appropriate emotional components of the crisis—anger, disappointment, suspicion, hope, love, aggravation—may now be considered. Actual and potential support systems are discussed; their positive and negative values weighed; and their entry and linkage examined. Present coping strategies are also explored and alternate possibilities are considered. Any of these strategies that seem perplexing to the client may be tested through role playing prior to wider use. They are all evaluated by client and practitioner after their testing.

At any point throughout this process, the client may be joined by the significant others of his or her support system. Their participation gives greater reality to the problem-solving sessions, extends the scope of possible solutions, and enlists the energy of all persons most interested in positive solutions.

At every point of the process, self-responsibility is emphasized. The temporary regression so common in many traditional mental health therapies is minimized. The consistent message is one of growth, capability, and normalcy. From the first communication, the practitioner takes care to clearly convey the confident expectation that the client will soon resume normal responsibilities of living and that through focused efforts, the crisis resolution will lead to adaptive growth.

ANTICIPATORY PLANNING PHASE

Although anticipatory planning is the final stage of the crisis intervention process, elements of its intention occur from the first. Anticipatory planning, or guidance, attempts to ease the transition between theory and actuality—that is, between working on crisis resolution with a crisis practitioner and living that resolution independently. With the practitioner's support, the client analyzes or rehearses future coping situations. Summation of the progress already made—the decisions and alternatives— enhances these efforts. Again, the client recognizes behavior patterns he or she has been using in response to sensitive events and the domino effect these behaviors have had upon others. Considered, too, are the likely response new strategies will elicit, as well as assessment techniques for this determination.

This shared summary precedes closure of intervention. Since the acute disorganization period is generally limited to between four to six weeks, this closure should occur by the end of that time span. As motivation for the hard work of change accompanies the stress of disorganization, so will lessened motivation accompany the establishment of a new equilibrium. Crisis work is done while motivation gives leverage, and its conclusion should coincide with the client's recognition of a newly attained stability.

Establishing a checkpoint for postevaluation ends the intervention cycle. Evaluation is essential to every intervention; it helps keep the crisis practitioner tuned into practicalities and it encourages clients' participation in services designed for their welfare. Postintervention evaluation can be accomplished through telephone calls, postcards, formalized self-assessment forms, or visits. The best approach is determined by client and practitioner; whichever is chosen, the evaluation centers upon further pitfalls encountered and progression made.

SUMMARY

Crisis intervention is a problem-solving approach for the acute disruptions of living. As a person perceives inadequacy in dealing with compromised needs, the disorganization of crisis may follow. Focused intervention can facilitate successful resolution of this upset. Success, in turn, enhances self-esteem and permits a higher level of function. The interventions are precise, fast-moving, and carefully focused. Their sequence matches the cycle of crisis, capitalizes upon its openness to change, and uses its disequilibrium for growth.

The philosophy and style of crisis intervention make it especially useful for practicing nurses. It is effective in the community in the clinic, in intensive care units, and in convalescence. The well, the worried well, and unwell respond to its approach. In each area and with each group of individuals, nurses have won recognition and personal entry. They function where crises happen and they are accepted as accessible health professionals. Theirs is a unique challenge to facilitate their clients' use of the positive element present in all crisis situations. And challenge, of course, is energizing.

REFERENCES

AUDY, J. RALPH. "Measurement and Diagnosis of Health." In P. Shepard and D. McKinley, eds., *Environ/Mental Essays on the Planet as a Home.* Boston: Houghton Mifflin, 1971.

AGUILERA, DONNA. "Sociocultural Factors: Barriers to Therapeutic Intervention." *Journal of Psychiatric Nursing* 8, no. 5 (September–October 1970).

CAPLAN, GERALD. *Principles of Preventative Psychiatry.* New York: Basic Books, 1964.

————, and KILLILEA, MARIE, eds. *Support Systems and Mutual Help: Multidisciplinary Explorations.* New York: Grune & Stratton, 1976.

ERIKSON, ERIK. "Growth and Crisis of the Healthy Personality." *Psychological Issues.* New York: International University Press, 1959.

FARBEROW, NORMAN L. "Crisis, Disaster, and Suicide: Theory and Therapy." In Edwin Schneidman, ed., *Essays in Self-Destruction.* New York: Science House, 1967.

HARRIS, M.R., KALIS B.H., and FRIEMAN, E.H. "Precipitating Stress: An Approach to Brief Therapy." *American Journal of Psychotherapy* 18, no. 3 (July 1963).

HOLMES, THOMAS H., MASUDA, MINORUS. "Psychosomatic Syndrome (Life Crisis-Illness)." *Psychology Today* 5, no. 11 (April 1972).

JACOBSON, G.G. "Crisis Intervention from the Viewpoint of the Mental Health Professional." *Pastoral Psychology* 21, no. 203 (April 1970).

LAZARUS, RICHARD. *Psychological Stress and the Coping Process.* New York: McGraw-Hill Book Co., 1968.

LINDEMANN, ERICH. "Symptomatology and Management of Acute Grief." *American Journal of Psychiatry* (1944–45).

KLEIN, DONALD C. *Community Dynamics and Mental Health.* New York: John Wiley & Sons, 1968.

McGEE, RICHARD K. *Crisis Intervention in the Community.* Baltimore, Md.: University Park Press, 1974.

McLEAN, LENORE. "Action and Reaction in Suicide Crisis." *Nursing Forum* 7, no. 1 (1969).

MITCHELL, CAROL EDGERTON. "Hazard Identification in Crisis Intervention." *American Journal of Nursing* (in press).

MORLEY, WILBUR. "Theory of Crisis Intervention." *Pastoral Psychology* 21, no. 203 (April 1970).

———. and BROWN, VIVIAN B. "The Crisis Intervention Group: A Natural Mating or a Marriage of Convenience?" *Psychotherapy: Theory, Research Practice* 6, no. 1 (Winter 1969).

PARAD, HOWARD J., ed. *Crisis Intervention: Selected Readings.* New York: Family Service Association of America, 1965.

RAHE, RICHARD. "Life Stress and Illness." In Robert O. Pasnau, ed., *Consultation-Liaison Psychiatry.* New York: Grune & Stratton, 1975.

ROSENBAUM, C. PETER, and BEEBEE, JOHN E., III. *Psychiatric Treatment: Crisis/Clinic/Consultation.* New York: McGraw-Hill Book Co., 1975.

SCHNEIDMAN, EDWIN, and FARBEROW, NORMAN L. *The Cry for Help.* New York: McGraw-Hill Book Co., 1961.

"Systems Approach to Mental Health Care in a HMO Model." Project Brief, R. L. Harrington, Principal Investigator. Kaiser-Permanente Medical Center, Santa Clara, Calif., August 31, 1974.

STRAKER, MANUEL. "The Psychiatric Emergency." In Robert O. Pasnau, ed., *Consultation-Liaison Psychiatry.* New York: Grune & Stratton, 1975.

STRICKLER, MARTIN, and ALLGEYES, JEAN. "The Concept of Loss in Crisis Intervention." *Mental Hygiene* 54, no. 2 (April 1970).

6. Working with Families in Community Health

Ruth Ann Terry
Teresa A. Bello

INTRODUCTION

A major theme in community health nursing has been the traditional emphasis on family-centered care in which the focus is on the family as a total unit and each individual is viewed within the family system. In such a service the family, not any one individual, is the nursing client. Many nurses will agree that this concept is very difficult to work with, especially when so much attention is paid to individualism and the importance of planning services to fit the particular needs of each client. Focusing on one individual client in establishing a relationship and planning for care is far easier than working with numerous family members as part of a group. Coming up with a global workable definition of family is even more difficult. A family is, after all, an idea or an abstraction with many different forms of reality.

Even if there is an agency philosophy concerning total family care, it is most often not the total family with whom most community health nurses actually interact on the job. Most contacts are made between nurses and the women of the family, usually the mothers. Health is often considered "women's work," and just as most nurses are women, so are most family caretakers women. Usually most fathers are at work during exactly the same hours we nurses are making home visits or holding clinics. And even if the male figure is unemployed, he often still considers health matters the woman's responsibility. Contemporary, narrow assumptions about responsibilities within the nuclear family often lead us to break a new mother's links with her extended family network of her own mother or her mother-in-law. And with school-age children away for many hours in the middle of the day, the nurse's family visit may thus include contact with only one adult—a new mother—and one child—her new infant.

Services to families cannot be delivered without taking into account the communities in which they are embedded. Nurses are plagued daily with the need to bring more continuous, positive linkage between the two. We have always thought of ourselves as advocates, but setting priorities to deal with all the social factors that confront our clients daily has become increasingly difficult. Which of the following should the nurse take into consideration?

Most nurses feel the increasing cost of the deductible many clients must pay for Medicare creates a hardship. Should we gather appropriate documentation and write our congressman voicing our concern?

Many nurses who work in inner cities realize that poor communities tend to be near the most polluted areas. These are often bounded by railroad tracks and freeways that increase the air and noise pollution and are away from parks and recreational areas. The children thus play in lots with broken glass and other hazards. Should nurses go to the planning department or to the city council to voice our concerns when we find a new housing project is being planned that will simply move the poor from an old to a new polluted environment?

Nurses working with families of school-age children are concerned with each child's school performance. Should we contact each school to determine the child's progress or lack of progress?

Many nurses are concerned about the kinds of recreational activities available for children after school or during the summer. Should we become involved in these programs by doing volunteer health teaching or rap sessions to a group of children in an effort to promote sound health practices?

Under what kinds of circumstances are the employed members of the family working? Are there potentially dangerous chemicals, toxic pollutants, or mechanical dangers? Should we be concerned about workers' health?

Nurses tend to have a great deal of knowledge about the major institutions within the community. What impact does the church have on the diabetic patient who fasts on Sunday? Should the nurse talk to the minister?

Many clients realize they should keep scheduled medical appointments, but often don't because of the long wait or the staff is unpleasant to them. Should the nurse intervene at the administrative level?

Unemployment constitutes a major health problem especially for black males, 20–40 years of age, and often results in family disorganization. Should the nurse take a role in trying to combat this problem?

Usually no one family or no one nurse is affected by all of these factors. However, these questions or problems may arise when we begin to make a complete family assessment. Families do not exist in isolation but are affected by the community in which they reside. Each family is interrelated within itself, its members, its community, and society in general, and each impacts upon the other.

Moving toward a more consistent practice of family care is important, if only because of the major influence doing so has on individual and community health beliefs and practices. In light of the review of theories of families and of crisis intervention presented in chapters 4 and 5, we would like to present some applications to real world clients in this chapter. No single theory can deal with the infinite complexities of actual family experience. However, looking at examples of families who often present more difficulties for nurses than do other types may be helpful.

A *well family* is defined as a family that is coping adequately, whether free from disease or in a stable state of chronic illness. The important consideration is that the family sees itself as in control. The nurse's efforts are directed toward supporting and strengthening the family's own maintenance program and only becoming involved if the family asks for assistance or experiences a crisis.

An *ethnic family of color* is defined as a family who belongs to a group that shares a common heritage, history, and culture, has experienced similar frustrations and anxieties, and aspires to similar goals and aims. Ethnic groups of color are defined as Asians, blacks, American Indians, and Latinos (Branch 1976). The family groups are not only influenced by their individual ethnic group but by the responses of the larger society as well. The nurse's role in working with ethnic families of color is to assist the family to maintain their optimum level of functioning by incorporating and reinforcing their cultural practices, traits, and strengths.

A *family in crisis* is defined as a family whose steady functioning state is disrupted due to an unexpected event or a series of bombardments that overwhelm their coping mechanisms. The family's normal relief-producing behaviors that have worked in the past are no longer effective. The nurse's role with the family is to assist them in regaining and then maintaining their optimum level of functioning.

THE WELL FAMILY

The primary goal when working with families is to assist the family and its members to function at their optimum level. The focus is at the level of health prevention and health maintenance. The ideal family responds in a flexible, adaptive manner to the needs of its members as well as their personal and external environment. We do not mean to imply that these families are without problems, but that they move through the developmental stages demonstrating prescribed, expected behaviors with mutual respect and emotional support. In one sense the family can be seen as a self-correcting system. The following case study is an example of how nurses can work with well families.

Case Study I

Mr. and Mrs. Green have been married sixteen years. They have three children, all girls fourteen, twelve, and three years of age. Mrs. Green called the health department requesting information about child health services. The community health nurse made a visit to discuss the program and inform the family of the services provided through the agency.

During the visit, the nurse assessed the family to be a close-knit unit that often shares many activities together. Mrs. Green stated that her adolescent girls are involved in numerous school activities and that only occasionally is there some discord within the family. Mrs. Green planned to place her youngest child in day care for a half day, two days a week, so she can pursue community volunteer work outside the home. Mr. Green is employed as a construction worker, and although he often comes home exhausted, Mrs. Green stated with pride that he always has time to spend with her and the children.

During follow-up visits the community health nurse took the opportunity to provide anticipatory guidance and reinforce the strengths noted in the family. So often we tend to focus on weaknesses or problems within the family without giving support and acknowledgment to the positive aspects we see in families. In assessing individual roles and interactions, the nurse discussed growth and development patterns for the preschooler and adolescent. Mrs. Green proved knowledgeable in this area; therefore, the nurse reinforced the information her client had.

The mother indicated her awareness that her preschooler is rapidly moving toward independence and becoming aware of her outside world. The nurse acknowledged that this process is normal and further discussed what to expect. The nurse noted the youngest daughter is always referred to as "Baby" and suggested lightly that this name might be inappropriate for such an active and growing child. Mrs. Green seemed to be looking forward to placing the child in day care. She and her husband have been telling the child what to expect (although they're not sure whether she understands). The nurse stated that preschool can be healthy; the child will begin to interact with children her own age and to learn new psycho-social skills in a positive way. For an example, the nurse went on to explain that as the child becomes involved with others around her, she may not be able to have everything when she wants it and will begin to develop the satisfaction of sharing. At this stage a child's conscience comes into play. The nurse also stated that the child may experience some separation anxiety, but children are very adaptable. The child initially may cry, hold onto her mother, and not want anyone to touch her, but this anxiety usually passes. The nurse reinforced that such anxiety is usually time limited. An important aspect is that the family pay attention to the child, by encouraging her to relate what went on at school, who her new friends are, and so on.

The nurse went on to discuss the adolescent period. Her focus continued to be on maintenance of the family functioning, by clarifying specific roles that each member plays, how these roles affect the family as a unit, how the family influences its environment, and how the environment affects the family. For many families this period is one of great stress—a push and tug between the adolescent and parents. The adolescent wants to be independent and at the same time dependent, which often results in conflict. Although the twelve-year-old is taller and heavier than the fourteen-year-old, the family seemed careful not to single her out or make fun. The nurse emphasized that adolescence is a period of increased physical growth. Mrs. Green stated in passing that she hates to see her girls grow up. This reaction is normal for parents in beginning to prepare themselves for their children heading for a life separate from theirs. The nurse also mentioned that in this period peer groups are a major part of adolescent lives. The tasks of the adolescent are expanding and developing during this period, and importantly, a balance should be maintained between mutual limit setting between the adolescent and parents and allowing a certain amount of independence. The nurse also discussed sex education for all the children and the family's feelings about dating.

The varied roles of both parents were discussed: The mother assumes the major responsibilities for running the house, meals, and shopping, and she provides emotional support to the family. The father is the source of economic support, and he helps out in the home. Mrs. Green feels that the girls' help in managing the home is important, and each girl has a list of household chores she must do before pursuing social activities. Mrs. Green also stated she and her husband sit down every week and go over bills and expenses they have. Although she is home every day, the children understand that child rearing is shared between the parents, which cuts down on "games" children may play on either parent. Both Mr. and Mrs. Green have hobbies and are active in their church and community. This family reflects the members' ability to share mutual support for each other while at the same time demonstrating their involvement with others outside the family system.

DISCUSSION

The nurse's approach with the Green family was based on knowledge of the normal developmental tasks each family member must complete and on how these individual developmental tasks affect the family's developmental growth. The nurse's interventions were aimed at helping the family understand and cope with changes and in so doing helped the total family master the family's passage from one stage to another. Two specific examples make this point clear. The nurse's helping Mrs. Green anticipate and understand the younger child's reaction to child care also helped the family work through the developmental task of "last child into school." The nurse's helping the mother understand the adolescents' behavior assisted the family through the "letting go" stage—when the children begin to move from childhood to adulthood. These examples are excellent ways of demonstrating how nurses can use the developmental approach with a family. The nurse's comment about referring to the youngest child as "Baby" implies an interactional framework that suggests what you call someone has a good deal to do with how that person will act.

We should note that in no way do we consider the nuclear family to be the only example of a well family. Single-parent families, both female-and male-headed households, are increasing in number, and many of these families are able to fulfill and nurture its members. Over and over we see constellations of family groupings that some people consider "nontraditional"—adults, same or opposite sex, unmarried couples, communal groups—who are able to more than adequately provide the love, socialization, mutual commitment, and personal satisfaction that fall within the traditional functions of "family." More importantly, the "nontraditional" family not only meets the needs of its members, but participates and helps to solidify the very institution on which our society is based.

In viewing the Green family, we find it able to meet the basic needs of its members and to respond appropriately to the environment. The primary role of the nurse was on developmental health education. The nurse was able to assess the individual roles of the members and the response of the members to each other in order to provide information to maximize the family's response to each other and to support the family's involvement with its environment.

ETHNIC FAMILIES OF COLOR

Much of the literature in nursing has focused on "normal," nuclear families. Only in recent years have cultural and ethnic characteristics been seen as a necessary and important component of family assessment. However, much of the information utilized focuses on problems or pathological conditions of these families.

Ethnic families of color tend to behave in a manner that fosters the survival of the family as a group in contrast to white middle-class values that foster individuality in its members. One of the responsibilities of the family is to socialize its members not only to their particular culture, but to the larger society as well. Culture is transmitted from one member to another and helps to build a common bond within the group. For a long time, we presumed that immigrants would shed their old ways, adopt the local culture, and thus become assimilated or "Americanized." However, we have recently become aware of the importance of acknowledging the value of various cultural heritages. Since maintaining traditions and continuity with one's forebears is less difficult when there are many others around who share the same patterns, ethnic groups of color in our society often have many similarities and differences that do not follow the pattern of their ancestors alone. These characteristics may be traced to the fusion of three components of cultural elements: those inherited from ethnic forebears, those derived from mainstream America, and those related cultural traits of other patterns absorbed from other ethnic groups in the same area (Cole 1970).

Due to factors such as racism and exclusion of cultural and ethnic components from the nursing curricula, many nurses lack adequate information or have never been encouraged to include cultural and ethnic considerations into family assessments and nursing interventions. Additionally, only recently has some of the literature begun to focus on assessing families in view of their strengths instead of flaws (Hill 1972; Otto 1973). Otto presents an initial framework for assessing family strengths in which he identifies thirteen criteria. While the framework has broad application for viewing families, his criteria must be modified to take into account the ethnic and cultural characteristics and structural variations represented in our diverse population. For example, one criterion concerns the parents' ability to grow with their children and recognize the children's openness and honesty as an important part of the parents' self-realization (Otto 1973). That particular behavior would usually be seen negatively in a Spanish-speaking family where the children are taught that individual needs are secondary to the family group as a whole (Murillo 1971). The children are not encouraged to be open and frank as such behavior may be viewed as a sign of disrespect. Children are to do as they are told and individuality is not frequently encouraged.

A student of one of the authors was resistant to working with a Spanish-surnamed family. When asked why, the student responded that in her past experience with one Spanish-surnamed family, the mother told the student that her attitude was arrogant and demeaning and that she did not understand the family's way of taking care of its own. The mother was upset that the student attempted to place "her values" on the family. The student realized that the mother's assessment of her behavior was correct since she tended to consider any family receiving public assistance as somehow deficient. The basis of her belief was the literature on welfare families she had read and comments from previous teachers. The student found herself in a bind: behaving in one way, yet being embarrassed because she received negative feedback about her beliefs. The student was fearful of having to face a similar situation. The instructor encouraged the student to discuss her feelings about the bind she felt herself in and then asked the student how she would like to handle the situation. On reflection, the student wanted to make the home visit because she felt she was now more aware of her attitudes and offensive behavior. The instructor assigned more current readings on ethnic families and discussed them in conference with the total clinical group. Although the student's attitudes could not be completely changed in one term, her self-awareness about attitudes and her sensitivity to all clients did increase.

The following case study illustrates the process one student nurse used to provide a growth-producing relationship with a Chinese family. The student attempted to incorporate cultural and ethnic considerations into the nursing care she provided.

Case Study II

The Fong family consists of seven members, including the paternal grandmother who was born and raised in China. The father, born in Hong Kong, was brought to this country at an early age, while the mother, born and raised in Hong Kong, came to this country as an adult. They have two sons, ages thirteen and eleven, and two daughters, ages seven and three years. The mother had been diagnosed with tuberculosis of the kidney several years ago and placed on Streptomycin, INH, and Myambutal. Her cultures were negative at the time the referral was received at the health department from the internist who felt Mrs. Fong needed assistance with the behavior problems of three-year-old Linda. She constantly had temper tantrums, and Mrs. Fong appeared fatigued much of the time. The family was assigned to the student nurse.

Prior to the initial visit, the student realized the necessity of seeking resources to increase her knowledge of Chinese culture and value systems. She read as much as she could find. Nursing literature was almost nil, so she went to other disciplines: history, anthropology, and sociology. The student also found a Chinese cultural center approximately twenty miles away that she visited and established contact with several of the workers there. She luckily was able to find a person who had recently visited China and who willingly showed her slides and shared the information he received while there.

On the initial visit, Mrs. Fong expressed a great deal of concern that three-year-old Linda was not acting "Chinese" and indicated her own fear of dying before her children became adults. In the course of subsequent conversations, the fact became clear that she equated tuberculosis with cancer. The student was able to reassure the client that tuberculosis was not cancer and by explaining what the negative cultures meant, that her chemotherapy had been effective. The student knew that although great advances have been made in terms of patients' rights to information, many people's illnesses are still not explained to them in a manner they can understand. Health professionals often forget to translate their own in-group jargon into language that clients can understand. We also have a tendency to make assumptions about how much knowledge our clients have without checking it out.

The mother showed many doubts about the helpfulness of health professionals and finally mentioned a specific bad experience she had had as an example of her skeptical outlook. She said her three oldest children had been born in a Chinese hospital, but Linda was delivered in an American hospital where her culture was not respected. According to Chinese tradition, for one month after the birth new mothers stay indoors and do not shower or bathe. Shavings of ginger are used in the water of a sponge bath to prevent illness. Custom also does not allow new mothers to wash their hair for one month postpartum except with this broth of water and ginger shavings. At the American hospital Mrs. Fong was forced to shower even though she protested and explained to the nurses there was a cultural reason for her not to comply. She mentioned specifically the traditional postpartum broth of ginseng, lotus seeds, Jerusalem artichokes, and small bits of reindeer horns cooked with chicken in water for eight hours, which was not permitted to be brought to her and obviously not available in the hospital. The reindeer horn broth is strictly a female food eaten for strength by women. Men are said not to need it because of their natural strength. After these foods, no sour foods such as orange juice, lemon juice, black vinegar, or carrots are to be eaten for one month. The thought occurred to the student nurse that the hospital in not allowing the mother to maintain her cultural practices was at the very least insensitive to a client's belief system and could be seen as infringing on the rights of the family. It also seemed possible that the mother's expressed concern that Linda, the youngest, was not acting "Chinese" may be a carryover from this bad experience.

Mrs. Fong expressed a great deal of anxiety over Linda's being a poor eater. As the student talked with the mother, she found that the child did not yet feed herself and usually disrupted meals by throwing food, demanding all the attention, and attempting to get down from her chair. The family used chopsticks at meals, and Linda appeared to be having difficulty manipulating them. Growth and development was explored in discussions emphasizing a three-year-old child's need to seek independence. The student also suggested that the child not be excluded from meals but a protective covering be placed on the floor to allow for freedom of the child and to relieve the mother's anxiety over having to clean up the mess.

The grandmother tended to take charge of Linda and spent a great deal of time with her. When Linda wasn't with her grandmother, she constantly whined and threw temper tantrums to gain attention. Mrs. Fong also expressed concern over Linda's hitting her siblings and peers. As they talked, the fact became apparent to the student that one of the difficulties was that the child only spoke Chinese and often became frustrated when she could not verbally communicate with her friends. Although the parents and the other Fong children could speak both Chinese and English, in deference to the grandmother only Chinese was used in family conversations. The student suggested that Linda's siblings teach her English so she too could be bilingual. The student also encouraged using a form of play therapy to deal with the hitting. The mother, being a good seamstress, made several dolls for Linda and emphasized that she could hit her dolls but not people. Mrs. Fong was also encouraged to be explicit about the demands she made concerning Linda's behavior and to be consistent in reinforcing these demands to minimize tantrum and "uproar" games. She was discouraged from using double-bind messages and encouraged to verbalize anger and/or disapproval. Perhaps increased touching and praise would decrease Linda's unsatisfactory methods of communication. Since the grandmother was an avid gardener the student suggested that a small area in the yard be given to Linda so she could garden with her grandmother.

The fact became apparent that the grandmother was revered both for her age and her role, next were the men of the family, and then the other women, all according to age. The mother looked toward her mother-in-law for guidance and felt they could mutually discuss the care of the family.

On one particular visit Mrs. Fong was upset that her own sister was acting strangely. As they talked, the student felt that the sister was demonstrating paranoid behavior. Mrs. Fong stated her sister had had two previous hospitalizations after her husband was killed in a robbery attempt. Mrs. Fong expressed shame over her sister's behavior. A great deal of time was spent discussing Mrs. Fong's feelings. The student emphasized that the sister was ill, as with a physical illness, and required medical care. The family preferred she see a Chinese therapist, and after several calls the student was able to locate a Chinese physician who would see her. Such referrals are often difficult to make since there are seldom proportionate numbers of ethnic professionals available.

The student continued to work with Mrs. Fong around Linda's tantrums and found they were beginning to decrease somewhat. The grandmother had tied Linda in bed in trying to "mummy" her. The student, without attacking the grandmother's actions, offered other alternatives for discipline. She also encouraged other family members' participation in providing Linda with activities she enjoyed. The mother, however, continued to feel Linda was not acting Chinese and had difficulties managing her. Her other children had not behaved in this manner; they had been obedient and respectful. Mrs. Fong expressed concern that her eleven-year-old son had also begun to question "Chinese ways." The parents and the grandmother were upset over the different values demonstrated by the children. The student tried to help the older members to be more tolerant of the assertive behavior of the children and accept their behavior rather than call it "less than Chinese." A great deal of discussion centered around the family being a part of two cultures and what aspects could be tolerated and assimilated between the two. The goal was to support the family in its efforts to retain strong cultural ties and yet encourage independent thinking by the children as signs of maturity and creativity.

On subsequent visits, Mrs. Fong expressed delight that Linda's tantrums were decreasing. Linda was playing outside more and took pride in "her garden." The student had given the mother a recipe for play dough, and Linda enjoyed playing "mommy" with the dough and her tea cups. The mother had allowed the child to use kitchen utensils and encouraged independent activity. Mrs. Fong perceived the child as being "more Chinese" at play. Her tantrums had decreased, she was quietly trying the role of adult female, and Mrs. Fong found Linda's dainty behavior more acceptable. On the last visit the mother told the student that Linda was to be baptized. The other children had received baptism before two months of age, and thus this decision was an important step in accepting Linda as "Chinese."

The student found the termination visit difficult, as do many nurses who have established a mutual relationship with a family. As the student was leaving, Mr. Fong met her outside and gave her an envelope inscribed in Chinese and containing money. The father explained that when someone helps the family, their custom is to pay. He was adamant she take it. Not wanting to offend Mr. Fong, the student accepted the envelope, but returned the money. She stated she was giving it to the family to buy Linda some gardening tools, but she would keep the envelope as remembrance of the family. The student wanted the family to feel that she was a helping person and her biggest reward came from their mutually working together.

In thinking back on the family, the student determined that each member had certain prescribed roles and expectations in the family. Linda's behavior caused concern because she was not behaving in a manner the family approved of. The eleven-year-old son threatened the customs and practice of the family by questioning "Chinese ways." The family was also going through a stressful period trying to maintain two cultures.

DISCUSSION

The nurse working with this family used concepts from the structural-functional framework as the approach to helping the family members deal with Linda, the three-year-old. Recognizing that this Chinese family lived by prescribed roles, the nurse was able to suggest ways that they could help Linda develop the acceptable behaviors. Knowledge of the family's ethnic and cultural beliefs and practices was essential for the nurse, as they dictated the prescribed and expected role behavior Linda was to play. Additionally the nurse pointed out how the predominant social structure affected the family structure in an attempt to help the family place Linda's and the older boy's behavior in perspective. In this way, the nurse's knowledge of structural-functional theory provided a framework for interventions that were appropriate to the family's framework of interaction, expectations, and norms.

When working with ethnic families of color, we nurses need to explore our own attitudes and beliefs about them and then seek added information. We should seek out resource persons who may provide valuable insight and knowledge about such families. As we saw with the student nurse, the resource people may include other nurses, community workers, a professional person from the same ethnic group, or workers in an organized community group of the particular community. Naturally, nurses' greatest source of information is the family itself, and we should not hesitate to check out our knowledge with the family to be sure they consider it applicable to them. Many families, although identified with an ethnic group, do not necessarily follow *all* of the practices that may be attributed to such a group. In other words, overgeneralization should be carefully avoided.

An illustration of this point may be seen in the following anecdote related by one of our colleagues. On a day for orienting new students, she and one student had just finished a postpartum visit to an unmarried black adolescent whose own family seem to be absorbing the new baby with ease when she became aware that the student had said absolutely nothing during or since the visit. As they were driving along to the next visit, the instructor tried to jolly the student into the easy conversational mood they had had before the visit, but without success. Finally the student blurted out, "But how could she do it?" The instructor tried a flippant tone and pretended to explain "the facts of life," but the student was clearly too upset to respond. It suddenly hit the instructor that the student nurse was also black and may, perhaps, have been appalled by what the family had revealed to her, a white nurse. The student finally said she was unable to understand how the client could even go through the pregnancy, let alone actually *keep* the baby. The instructor tried to suggest that they did not have any information about why the young mother had gotten pregnant, so the best they could do was try to figure from their own perspective. "Now I can imagine myself getting pregnant and entertaining the idea of keeping the baby. But I live alone. And my landlady won't permit children! I have a full-time job that I have to keep to support myself. I have all kinds of career goals that being a single mother would make much more difficult. So, I can't imagine myself keeping the baby," the instructor stated. "But this young woman has family support; her own mother is giving her all kinds of lessons in child rearing and making it possible for her to go back to school next semester and finish." The student nurse was still tense and unconvinced: "If I did that, my father would kill me! And I'm sure my mother would never mention my name again!" The instructor and student talked on about how hard it is to guess how parents *actually* would act when disaster strikes a child, and the student became somewhat more relaxed, if still dubious.

Later, the instructor talked the incident over with a sociologist friend who pointed out that the student's reaction as well as the young mother's decision were probably examples of attitudes learned in families with different value systems, which may or may not be related to social class or ethnic background. The student's background was clearly more similar to the instructor's than to the young unwed mother who was economically disadvantaged.

Possibly, there has been some relaxation of judgmental attitudes toward others' behavior in our society today. Certainly we are all more aware that many single mothers are keeping their babies. Because of differences within as well as between ethnic groups, as well as rapidly changing family patterns, we caution against making hasty overgeneralizations with regard to family practices and attitudes.

FAMILIES IN CRISIS

Crisis can be defined as a person's sense of acute disruption suffered in response to overperception of an external event, or stressor (see chapter 5). Many families may experience disruption because their usual coping resources fail to relieve either the internal stress or the external source of stress. An event can be considered a crisis when it is a threat to the family's life goals or basic integrity. It may also be a series of otherwise manageable stresses that finally exceed the adaptive abilities of the family, which thus finds it is no longer able to cope and in some instances may resort to maladaptive means of relieving the stress. In any case, the event is different from any that has previously occurred. As the family struggles to cope with this novel event by using past learned coping behaviors, they can find no relief from the disruption and discomfort of the event. Hence, the struggle continues and the family is considered to be in a crisis.

Many theorists agree that a crisis can promote maturity in dealing with life problems. Even in a person with tremendous ego strength, however, a crisis may bring about disorganization and maladaptation. The community health nurse must make a careful assessment before labeling any coping behavior as maladaptive. Some behaviors, while not generally acceptable on the surface, may represent the best possible solution to an overwhelming problem. The role of the community health nurse is to help individuals and families regain and strengthen their coping behaviors in an effort to increase their functioning.

An important consideration in working with persons in crisis is that their families constitute a major supportive resource. When a family in crisis constitutes the client, other relatives or close friends can provide support if there is a mutually caring relationship. Sometimes there is a time lag, however, before distant contacts can be mobilized to provide the needed support. In such instances, the community health nurse may be able to provide temporary support while she determines with the family members which relatives and friends could be involved in a helpful way to regain emotional equilibrium.

A crisis can occur at various stages of a family's life. It can result from an *unanticipated* life event that occurs when the balance between a person's internal ego adaptation or homeostatic state and the environment is disrupted (Burgess and Lazare 1976). These are usually events such as the illness or death of a loved one. A crisis can also be an expected event such as *developmental* crises that often occur during adolescence, pregnancy, or menopause. These are internal disturbances that are psychological and physiological in nature. External social events, such as difficulties with housing or finances, may also precipitate a crisis state. Case Study III illustrates an example of an unanticipated life event, and Case Study IV represents a family experiencing a developmental crisis, a birth, and a recent separation.

Case Study III

A referral for community nursing followup was received from the teacher of the district day care center: Four-year-old Tommy Zelda had recently been acting "nervous and withdrawn." The teacher was aware that Tommy's mother was under some kind of major family stress and requested a nursing evaluation of the causes of Tommy's behavior changes. The community health nurse experienced some difficulty in arranging a home visit with Mrs. Zelda. Finally, arrangements were made for the nurse and Mrs. Zelda to meet early one morning at the day care center.

Mrs. Zelda was defensive. She thought the teacher should have discussed the referral with her before she contacted the nurse. The teacher related to Mrs. Zelda that she did inform her and she had agreed. Embarrassed, Mrs. Zelda stated she did not remember the conversation. She added she had noticed that her memory had gotten poor lately. The teacher discussed the child's behavior change she had observed and told Mrs. Zelda of her attempts to deal with the child. The mother stated she saw these changes too, but didn't know what was causing them. Mrs. Zelda seemed reluctant to express herself. Sensing this, the nurse suggested another visit be scheduled during a less hectic time, since the noisiness of the children was deafening. Mrs. Zelda agreed, took the nurse's card, and left.

Two days later, Mrs. Zelda called the nurse to ask whether they could visit over lunch. The nurse agreed to meet her in the nearby park. With very little preamble, Mrs. Zelda blurted out that her brother, a first-year medical student, had just been found to have an inoperable brain tumor. She cried profusely as she described her own feelings about his condition to the nurse. She felt hopeless. She couldn't handle the thought of her brother dying, and at the same time she was trying to be a support to her parents. She also stated that her parents constantly argued and blamed each other for the son's illness. As the oldest child, she had always played the role of mediator in family fights. Now she just couldn't do it! The nurse explored with Mrs. Zelda the feelings she had concerning the obligations of being the oldest and what a burden these responsibilities must be. Mrs. Zelda had not previously thought about how overwhelmed she felt at times and by discussing her feelings, began to reassess her role and responsibilities to her family. The nurse, in an effort to assess this client's own resources and support systems, asked how Mrs. Zelda had tried to handle previous difficult situations. As she talked, Mrs. Zelda indicated that she was feeling so overwhelmed that she had not used the supports that were available to her—her husband and her best friend—but instead drank to drive out the pain. Suddenly, Mrs. Zelda glanced at her watch and exclaimed she had to return to work. The nurse and Mrs. Zelda agreed to meet for lunch the next day.

As so often happens, the nurse realized that although Tommy Zelda's behavior problem was the reason for referral, it was not the central crisis issue. Even though Mrs. Zelda had indicated that her parents considered their son and his fatal tumor to be well managed by the hospital staff, who seldom see the fallout of stress in the lives of many families, the nurse knew a crisis could upset the equilibrium of those beyond the group immediately involved in the problem. Thus the case actually represented three family configurations in crisis: the sick son and parents, the sister and her parental family, and the sister and her own family, including the child Tommy. The extreme psychological impact of the imminent death of the beloved son/brother of the families strained what in less dire circumstances may have been adequate coping behavior. Mrs. Zelda was clearly attempting to handle her emotional pangs with alcohol, while whatever problem-solving approaches the parents had used in the past were obviously not adequate to deal with this situation. Their difficulty in coping was reflected in the disorganization of both families.

The community health nurse returned to the office and mulled over the visit. She decided that Mrs. Zelda was attempting to cope despite her use of alcohol. The nurse was aware that alcohol and other sedatives are often reasonably effective ways of relaxing from moderate tensions and only when their use begins to interfere with daily life, do they become a problem instead of a solution to other problems. Mrs. Zelda continued to work and take her child to the day care center. She had noticed the change in her child's behavior and she did seem concerned about her own family, her brother, and her parents. Thus the nurse decided to continue discussing Mrs. Zelda's feelings and her behavior in this situation. The nurse knew it was important for her own attitude to be nonjudgmental and above all that if she were patient with Mrs. Zelda, the resolution of this crisis could be a growth-producing experience for all.

Case Study IV

A referral received from social services requesting nursing followup stated that the father, Mr. Brown, was left by his wife to care for their five children. Mrs. Brown's whereabouts were unknown at the time. The

Brown family consists of the father and five children, ages seven months, two, six, seven, and eight years. Mr. Brown has been separated from his wife approximately six months and works the night shift. The family lives in a three-bedroom home; the three older children attend the neighborhood school.

The nurse initially was not quite sure how to approach the family. She was accustomed to working with women and had very little if any experience providing health services to men. To be honest, she was a bit nervous. The nurse was aware, however, that many men are taking on the responsibility of rearing their children alone, but how do you explain to a father the fine points of child-rearing procedures or meal planning?

On the initial visit Mr. Brown told the nurse that a physician had recently seen the infant for a rash and diarrhea, which were diagnosed as an allergy to the original formula. The milk was replaced by a soybean formula. The father stated that it was too expensive and that the lady next door recommended evaporated milk. Mr. Brown also stated he was having difficulty toilet training the toddler; the child had been doing fairly well but now seemed to be forgetting what he had learned. The use of additional disposable diapers also added to the expense of the household budget. Mr. Brown said he had been feeling "bone tired" for the last several months. He just wasn't used to managing five children, working, and running a house too. Finally he said rather distractedly that he just didn't know what he was going to do.

During the initial visit, the nurse recognized the importance of Mr. Brown's ventilating and expressing his feelings of frustrations. Mr. Brown seemed so overwhelmed with his present situation he had difficulty in managing even minimal tasks in the home. The first priority the nurse thus focused on was helping Mr. Brown to decrease his feeling of being overwhelmed. The nurse encouraged Mr. Brown to talk and was careful to avoid placing blame, but instead to move toward active problem solving.

As Mr. Brown began to talk, he expressed resentment at having to rear five children alone. Mr. Brown felt he and his wife were unlikely to reconcile. As he talked his resentment over the separation increased. He talked openly about the difficulties he and his wife had experienced. He kept blaming himself and said that he should have paid more attention to her. Later, he alternated self-reproach with anger both at her and, by extension, to all women. This anger surprised him and he quickly acknowledged that he liked women too well to wipe them off his list. As he continued to talk about his marriage, the nurse pointed out areas of disagreement where he had no control and tried to help him understand that he was not the sole reason the marriage was breaking up. The nurse agreed that the feeling of hurt and failure would take some time to resolve, but discussing it would help.

During the first visit, the nurse tried to identify what support systems Mr. Brown had. His widowed mother had been staying at their house overnight while he worked, so the children's safety was already being considered. Mr. Brown then thought of a friend whose daughter could come over after school to care for the children and give him a chance for rest before leaving for work. On her second visit, the nurse brought a number of sample cans of soybean formula from her agency and showed Mr. Brown how to reconstitute them for the baby's needs. Within three days, the infant's diarrhea and colic had subsided, and Mr. Brown was easily convinced that there was a direct connection with the new formula. Even though its expense would strain the budget, he felt the improvement well worth the cost. The nurse decided to discuss cow's milk allergies at later visits when Mr. Brown had more energy to learn new material.

On subsequent visits, the nurse and Mr. Brown mutually agreed on the areas they could work on: more permanent child-care arrangements, safety, normal growth and development, meal planning, and budgeting. They also agreed that the toilet training of the toddler could wait until the child adjusted to the younger baby and the absence of his mother.

DISCUSSION

In Case Studies III and IV, the nurse took a direct, nonjudgmental role in assisting the families through crisis until each was able to assume more responsibility. The nurse assisted each family to identify and utilize support systems and resources available to them. With consistent, positive actions the families were able to use their crisis as growth-producing experiences.

In addition to the use of crisis theory, the nurse used an interactional framework in approaching both families. Each family member was viewed as the member of a unit in which roles were played in terms of other roles. Roles were not fixed, but were enacted in relationship to how the other members behaved. Behaviors had meanings and in turn prescribed how each person performed. For example, for Mrs. Zelda, her brother's impending death due to inoperable cancer had meaning that she could not handle. Added to this inability were her feelings about expectations laid on her by her parents because she was the first born. For Mr. Brown, in Case Study IV, the job of assuming both parental roles was overwhelming. In his attempt to mother as well as father, he found he had no time for sleeping. Even though Mr. Brown had placed first priority on his responsibility to provide for his children, their needs and demands were more than he could meet. In addition, having to deal with both expressive and instrumental aspects of roles was painful for him. The nurse later admitted privately that she was also confronted with her own inexperience in relating to men as parents and homemakers.

With both families, the nurse focused on what meaning the situation had for the family member and then sought to assist that family member in finding ways to deal with the situation by considering available resources. No other framework would have worked as well as an interactional one.

SUMMARY

Working with families in community health nursing, while often rewarding, can be a very complex activity. The shift of focus from individuals to families as the client is often difficult. The variety of configurations found in contemporary families also makes it difficult to see common characteristics among them. The families with whom nurses most often come in contact are usually under some degree of stress or even in crisis, thereby making our understanding of the ways families work even more important. We have attempted to illustrate in this chapter both the complexity of families and some of the theories presented earlier. Such case examples are representative of those with whom many of us often work, but for whom we may experience some difficulty in providing appropriate nursing care.

The primary goal of the community health nurse is to assist clients to reach and maintain their optimum level of functioning. We can do this best by being knowledgeable about the backgrounds of our client-families and by utilizing appropriate theoretical frameworks and community resources to assist us in the effort to support, strengthen, and facilitate optimum family functioning.

REFERENCES

ADAMS, D., BELLO, T., et al. "Models for the Curriculum." In M. Branch and P. Paxton, *Providing Safe Nursing Care For Ethnic People of Color.* New York: Appleton-Century-Crofts, 1976.

BRANCH, MARIE, and PAXTON, PHYLLIS. *Providing Safe Nursing Care for Ethnic People of Color.* New York: Appleton-Century-Crofts, 1976.

BURGESS, ANN, and LAZARE, AARON. *Community Mental Health: Target Populations.* Englewood Cliffs, N.J.: Prentice-Hall, 1976.

CHUNG, HYO JIN. "Understanding the Oriental Maternity Patient." *Nursing Clinics of North America* 12, no. 1 (March 1977):66–75.

COLE, JOHNNETTA B. "Culture: Negro, Black and Nigger." *The Black Scholar* 1 (June 1970): 41.

HEISS, JEROLD. *Family Roles and Interaction: An Anthology.* Chicago: Rand McNally, 1976.

HILL, ROBERT. *The Strengths of Black Families.* New York: Emerson-Hall, 1972.

MURILLO, NATHAN. "The Mexican and American Family." In Nathan N.

Wagner and Marsha J. Haug, eds. *Chicanos: Social and Psychological Perspectives*. St. Louis: C.V. Mosby Co., 1971.

OTTO, HERBERT A. "A Framework for Assessing Family Strengths." In Adina M. Reinhardt and Mildred D. Quinn, *Family-Centered Community Nursing*. St. Louis: C. V. Mosby Co., 1973.

SUE, STANLEY, and WAGNER, NATHANIEL. *Asian American: Psychological Perspectives*. Palo Alto, Calif.: Science and Behavioral Books, 1973.

SUSSMAN, MARVIN B. *Family Systems in the 1970's*. New York: McGraw-Hill Book Co., 1973.

"Symposium on Cultural and Biological Diversity and Health Care." *Nursing Clinics of North America*, 12, no. 1 (March 1977).

TAO-KIM-HAI, ANDRE M. "Orientals Are Stoic." In J.K. Skipper and D. Leonard, eds., *Social Interaction and Patient Care*. Philadelphia: J.B. Lippincott Co., 1965, pp. 243–55.

7. Family-Focused Community Health Nursing Services in the Home

Carol A. Lockhart

INTRODUCTION

Self-care and care provided by health professionals in the home account for the greatest portion of health care provided in this country today. The time a person spends in the hospital receiving care for acute conditions occupies less than 10 percent of his or her life. Thus we are realizing the need to prepare people to care for themselves through understanding their bodies, the meaning of health, and what they can and, indeed, must do for themselves. Skyrocketing costs and ever-earlier discharge from acute care facilities are making the family an increasingly major focus for providing care to its members as well as for promoting each member's optimal level of functioning. The community health nurse's roles as advocate, caregiver, coordinator of services, facilitator, teacher, and change agent are all of crucial importance in helping families assume and discharge these responsibilities for themselves and their members.

As community health nurses, we are in the position to help families identify and receive appropriate care, education, and services. This chapter provides information on assessing client and family coping abilities, developing client-nurse contracts, and actively involving clients in all phases of planning, delivering, and evaluating care. The case study herein presents one example of community health nursing care with one client. Hopefully, the discussions will help you to identify your roles with your clients.

152

In this chapter as throughout this book, *client* is defined pluralistically in the systems context: Each contact with a client is a contact with a person and the significant others involved in the person's life. A person cannot be viewed outside of the context of the family system and community. Disruption for one member of the family system automatically affects all others in the system. The effect varies, but a disruption cannot be seen as an isolated event for an isolated person. Family-centered care, holistic care, or any other term must refer to the network of relationships entwining people's lives.

With the practice of early hospital discharge, clients or their families have assumed responsibility for much of the needed health care. The United States, however, has experienced an increase in the number of small nuclear families, and as family size has decreased, the stress experienced with an ill member has increased. No longer are large numbers of family members available to assume health care responsibilities. Such a change makes today's family a weakened base for the increased responsibility of home care (Craven and Sharp 1972). Health professionals and families need to acknowledge these stresses and devise support systems that can strengthen the individual, family, or group.

CASE STUDY

On her first day back to work, Lillian Gray felt great. Two months had passed since she noticed a lump under her right arm. Two days later she had had a radical mastectomy. The initial shock had been great, but being a Licensed Vocational Nurse (LVN) and understanding her condition helped Lillian get life back into perspective. The loss of her breast was not easy to accept. She had seen many other women who had had mastectomies and had seen them make adjustments. She was learning to make adjustments too.

The doctor had not wanted her to return to work quite this soon, but twenty years of working in the hospital had become a life pattern for her. She did not like to cook, and besides, her husband did most of the cooking. Housework had never been a favorite pastime either. With only the two of them in their second-floor apartment, there just was not enough to do to keep her busy. Working in her nursing organization, bowling, or attending baseball games filled most of her time. Life did not revolve around home.

The morning's work went well, but Lillian began to feel weak as the day passed. Maybe the doctor was right about two months' being too soon to return to work. By 4 PM Lillian's legs were even weaker. By dark she was unable to walk. The doctor was as confused as were Lillian and her husband. No hospital beds were available, but the doctor assured her that if she were not better by morning, she would be admitted somewhere. By morning, Lillian was paralyzed from the waist down.

The paralysis continued to spread. A tracheostomy was done the afternoon she was admitted to the hospital. By the second night Lillian was unable to move. The diagnosis was Guillain-Barre Syndrome, and Lillian began a three-month stay in the hospital intensive care unit followed by three more months on a medical ward.

On a day some months after admission to the hospital, the phone in Lillian's room kept ringing. Unable to reach it, she became more and more angry as she struggled to sit up in bed and pull the phone toward her. She forgot her inability to lift the weight of her body. Only after she was actually talking on the phone did she realize what she had accomplished in her anger. She had made her first independent movement in months.

Six months of hospitalization left Lillian feeling defeated. No matter how often she went to physical therapy, nothing seemed to happen to her legs. They grew stronger but responded no more than before. The neurologist could not say with certainty whether Lillian would or would not walk again. Lillian believed that she would walk again. With months of paralysis had come a large sacral decubitus ulcer that extended to the bone. It was not responding to treatment. Skin grafting was considered, but thought to be too uncertain at the time. Lillian was simply not recovering. Even though Lillian still needed intensive care, both she and her husband wanted her home. The doctor agreed to the discharge if Lillian had twenty-four-hour care. The hospital's home care coordinator worked with Lillian and her husband as they began to plan for discharge.

Mr. Gray arranged a month's vacation from his job to allow him to care for Lillian at home. After the month they would make plans according to the needs still existing. The community health nurse visited Mr. Gray at home before Lillian's discharge to assess any changes that might have to be made in the home setting. The bedroom was situated off the kitchen, while the bathroom down the hall had entrances from the hall and dining room. To make care easier, the bedroom was moved to the dining room and an electric bed was rented. It was paid for by the insurance company. The insurance company also agreed to install an electric elevator chair since Lillian was still unable to walk the long flight of stairs to the apartment. The community health nurse scheduled visits to teach Mr. Gray to change the dressing on the sacrum and give Lillian care. Daily visits from the occupational therapist and physical therapist allowed for needed exercise and the teaching both Mr. and Mrs. Gray required to supplement the therapists' regular visits.

Lillian progressed rapidly at home. With her own knowledge of nursing care and that of the nurses and therapists visiting her, she was able to get care and support for each of the problems confronting her and her husband. Mr. Gray became skilled at providing for his wife's needs. Within three weeks of discharge, granulating tissue began to fill the decubitus. Within five weeks of discharge, Lillian was able to walk a few paces without the aid of leg braces. When Mr. Gray returned to work, Lillian's sister stayed with her during the day. Six weeks after discharge Lillian was well enough to care for herself during the eight hours Mr. Gray was gone.

Lillian made steady progress with fewer and fewer health team visits needed. Within a year of discharge from the hospital, Lillian ambulated on crutches, walked short flights of stairs, and did independent bed and tub transfers. At this point she was discharged from the home care followup and was maintained only by her routine appointments with her physician.

Three months after discharge from the home care program, the district public health nurse, me, made a series of nursing visits that revealed three continuing concerns: nutrition, evacuation, and exercise. Lillian had continued to exercise but only once a day. When walking more than the length of one room, she noticed a weakness in her legs. Because of constipation, she had to take two ounces of milk of magnesia every night. The doctor wanted her to lose weight because of a forty-pound weight gain since the onset of her illness.

Lillian and I developed a client-nurse contract. For the next four weeks I would visit once a week. In that time we would concentrate on the three areas that we identified and agreed upon as continuing problem areas. In reviewing each problem and its effects on her body, we decided that her need for increased exercise was the first area to be worked on directly. Lillian would use her exercise bike (provided by insurance) for five minutes three times a day for one week. I would visit at the end of that week.

After the first week, Lillian felt the strength in her legs improved enough to increase the time of each exercise session. With every passing week Lillian increased her exercise time slightly, and each week we noticed increasing strength in her legs. During each visit Lillian and I discussed diet and nutrition. In between visits Lillian tried to watch her diet and control her intake. No great weight change took place, but Lillian did feel well and paid more attention to the family diet.

At the end of the four weeks we decided to decrease the visits to every other week. By the end of the next four weeks, Lillian had made changes both she and her husband were proud of. Lillian was now exercising fifteen minutes two to three times a day and increasing the resistance level settings on the bicycle. With the increased exercise she was able to do more about the house and even fix an occasional meal—a task she was beginning to find interesting. She was now able to shop on crutches and proudly related the experience of walking the entire length of a shopping mall with only one rest period. Lillian had decided to attend home games during the next baseball season. She felt that by packing a lunch and taking the streetcar early, she could avoid the crowds and wait for the game to start while others were finding their seats. With all her increased ability, she had also reduced the dosage of milk of magnesia from two to one ounce a night, and a recent visit to the doctor had shown a beginning weight loss of two and a half pounds. Lillian and I agreed there was no need for me to continue visiting her on a regular basis. We set a return visit for three months later to allow another evaluation of changes and needs. If Lillian needed me before that time, she would telephone the department and request that I visit.

Both Lillian's and her husband's lives have changed. They know she will not work again. Both look for interests and activities they can adapt to their new lifestyle. Fixing dinner is a source of excitement and a feeling of accomplishment in Lillian's life; such achievement gives her husband a feeling of satisfaction, too. Mr. Gray does most of the housekeeping and takes the laundry to the laundromat. Lillian does the things she can and is trying to do more. She continues on medications to assist with bowel and bladder retraining and must practice a rigid schedule for both. The problems are not gone but Mr. and Mrs. Gray know the limitations placed on their lives and are living within them. Mr. and Mrs. Gray are coping. Should something occur to disrupt that coping ability, Lillian or Mr. Gray know where to call to reach the nurses, doctors, and others who have helped them thus far.

ROLES OF THE COMMUNITY HEALTH NURSE

Community nurses act as facilitators, coordinators, advocates, caregivers, teachers, and change agents. Which role and how long we occupy it depends on what transpires between us, our clients, and our clients' families. Community nursing requires that we be involved and willing to assist people in areas that are mutually defined as needful. People's needs, which occur twenty-four hours a day, seven days a week, require community nurses to reexamine the nature of their commitment to the individual person, family, and community. Services offered between 8 AM and 5 PM, Monday through Friday, are not adequate. Consumers are demanding greater availability of health services. Community health nurses must support these expanded schedules and then be willing to staff them.

Roles are developing that allow the community nurse to provide broader services for the client. One such role places the community health nurse in the position of coordinator of primary care services. Clients maintain contact with the nurse who arranges and coordinates all needed services. For example, they receive services—all coordinated by the community health nurse—from physicians, nutritionists, dentists, social workers, indigenous community workers, and other specialists required to meet their needs.

A second role of the community health nurse is as the provider of primary care. Within legal limits, the nurse gives the care and evaluation needed by clients. Specialized knowledge is available through other members of the health team. Outside expertise provides interdependent and guided decisions beyond the primary care functions of the community health nurse (Brunetto and Birk 1972:785–94).

In either of these roles the community health nurse must be proficient in the delivery and teaching of nursing care. A client may be an individual person, a family, a person within a social unit or family, or a person cared for by a paid attendant or caretaker. In each situation we must be able to perform, demonstrate, and teach the care required.

The nurse may enter a situation as a care provider, as I did in the case study. By acting as a teacher and role model, I was able to help Lillian and her husband learn what she needed. As they demonstrated their ability to provide needed care, I moved to a support position, with the family assuming ongoing responsibility and independence. Lillian's nursing knowledge allowed the transfer to take place rapidly. Her advances in abilities to function were largely due to the knowledge she and her husband possessed and the care responsibility they were able to assume.

Another role of the community nurses, that of facilitator, is to assist or make something easier for clients. Community nurses can assist people in every life situation. The assistance we give depends on our own willingness to invest ourselves in meeting others' needs. Nurses' knowledge of community resources may open avenues of service that clients did not know existed. For example, referral to an agency can begin care that has been needed, but which the client thought impossible to obtain. A community health nurse may also be able to explain ways clients can more smoothly deal with agency procedures in the complicated and confusing present-day American health care system.

Just as the facilitator role depends on the nurse's involvement and commitment, so does the role of advocate. An advocate speaks for or in favor of a person or cause. This role may be interpreted in a militant manner, but a preferred definition involves use of the nursing knowledge to bring about changes in the system to help the client. For example, an essential nursing function may be to pressure agencies into modifying policies or to educate clients and their families in ways to overcome needless restrictions. If we speak of an optimal level of functioning as a goal for clients, then we must act to help achieve that level. Nurses committed to a community and its well-being cannot allow health issues and problems to go unnoticed; we must involve ourselves and our skills. The effort needed to allow a client to remain at home rather than be transferred to a nursing facility may require a lot from the community health nurse. Lillian was a vocal client and had the knowledge and family support to permit her discharge from the hospital even though she needed extensive care. Others might not have the choices open to Lillian and will need extensive intervention and support from the community health nurse.

The community health nurse is also a change agent. Each time an idea or action is introduced into a situation, we bring about change, no matter how small. In chapters 2 or 3, the influences of the ecosystem on the optimal level of functioning are well described. Community health nurses need to know these influences, how each affects the other, and where and when one is dependent on another. Unless we recognize, accept, and use these parts of the ecosystem in our efforts to influence and change the level of health, we will be ineffective. Community health nursing is that broad scope and understanding that incorporates the entire ecosystem into planned nursing action with clients and families.

Community health nursing's roles and actions are interdependent, not discrete. Whether we are acting as change agent, caregiver, teacher, coordinator, facilitator, or advocate, we act with the client and with objectives that are meaningful to the client.

CLIENT-NURSE COMMUNICATION

The ability to communicate is the ability to exchange thoughts or messages with another person. The client and nurse are engaging in an exchange in an interview situation. The effectiveness of the transfer depends on the perception each has of the other. Perception of others is the forming of judgments by people about people. It concerns the reactions and responses we have to each other in thought, feeling, and action. Inaccurate inferences and intuitions are too frequently the basis on which we decide our perceptions (Cook 1971). What Jourard states about general medical practice is equally true of nursing:

> The more that you experience as a person, inside a sickroom and in outside life, the more progress you make toward general practice. The more suffering, enjoying, sinning, being afraid, becoming psychotic and recovering, being sick, reading books, having babies, fighting and arguing, loving and making up, daydreaming—in short, living and learning about yourself—the more you move toward general practice [Jourard 1964:137].

Understanding and accepting ourselves can help us understand and accept other people and allow them the freedom to be different. Gail Sheehy speaks of the predictable crises of adult development in *Passages* (1976). Such insights help us deal with ourselves and others.

Each client-nurse interaction is unique. The special knowledge and experience of a lifetime comes with the persons involved in the exchange. No two persons are identical nor does the same person behave the same from one encounter to another (Ittleson and Cantril 1976). The community nurse and client respond to each other according to the cues in their interaction.

The first meeting of the nurse and client is significant for the future relationship. Initial impressions and judgments made by either one will influence the other's responses. The community health nurse is a guest in the family's home. The nurse must convey acceptance of the client and the family as they are in their life setting. Numerous health issues may exist, but until they are a concern to the client, the nurse must work with the issues the client and family identify as important to their lives. Once the initial contact is made, the progress of communication will depend on the community nurse's skill at maintaining rapport and positive client-nurse feelings.

Rapport, harmony, and *vibrations* are all words we use to describe the "click" between people when they meet. Rapport may take months to establish; often it happens in minutes. Sharing, understanding, and trust take time, but most often the tone of the relationship between us and our client is set, if not at the first meeting (when everyone is a little nervous), then at the second. Not only our knowledge or skill as a nurse determines rapport, but also our caring and ability to respect and involve the client and family in the events taking place.

Communication attuned to the client's needs is the goal of the client-nurse exchange. Too often, however, we develop a routine or style and use it with every client. Such ritualized behavior produces ritualized responses from the client and family (Mayers 1973). Nothing is accomplished between nurse and client unless each is able to perceive one another as unique people with particular needs, ideas, and values. Communication skill requires us to be open to the client. Payne's *The Art of Asking Questions* can help us learn how to ask a question, but we must be able to hear the answers (1973). The ability to attend to verbal and non-verbal messages sent by both the client and ourselves is our greatest interviewing skill.

As community health nurses, we must also be attuned to our own assumptions about different groups of people. No matter where we were raised, we have certain "assumptions" about what is appropriate expected behavior from a person, family, or group. When someone does or does not conform to these expectations, we may show approval or disapproval through verbal and nonverbal communications without even trying.

Sensitivity to our assumptions does not necessarily mean we will change them or that our behavior is wrong. It simply means we are conscious of their influences on interactions with others and that we can weigh their relative merit on the assessments and judgments we make about other people's behaviors.

The following are only a few of the areas in which we make assumptions about expected behaviors. We should be aware of how we, as well as our clients and their families, feel about the meaning of:

1. Time and its use (scheduling, promptness, and so forth);
2. Cleanliness;
3. Health and illness and their causes;
4. A right to health and health care;
5. Independence of a person and family and a person within a family;
6. Decision making in a family and who is responsible for it;
7. Achieving and upward mobility;
8. The role of a man and woman within and outside of the home.

We can add to the list as we identify other areas where assumptions about expected behavior influence us in interactions with particular clients and families. The more aware we become, the more our client-nurse communications will be constructive interchanges.

CLIENT-CENTERED CARE

ESTABLISHING GOALS AND OBJECTIVES

Client-centered goals and objectives are established through interactions between client, family, and nurse using client-defined needs and values as guidelines. The nurse's knowledge and skill provide information and assistance in attaining specific objectives en route to reaching the overall agreed-upon goal. Thus the goal of client-centered care is the long-range outcome that client and nurse have agreed they want to attain. The client's wishes must be central to these decisions. Client and nurse may have differences of opinion about what needs to be done or what the priorities of the situation are. If mutually agreed-upon goals and objectives cannot be reached, the nurse must work with those the client has chosen. Once these are achieved, or even during the process, the nurse can help the client and family broaden their understanding of the situation and the large selection of options open to them.

At times nurses visit homes with a hidden agenda of short- and long-term objectives. The client has not assisted in formulating these objectives or been informed of their existence (Mayers 1973). This approach precludes client and family involvement, with the result that few of the changes chosen by the nurse are implemented. As noted in chapter 3, clients are disinclined to tolerate a lack of involvement on their part in decisions affecting them.

Objectives need to be stated in terms both the client and the nurse can make operational. The objective must state in measurable terms how the client or the situation will have changed when the objective is accomplished. The behavior expected of both the client and the nurse must be made clear. Thus, stated objectives help in the assessment of and evaluation of progress being made toward attaining the overall mutually agreed-upon goal (Mager 1962).

In the case study cited earlier, Mrs. Gray had three continuing problems: nutrition, exercise, and elimination. She was able to identify her concerns, and as community health nurse, I was able to guide her choice of short-term objectives. Increasing the time spent in daily exercise was another objective. A long-range goal was to permit Lillian to be able to return to independence. The short-term objective gave Lillian immediate feedback as she felt the strength in her legs increasing. The long-term goal was partially achieved, but it remained a goal as she attempted to achieve her optimal level of functioning.

Objectives give direction to the continuing client-nurse interaction. They act as signposts in the ongoing health care. Objectives change as the client's needs change. Frequent review of objectives keeps the client-nurse interaction meaningful and related to identified needs. If objectives are not reached or if the client is unwilling to actually do the things necessary to progress toward the goal, both the client and nurse must reevaluate the purpose and direction of their exchanges.

THE INFORMED CONSUMER

The health care consumer is any client receiving or needing services. It is the public. When clients seek services from the health care system, they are asking for assistance; they are not abdicating their rights as individuals. Medical care cannot be treated as mysteries whose decisions and meanings are kept from submissive clients. Clients and families must be assisted to participate actively in decisions affecting their health status. Health education needed for knowledgeable decisions is an essential part of every community health nurse's activities (see chapter 10).

The community health nurse's position allows contact with the client and family on a continuing basis. Through sustained contact the community health nurse is able to explain and explore opportunities and alternatives with clients. Clients therefore are able to choose situations that meet the needs and responsibilities of their broader life setting. They are also able to give informed consent to health care providers to institute understood and agreed-upon interventions. Helping clients make informed choices is a community health nurse's most meaningful and essential action. As clients become informed consumers, they work in cooperation with health professionals toward their optimal level of functioning. If changes occur requiring intervention, the informed consumer can request and receive support early in the situation. A crisis situation is therefore averted.

Informed consumers are cognizant of health issues to such a degree that they are able to identify life changes that are needed. Clients seek assistance in a health care system they understand and can use to meet their health requirements. They are independent actors because of their knowledge.

The emphasis in health care is changing. Hospitals are dealing with acute medical episodes in shorter periods of time. Chronic diseases account for more and more hospital days since medical technology enables much of our population to live with one or more chronic diseases. Rising hospital costs contribute to early discharge of clients. Ambulatory care centers and primary care centers located in strategic areas in the community provide on-site medical care. Community health agencies are becoming more involved with pathology-focused care and providing less and less preventive medicine. Each of these developments demands informed clients who are able to identify health issues in their own homes. Preventive health measures are something the community health nurse must teach clients for without this information they are unable to use their own resources and the community's to their benefit. The rise of the holistic health movement and the vast variety of alternative care patterns in the past few years are positive steps toward helping people to promote and protect their own optimal level of functioning. Many community health nurses have become involved in these kinds of education and service delivery systems (see chapters 1 and 2).

CLIENT-NURSE CONTRACT

Nurses have always identified a direction for their interactions with clients. Using a contract simply acknowledges the direction and involves the client in the problem solving done to reach a goal. The client-nurse contract is an agreement to work toward stated objectives in a specified time. The frequency of visits and the work done during and between visits is specified for both client and community health nurse. The use of a contract agreement makes the client and the community nurse accountable for the effort and time invested in their interaction. Responsibility for change is placed with both. If either party does not live up to the agreement, the other can request a reevaluation of the agreement.

The agreement may or may not be written, but either way it should be clearly identified. The client may wish the objectives written and the times noted as a reminder of his or her responsibilities. The nurse's notes of the visit should record the decisions agreed upon. The care plan can be and often is the contract in written format (Blair 1971). A client-nurse contract may sound formal, but it is only as rigid as the manner in which it is presented. In the case study, the contract between Lillian Gray and myself was verbal. We identified three areas of concern with objectives established for each, and weekly visits allowed review of the progress made. At the end of four weeks, we reevaluated the time needed for client-nurse visits and changed the frequency to every other week. The objectives remained the same.

Dates for review of an agreement and the objectives should be set at the start. Intervals between reviews are determined by the severity and complexity of the health issues. The more changes occur, the more frequently the reviews are needed. If objectives do not need revision, they can be carried into the next time period with the new times specified.

The number of objectives and the changes made in them are determined by the nurse and the client. Together, decisions are made on the frequency of visits and the amount of support needed by the client. Just as client responsibilities influence the scheduling of visits, so too do the responsibilities of the community health nurse. When personal visits are not possible, the telephone allows sustained contact and promotes the feeling of mutual concern and assistance needed in any joint agreement.

ASSESSMENT OF FAMILY COPING ABILITY

At a time of stress the family and the person requiring health care must continue to cope. If clients and families are able to keep from being overwhelmed and maintain function in the face of stress, even if the methods seem unusual, coping mechanisms can be considered effective (Fond 1972).

If community health nurses can give assistance that enhances coping mechanisms, a need for service is identified. If our presence as nurses brings no change or causes resistance, even though a need exists, we cannot force our intervention onto clients. (*Family Coping Index* 1964). The ability to change lies within the client. The community health nurse can only offer assistance; whether the assistance is accepted is the client's choice. Dealing with refusals is difficult for health professionals, but unless the client wishes to change, no nursing pressures will alter behavior. Nurses hesitate to "close" a family even if the family is resistant or unwilling to engage in activities that work toward mutually identified goals. We somehow believe in the power of our presence and go on visiting families years after our visits have ceased to display any impact, changed behavior, or outcomes. In community health, nurses must accept clients' rights to make their own decisions, help prepare them to face the consequences of their decisions, and help them identify how and where to get help when it is needed or wanted (Blair 1971).

When nursing intervention is accepted as an aid to maintaining or enhancing the client's coping mechanism, the strengths and weaknesses of the family are evaluated. Identifying these gives direction for establishing objectives. Assessment of strengths and weaknesses relates to the client's ability to deal with health problems, not the relative illness or wellness of the family. How a family handles stress and the day-to-day needs of its members is what must be evaluated (*Family Coping Index* 1964). Assessment of coping ability requires appraisal of total functioning, not just health needs or lacks. Anything impinging on a family has some influence on its ability to deal with stress. Unemployment, educational problems, and social strain can affect families' ability to deal with specific episodes or series of episodes.

In chronic disease conditions, the disease trajectory may be one of slow decline. Understanding the disease and dealing with the situation it creates indicates ability to cope. In the case study, Lillian and her husband were evaluated for their coping ability before Lillian's hospital discharge. As her condition changed, they learned how to deal with the limits it imposed on their lives. As informed consumers, they were able to cope with a variety of problems. Lillian has chronic limitations but she and her husband cope with them. Mr. and Mrs. Gray function at a high level of well-being and therefore require minimum assistance from health professionals.

Suggested Categories and Questions for Assessment of Family Coping Ability

ECONOMIC STABILITY

Is there enough money to meet the family's needs? (The response to this question can vary widely since people interpret "needs" differently.) Are sufficient food, clothing, and shelter available? Who provides the income in the household? Is the income regular or sporadic? Is official agency financing needed at intervals? Are resources available to enhance the family income? Does the family know how to seek assistance? Has asssistance been sought?

PHYSICAL/SOCIAL SETTING

Are living arrangements adequate for the number in the family? Are play areas or recreational programs available for the children? Do racial or ethnic conflicts exist in the area? Does the physical structure limit the activity of one or more family members? (Are there architectural barriers?) Is other housing available if the family wishes it? Does the family require assistance to bring about a move? Are water, heat, and electricity available in the home?

SAFETY

Is housing structurally safe? Do fire hazards exist in the dwelling? Is paint in good repair? Is paint peeling where children can reach it? Are rodents and harmful insects present in the home or surroundings? Have efforts been made to eradicate them by the family and/or city? Are children and adults safe on the street?

EMOTIONAL CLIMATE

Are family members able to support one another in their daily lives? Is stress evident among members or between specific members? How does the family react to stress of health/family problems? Are health/family problems realistically evaluated? Do the family members have adequate knowledge to evaluate the problems? Does one member of the family provide the emotional support needed in the family unit?

HEALTH PRACTICES

Does meal planning show a knowledge of nutrition? Does the family understand and use health services in the community? Do the members use services appropriate for their problems? Are preventive medical and dental care provided regularly? Do family members obtain adequate rest? Are there appropriate sleeping facilities for the number in the family? Is there a designated room for sleeping? Do washing habits maintain the integrity of the skin and prevent the spread of disease? How is health care provided? From what sources does the family obtain health care?

UNDERSTANDING HEALTH PROBLEMS

Is the family able to identify health changes requiring care? Is care sought? Do family members have appropriate knowledge of health problems in the home? Is the need for changes in roles and responsibilities during illness identified and understood by all family members? Are family members able to identify changes in the status of an ill member, particularly one with a chronic disease? If changes are noted, is care sought? Is care sought from appropriate sources?

RESPONSES TO HEALTH PROBLEMS

Does the family select with discrimination among the resources available for health care? Are health problems seen as a body response or as an indication of sin or punishment? Are appointments for care kept or does the family discontinue care once the pain or acute symptoms disappear? If a family member is ill, can the family (including the ill member) be maintained at an optimum level? Are treatments, medications, diets, and so on done correctly? Do family members understand the why and how of care given? Do family members share responsibilities in the home (including the ill member)? Is self-care possible for the ill member, or does the ill member need assistance? Who provides the assistance? Is the responsibility shared or can it be shared? Does the ill member feel he or she is a burden on the family or, rather, a part of the family unit?

The strengths a family possess, no matter how few, are the bases on which the nurse and the client build toward increased coping abilities. The direction for that building is determined together.

COMMUNITY HEALTH NURSING—CONTINUITY OF CARE

The ability to evaluate a client's level of functioning enables the community nurse to play a key role in the health care planning. Planning is continuous, whether the client is in the home, hospital, or an extended care facility.

In the hospital, discharge planners, home care coordinators, and liaison nurses function as coordinators for services the hospitalized client and family will need on the client's return home. Such coordinators may be employed by a hospital or a community agency, but all work to ease the transfer from one manner of care to another. The discharge planner acts as a constant reminder to hospital personnel of the need for planned client discharge. Each client in an acute care facility is evaluated as to potential need for services in the home setting. If need is identified, a referral for followup by an agency providing care in the home is indicated (see chapter 19).

The community health nurse is the home contact for clients and must be aware of their life setting and the constraints imposed by it. Clients discharged with continuing care needs require an evaluation of family coping ability and the needy member's ability to function in the home setting, if there is a home to return to. Visiting the client while hospitalized gives the community health nurse the opportunity to assess treatments, limitations, and problems that will require attention after discharge. A predischarge home visit allows the community health nurse to speak with the family and evaluate the home for its ability to provide the care needed. During the visit the nurse can help the client and the family plan and discuss problems they identify. The information obtained by the community health nurse is then shared with the discharge planner who can arrange teaching or other interventions.

Arranging home care for a client involves the coordination and cooperation of the client, family, hospital staff, and community health professionals. Each provides information to the discharge planner who evaluates the data and seeks assistance from the most appropriate person in solving problems identified. The more complete the information and planning before the client's discharge, the smoother the transition from hospital to home or vice versa.

The discharge planner and the hospital nurses need to be sure the client has had opportunities to learn skills and procedures needed at home. Many home care nurses are frustrated to find out that their new client has never practiced colostomy irrigation or self-injection of insulin despite lengthy hospital stays. Conferences, involving all the parties, before and after discharge allow for attention to changes and problems before they are unmanageable. Supplies for treatments or appliances are arranged to allow a ready stock for continued use. Return clinic appointments or doctor's visits are scheduled before discharge and should include arrangements for transportation.

Home Assessment

Clients discharged from the hospital, but still needing care, require appraisal of their living situation beyond that of the family coping ability. The physical setting clients return to determines many aspects of their care. Physical/social and safety categories of assessment are expanded to include appraisal focused on clients' physical limitations or increased needs. The community health nurse's knowledge of clients' level of functioning in the hospital allows for appraisal of the home in terms of ease of care and possible barriers to care. Modifications to the environment are well described in Lawton's *Activities of Daily Living for Physical Rehabilitation* (1963). The *American National Red Cross Home Nursing Textbook* (1963) also provides many practical suggestions that can easily be implemented in the home.

SUGGESTED QUESTIONS FOR HOME ASSESSMENT

Is there a home for the client to return to for care? Is the home on ground level? Are there stairs at any point? Is there an elevator? What is the width of the doors? (Wheelchairs need thirty-six inches.)

Is the bathroom large enough for a wheelchair? Can the wheelchair be positioned to allow transfer to and from tub/shower and toilet? Are safety rails present in tub/shower and at the toilet? If not, where can they be attached?

Are the client's bedroom and the bathroom on the same floor? Is the bath readily accessible? Can a chair or stool be positioned in the tub/shower to allow bathing? If the client is confined to bed, how can the height of the bed be raised to make giving bathing care easier?

What is the height of the toilet? Is the client able to get up and down alone or with assistance? Would an elevated toilet seat allow easier transfer? Are bedpans, urinals, overbed tables, and back rests available if indicated? Can they be improvised or purchased?

Does the client have a private bedroom? Does the client live alone or with others? How many? If the client is unable to provide self-care, are persons in the home to assist in the care? Is a paid attendant or caretaker needed or can other arrangements be made to provide services?

Is the client able to prepare meals? Are outside services such as "Meals on Wheels" or help from friends and neighbors available? If the client will be cooking, are facilities accessible from a wheelchair or while using a walker/cane/crutch? Are rugs secure? Are floors highly polished or slippery?

Is there hot and cold running water in the home? Are adequate heating and cooling available if indicated? Is a laundry present in the home? Is a laundromat used? Is the client able to use the laundromat or can family, friends, or housekeeping services do laundry? Is the client able to shop and clean, or can these chores be done by a family member? Are homemaking agencies or services available?

Are special adaptations needed to allow independent eating, dressing, and so on? Will devices be developed while the client is in the hospital or after discharge?

The questions continue as long as any area of care or service remains unresolved. The more prepared the home and family, the easier the adjustments will be for all involved.

RECORDING HOME VISITS

The interaction between client and community health nurse is recorded by the nurse after each visit or after each action taken on behalf of the client between visits. Accurate, clear recording gives the community health nurse and other health professionals a continuing picture of the level of functioning maintained by the client.

Records in most community health agencies are kept in a "family folder." Sheets of nursing notes are arranged in sequence with the most recent date on top. At each visit, the names of family members seen are indicated. After each member's name is recorded the information about the person obtained on that visit. Even though every member may have been seen, care may not be considered family centered until the interaction and appraisal of the family as a unit is considered. As noted earlier, a person is not isolated in a living situation. Each person's actions and those of family members toward the person must be evaluated to give a total picture of family functioning.

Objectives and/or care plans for a family may be noted within nursing notes or on a separate sheet. Family assessments and home evaluations may also be presented on readily accessible individual sheets with current information. Either way, the goal is to present visible reminders of plans for action that will lead to an optimum level of functioning.

Identifying objectives for each member of a family and the family as a unit promotes a coordinated approach to family care. The use of problem-oriented medical records seems a useful adjunct to such an approach. Problems are identified and given a number. The number represents that problem throughout the record. Each action taken toward solution of the problem is recorded under the same number to enable easy identification of the problem. When the problem is solved, the date of closure is noted beside the problem on the problem list kept in the front of the record folder (Weed 1970).

Accurate documentation of actions and observations by nurses are assuming an increasingly important role in health care. Law suits are on the rise, and nurses must make concise and precise statements of care offered. Inaccuracies, alterations, or failure to indicate that medical orders were followed by nursing personnel may bring judgments against nurses (Hershey and Lawrence 1976).

All notes, objectives, problems, or evaluations are simply tools to provide guides to care. The more clearly each is written, the easier is working toward identified goals and levels of performance desired by the client. Records should be accurate reflections of observed realities, evaluations of events, or judgments about them. Being completely objective is not possible for any of us. Thus subjective impressions can appropriately be included in a client's record when they influence the client-nurse interaction, but such subjective observations should be noted as such.

As noted in chapters 1 and 2, the complexity and fragmentation of the health care delivery system in the United States make the community health nurse's coordination and liaison functions more important now than ever. Members of many provider groups and from a plethora of public and private agencies are offering services to clients and families in their homes. Often we community health nurses are the only providers with whom the client and family have a longitudinal relationship. Our responsibility, therefore, is to see that appropriate services are obtained, provided, and evaluated. Many community health nursing agencies are developing interdisciplinary problem-oriented recording systems such as the one used at the Tacoma-Pierce County Health Department (Kelly and Ressler 1976). These kinds of recording systems not any assist in assuring continuity of care but also facilitate auditing procedures required by governmental and other third-party reimbursing agencies (see chapter 12).

CLIENT TEACHING

Shifting care responsibilities from a visiting health professional to the client or family places the community nurse in the position of a teacher and supporter. Rather than performing care on a continuing basis, as nurses, we instruct clients and their families in procedures and treatments. As proficiency is demonstrated by the clients, we relinquish our direct care-giving responsibilities and act as resource persons to ensure a sustained level of care. Only with exceptional procedures or the early demonstrations of new ones do community health nurses provide direct care.

The ability to teach requires that we understand learning principles and apply them to client teaching. People learn what they feel is important to learn. No one can force others to learn if they do not see the thing to be grasped as significant to their own experiences or needs (see chapter 10). Earlier, the need to establish goals and objectives that are meaningful to the client was mentioned. Similarly, teaching requires shared appreciation of the relevance of what is taught. At times the community nurse may need to assist the client and family to understand how a specific thing relates to their well-being in order to help them become informed consumers. When objectives are decided upon together, the client is motivated to work toward their accomplishment. Nurses often become frustrated and refer to a family as "difficult" or "lazy" when the difficulty is in the nurse's ability to translate health objectives into terms meaningful to the client. Until they are meaningful to the client, there will be no change in behavior.

Once a meaningful objective is identified, the client and community nurse begin the second step, the actual teaching-learning process. Teaching skills and ideas become part of every client-nurse contact. Seeing a procedure done by the community health nurse and then doing it in the nurse's presence and receiving praise for doing it correctly and safely gives the client the confidence needed to undertake the procedure when alone. Repeated visits by the community nurse allow questions to be answered and procedures to be reviewed as necessary. The client can display progress or changes. If there is no progress, the community nurse is there to explain and console as needed. Through explanations, demonstrations, and answering questions the community nurse helps the client achieve objectives.

Remembering a procedure or explanation may be impossible for listeners with "emotional noise" or interference dividing their attention. Clients who are preoccupied with money worries, a sick child, or other events in their lives have difficulty retaining the full content of information they may be given. Thus attention must be paid to their immediate needs so that once these are met, the clients can again listen. Until clients are able to explain or do procedures or exhibit any other health related behavior, the community nurse needs to repeat the information or demonstrations until the clients and their families become comfortable with what is being taught.

In the case study presented earlier, Lillian's initial care needs were extensive, as were her learning needs. Daily personal care, dressings, transfer and walking techniques, plus bowel and bladder training required numerous home visits on my part as her community nurse. At the time of the second series of nursing visits, Mr. and Mrs. Gray wanted to know the reasons for physical changes and how to deal with them more than they wanted direct nursing care. At each visit, we reviewed the effects of exercise and nutrition and discussed ways to modify them. Sometimes all the Grays really wanted was a sounding board for their ideas and questions. My response to their needs involved teaching. Because of mutually agreed upon objectives, changes took place.

CLIENT SUPPORT SYSTEMS

A support system is a network or set of services to provide harmonious, orderly care that will enable clients to function optimally. Coping with acute or chronic conditions in the home requires the resources of a support system. Informed consumers are their own best resource for support. Clients who know how and where to get services can work to insure their own level of functioning.

Extensive systems of support can be built by individual clients and the people around them. With appropriate health care knowledge, the persons living with or close to an individual client can provide effective planning care. Visits and services by family members, friends, and caretakers can allow a client with limited abilities to live alone or in a family without placing the burden of care on any one person. A neighbor watching for raised or lowered window shades every morning and evening may be enough support to allow an elderly person to remain alone and know attention will be quickly received if it is needed.

When intervention is needed the clients must know how to choose and obtain professional services. Providing this knowledge is part of the community nurse's role as a resource person assisting the client to be an informed consumer. Should the client be unable or unaware of how to reach assistance, a central referring agency can assist in identifying and obtaining appropriate care. Planned followup of acute or chronic conditions by community health agencies provides the client with professional resources. Scheduled visits with long-term clients allow periodic review of gradual changes that may be leading to either loss of function or improved function. A home visit by the community nurse enables reevaluation of functioning and reorientation of client and family to continuing or new objectives for care. If the client and community health nurse identify no further need for nursing followup, care is terminated. Part of termination, however, is providing the client with a means of regaining contact with a specific community nurse or community agency. Telling a client to "give us a call" does not give adequate guidance. Suggesting specific or general circumstances that might necessitate renewed services and providing information on who to call, what department to ask for, and how to present a problem or question are ways to leave the client with readily available help. No client should be "closed" to followup without this information.

Other resources for client support are the official and nonofficial agencies providing information, care, or financial assistance. Governmental, proprietary, and voluntary agencies can supplement or provide a major portion of the client support system. A national office and city or county level branch offices exist for most nationwide organizations. Locally created agencies, such as free clinics, church relief, and community self-help groups, are valuable resources.

In the case study presented, a support system was evident. Lillian, her husband, and her sister all provided her with direct care after her hospital discharge. The doctor, hospital discharge planner, community nurse, physical therapist, occupational therapist, and insurance companies provided support when needed. Later, Lillian and her husband continued to provide for her care; relatives and friends still visited and did errands if needed. These resources could be reached by Mr. and Mrs. Gray in minutes by telephone, the value which as a link in support systems is often underestimated or forgotten. Other clients use smaller or larger systems of support, but all need consistent methods by which daily needs are met by or provided for the client.

Resources for care are not learned from a book. They are learned by interaction with people and organizations in each of our communities. A beginning list of resources is given in the community nurse's "yellow pages" section of this book (chapter 15). This section is provided just to get you started. Each time you interact with clients, the search for resources to meet their unique needs will begin again. The more you learn of your own community's resources, the broader will be the scope of care you can provide. Seeking resources is an unending game of problem solving that will continue for as long as clients' or families' needs exist.

SUMMARY

Nursing in the community requires broad skills and knowledge. By offering assistance to clients in the home, the community nurse is placed in the roles of caregiver, change agent, teacher, facilitator, coordinator, advocate, and as many others as situations may demand. Each interaction between nurse and clients is unique, for each client and his or her problems are never duplicated. The responses to each must therefore be created out of the verbal and nonverbal communication between the client and nurse. Intentioned listening and sensitivity to expectations people possess provides the cues needed for building rapport and a working relationship. The ability to communicate allows both the client and nurse to identify client-centered objectives. Simply stated objectives describe the behavior the client is to achieve. They tell the client and nurse where they are headed and why.

Clear recording of objectives, plans for care, and client-nurse interactions allows easy review and communication with other health professionals. The use of problem-oriented medical records permits identification of a specific problem according to a number assigned to the problem and each action taken on it thereafter. These records also facilitate audit and other quality assurance procedures.

The more clients are involved in their own care, the more they are able to maintain a desired level of functioning. Informed consumers or clients take responsibility for their own health needs and turn to appropriate professionals to provide the required expertise. Client responsibility is also outlined in the client-nurse contract that presents objectives to be worked toward during a specified time period. Responsibility for the outcome is shared by the client and community nurse.

Clients are part of their families and their communities. One cannot be affected without disturbing the others. The community health nurse deals with each client, a single person or a family, as part of the larger social setting. In relations with clients, the community nurse must also assess the family's ability to cope with the stress of its environment. Assessing economic stability, physical/social setting, safety factors, emotional climate, health practices, understanding of health problems, and responses to health problems provides a base from which to determine health needs and objectives.

The needs of a client direct the care and services offered, whether in acute care facilities or the home. Client movement from one to the other requires the coordination of all health professionals. Discharge planners are hospital based but coordinate information between hospital and home. The community nurse continues the assessment process beyond the family's coping ability to the ability of the home to meet the continued care needs of a client. Appraisal is primarily directed toward the physical/social and safety requirements set by the physical needs or limitations of the client.

Coordination of care offers the client planned assistance. The community nurse offers assistance by teaching the care necessary to sustain the client at home. The things or objectives the client feels are important to learn direct any teaching-learning activity taking place. Demonstration, repetition, explanation, and question answering lead the client to the position of informed consumer.

To maintain their own level of functioning, clients need the support system or network of care offered by family, friends, health professionals, and various agencies. The people or organizations in the system may change over the years, but informed consumers work for themselves and with others to maintain an optimum level of functioning.

REFERENCES

American National Red Cross Home Nursing Textbook, 7th ed. Prepared by Nursing Services, American National Red Cross. New York: Doubleday & Co., 1963.

BLAIR, KARYL K. "It's the Patient's Problem—and Decision." *Nursing Outlook* 19 (September 1971):587–89.

BRUNETTO, ELEANOR, and BIRK, PETER. "The Primary Care Nurse—The Generalist in a Structured Health Care Team." *American Journal of Public Health* 62 (June 1972):785–94.

COOK, MARK. *Interpersonal Perception*. Baltimore, Md.: Penguin Books, 1971.

CRAVEN, RUTH F., and SHARP, BENITA H. "The Effects of Illness on Family Functions." *Nursing Forum* 11 (1972):186–93.

Family Coping Index. Developed by JHSHPH and Richmond IVNA—City Health Department, Nursing Service. Mimeographed, Richmond, Va., January 1964.

FOND, KAREN. "Dealing With Death and Dying Through Family-Centered Care." *Nursing Clinics of North America* 7 (March 1972):53–64.

HERSHEY, NATHAN LL.B., and LAWRENCE, ROGER. "The Influence of Charting Upon Liability Determinations." *Journal of Nursing Administration* (March–April 1976):35–37.

ITTLESON, WILLIAM H., and CANTRIL, HADLEY. "Perception: A Transactional Approach." In Floyd W. Matson and Ashley Montague, eds., *The Human Dialogue*. New York: The Free Press, 1967.

JONGEWARD, DOROTHY, and SCOTT, DRU. *Women as Winners*. Menlo Park, Calif.: Addison-Wesley Publishing Co., 1976.

JOURARD, S.M. *The Transparent Self*. Princeton, N.J.: D. Van Nostrand Co., 1964.

KELLY, MARY E., and RESSLER, LINDA M. "Development of Interdisciplinary Problem-Oriented Recording in a Public Health Nursing Agency." *Journal of Nursing Administration* VI (December 1976):24–31.

LAWTON, EDITH BUCHWALD. *Activities of Daily Living for Physical Rehabilitation*. New York: The Blakiston Division, McGraw-Hill Book Co., 1963

MAGER, ROBERT F. *Preparing Instructional Objectives*. Belmont, Calif.: Fearon Publishers, 1962.

MAYERS, MARLENE. "Home Visit—Ritual or Therapy?" *Nursing Outlook* 21 (May 1973):328–31.

PAYNE, STANLEY L. *The Art of Asking Questions*, 10th ed. Princeton, N.J.: Princeton University Press, 1973.

SHEEHY, GAIL. *Passages*. New York: E. P. Dutton & Co., 1976.

SPRADLEY, BARBARA WALTON. *Contemporary Community Nursing*. Boston: Little, Brown and Co., 1975.

WEED, LAWRENCE L. *Medical Records, Medical Education and Patient Care*. Cleveland: The Press of Case Western Reserve University, 1970.

PART III

Tools for Community Health Nursing

EDITORS' INTRODUCTION

The eight chapters in this section deal with a number of tools we believe are essential for community health nurses to understand and be able to use with or on behalf of our clients. The authors define, describe, and give examples of the tools so that you will feel more competent and confident in beginning to incorporate them into your own practice.

Chapter 8: Research for Community Nursing
Ruth P. Fleshman maintains that research is a tool to harness your natural curiosity to answer nursing questions systematically. Even as a person, you can carry out investigations of problems that concern you. She discusses field methodology and questionnaires—two techniques especially useful in community settings. Writing up research is also covered since that is often so hard for us to do. Short mention is made of research critiques as well as of such research issues as informed consent, participant risk, and duress.

Chapter 9: Epidemiology and Some Applications to Primary Prevention
Basic epidemiologic principles and the role community health nurses often play in epidemiologic investigations are illustrated in the opening case study of infectious hepatitis in a nursing school's dormitory. Sarah

177

Ellen Archer and Ruth P. Fleshman discuss these principles and explore the changes in leading causes of death for the U.S. population during the twentieth century. Diseases and conditions are classified into four groups: acute infectious, chronic infectious, acute noninfectious, and chronic noninfectious. Examples of each of these kinds of diseases and conditions are given along with specific primary, secondary, and tertiary preventive measures for each one. Particular emphasis is placed in primary prevention of chronic noninfectious diseases and conditions since these are increasingly responsible for disability and death in the United States. We stress the facts that primary prevention has traditionally been the responsibility of public health and that if we in public health do not reassert the importance of primary prevention, it will continue to get short shrift to the detriment of us all. A number of terms are defined and rate formulas are given in the chapter's appendix for your use as a future reference.

Chapter 10:   Aspects of Health Education in Community Nursing
Clients make better health decisions if they operate from a firm base of knowledge. Nurses need to share health information with their clients. Ruth P. Fleshman illustrates why and how by setting out examples of health education in schools and for adults, education of consumers, and illness teaching—all distinctly different kinds of education. She presents a model for planning client-centered health education that stresses the need for incorporating clients into the process from the very start instead of deciding that we know best what they need.

Chapter 11:   Politics and Economics: How Things Really Work
Political tradeoffs and power struggles between vested interest groups are the rule as they vie for the right to make policy decisions that will affect health and medical care in the United States. Sarah Ellen Archer points out that although nurses' participation in politics has increased in recent years, we still have a long way to go before nurses have a voice in health decision making at all levels. Playing a larger role in determining what happens is in our own best interests as well as our clients' interests. Before we can play this role, however, we must understand some of the rules and the stakes. Politics determines who gets to play the decision-making games, and economics deals with the resource allocations that are outcomes of these games. Community health nursing examples are given related to the political and economic concepts described.

Chapter 12:   Health Insurance: How the United States Pays for Health Care
Sarah Ellen Archer goes to *great* length to provide background information on health insurance practices and some of their relationships

to medical care in the United States. Many terms and processes that our experience shows nurses generally do not know are discussed in this chapter. These definitions are included for ongoing reference. We need to know about health insurance to be sure that our own coverage is adequate to our needs and to be able to answer clients' questions. In many instances unless the community nurse helps clients cope with health insurance, no one else will either. A number of principles for use in evaluating the many national health program proposals that are being and will be considered during the next few years are discussed. National health service and national health insurance proposals are compared and contrasted using some of these principles. We note that this chapter is particularly dull reading for the most part and so should not be undertaken after noon or on a full stomach.

Chapter 13: Quality Assurance Programs for Health Care Delivery Systems
Patricia Porter discusses the development of quality assurance programs that have evolved both from the federal government and from professional organizations. She defines structure standards, process standards, and outcome standards as the benchmarks for developing a quality assurance program in community health nursing. She shows how the implementation of an audit system based on the standards of care developed can serve as a comprehensive evaluation tool for quality assessment and assurance. Protocols or standards and the audit tools developed from them are included as models to assist you in devising similar quality assurance aids in your own setting.

Chapter 14: Community Health Nurses in Action: A Case Study
Rural Pomo County is the setting of this case study illustrating the application of many of the concepts and tools discussed in Parts I, II, and III and operationalized in a nontraditional approach to community-based nursing. Ruth P. Fleshman's and Sarah Ellen Archer's discussion points to the importance of the wide variety of colleagues involved in community work, issues of professional and lay groups' territoriality, as well as community characteristics and how to learn about them. The chapter illustrates the interrelationships of all of these variables on the development of community health nursing services.

Chapter 15: The Community Nurse's Yellow Pages
Here Ruth P. Fleshman and Sarah Ellen Archer take on part of the monumental task we all face of finding ways to get resources and information. We suggest a basic library of books that are particularly pertinent to community health nursing. Literature review has shown which journals from the United States and other countries carry the

greatest number of community health nursing articles. We pass this information on to you. You may want to subscribe to some or all of them if they are not available in your library. Guides for using some of the common information and retrieval services are also included. Our purpose is to help you cope with the information explosion without either going broke or into orbit.

8. Research for Community Nursing

Ruth P. Fleshman

INTRODUCTION

A constant exhortation within nursing is the demand that nurses do more research so that our profession may extend its own body of knowledge. Nursing practitioners are urged to engage in or at least endorse and support nursing research activities. Students at all levels are exposed to elements of research with the suggestion that these somehow be incorporated into their subsequent work. As part of their jobs as well as a major criterion for advancement within higher education, nursing educators are expected to carry out research projects in their area of expertise for the generation of nursing theory and the advancement of the scientific basis of the practice of nursing.

There are many kinds of and methods for doing research, and the practice of lumping them all together makes talking about research difficult. Few nurses have careers as researchers and many of these actually work within someone else's project. Such nurses do not often deal with the overall plan of the project and are frequently not involved in the entire process from start to finish: proposal, funding, administration, data gathering, analysis, and reporting.

If we begin to think about how individual nurses can make use of research, the topic becomes more manageable. Instead of considering it as confined to large-scale projects, but as a way of thinking about problems,

181

we realize that research is, after all, only a way to go about asking questions that are the direct descendents of every curious child's "Why?" The main differences between research and curiosity are that research is more systematic and follows rules of logic to ask the questions: What's going on here? Why does it happen? What happens if I do this instead of that? Research is *not* fancy equipment or elaborate multiple choice questionnaires, microscopes or telescopes, rat mazes or traffic counters. It is, rather, a basic philosophy that tries to ask questions in ways that can be systematically answered so that the information can also be available to anyone who looks in the same way for the answers to those questions. Few of us involved in community nursing plan to develop careers as full-time researchers. The overriding goal of most nurses is after all related to health care for clients. Most nurses are irremediably committed to doing something about situations, not simply studying them. Thus most of us are not generally concerned with developing theories or grand conceptual frameworks for the work world we are in. However, a common criticism of nursing, as well as other action-oriented, science-based disciplines, is that we fail to use the rational tools available to us and proceed on an intuitive level. Operating this way may result in helpful courses of action but hardly contributes to the systematic improvement of either the care we deliver to our clients or our occupation. Intuition cannot be replicated.

My own experience leads me to believe that individual nurses or at the most a small group of colleagues are quite capable of identifying a researchable question and studying it on their own. In community settings there are simply too many factors operating for us to be able to carry out tightly controlled experiments and thus manipulate some manageable number of variables to test some tidy theory about human health behaviors. I find a more utilitarian approach in the kind of careful observations and descriptions of a field research approach. I can arrive at a better understanding for making my clinical decisions in community nursing if I describe and analyze what is going on than if I just wade in with a set of memorized principles of nursing intervention or with vague intuitions about what needs doing. My distrust of either rigorous experimentation or wide-ranging sensitivities as the basis for nursing actions has gotten me into trouble with some of those wholeheartedly invested in those processes. I believe neither one can solve the problems that bother me in community health or answer the questions that engage my curiosity.

We begin this discussion of research with some of the field notes and memoranda recorded by a nurse colleague in her research on nursing in one work setting, a school system. These examples show the progression she made from early observation, through some of the checking out process, to a stage of conceptualizing what she found, including some outcome recommendations for action to deal with the identified recurrent theme.

In this case, the *observation notes,* which are limited to direct observations and interview content, are typed on plain paper with a wide left-hand margin in which later comments can be recorded or in which identified themes can be noted. Attached separately on different colored paper are the other kinds of notes in the form of memos. Because this study was conducted by a nurse concerned with improving the situation for nurses, she created a category of memos labeled here *action notes.* These notes contain ideas that occur to the researcher to resolve some of the newly identified problems observed. *Theoretical notes* represent the beginning development of concepts from the events being observed, including the current speculations about what seems to underlie what's going on. *Methodological notes* are reminders the researcher records about things that need checking out or doing at some future time, or they may be comments about what tactics are being or should be used. *Analytic memos* are kept separate from any set of observation notes, although they contain keyed references to the various notes that have gone into the thinking involved. Their content is often the conceptual summation from a number of observations and theoretical notes already written. These represent the current thinking about what's going on and may well change with further work.

In the actual research project a great deal more material was written than is included here. Field researchers regularly leave their observations to spend many more hours writing down as literally as they can what has been seen and heard. Keeping detailed, concurrent narrative reports captures the immediate event for later use in considering the particulars that are the focus of the research. It is crucial that the notes—theoretical, methodological, and action—be recorded as soon as possible after they occur to you, since there is a tendency to forget or absorb ideas into your thinking in such a way that they can never be retrieved for later consideration. These notes are one way to keep a process record of how your thinking got from There to Here and what false leads you may have entertained along the way, as well as what incidents stimulated you to think of each as you went along. This method of recording is a tool of field research, a method especially used by anthropologists and sociologists studying groups of people in their own territories. It is also useful in looking at work environments, since many things go on that do not necessarily strike you at first, but after a few repetitions as in this instance, you become aware that the theme is one that has some importance to the folks on the scene.

An especially important aspect is to keep clear those observations that are filtered through our professional judgments (the action notes) and all those others that are less tainted by our nurse role. It is very hard to stop being a nurse, but as a researcher, we must be aware of when that role begins to interfere. This point is discussed again later in this chapter; we can't urge you strongly enough to try to see things with the eyes of a stranger, even on your own turf.

FIELD NOTES—SCHOOL NURSE ROLE TRANSITION STUDY

OBSERVATION NOTES

February 5: District School Nurses' Meeting with Their Supervisor. (The new program has been in effect only since the start of the school year, and although some of the nurses are holdovers from the prior system, many are new, including Mrs. Brown, the supervisor. This session is their sixth staff meeting.)

1. Mrs. Brown reports to group that another resource for getting E. H. physicals done is the Flatlands Free Clinic. Both the local health officer and the health educator had brought this possiblity to Mrs. B. Clinic hours were listed and the request that although there is no charge for patients, they are asked to give what they can.

2. Mrs. Brown next reports phone call from Mr. White, principal of City High re availability of nursing service (for accidents). Quite upset; apparently a student was injured during P.E. School secretary gave first aid then called both central administration and Mr. White (see previous notes re her wielding power). Marian felt the secretary "brags about it while she's doing it, then complains later." Janet added that "Dr. Chryst has been battling this for years. Mr. White wants us there for first aid and to hell with health ed!" Many others joined in agreement; only Anna did not. General feeling was that most (?) many (?) teachers and administrators consider that top priority for nursing time use is first aid. Several used the term "priority" to indicate that there wasn't total opposition to health ed. but that the first and most important use of nursing time is to take care of minor problems, then referral and/or defect follow-up, and then if there's any time left over, health ed. Millie added with much heat, "Mr. White said we don't need any more *socialization.* We have psychologists and guidance people socializing all the time; we don't need any more people." This met with quite an outcry from the rest of the group. "Is that what he thinks we do?" "Socializing?!" "What?!" etc. Mrs. B. indicated that she planned to meet with all the secondary principals next week because a number of them seem to feel that first aid is the top priority. "I expect a bloody battle! I'm going to take on my boss." (One of the nurses asked "Who *is* your boss?" and Mrs. B. explained.)

3. Discussion of just-ended hearing and vision screening program;

nurses complained testers worked too quickly, did not give child time to respond with different pictures than they had been prepared for. Failure rate of 20 percent in vision tests was judged average in screening. Hearing tester reported rude to children and parent volunteers although some nurses (Linda and Millie) agreed behavior of children justified firmness.

4. Discussion then turned to interminable consideration (1 hour +) of report from the "Sunshine Committee." They wanted $10 limit for gift at each staff illness . . . .

ACTION NOTE

Memo: Is there possibility that if a nurse was able to convey to staff that she is not opposed to doing first aid and will do it on a screened demand but that priority rankings might be reevaluated *together,* that it would foster some resolution of what seems to be a role conflict?

THEORETICAL NOTE

Memo: There seems to be little communication between school staff and individual nurses in terms of working out problems of role perception. When there is dissatisfaction, a call is made to supervisor or central administration rather than approach the nurse herself.

METHODOLOGICAL NOTE

Memo: Need to verify this pattern. May want to ask nurses hypothetical question; ask Mrs. Brown directly.

OBSERVATION NOTES

March 12: Interview with Nurse #9. . . . Sometimes the secretary does have to take over for band-aiding things but if I let her gripe at me personally then she doesn't complain to the principal.

April 21: Interview with Nurse #17. . . . This principal feels that my primary responsibility is first aid. He doesn't mean that I should be here to give it all the time, but that it's my responsibility to see that someone is there at all times who can. As long as that runs smoothly, I can do anything else. *But as soon as that breaks down then he sees the other things as inappropriate.*

ANALYTIC MEMO

Memo: At this stage of developing the new nurse role, they were trying to teach first aid classes to school staff who were, after all, on the site all the time the children were, unlike the nurses who rotate among three or more schools.

ACTION NOTE

Memo: Need for Assistant or Delegation of First Aid. If the nurse is to operate in program planning, developing health ed., serve as resource, get acquainted with staff and community, it was felt that it is essential to have some form of assistance in the health office to relieve the nurse from the innumerable demands on her to take care of minor cuts and bruises, excuses, sending home of ill students, etc. This was seen as a necessary part of a health office as perceived by some (not all) of the nurses and almost all of the school staff, therefore cannot be ignored. As long as this is taken care of, the nurse can utilize her time in other areas more appropriate to the program directions.

ANALYTIC MEMOS

Memo: Health Assistant Job Priorities. So far, of the three interviewed, "first aid" was mentioned first. The idea seems prevalent that the health assistant is a "catch all" for problems, needs, advice, praise, interest re: children, etc. Minnie seemed to feel that teachers can do more to screen before sending children. Marian feels this serves a more basic need and a natural part of the nurses' office function; she called it a "comfort station," particularly when the school district is undergoing educational changes, program trials, integration, etc.

Memo: Role of Health Assistant. Minnie feels they are "closer to the children" and "impartial" because they do not evaluate the children as do the teachers. So this may be the reason children feel free to approach them with problems. "We do anything that will meet the needs of the child." (Including letting them use phone for personal calls, sewing torn clothes, etc.) The idea comes to my mind that a nurse and/or the assistant may be thought of as a "child advocate" or a "pupil advocate."

Memo: Job Priority of Health Assistants as a Group. Since interviewing eleven of the twelve permanent health assistants (one is temporary and one is out with oral surgery, but will interview her as soon as possible).

First aid or minor ministrations for injuries and common ailments (which they all seem to lump under the term "first aid"), is seen to be the main reason for the health assistant to be in the nursing office in the schools. This was not necessarily seen as part of relieving the nurse for other responsibilities but rather the primary reason for being there. They are aware that the nurses should be contacted if an extreme emergency arose that they could not handle. But this was fairly rare as parents are always called to take responsibility for seeking medical care for anything too severe to be within the health assistant's purview.

DISCUSSION

This particular project went on for many more months and covered a great deal of the interactions between nurses and their hierarchy, the school system, the students and their parents, and the community in general. These small elements from within a larger set of observations were chosen to show how a theme can be followed over time. The first action memo suggested one possible idea of how to resolve an issue of role conflict, but as was apparent later, this solution was not seen by the nurses as the way to go. The methodological note included the researcher's instruction to herself to check out a pattern she thought was emerging, and before long, she learned more from another nurse of one way to keep the flak under control. By the end of the first year of the new program, clearly neither the nurses nor the principals could reach consensus on a nurse role that does not take into account the administration of first aid. There were many sessions when the nurses tried to explain that if mothers can band-aid their children, any school staff member should be as well qualified with a short course on minor emergencies. But with a few exceptions, this solution was not acceptable; hence, the suggestion in the next action memo for someone designated "first aider." After that program was proposed, funded, and initiated, the researcher began to look at how these new workers defined their jobs.

Unlike the response to the innovative nurse role, there was quick and complete agreement that first aid (however that was defined) was the main job of the health assistant. There was no conflict here: The nurses didn't want to do it, the health assistants did, and the school staff had someone around all the time to whom they could send all the minor health problems they didn't want to deal with. Also of interest was seeing a new theme emerge from the interviews and later become a large element in understanding why nurses are often used by the children as nonjudgmental sources of solace. The health staff, like the school janitor who is also another major mental health resource for pupils, are not in the business of grading students or, for the most part, in sending reports home to parents about student problems. Thus, the researcher could begin to establish the attributes necessary for a successful advocate within the school system.

THE RESEARCH PROCESS

We would be foolhardy to try to present a recipe for research in such a brief space. The language used is often specific to various forms of research and the details of procedure, sampling, measuring, and evaluating are far too weighty for justice to be done them here. Instead, in this chapter we want to try to generalize the process as it might occur for any community nurse. The examples from my own experience illustrate how it actually did. Although some projects begin with formation of hypotheses, proposing something quite that formal, especially in community settings, often seems premature. This reason is why field research that tries to describe complex, ongoing situations is a method that appeals strongly to my own sense of how to find out enough to get about the business of being a community nurse.

BEGINNING QUESTIONS AND ENTRY

The decision to carry out any research project almost always starts from some question or set of questions that are bothersome because you can't come up with easy answers, or the answers that are usually given don't quite fit. You've found an "intellectual itch" that's hard to scratch. Once you decide what the question really is, you start looking for ways to find answers. This process often leads you to realize that the original question isn't quite "it" or that there are other questions that need answering first. Sometimes discovering the other questions can be done simply by thinking through the logic of what you want to answer. Some questions are simply not amenable to research. This is particularly true of questions involving philosophical or moral issues: "Should we keep severely handicapped people alive?" "Is premarital sex right?" As immediately becomes clear, such questions cannot be answered short of direct revelation. However, it is possible to rethink them in terms of "What groups of people believe what different things about the various aspects of whatever issue is being studied?" or "What are the various arguments used for, against, or around an issue?"

Similarly, the kind of question asked may be generated from thinking about some larger problem. In one graduate research project, I was, for instance, concerned about ways to improve the service delivered to health care clients. We decided that a frequent barrier might be the difference in social class between clients and health professionals. We asked the question, "If we wanted to look at this phenomenon, where would we try to observe it?" Clearly, asking clients and professionals directly would not be helpful for a number of reasons, including the time that would be needed to define and defend the notion of social class. Direct observation of interactions between physicians and clients of lower social class would reveal data that could be contrasted with such interactions with clients of similar social class. Where, however, would such interactions be observable? Physicians' offices are not easily accessible to casual observation. Besides, physician-client exchanges are privileged communications. Further, my own experience with outpatient services might interfere with the freshness with which I might be able to view interactions. So some hospital setting seemed appropriate and a county emergency service the most productive of a wide range of clients of various social origins.

LEGITIMATION

It is one thing to select a possible site for research and quite another to make your way into it. The first step is a thinking process that proves to yourself the legitimacy of trying to do such a thing. For example, in my project described above, as a learner, I could justify that I needed practice in field observation within a medical institution (since all my prior exercises had been deliberately carried on in entirely different settings to prevent clouding my observations with old assumptions about what was going on). I would know enough as a nurse to keep out of the way when things got really frantic; occasionally I have been bothered on my job by naive researchers getting underfoot when I had better things to do than deal with their priorities. At the county hospital I could honestly claim enough ignorance to prevent being pressed into service since I was indeed on strange territory. After thinking this through, I presented myself to the director of nurses and explained my purpose: to observe what went on between patients and professionals in an emergency room. Her commitment to teaching students led her to approve my proposed period of observation with the clear understanding that I was to avoid participating in any care because I was not employed by that hospital. It was agreed that open explanation of what I was observing would alter the behavior of those I wished to observe, so when she introduced me to the unit's head nurse, the purpose she stated was even more general than the one I had given her. I was planning, she said, to observe patient behavior in emergency situations, which carefully omitted the professional half of the interaction. Making such observations in a formal research project would be far more difficult if not impossible today because of the stress laid upon the rights of subjects to approve being used for research. I think such a learning exercise is as legitimate an enterprise now as it was then, especially since no action was ever taken on the basis of the observations I made and recorded.

I always wore a white lab coat with a name pin identifying me only as Mrs. Ruth Fleshman, R.N. I carried a clipboard with note paper since I knew there would be long stretches of time when I could not leave to catch up with my field notes. Thus I could jot down topics, key phrases, and other memoranda that would help me later to call the scene back into memory. I did not expect my standing around writing to be seen as unusual since many other people made notes on a variety of subjects as part of their own jobs around the hospital.

Having come through proper channels and having been endorsed by the administrative hierarchy seemed to confer acceptance. Staff people were introduced to me by name with no notion of my mission. It was only after I had been hanging around about two-and-a-half weeks, asking casual questions, becoming part of the landscape, and appearing on all the shifts for long enough to get to know the staff members, that a few of the staff began to realize that they didn't actually understand what I was there for anyway. Only then did I begin to get questions that, interestingly enough, followed the pattern, "Now what was it you said you were doing?" even though I had never said anything. I always carefully avoided the word research since I considered that to carry a threat; I stressed that I was a graduate *student* (students are always harmless), that I was carrying out a project (projects aren't *real*), that I was studying patients (and everyone knows how important *they* are). Almost any one of these answers sufficed, and seemingly a reassuring tone was more important than the content of my answers. The fact that nothing bad seemed to happen as a result of my hanging around added to their feelings of reassurance. That I always deferred to their expertise put them in a one-up position over me so they could teach me what they felt was "really going on," which thus provided a great deal of information about the ways they viewed their patients. Observing the ways they treated various kinds of patients also showed the ways in which they either reinforced or masked their privately revealed beliefs. Thus, although I could not give them any direct benefit from my presence, I could provide a chance for staff members to teach me, which is often an ego reward in itself. I provided an opportunity for the various professionals to blow off steam about events, individuals, or other work groups they were upset about. Even unit nurses had the chance to feel superior to another nurse who obviously didn't know anything about what they knew, even though she was a graduate student. Playing the one-down to their one-up was no threat to me since I wasn't in competition with them for status in that system. By remaining an ambiguous figure, I could be relatively invisible; adopting the multipurpose lab coat uniform made me seem a part of the system even though the R.N. on my name tag made clear I was not a part of that hospital's image of nursing. I frequently discussed work-based examples from my outpatient experience so there was never a sense that I was a rank beginner. Doing so gave me some credibility and reduced my getting the kind of putdown that undergraduate students often experience. As an identified student, however, I could also enter into casual conversation with the two senior students on affiliation from a nearby hospital school and draw them out about their views of the doctor-patient interactions.

Now, of course, I can no longer use the marvelously nonthreatening passport of studenthood to aid my entry. However, I have learned the similar value that most people attach to that other identity that is mine to use: being a nurse. There are times when I cannot accept the one-downing that occurs when told I'm *"only* a nurse" or that I "seem smarter than *most* nurses" or even "what kind of a nurse *are* you?" Most people perceive nurses as thoroughly helping people, will openly discuss the widest range of intimate personal and social problems, and ask the most revealing questions. However, they seem to expect that nurses will have wonderfully expert advice to give not only for things physical but for a whole array of experiential matters generally not recognized as a part of the art and science of nursing! By the time they realize I'm not the white cap and starched uniform type, it's already too late. That I am studying health problems that seem to be a bother to them is seen not as a snoopy research project, but as the probable base for some future action to be taken to make things better for them. In addition, my being a nurse enables me to pay back their openness and hospitality with useful information about how to deal with problems they have right now. A sociologist friend admits he envies my profession since he feels "advancement of knowledge" is a pale excuse for his research into the lifestyle of commune dwellers.

FIELD NOTES

RECORDING

While the situation you've observed is still vivid in your mind, it's vital to get as much as possible down on paper in full detail. Of course, it's not possible to record everything—even a tape recorder on the scene won't catch the visual images or the interactional patterns. But the sooner you record your observations, the less likely you are to lose content. The human mind begins to try to organize events on the basis of its own past definitions and, given a chance, will try to do so with observations of new and wonderful events. For this reason newcomers to any scene don't see things the same way oldtimers do. New nurses in their attempts to question procedures and methods are often put down as naive, inexperienced, and unthinking. Experiencing things from a research perspective suggests that, contrary to what they believe, often the oldtimers are the ones who don't understand what's really going on. Newcomers have a fresh perspective that can provide the basis for insights, or at least searching questions about situations that might benefit from being rethought. (It is often unwise, however, to come sailing into a new job full of bright notions about how things *ought* to be done and believing that as a change agent you can get them that way; this approach is sure to create trouble!)

Field notes, especially in the beginning of a project, should contain as much as possible of what you observed in using your full array of senses. Even when you don't understand the meaning of details, they can often later prove to be rich sources of information since you won't be imposing your own definition and may well catch details that no insider would have looked for. For the school district nurses discussed earlier, first aid was only a recurrent annoyance, a disliked task that kept interfering with the professional tasks they valued more highly. The researcher, however, could identify first aid as an issue that exemplified role conflict between the nurses and the perceptions of how nurses ought to operate held by the school staff members.

In addition to actual observations, it is important to keep notes on the various strategies used to get at the observations. It has been a matter of great interest to me to see the value of costume in gaining entry. In studying the conflicts between a county health agency and an illegal communal group, for example, I adopted two separate images—little-old-lady clothes and jeans-and-workshirt—as my passports to acceptance in each area. In the emergency room situation, a white lab coat and clipboard made me almost invisible to the entire staff there.

Emerging ideas of explanation for events should also be included as they occur but kept separate both in your thinking and your recording. In the examples presented earlier, the theoretical note at the end of the first staff meeting recorded such material.

At first, getting even a part of the events down is very hard, but after a while, your memory begins to improve. In my own experience, I have noticed that I almost begin to feel as if the images were flowing straight out of my memory through my fingers to the typewriter. It takes a lot of both time and energy to do such intensive recording, so it's vital not to overload in the field situation. At first, an hour or two seemed all I could manage and still get the recording done. The temptation is to stay "just a little bit longer," but you soon learn what your limits are. Procrastination in recording notes is attractive since field notes are so time consuming. But it defeats the whole purpose of observing because a later attempt to recall is irremediably colored by your present stage of understanding of what's going on.

Technically, the notes should be typed since legibility is so important. Dictating onto tapes can be a time-saver, but these must be transcribed, which is costly in time or, if a typist is hired, in money. As with any motor skill, you can learn to type at least as fast as you can write, with the added benefit of having your notes readable by someone else. Leave wide margins on the left side since you will be making notes, comments, and code entries there. Be sure to double space the typing, since reading single-spaced material is killing on the eyes. Make at least two copies, one of which is left unmarked for future reference and in some place other than the first copy. One copy should be designated for use in analysis. The reason for the second copy may seem pretentious, but all researchers know of at least one heartbreaking incident of someone's lifetime of data being wiped out by a fire, burglary, or overzealous housecleaning. More than one copy means a copious supply of paper, which may seem wasteful, especially if you're on a tight budget. But there's a world of recyclable paper that can be reversed and used to good economy and good ecology!

The necessity of recording field notes also requires you to pull back from the field, which can be a welcome aid to your mental health. Too prolonged exposure to an emotionally loaded field experience can be so draining that a fair amount of time is needed to recuperate. During my four-year study of communes and health education, our sojourns to country locations were almost always followed by a week or so of R & R while we healed up in preparation for the next foray. One of the reasons I bought a battered camper for my own use was to provide an on-site spot of privacy from the overwhelming togetherness. I could also use it as a place to record my field notes as well as hit up a little meat before joining the vegetarians in the commune for their soybean dinners.

Gradually, as observations continue, that human trait of pattern making begins to emerge and the curious researcher begins to come up with themes, common or similar events, and a growing feeling that certain things go together. These notes differ from the sort of thing you were including within the field notes in that they are more inclusive, perhaps by beginning to be more clearly thought out, and will incorporate material from more than one set of observations, as a rule. Thus they are attached to no one set of field notes but are properly a separate part of the analysis process. One method often used to keep these separate is to type such memos on different colored paper (again two copies at least) and file them separately from field notes and each other. Cross-referencing these memos to the specific field notes is important so that later the observations on which they were based can be located. I head all my notes with the date and locale and, if significant, the time of day and people involved.

TALKING ABOUT DATA

The emergence of themes is hastened by regular review of notes and their discussion with someone else. Verbalizing about raw data often improves the likelihood of detecting interesting or useful patterns. That other person, however, can't just be any old somebody. Relying on someone who is a part of the "field" being observed is not helpful and may prove harmful. Their perceptions of events are restricted by their having an insider's definition of the situation and would only tend to repeat interpretations of observations already gathered. It might also lead to feedback into the field that could jeopardize your ability to continue to observe or might well create changes in behavior of others in the field. When studying turnover rates among hospital nurses, for example, I identified a pattern I labeled *touristry*—that is, the ability to move among attractive areas of the world by relying on a certificated job skill in high demand (Pape 1964). I found I could not talk about the emerging concept with other nurses since they considered it pointless to analyze something that "everybody already knows about." My sociologist colleagues with whom I did discuss it found touristry a fascinating example of geographic mobility.

The other person should not be someone who is in a position to interfere with the flow of events in the field. One hope of the field observer is to be as invisible as possible so as to exert little effect on the "natural" course of action. Of course, the mere presence of an observer or even another body has some effect, but a field researcher should try to minimize this effect or at least take it into account. In one instance, I had been studying the conflicting views between an official health agency and a community whose lifestyle violated some of the county health ordinances. I had thought to use one of my neighbors as a sounding board since he was neither a part of the community group nor a part of the local health system. However, he became so enraged at what began to look like an impending crackdown that he began to talk about pulling a Paul Revere act and rush off to save the people. With some difficulty I talked him out of that and found someone else for subsequent discussions. Needless to say, the other person must understand the need for confidentiality and be able to avoid talking about your research with others. In addition to these limits, the co-discussant should be able to understand the research perspective and differences between it and the usual way nurses operate.

In pursuing research in its pure form, the researcher attempts to gather data without influencing the course of events—to be an observer without participating in the activity—which is, of course, impossible except in theory. On the other hand, nurses are committed to intervene in the health concerns of clients whenever there is some quantity of information to indicate in which direction action would be most helpful. On a simple level, nurses and other practitioners must generally act on the basis of incomplete data or risk never acting at all. Researchers only have a commitment to gather as much information as possible. For them, data gathering can go on a lifetime without any necessity of devising an intervention from it. There can be a problem when nurses adopt a research stance and are then confronted with a situation when they must choose between observation and participation. My three-month observation stint in an emergency room highlighted this dilemma for me since many events were going on which I alone observed and about which, as a nurse, I felt a pull to take action. For example, I felt a nursing obligation to report the time at which an unattended dying man finally ceased breathing. Since I was, however, an observer and not a staff member, I considered it more productive to wait to see how long it was before the staff noticed and what processes they went through in deciding how to fill out the necessary forms. In struggling with the decision, however, I had to ask some hard questions about what difference any action on my part would make, and deciding there was nothing important I could do anyway, I opted for the nonintervention tack.

On the other hand, visiting a commune where a child was clearly very ill, there was no question in my mind of leaving the process unimpeded, and I spent a lot of time persuading the parents and other family members of my concern for the safety of the child and eventually got them to accept my definition of the situation, at least to the point that they took the child to a local physician. That they did not follow up on his referral for heart surgery and instead chose to pray over the baby until it died upset me. But, in view of the realistic alternatives open to me, I considered I had made the best contribution I could to the parents' decision, and they as well as I had to accept the outcome. They, at least, had a continued religious faith to justify their actions. Having a sociologist as preceptor was often helpful in maintaining the research view in the face of my own pull toward intervention. However, he could not always understand the strength or direction of this pull since he did not share my perspective as a practitioner. In this instance, I was exceedingly fortunate to have a nurse-sociologist available to me to help wrestle through to an understanding of the dilemma. Having experienced the dilemma herself, she not only helped me interpret the experience but provided me with methods of coping with its impact.

ANALYZING FIELD DATA

Purely descriptive material risks being regarded as merely anecdotal unless steps are taken to move from specifics to varying levels of abstraction. Processes by which this move may be accomplished are described in a variety of references from anthropology and sociology (Narol and Cohen 1973; Glaser and Strauss 1967:61–115; Schatzman and Strauss 1973:108–27).

The rich material recorded by Terkel in *Working* (1972) and by Lewis (1961, 1968) in his books about poverty families is only focused by the selection made of what was to be printed. Lewis, at least, includes methodological notes and has the implicit assumptions of anthropology to aid in explaining his records. Part of the exhilaration of reading unanalyzed field notes, however, is the "ah-ha" phenomenon that accompanies the awareness of one's own insights; the "analysis" is left to the reader's own ability to see patterns.

In general, analysis is the process of imposing logical patterns on the mass of observed action and maintaining records to enable these patterns to be tried out on still other examples of action. Such analysis, in essence, is the way that hypothesis-formation and prediction can be seen in field method. If your explanatory pattern does indeed reflect what's actually going on, you should be able to look for other field experiences where it would also hold true. In my analysis of turnover rates among hospital staff nurses, I identified what seemed to me to be occupational conditions that made touristry possible for nurses. To test these, I looked for the same conditions in other occupations whose members could also travel on the basis of their work skills (Pape 1964).

At the first level of abstraction, analysis aims to identify categories or classes of events by tying apparently disparate actions into groups that share certain identified characteristics. Thus, making a first home visit to a new family, figuring out a way to become a volunteer in a community agency, and persuading research subjects that you are not dangerous to them as a researcher are all events in the category of "entry into a field." Once this notion is clear, you can look for its attributes and detect conditions that ease or make it more difficult—in the situation, in the enterer, or in the persons whose territory is being entered. Considering other examples of the same class of action, entry, can both sharpen the delineation of that category and reveal unexpected attributes that had escaped earlier notice. Analysis is where those lengthy field notes really pay off, because you can go back and see recorded behaviors or events that were not meaningful at the time, but that now contribute to better understanding of the abstracted event you have just identified. These are the early stages of the processes that generate grounded theory (Glaser and Strauss 1967).

Although research reports may give vast amounts of information about final conclusions reached from a project, they seldom give any inkling of the process gone through to arrive at those conclusions. Many writeups sound as if the researchers knew exactly what they would end up proving and just set about methodically doing so. This process is simply a convention of scientific reporting—no project I have ever heard about proceeds from sure knowledge to sure conclusion in any significant area of research, or there would have been no need to do the study in the first place. Some other researchers give the impression that they went into a strange field with absolutely no prior assumptions, which is actually a human impossibility. Even anthropologists studying the most alien or primitive cultures come with overriding assumptions and theories of their trade or they wouldn't even know where to begin their study. For example, "learning language is the essential tool in understanding interactions," is already a research assumption, since they know that is not why babies learn to speak or, for that matter, why diplomats and businessmen learn another tongue.

Most field method studies, however, include only enough material on methodology to suggest the successful strategies used to get the material reported. In some instances unsuccessful ones are recounted as well, thereby providing negative examples for all our profit. In any case, it is likely that the kind of research we are doing as community nurses has some relationship to our clients' functioning levels or the institutions in which they are receiving their health care. We may unearth fascinating discoveries during research, but our overriding assumptions are tied to our professional goals that are very hard to eliminate.

WHY DO RESEARCH?

Our exploratory or descriptive research can have a number of possible outcomes. At the first level of abstraction, it can provide one answer to the question "What is going on here?" The response can be directly used as the data base for action in the health care arena. We are after all committed to some intervention and need to get on with the job. Such descriptive material may well provide a base for planning change in the studied community since we can continue to gather information about changes as they occur and the adaptation needed to deal with them, both by client groups and workers.

These kinds of data can also provide the beginning from which hypotheses may be generated for more formal or extensive testing. This process comprises a respectable portion of the research game and is often part of academic preparation for advanced degrees or teaching roles in universities. Clinical research in communities, however, cannot generally be subjected to the rigorous controls deemed necessary for high level scientism. Thus, you might guess that there is some conflict between experimental and descriptive researchers and you'd be right. The same goes for the differences between "pure and applied," "laboratory and field," "quantitative and qualitative." But that's one of the things that makes research interesting; if we all thought, investigated, and wrote alike, wouldn't the world be dull!

WRITING UP THE STUDY

Even when the whole process of investigation, recording, and analysis has been completed, there is still one more stage before your project can be considered complete. Up to this point, what has been described is simply a variation on problem solving or nursing process or whatever jargon term is used to describe how any practitioner goes about attempting a rational approach to practice. If you are simply satisfying your own curiosity, you now go on about your business and use what you have found. The stage that finally converts your project to some bigger arena is that of sharing the whole thing with interested others. A project small in scope—a more effective nursing tool, a particular intervention applicable to local circumstances, and so on—may be shared with fellow workers in a single unit. Nursing is not, however, only a local profession and there are people involved in similar activities nationwide. Hence, the most common way of sharing information is writing about it and getting it published. All you have to do is scan the nursing journals to realize that their contributors are not professional writers. Even educators who get special points for publishing tend to be stylistically anesthetic. The writing of nurses working in service settings is technically precise but seldom stimulating. This situation is not entirely our fault since the scientific writing market quickly squelches any attempts by writers to do anything but present information in a bare-bones style.

As with all the communication media, there has been an exploding number of professional nursing journals, each geared for somewhat different audiences. All look to nurses for content. But writing is another area where nurses have inordinate problems. Editors, literate educators, and nursing writers all complain about the difficulties nurses have in producing written materials. In what may seem a long jump from research, let's look briefly at why this situation may be so.

Consider the major writing activity that most nurses engage in: nursing notes. Nurses are drilled in keeping them thoroughly devoid of personal style, reducing them to a minimum of language, and sacrificing grammar, punctuation, and logic for a ritual formula of nonevaluative reporting. Students are well known and often criticized for writing too much, and the goal of nursing notes seems to be the irreducible minimum that proves somebody noticed the patient on each shift or proves that the nurse did visit and give service for which the agency can be reimbursed. The role of nursing notes in contributing to patient care is clearly demonstrated by such facts as follows: They seldom form a part of the required reading for physicians or other nurses catching up on patient progress; they are usually removed from the patient's file when it is permanently stored; charting is one area consistently raised by nurses complaining about job dissatisfactions. Such factors as these make charting a devalued activity, which further diminishes the effort expended on it. The quality of charting spills over into the entire area of writing as far as most nurses are concerned.

Communication skills and problems are repeatedly identified as dilemmas in nursing (as well as the rest of the modern world!) but stress is continually placed on the verbal portion of communication. One-to-one, nurse-patient interactions are so heavily emphasized that face-to-face conversations may seem to be the major content of nursing, to the extent that telephone discussion of health problems has become less legitimate than the same content transmitted in a home visit—time consuming as that may be. Concentration on spoken communication may well detract from the ability to present material in the formal, academic, or even journalistic format since conversation depends on interactional cues from the other person and does not proceed from start to finish along an internally consistent path. A written article requires an introduction, presentation, exposition, and conclusion. It must present all the points concisely and clearly so as to be understood by a reader who does not already know what the author is trying to say. Unlike in a conversation, a reader cannot express lack of understanding or ask questions. Due to conditioning, many nurses appear unable to sustain a single line through a whole article without receiver-feedback.

Some part of this problem may be due to the need for nurses to find validation in the willingness of others to continue listening. Many nurses feel their knowledge is of low value—"if *I* know it, everybody else does too"—because of the usual location of nurses with the hospital hierarchy. So many more important people seem to know so much more than most nurses in a given situation that it is easy to extrapolate to the whole world. You may harbor this illusion until you discover how little people know about health when you get to teaching them (see chapter 10).

Another factor is the lack of reward for writing in the usual nursing system. A few universities are rethinking the publish-or-perish dictum, although nursing educators may be the last to find out. Student papers generally are written only to meet the criteria of particular faculty assignments, and few are even considered for a wider audience. This result is especially likely if students are assumed incapable of original or creative thinking, and are required to search the literature for documentation of every thought. Service agencies are geared even less to writing than to the reflective time needed for research. Even when there is value attached to sharing information or expertise with one's peers, agencies often assume these are limited to those within the agency and so communication can be done face to face in that oral route that is travelled in a conference or, at most, a nursing workshop. Any writing, in the majority of nursing jobs, is to be done on private time and fueled entirely by internal drive. This factor and the emphasis on conversationality may be reasons there are so few role models for readable yet communicative nursing literature; material is either dully academic or trivially chatty and consequently is rarely read, let alone incorporated into nursing practice.

There are two approaches to learning to write that may be helpful in different ways. There are books dealing with the technicalities of writing: proper citation format, construction of sentences, paragraphs, sections or chapters, punctuation and spelling, and so on. These are especially valuable references for preparing footnotes and bibliographies since they indicate the different arrangements used by various disciplines, including scientific journals. Among the easiest and clearest is Strunk and White, *Elements of Style*. For another reference, consult the University of Chicago Press, *Manual of Style*. But if by style you mean those distinctive elements that suggest the individuality of the writer, manuals are little help. Individual style is developed only with time and practice. To begin, look widely at excellent prose in a variety of forms: novels, plays, essays, and so on. If you know one author really well, compare that one's writings with another's on the same subject, and you'll begin to get a feel for the ways "real" writers express their personalities with words. Long-time writers also suggest that there is a strong factor in practicing; they advise young aspirants to write some set amount every day, even if it's only a diary account of events.

Even if you develop an appreciation for good writing style, you may find few professional journals are interested in it. However, to help decide where you might like to be published, you should scan the journals serving audiences you would like to reach. Leafing through a few issues of each will show you the layout of articles and topics each is publishing, as well as the particular style each considers appropriate. Go and do likewise.

A traditional approach in writing about research is to avoid employing personal identification by whatever means necessary. When a person *must* be referred to, awkward terms like "the author" or "the investigators" are preferred. Actually the standard method is to use the passive voice. In this form, the sentence does not have an active subject—not "I searched the literature for . . ." but "the literature was searched for . . . ." It is almost impossible to carry off this style of writing without using many more words to end up making the same sense you would otherwise. When writing research studies, the passive tense is nevertheless the preferred construction. But because it is stylistically tedious, you should try to avoid it at all other times, partly because it is awkward and partly because we tend to get wordy anyway and passive voice doesn't help that. Other writing conventions can be garnered by watching for them as you read the journals.

Nursing journals and publishers of nursing texts do receive unsolicited manuscripts and publish them. A colleague calls these "over the transom articles." This way of proceeding, however, is usually not the most efficient, unless your burning urge to write cannot be extinguished by rejection letters. Editors suggest instead that you write to appropriate journals, for example, with a clear outline of the article you wish to write and ask whether they would be interested in examining the article itself with an eye toward publishing it. This procedure cuts down on the time needed to make a successful contact since sending a single manuscript to more than one possible publisher at a time is not ethical, while many letters of inquiry can go out. The result may be a number of positive replies, which happy situation would permit you to choose the best possible one, if quality is your aim; if quantity is a goal, you could write separate articles on the same material but aiming for the particularities of the different audiences served by each specialized journal.

The notion of audience may not always be kept clearly enough in mind. You should consider the different perspectives brought to reading an article by a nursing administrator, an operating room staff nurse, a nurse-researcher, or a public health nurse. Difference of perspective is one reason why each of these would, hopefully, read the particular journals directed to their specialty. Each journal contains information in very small type somewhere near the front about addresses to which letters or manuscripts may be sent. Some contain specific instructions to authors about preparation of manuscripts: width of margins, footnote and reference style, charts and illustrations. If this information is not specifically indicated, check several issues to get a clearer idea of these technicalities and of the areas of current concern and the probable biases in the journal's audience. Certain research publications, for example, are routinely cluttered with graphs, charts, and mathematical symbols. Others deal with case histories, patient examinations, and clinical specifics. Neither one would be the most appropriate recipient of a report about nurse role conflict such as came from the data recorded at the start of this chapter. In all certainty, a journal will reject material that is old hat to its audience. An article that presents a completely opposite viewpoint to the orthodoxy of the audience might also have a hard time being accepted. For example, the *American Journal of OB-GYN* would be unlikely to take an article advocating home deliveries! Very few journals pay contributors (although some will give a limited number of free reprints), so don't plan to make a living doing journal articles.

A problem for novice writers is overattachment to their own deathless prose. Editors' suggestions for revisions or, worse yet, deletions can become a major trauma. There seems to be a general expectation among many beginners that producing the first draft is the last effort that must be made. Actually, that draft should only be viewed as the first of many steps of rewriting, and the editing process in general should be seen as polishing and trimming to an eventual end product. The white heat of inspiration may do for poets and humorists, but even the best of those rewrite to achieve the appearance of an off-hand style. Some of my casual acquaintances are sure I write chapters like this one straight from my own conversation. Actually, arriving at such a casual tone has taken many agonizing rewrites!

Few people write easily. If the services of a professional editor are not available to you, giving your more-or-less finished material to a couple of other people to read is of some help. Another nurse may be helpful since there are times when you get so close to material that it no longer makes sense to someone else in the profession. Questions to ask then would be: "Does it make sense?" "Am I telling you what I want to say?" "Are there giant holes in my logic, obvious things I didn't think of?" Another person can help with the more general task of checking your manuscript for proofreading problems (I sometimes think nurses are among the world's worst spellers). With either task, someone fresh to your material provides a better evaluation than you or someone else equally immersed in the topic can.

Once you get past the shock of someone else chopping at your material, you can often see the value an incisive editor can bring—by rearranging the order of your points, by eliminating redundancies, and by suggesting more precise or attention-getting synonyms. Sometimes simply asking what your intention is becomes necessary since it is unclear as written. We often recommend that our students read and edit each other's papers before they do the final copy which will be submitted.

We all realize that writing is often difficult and tedious. However, it is one of our major ways of communicating ideas economically to people over a distance. Too many of us have been conditioned to believe that we cannot write. Writing, like other skills, comes with practice. Many nurses have excellent ideas and experiences that need to be made available to others. We have a professional and personal obligation to communicate these ideas to advance our profession. Further, it is incumbent on each of us to help our colleagues improve their skills and gain confidence in writing, through our support and constructive criticism. All of us were beginners at some point; some of us were assisted in our endeavors by teachers and colleagues. Others of us continue to write in spite of less than helpful and sometimes destructive comments from other nurses. We hope *you* find helpful colleagues. Good luck.

QUESTIONNAIRES

There are a multitude of research methods appropriate to many different research questions, and theoretically we should be equally prepared to use whatever suits the situation. Reality doesn't often work out that way and some researchers become so comfortable with a few methods that they are limited in the kinds of questions they can even ask. Gathering data to plan community services or learning specific facts from a large number of people are examples of research that really cannot be done with in-depth interviews or field observations, if only because of the numbers involved. Questionnaires are a valuable tool for this aim, and the need may arise to use one. Examples of such times in community nursing include gathering and updating facts from agencies for an information and referral service or agency directory, collecting data on client needs, attitudes, practices, and reactions, or randomly surveying selected clients to evaluate the services they have received. Questionnaires may be sent and returned by mail or administered face-to-face or by telephone.

Many novices think it very easy to go after bulk information by jotting down a list of questions and passing them out to everyone in sight. But a lot of projects founder on such misconceptions. Again, giving you all the details in a short space isn't possible; whole chapters in methodology texts are devoted to test construction alone (Payne 1951; Seltiz et al. 1965).

Designing the actual form is probably the hardest part of the whole process. Importantly, the wording should be clear, unambiguous, simple enough to be understood by the expected audience, able to reveal real differences among respondents, and unlikely to offend or otherwise cause harm. The only way to find out is to test the questionnaire with people much like those who will be taking it. That means trying it on someone else, because even though *you* can easily understand what you mean, the ability of an outsider or a nonprofessional to figure out what you're asking is a whole different thing. The questions must allow people to have a real choice among answers; the response choices must not put down people with different beliefs or practices from what you would prefer. Keeping the questions simple is also very important; be sure you don't ask two or more questions in the same item. We've all had the experience of finding a question we have to answer true or false when part is true and part is false, and that's the kind of question that doesn't get answered! Many people find multiple or forced choice questionnaires to be a depersonalized way to give information and may resent the lack of opportunity to express their own opinions or unique perspective. This problem can be avoided sometimes if you include one or more items that solicit their comments about whatever is being considered, if only about the test instrument itself.

Once you get past a very few questions or a very small number of respondents, the problem of analyzing the responses often becomes far too complicated to manage without the aid of computer technology. Simply counting responses is fine, but if you want to begin to compare and contrast answers and the kinds of people who gave different answers, you can't possibly juggle enough little pieces of paper. As a student, you may have chances to learn to use your school's computers, which may have built-in programs that can be used for any variety of data. However, the important thing is to know about these *before* you administer or even really design your questionnaire. This kind of information makes possible setting up the questions and responses to fit the programs available.

There are many opportunities to learn all the stages of data processing beginning with that super-dull work of key-punching coded responses onto data cards. The actual process of running the cards and getting miles of printouts with counts, correlations, and tables can be done very rapidly and for very little expense if the built-in programs are used. Some schools provide this service to students without charge as part of their educational process. However, computers can't make sense out of the material; only you can determine whether the relations you ask the machine to make are meaningful. It is reassuring to know that we still need the human brain to understand data! Learning to use the computer can help you overcome the awe a lot of people have for such a complicated piece of equipment. It often turns out to be very useful!

Once again, any thorough plan for administering a questionnaire will take far more planning than can be presented here. Even the best laid plans, however, have a way of going awry. To give you a hint of some of the problems, in table 8.1 we share experiences some of us have had in trying to carry out various questionnaire projects.

CRITIQUING OTHER PEOPLE'S RESEARCH

Not everyone wants to or needs to do research. It presents a variety of problems for nurses, and one of them is the difficulty most of us have in figuring out the value of any given piece of research on the basis of its published report. There are two common reactions: complete avoidance or cowed acceptance. As more research is being produced in nursing, it becomes less possible to avoid dealing with it somehow. But despite the fact that printed information somehow assumes an authority all its own, some projects are so clearly inept that we couldn't possibly take them seriously.

We need to begin asking questions of any given report in order to develop a healthy and informed skepticism about research reporting. Fortunately, as nurses in practice, we have a base of experience that tells us that many of the idealized models of studies cannot possibly work out as smoothly as planned. In spite of all the putdowns nurses encounter, we have an expert knowledge of the realities of many client-community situations. One nurse lost much of her awe for a bright young sociologist who proposed a two-hour interview schedule to be administered to the mothers of newborn babies. Her experience told her that no new mother would have the time, patience, or willingness to sit still for that kind of marathon.

By looking for holes in the planning, gaps in the logic, leaps of faith in

TABLE 8.1 *What Can Go Wrong with Questionnaires—and Usually Does!*

The Ailment	Possible Reason	Possible Solution
They don't return the form.	—Takes too much effort to get it back.	—Make it easier; send a stamped envelope. If local, make the return point as central as possible or pick them up yourself.
They didn't even *do* them!	—Folks have a right not to participate.	—Accept.
	—May not be as interested in the topic as you are.	—Jazz it up. —Try to increase their motivation to participate.
	—Didn't understand what you wanted.	—Keep things as clear as possible—people don't struggle to understand; it's just easier to throw it away. —Really good pretests would have shown a problem here.
They didn't follow the instructions.	—Maybe they weren't all that clear.	—Try forms out on coworkers, friends, small groups of strangers, small groups of the kind to be used as subjects—ask for feedback, suggestions. —Expect there will always be some like this. Dolts!
They didn't answer all the items.	—Not time enough?	—Don't rush them. —Don't ask too many questions for the time allowed or for the effort it takes.
	—Maybe some were too uncomfortable to answer.	—Try to eliminate unnecessary hot items. —Soften necessary ones with several cool, unloaded items on either side. —Try wording uncomfortable items to minimize the reaction. —May not be able to get at crucial stuff in this way; may need a relaxed, trusting interview.

TABLE 8.1 (*Continued*)

The Ailment	Possible Reason	Possible Solution
	—Maybe they didn't know what to answer; not enough information or had no opinion.	—Offer a "don't know" choice. —Be careful to ask items your sample could be expected to know.
	—Maybe you didn't give them the choice they wanted.	—At least at pretest, and if possible at test, leave one space for "Other (specify) _____."
They cut off my secret identifying code.	—People aren't as dumb as they used to be.	—Be open with your identification. —Ask them to sign; but it has to be voluntary. (You risk getting fewer returned.) —Don't bank on knowing exactly who they are.
They marked too many answers.	—Maybe the choices you gave weren't mutually exclusive.	—If the choices are of the same kind, try to combine them into a single answer that reflects both parts.
	—Some answers depend on different circumstances.	—Sometimes you can ignore the second answer. —Sometimes you can figure out which is the more likely answer. —Be prepared to have to jettison items or whole forms for those problems.
	—Your directions were not clear.	—Be sure initial directions and even each page or items says how many to mark. —But some folk just won't follow anyway!
They added an answer to the list of choices.	—Maybe you forgot a whole category of answer?	—Hope you can include that on the next go-round. —It's better to get this on the pretest but you can't always be so lucky.
Everybody marked the same answer.	—You picked a skewed sample.	—Unless it's contraindicated, look for balance in other groups.

TABLE 8.1 *(Continued)*

The Ailment	Possible Reason	Possible Solution
	—You didn't break the answers down far enough.	—Remove the item for reworking, pretesting, etc.
	—You asked an obvious question.	—Dumb!
	—You've just confirmed a major trend.	—Publish your finding fast!
I don't think they answered honestly.	—May be hostile to tests, the situation, you, etc.	—Try to win their cooperation. —Be ready to toss out obvious goof-ups.
	—May have a sense of humor, be drunk, etc.	—Ditto.
	—May be guarding confidential material.	—If it's vital to know, use double items to check reliability (same or similar one at different spots). —Be prepared to lose items. —Try to figure out why they'd want to lie and judge what to do accordingly.
Why didn't I think to ask just that one other question?	—Even researchers aren't omniscient!	—Try a new form. Set up dummy conclusions as completely as you can *before* you give the test; using your imagination this way can often suggest an omitted item. —Try a new group with it added. —Better luck next time.
They didn't return it for so long.	—You didn't put a return date on it.	—Place the date by which you need it where it's sure to be seen. —Send a reminder a week or so after the due date to remind those who have yet to return them. (This is where it pays off to know just who's who, by code or open identification.)

the explanation, and failures to ground explanations in actual data, we can all develop skills in critiquing research studies. By refusing to accept research reports as gospel, we can become astute assessors of the reliability and usefulness of much research that applies to our areas of practice. Such a critical approach should make possible selecting with greater discrimination which studies have potential for use in our field either as presented or as adapted by us to suit the special needs of our own clients and communities. It may also provide a helpful starting point for us; by observing the mistakes of others, we may avoid a few of them in projects of our own. For further suggestions, see Fleming and Hayter (1974), Fox (1970: 287–309), or Leininger (1968).

INFORMED RESEARCH CLIENTS

An issue in research, especially in areas related to medical and health services, is the importance of the research subjects' being fully informed about what research they are participating in, knowing as much as possible about the possible risks the research exposes them to, and agreeing knowledgeably to participate in the research process. In addition, research subjects must be provided with every chance to remove themselves from the research at any stage they wish to. If you think about some of the projects for which people have volunteered—testing unknown vaccines, cancer transplantation, being inoculated with possible disease-causing organisms—you can't help admiring their bravery—or foolhardiness—for being a part of the advance of medical science is exciting. But on the other hand, you might wonder whether the participants really understood what might happen to them if the experiment turned out wrong.

From the standpoint of medical ethics, it is not possible to deprive an individual of all the life-saving or life-enhancing therapeutic approaches that are available. This stance, however, is very hard to reconcile with the researcher's desire to establish clearly the effects of single actions or interventions. The conflict between research and therapy broke into public awareness with the news stories describing a forty-year study by the U.S. Public Health Service of a number of untreated syphilitic men. In spite of the research goal of learning the long-range effects of nontreatment, it was publicly unacceptable that such men should have been deprived of possible aid after the benefits of penicillin had been discovered. There have also been exposés of health workers' leading individuals to consent to sterilization by the use of threats of withdrawing services or outright lies about the nature of the procedure to be done.

Even before such incidents were reported, Congress and HEW, major sources for funding of health research, were concerned and had moved to establish guidelines to protect human subjects in any research for which the government paid, with the implication that such guidelines would be appropriate to any research involving humans, regardless of funding source. These guidelines are constantly being revised and toughened, but basically include devices to insure that all possible risks to subjects are identified clearly beforehand to both the researcher and the subject, that the value to the individual client outweigh the possible harm, that the subject may withdraw consent and refuse to participate at any time without bad consequences, and that no duress be applied to "persuade" a subject to agree. One stipulation requires that all research funded by the government must have the approval of the institution within which the project is administered. The mechanisms for establishing this approval are generally left to the institution, but the government must be satisfied that its method of overseeing research is adequate to protect the rights of research subjects. In some cases committees made up of researchers and people involved with medical ethics and medical law may be established to evaluate the risk and protection from it within all projects carried on by the institution. There is some feeling that potential research subjects— laypeople or clients—should also have a voice at this level of decision making.

RISK

Much research has tried to advance knowledge for some broader social good at the cost of great risk to some people. Our Constitution supports the ethic that individual rights cannot be sacrificed to the common good, in contrast to the excuses for Nazi experiments exposed in the Nuremberg trials. Persons may still agree to take part in risky research, but they must understand clearly what they are doing. The benefits of research must also outweigh the harm it might do to subjects. This guideline has complicated community health research; controlled studies are ethically impossible when they entail depriving someone of interventions of even potential life-sustaining value.

It is easy to look for possible harm in physical actions, such as drugs, radioactive isotopes, surgical procedures, and so on. But risk also includes emotional and social harm that may occur. Thus the possible stress the research may cause the persons involved, the harm that may follow to their reputation were their identity revealed, or in cases of research dealing with illegal behavior, the possible legal repercussions, are all examples of risk. Studies of individuals, groups, or communities must make provision for guarding against invasion of privacy, a basic right that cannot be waived. Common devices include the use of pseudonyms (which everyone then tries to identify), masked photographs, composite descriptions, or merged statistics, depending on the method of reporting findings. For example, all the places and subjects mentioned in the field notes at the start of this chapter have been renamed.

Researchers must also be concerned about the psychological impact of participation on subjects. Interviews may deliberately or inadvertently delve into areas that one or more individuals might wish to leave forgotten; opening touchy subjects places a responsibility on the researcher who opens it to deal with the emotions as well as the content of the answers. Examples may be seen in postabortion followup studies of women who may wish to forget that they were ever pregnant and for whom even the recollection is emotionally loaded. Privacy often depends on the ability of self, family, and neighbors to forget; researchers and their never-forgetting computers may interfere with this process. Present court rulings demand enforcement of a research ethic that protects people from undue invasions of their present lives.

Few research enterprises are ever totally free of risk but subjects must, under terms of HEW guidelines, be informed fully of any risks they might encounter. To be certain that the explanation of risk doesn't become another case of medical jargon that is incomprehensible to laypeople, the usual requirement is that the explanation be written as well as verbal and the subject sign the explanation to indicate it has been read and understood. That, of course, invalidates those sweeping consent forms that give hospital research people the right to do anything to anybody.

DURESS

Although research subjects may be reimbursed for participation, it is not legitimate to lure them into unforeseen or unreasonable risks with excessive promises or threats. The physician who threatens to withhold service if a patient refuses a procedure or the researcher who suggests early parole to a prisoner-"volunteer" both violate research ethics. A payment of $200 may lure very poor persons to accept risks they would not take for $20. The basic stance is that individual protection must be "above gold." Payment may be seen as constituting a promise, and not paying someone who wishes to withdraw consent seen as a threat. Further, false information, either in predicting benefits or in omitting risks, is not only unethical but also illegal.

The all-too-human ability to persuade ourselves of the purity of our own motives has led HEW to propose that institutions taking research funds from the government must set up some review process through which research projects must go to be evaluated for risk to and protection of human subjects. Many places have extended the criteria to all research being done there whether funded or not. The intent is to try to make researchers aware of the rights of research subjects to understand as fully as possible beforehand what they are agreeing to do—that is, the right to decide whether to participate on the basis of thorough knowledge of what is entailed.

CONSENT

The issue of informed consent may seem like an easy one for nurses to avoid, but an example should bring it very close to us all. Nurses are the ones who generally are called upon to sign as witness to the consent forms stating that the patient understands the experimental nature of the procedure to be done. That witness signature can place the nurse very firmly in court when the late patient's family sues the physician. The nurse is also the one to whom patients often turn later to say that they really didn't understand what they were just told but didn't want "to waste the doctor's time further when he's so very busy."

This situation places the nurse squarely in a double bind: If you suspect or know that the patient has not been fully informed and insist that this be done, you stand in jeopardy of losing your job. If you shield the researcher from fulfilling this obligation, you can stand as a principle to the fact and must share a joint responsibility in court. Lawyers have no trouble with this dilemma: They tell us to inform the patients that they may refuse or insist that the researcher explain again. Physicians tell us to mind our own business and leave it to the physician in charge of the case. As nurses, each of us must wrestle this one through on the basis of our own ethics. Although the decision will have to include many particularities of the situation, it must also include some notion about whether each of us sees part of our particular job responsibilities as the protection of the patient or the protection of the physician, researcher, or institution.

Although the researcher has basic responsibility for guarding the subjects' rights, it is also important that the agency or institution in which any research is carried out insure that protection. At the level of nonresearcher, whether in a unit administering experimental drugs or when hired to carry out some portion of a research project, the nurse has a legitimate obligation to be certain that research subjects have indeed given informed consent, particularly if the nurse must serve as a witness to a subject's consent. Such an obligation may be fulfilled simply by inquiry into the procedure by which subjects are informed, although there are times when how thoroughly subjects have really understood the project will be dubious. If ethical standards of research are clearly not being carried out, our obligation is to treat that as seriously as we would any other conduct that endangers client health or safety.

The need to understand informed consent for research subjects is important for students as well as graduate nurses. Ethical standards that apply to professional research also apply to that conducted by students. Thus, keeping this fact in mind is important when given an assignment that requires you to carry out a research project of any kind involving humans. That a project is done as part of classroom learning does not make it any the less research and subject to the same constraints as projects that are funded by HEW or carried out by academic researchers. In addition, you should also remember that much academic research is carried out on students, a convenient captive population that has been the basis for classic research for decades. Although not all research is required to conform to the HEW guidelines, an interesting project may be to find out how your own institution deals with ethical issues applying to research being done by its own faculty or on its own students.

Agreeing to participate in research establishes a contract between the subject and the investigator. The ability to agree to any contract demands the capacity to reason. Obviously, an unconscious person cannot give consent to anything. (There are legal processes for administering emergency procedures in exactly such circumstances, but present laws insist these can never be experimental nor may they be continued after the patient regains the ability to give consent and does not wish to do so.) Persons considered legally incompetent may not give consent either. This group includes the mentally ill, children, and those not in possession of their civil rights, such as prisoners. These three categories of people present thorny issues in both law and research since all three are frequent research subjects.

SUMMARY

Research is both a tool and a frame of mind that enables nurses to clarify questions, systematically look for answers, and present them within a logical framework for the scrutiny of others. Community experiences are seldom amenable to laboratory manipulation and are most readily studied with exploratory, descriptive methods and qualitative analysis of data. Recording extensive field notes that form the basis for constant comparison analysis can produce unexpected and productive answers to significant questions in community nursing practice. Unlike more elaborate research procedures, such a method is also within the scope of a single nurse-researcher.

An important point is that all nurses utilize a research stance for both problem solving and improving client services and that they communicate their findings to others involved in similar situations. Writing for publication, therefore, is a vital part of the research process. Ability to critique other people's reports can improve our ability to assess the general validity of research findings as well as improve the selective use of such findings or of some of the tools and methods used by a particular researcher.

Concerns for client autonomy as well as exposés of research abuses of subject safety and welfare have led to federal restraints on research involving human subjects. Issues of risk and protection from it are involved in preparing for research; subjects must be fully informed before giving their consent to cooperate. Client-advocates must concern themselves with a subject's well-being regardless of who is carrying out the research in question.

REFERENCES

ABDELLAH, FAYE G., et al. *New Directions in Patient-Centered Nursing*. New York: Macmillan Co., 1973.

BABBIE, EARL R. *Survey Research Methods*. Belmont, Calif.: Wadsworth Publishing Co., 1973.

BAKER, ROBERT, and SCHULTZ, RICHARD, eds. *Instructional Product Research*. New York: Van Nostrand Reinhold Co., 1972.

BROOK, ROBERT H. *Quality of Care Assessment: A Comparison of Five Methods of Peer Review*. Washington, D.C.: Government Printing Office, HEW Publication No. HRA74–3100, July 1973.

CAMPBELL, DONALD T., and STANLEY, JULIAN C. *Experimental and Quasi-Experimental Designs for Research*. Chicago: Rand McNally & Co., 1963.

DIERS, DONNA. "Finding Clinical Problems for Study." *Journal of Nursing Administration* 2 (November–December 1971): 15–18.

DOUGLAS, JACK D. *Investigative Social Research*. Beverly Hills, Calif.: Sage Publications, 1976.

DYER, ELAINE, et al. *Improved Patient Care through Problem-Oriented Nursing*. New York: Springer Co., 1974.

FESTINGER, LEON, and KATZ, DANIEL, eds. *Research Methods in the Behavioral Sciences*. New York: Holt, Rinehart and Winston, 1953.

FLEMING, J.W., and HAYTER, J. "Reading Research Reports Critically," *Nursing Outlook* 22 (March 1974): 172–95.

FOX, DAVID J. *Fundamentals of Research in Nursing*. New York: Appleton-Century-Crofts, 1970.

GANS, HERBERT. *Urban Villagers*. New York: The Free Press of Glencoe, 1962.

GLASER, BARNEY G., and STRAUSS, ANSELM L. *The Discovery of Grounded Theory*. Chicago: Aldine Publishing Co., 1967.

GOFFMAN, ERVING. *Asylums*. New York: Doubleday, 1961.

GORTNER, SUSAN, and NAHM, HELEN. "An Overview of Nursing Research in the U.S." *Nursing Research* 26 (January–February 1977): 10–33.

JUNKER, BUFORD H. *Field Work*. Chicago: University of Chicago Press, 1960.

KERLINGER, FRED N. *Foundations of Behavioral Research*. New York: Holt, Rinehart and Winston, 1964.

KESSNER, D.M. and KALK, C.E. *A Strategy for Evaluating Health Services*. Washington, D.C.: Institute of Medicine, National Academy of Sciences, 1973.

LEININGER, MADELEINE. "The Research Critique; Nature, Function and Art." *Nursing Research* 17 (September–October 1968): 20–32.

LEWIS, OSCAR. *The Children of Sanchez*. New York: Random House, 1961.

—— *La Vida*. New York: Vintage Books, 1968.

A Manual of Style, 12th ed., rev. Chicago: University of Chicago Press, 1969.

McCLOSKEY, JOANNE. "Publishing Opportunities for Nurses: A Comparison of 65 Journals." *Nurse Educator* (July–August 1977): 4–13.

MILLER, DELBERT C. *Handbook of Research Design and Social Measurement*, 2nd ed. New York: David McKay Co., 1970.

NAROL, RAOUL, and COHEN, RONALD, eds. *A Handbook of Methods in Cultural Anthropology*. New York: Columbia University Press, 1973.

PAPE, RUTH H. "Touristry: A Type of Occupational Mobility." *Social Problems* 11 (1964):336–44.

PAUL, BEN. "Interview Techniques and Field Relationships." In Alfred C. Kroeber, ed., *Anthropology Today*. Chicago: University of Chicago Press, 1953.

PAYNE, STANLEY L. *The Art of Asking Questions*. Princeton, N.J.: Princeton University Press, 1951.

"Research in Practice Areas." *Nursing Reseach* 26 (May–June 1977).

ROSSI, PETER H., and WILLIAMS, WALTER, eds. *Evaluating Social Theory: Practice and Politics*. New York: Seminar Press, 1972.

SCHATZMAN, LEONARD and STRAUSS, ANSELM L. *Field Research*. Englewood Cliffs, N.J.: Prentice-Hall, 1973.

SELTIZ, CLAIRE, et al. *Research Methods in Social Relations*, rev. ed. New York: Holt, Rinehart and Winston, 1965.

SIMON, JULIAN L. *Basic Research Methods in Social Science*. New York: Random House, 1969.

STEELE, SARA M. *Contemporary Approaches to Program Evaluation*. Washington D.C.: Capitol Publications, 1977.

STRUNK, W., JR., and WHITE, E.B. *The Elements of Style*, 2nd ed. Riverside, N.J.: Macmillan Publishing Co., 1972.

SUCHMAN, EDWARD A. *Evaluative Research*. New York: Russell Sage Foundation, 1967.

TERKEL, STUDS. *Working*. New York: Pantheon Books, 1972.

WEISS, CAROL H. *Evaluation Research*. Englewood Cliffs, N.J.: Prentice-Hall, 1972.

WHYTE, WILLIAM. *Street Corner Society*, 2nd ed. Chicago: University of Chicago Press, 1955.

9. Epidemiology and Some Applications to Primary Prevention

Sarah Ellen Archer
Ruth P. Fleshman

INTRODUCTION

Epidemiology is both a field of knowledge and a tool in the practice of community health to study the distribution of diseases and other conditions in an entire population. Epidemiologists proceed with any tools available to them to determine the what, why, where, how, when, and who of the matter being investigated.

The chapter begins with a case example of illness in a nursing school dormitory as an illustration of the use and process of epidemiology in tracking the origin and distribution of a disease as well as pertinent preventive and treatment measures. Epidemiology and its uses are defined and discussed. Primary, secondary, and tertiary prevention measures based on epidemiologic data are presented for acute and chronic infectious and noninfectious conditions. Particular emphasis is placed on chronic noninfectious conditions since these account for seven of the ten leading causes of death in the United States and their epidemiological study is much more complex than is the case for most acute infectious diseases. The glossary at the end of the chapter contains a number of definitions of terms, and the appendix contains formulas for computing various rates used in vital statistics.

CASE EXAMPLE

Crowded living arrangements, such as barracks and dormitories, put many people close together who are more or less strangers to each other. Unlike family members, these strangers have not had close contact long enough to build up resistance to one another's various pathogens. Thus, not surprisingly, especially at the start of the school year, various minor illnesses make the rounds of the dorms. The staff in the student health service can tell from their census counts what the calendar will say: start of the semester, first big weather change, midterms, and finals. Students have no one else to turn to for health care when they are living away from home, and so even minor ailments that would have been treated within the family are taken to the student health service.

This particular year there were indeed the usual numbers of upper respiratory infections at the opening of school. Some of the new students complained about bug bites as they began to get used to the local insect population that the natives were practically immune to. A few last warm weather picnics brought contact dermatitis from the local poison ivy plants. At the start of cold weather, a mild flu began going around but was easily treated with aspirin, rest, fluids, and a little paregoric.

Along about October there was a rise in complaints from one of the nursing dorms but no one had any really definable disease: rundown feeling, loss of appetite, tiredness. Unfortunately most of the complaints could be tied to nervousness about upcoming first midterms and were given only cursory attention by the center's staff. The situation changed, however, when an early morning phone call from the house manager reported a student severely ill, vomiting, feverish, and bright orange. Brought to the hospital admitting unit, the twenty-two-year-old woman was indeed clearly jaundiced, very weak, and retching. Her temperature was 39.7 (C) and her liver was enlarged and tender. She told the examining practitioner that she had been ill for several days but thought it had been little more than what the others in the house had been complaining of, although she had thought vomiting over midterms was a bit unusual. Lab tests of her blood and urine both confirmed that she had hepatitis. The only questions that remained were where did she get hepatitis and who else had been exposed to it?

After she had been admitted to the communicable disease unit, she was placed in enteric isolation to keep her own organisms under control. Because hepatitis is listed as a reportable communicable disease, the unit clerk was instructed to notify the county health department by phone as well as by filling in the mandatory report form. The local health department's policy was that reports of viral hepatitis are to be followed up within twenty-four hours. Quick investigation was especially urgent in this case since the patient lived in a dormitory and had been in close contact with a number of her classmates. She also had been in contact with sick people in her work at school.

The same afternoon, the district public health nurse (PHN) arrived at the hospital unit with her epidemiological investigation form in hand. In addition to the usual personal information, she asked the names and ages of those sharing the same household. The fact that there were twenty-four other women on the student's dormitory floor created a bigger interviewing job than she had anticipated! The patient was not sure which if any of these dorm-mates had had any of the more subtle symptoms of hepatitis in the past month although several of them had had vague complaints. Certainly no one in the dorm had been jaundiced. The PHN asked specifically about injections of many kinds: blood or blood products, halothane anesthesia, medicines including INH, vaccinations, blood or skin tests (which of course had been a part of the entrance physical exam for school), any dental work, acupuncture, or tattooing. All of these can be a source of injecting the hepatitis virus into the victim unless the greatest attention is paid to the care of needles and instruments, which is thus one of the reasons for using disposables as much as possible since killing the hepatitis virus is really very hard.

Because this virus is also spread through ingestion of fecal and urine contamination, the PHN asked about the water supply of places where the student had been during the two months just past. Had she been swimming or surfing or wading in creeks or lakes? Where had she traveled and what was the state of sanitation there, especially involving drinking water and toilet facilities? What was the sewage disposal method and had there been any overflow while she had been there? Had she cared for any sick animals? Had she eaten any raw clams or oysters?

The PHN learned that the patient had spent the past summer in rural Pomo County, working with a local community project (see chapter 14). She had stayed with a group of other students in a farmhouse with its own well and indoor plumbing. She wasn't sure whether there had been any problems with the sewage overflowing, but she doubted it since there had been no discussion about that in the household. None of the farm animals had been sick, and she couldn't recall coming into contact with any sick animals anywhere else. She had gone swimming several times with the others at the local river, but they had been careful to swim upstream from the large informal campsite that young travellers had set up near the highway. She had eaten out a number of times during the summer and more recently since starting school and could recall only a few of the places. Most were perfectly usual restaurants, both here and in Pomo.

Sometimes she had eaten at friends' homes, and she was sure there were other times and places that escaped her mind right now when she was feeling so crumby. This intensive questioning was difficult to carry out when the person being questioned had to interrupt apologetically to retch and vomit, but the PHN was sympathetic and gave no evidence of impatience. The student tried very hard to answer all the investigation questions; she was absolutely sure she had eaten no raw shellfish since she hated the things!

After leaving the hospital unit, the public health nurse went directly to the dormitory to begin arranging for interviews with all the other student nurses on the patient's floor. A few were in, and she was able to begin the first of the twenty-four interviews that needed to be done. None of these students had had any discernible illness in the past two months except for one case of poison ivy dermatitis. All were notified to go to the student health service, their own physician, or the local health department for prophylactic injections of immune serum globulin.

The next day, the PHN reported her findings to the disease control unit of the central health department, and when the medical officer heard of the student's residence in Pomo, he phoned the medical officer of that county's health department. The Pomo medical officer reported the area was also experiencing an outbreak of viral hepatitis that had been tracked to the local water supply drawn from wells, most of which were grossly contaminated with fecal organisms. Since the nursing student had been living at the edge of the community most involved in this outbreak, she had undoubtedly received a number of exposures during the summer she had spent there. The Pomo health department had also established that the outbreak was Hepatitis A, infectious hepatitis, rather than Hepatitis B, the more serious serum hepatitis. Of course, both were diseases of long-term consequences for their victims, but recovery was usually less problematic for the A type hepatitis. (The hospital antigen studies confirmed the specific form of hepatitis in the student.)

An integral part of each interview with the student's contacts had been an explanation by the PHN of the nature of the disease, what could be done to prevent it, and what should be done during the period of time it might be incubating in anyone actually receiving a sufficient exposure: Trying to insure that dormitory sanitation was tip-top and that everyone paid special heed to breaking the link between contaminants (urine, feces, and blood) and the humans in the environment. There was no trouble persuading everyone to be rigorous in handwshing after using the toilets. (The use of hand towels and soap in fact rather taxed the dormitory supplies.) A few of the more anxious students even started keeping daily records of their temperatures, although the novelty of this exercise soon tapered off as the weeks passed. For the most part, the other students were most reassured when the PHN explained that being exposed to enough hepatitis viruses in the usual course of things to come down with the disease is really rather hard.

About three weeks after the student had first become ill, her roommate awoke one morning with a very tender abdomen, nausea, and vomiting. She was immediately sure she was the next victim and sought care at the student health center right away. However, her problem turned out to be a bad case of menstrual cramps, and she was embarrassed after the first day passed. The rest of the two months' incubation period passed uneventfully; no other case developed as a result of exposure by the student nurse. Although many people were certain the reason was the prompt use of immune serum globulin, it more likely was the relative difficulty of being exposed to the disease and to the basic reservoirs of resistance among the student population.

DEFINITION AND USES OF EPIDEMIOLOGY

Most of what we do in nursing and medicine is focused on individuals, mother-child dyads, and, occasionally, families. This one-to-one emphasis is known as clinical or case nursing or medical practice. This approach is microscopic in that we look at the individual's psycho-social and physical history and symptoms with the objective of diagnosis and treatment of disease in that person. Epidemiology is macroscopic in that it looks for the distribution of diseases and injuries and their determinants within the total population. Thus epidemiology is the study of total populations' disease and disability patterns, while case or clinical nursing and medicine deal with individual's disease and disability patterns.

As an applied science, epidemiology is both an academic field of study and a tool used widely in community health. Epidemiologic studies provide information on the incidence and prevalence as well as the severity of disease and other conditions that cause morbidity and death in the population in general as well as within specific age, sex, racial, or other subgroups. (See the glossary and appendix at the end of this chapter for a number of terms and rate formulas.) These kinds of data are essential for health planners to determine what facilities, services, and person power are needed to meet the population's needs adequately. With these data, planners can discern changes in the pattern of diseases or conditions in their communities and begin to look for etiological factors influencing these changes. For example, we are currently seeing an increase in lung cancer and heart disease rates in women approaching those for men.

Etiological factors include changes in lifestyle and stress levels for women. Until this trend can be reversed, an increased need for medical services for this greater number of illnesses must be anticipated.

From a disease-oriented system we might expect ever-larger amounts of funding to be poured into treatment centers. Better preventive measures could begin to reduce the occurrence of these diseases. Epidemiology can help in choosing between these approaches, not only by providing information about what could be done but also by defining especially high-risk groups for preventive and treatment measures. The epidemiological investigation conducted in the case study of hepatitis in a nursing school dormitory is an example of how these kinds of data are gathered and used. The National Health Survey carried out continuously by the Health Resources Administration of the U. S. Public Health Service provides a variety of epidemiological information on a carefully selected sample of the total population.

In the course of studying the distribution of diseases and conditions in a population, the epidemiologist learns a great deal about their natural history. Case medicine practitioners generally see only the relatively few severe or moderately severe cases of any given condition that develop within their client population. They know a great deal about those few cases but very little about what is happening in the rest of the population. They see only part of the tip of the iceberg. For most infectious diseases, the majority of cases are mild or subclinical and thus may not even be noticed by the person, much less brought to the attention of the physician. These cases go unnoticed and unreported. In some epidemiological investigations, antibody titers are done on entire groups. These data in conjunction with detailed histories and physical examinations reveal disease severity patterns like the one illustrated in the iceberg in figure 9.1. Without these kinds of studies, the natural history and real distribution of a disease would remain unknown. Epidemiologists use whatever research methods are appropriate to obtain needed information. In our case example, interviews revealed the clue that a simple phone call confirmed regarding the source of infection.

For example, had antibody studies been done on all the student nurses in our dormitory and all of the people in the Pomo County communities where the hepatitis outbreak occurred, a pattern of disease distribution similar to that illustrated by the iceberg in figure 9.1 would probably have emerged. The case fatality rate—that is, the proportion of people who have the disease and die from it—is relatively low in hepatitis, presuming adequate treatment is available. This statement is supported by the fact that no one in the dormitory or in Pomo County died as a result of the hepatitis outbreak. Less than 10 percent of the people known to be exposed in Pomo County came down with clinically demonstrable dis-

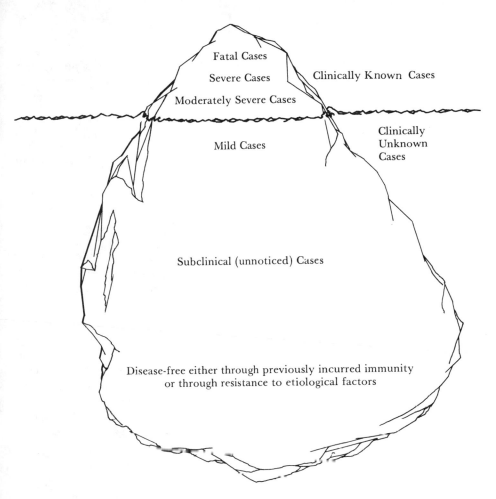

Fatal Cases

Severe Cases   Clinically Known Cases

Moderately Severe Cases

Mild Cases   Clinically
                              Unknown
                              Cases

Subclinical (unnoticed) Cases

Disease-free either through previously incurred immunity
or through resistance to etiological factors

9.1   *Iceberg Epidemiological Distribution of a Disease in a Population at Risk*

ease. Our student nurse was unfortunately one of them. The other 90-plus percent either had mild cases of hepatitis that were ignored as minor stomach upsets, had no symptoms at all although they were infected and did develop some antibody reaction, or were not infected at all. This last group of people who were not infected at all either were already immune through previous antibody development or were too innately resistant to become infected. The other students in the dormitory with exposure to the student nurse were provided with temporary passive immunity through the use of the immune serum globulin injections to supplement their innate resistance to infection.

Epidemiology is also useful in studying the etiology of diseases and in testing measures to control their incidence. The hepatitis case example will again help to illustrate this use of epidemiology. Classical epidemiological studies of infectious diseases have shown a relationship between host, agent, and environment, as illustrated in figure 9.2. Investigations, histories, and direct observations have identified the ways in which these three factors are related and particularly how the host becomes infected with the agent. In the case example, our student nurse is the host, Hepatitis A virus is the agent, and Pomo County and the school dormitory are the environment. The mode of transmission, or how the agent reaches the host, in Hepatitis A is known to be via food, water, and other articles or fomites contaminated with feces, urine, and saliva from a person already infected with the Hepatitis A virus. There is evidence that some people who have recovered from hepatitis can still be carriers and so are potential sources of infection for others although they themselves have no signs or symptoms of the disease. Hospital personnel who are known to be hepatitis carriers are increasingly being barred from working on renal dialysis units because of the patients' extreme vulnerability to infections. This measure is one method of interrupting the transmission of the agent to the host.

Other ways of preventing the agent from reaching a host were illustrated in the case example. The student nurse–case was placed on enteric isolation to prevent her contaminated urine, feces, leftover food, and other secretions from endangering others. All dormitory residents were urged to be particularly diligent in their handwashing after using the toilet. All sewerage and water systems in the dormitory were carefully checked for leaks and cross-connections. In Pomo County the health department went through these same procedures on a much larger scale in the communities where the outbreak occurred. Another preventive measure was to administer immune serum globulin to potentially infected contacts of known cases, such as the other students in the dormitory. This measure

9.2   *Host, Agent, and Environment Relationships*

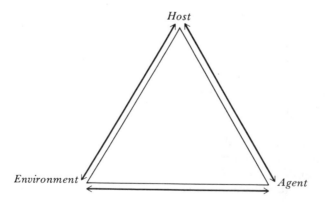

increases the resistance of the potential host to the invasion of the disease agent.

The foregoing discussion of means of preventing the agent from infecting the host and of increasing the host's resistance to that invasion are illustrative of the important role epidemiology plays in determining the etiology of a disease—that is, the host, agent, and environmental factors that are characteristic of the disease—and then using this knowledge to prevent or control the disease's spread. The illustration we chose to use was that of an acute infectious disease, hepatitis, because, as is the case with many of these kinds of diseases, the relationships of the etiological factors are relatively clear. These relationships are far more complex and less clear in chronic, noninfectious diseases and conditions, as we shall see later in the chapter.

Briefly, then, epidemiology is an applied science that is eclectic in its use of research methods to study the distribution of diseases and other conditions, such as accidents, and their determinants in a population. Epidemiological information is put to many uses: Identification of host, agent, and environment factors are used to predict, prevent, and control the occurrence of diseases and other conditions; to supply information to planners and administrators to aid them in making decisions about the most effective and efficient use of limited resources; and to learn about the natural history of diseases and conditions through study and observation. Epidemiology deals with diseases and conditions that affect entire populations and seeks to obtain a macrocosmic view of the entire distribution of the disease or condition as illustrated in the iceberg analogy in figure 9.1. In these ways, epidemiology differs from case or clinical medicine or nursing, which focus on the diagnosis and treatment of fatal, severe, or moderately severe cases of specific diseases.

CLASSIFICATION OF DISEASES AND CONDITIONS

Diseases and conditions that affect the population can be classified into four groups based on two major variables: duration and etiology. This division with examples is shown in table 9.1. As we noted in the previous section, acute infectious diseases were much more prevalent and lethal for the U.S. population than they are now. We chose to use the example of hapatitis to illustrate host-agent-environment relationships because these relationships are often much clearer in such diseases than in other diseases or conditions as we shall see. Again, many of the acute infectious conditions are now preventable by immunization, provided that the proportion of the population that is immunized is large enough to prevent the spread of epidemic diseases and thereby protect the unimmunized

TABLE 9.1 *Classification of Diseases and Conditions in Terms of Etiology and Duration*

Etiology	Duration	
	Acute	Chronic
Infectious	*Hepatitis,** measles, chicken pox, cholera, diphtheria, polio, pertussis	*Tuberculosis,** rheumatic fever following streptococcal infections
Noninfectious	*Automobile accidents,** other accidents, poisonings	*Hypertension,** diabetes, arthritis, cirrhosis due to alcoholism

*Conditions discussed in the text.

members of the population. In the late 1970s this so-called herd immunity dropped to dangerously low levels. All community health workers must take every opportunity to teach about the value of immunizations and urge people to protect themselves and their children from acute infectious diseases.

Examples of chronic infectious diseases include tuberculosis and rheumatic fever following streptococcal infections. Although these diseases are caused by infectious agents, their duration is long term and so require continued treatment and surveillance. According to estimates, over 90 percent of all new cases are really activations of dormant disease in previously infected persons (Mauser and Bahn 1974:295). As we shall see later in the chapter, improvements in general living standards and the development of antimicrobials have removed tuberculosis from among the leading causes of death in the United States. Another reason is the work of tuberculosis control units in health departments that monitor known cases and conduct screening programs to enable early diagnosis and prompt treatment of new cases.

Acute noninfectious conditions such as accidents, other forms of trauma, and poisonings are on the increase. The causative agent in these conditions includes automobiles driven recklessly, too fast, or under the influence of alcohol; guns, knives, and other weapons; and chemical agents such as pesticides, cleaning agents, solvents, drugs, lead-based paint, and other compounds. Nowhere is primary prevention through health promotion and specific protection more needed than in this classification of conditions that disable and kill so many of our people. Community health nurses can have a considerable impact on the incidence of home accidents and poisonings by careful home assessments and discussions with families about home safety precautions such as keeping dangerous chemicals and sharp objects away from children; making sure stairs have rails, good treads, and are well lighted; putting no-skid materials on shower and tub bottoms; securing rugs so they do not curl or slide; and adequately venting gas stoves and heaters. All too often people are not aware of these kinds of hazards in their home environment until someone else points them out and suggests ways to correct them.

The incidence and prevalence of chronic noninfectious diseases and conditions in the U.S. population is increasing as reflected in the listing of the ten leading causes of death in 1976 (table 9.2) and the discussion of health indicators in chapter 2. Later in this chapter we shall discuss some of the challenges community health workers face in primary, secondary, and tertiary prevention of these conditions. Because most of these chronic noninfectious conditions and diseases are incurable, we must find ways to prevent or at least forestall their development as well as developing methods for their treatment, which as we shall see, is no small order.

Again we must acknowledge that although table 9.1 as presented looks nice and clean with the diseases and conditions comfortably assigned to their respective boxes, reality is not so easily classified. A few examples will illustrate the complexity. Most cases of hepatitis are of short duration and then leave no residual effects; others result in necrosis of the liver and long-term consequences. Tuberculosis can have acute episodes and rapid

TABLE 9.2 *Comparison of the Ten Leading Causes of Death in the United States, 1900 and 1976, for All Age Groups*

1900	1976
1. Influenza and pneumonia	1. Diseases of the heart
2. Tuberculosis	2. Malignant neoplasms
3. Gastroenteritis	3. Vascular lesions of the central nervous system
4. Diseases of the heart	4. All accidents
5. Vascular lesions of the central nervous system	5. Influenza and pneumonia
6. Chronic nephritis	6. Bronchitis, emphysema, and other chronic obstructive lung diseases
7. All accidents	7. Diabetes mellitus
8. Malignant neoplasms	8. Cirrhosis of the liver
9. Certain diseases of early infancy	9. Arteriosclerosis
10. Diphtheria	10. Birth injury, difficult labor, and other causes of early infant mortality

Source: U.S. Department of Health, Education and Welfare, Public Health Service, Washington, D.C.

course in some people, which is what used to be called "galloping consumption." Traumatic accidents and poisonings may have an acute onset but can and often do have protracted sequelae. Diabetic coma or insulin shock, stroke, and myocardial infarct are examples of acute episodes of chronic noninfectious diseases and conditions. These kinds of limitations must be borne in mind regardless of the kind of classification of diseases and conditions we choose to use. We must be constantly aware that the complexities of a multidimensional world can only be partially represented on the plane surface of a page.

CHALLENGES TO MODERN EPIDEMIOLOGY

CHANGES IN LEADING CAUSES OF DEATH AND DISABILITY

Dramatic changes in the leading causes of death for all age groups have taken place during the twentieth century as illustrated in table 9.2. In 1900 the top three killers in the United States were acute infectious diseases: influenza and pneumonia, tuberculosis, and gastroenteritis. By 1976, tuberculosis, gastroenteritis, and diphtheria were gone from the list, and influenza and pneumonia had dropped to fifth. Their replacements are all chronic noninfectious conditions. Diseases of the heart, malignant neoplasms, and vascular lesions of the central nervous system are now the top three killers of the U.S. population. They have been joined on the list by four chronic, noninfectious newcomers: bronchitis, emphysema, and other chronic obstructive lung diseases; diabetes mellitus, cirrhosis of the liver, and arteriosclerosis. All accidents have risen from seventh to fourth on the list of killers for all age groups and are the number one killer of people under the age of thirty-five.

Why the changes? Many factors have contributed. Diphtheria and its fellow epidemic infectious diseases such as pertussis, measles, and mumps have been greatly reduced through the development and use of immunizations. As of the time of this writing, however, the fact that the immunization rates of children entering school for the first time have reached a dangerous low gives rise to increasing concerns about the potential for resurgence of epidemics. General food and restaurant sanitation, including restaurant inspections, food handler training, automated high temperature dishwashing as well as animal, farm, slaughterhouse, and packing plant inspections and better medical care for animals have all played their parts. Perhaps the most significant environmental changes have been in the area of the sanitary disposal of liquid and solid human, animal, and industrial wastes as well as the provision of generally safe drinking water. Although we cannot afford to neglect the improvements still needed in environmental sanitation, the fact remains that we have come a long way since 1900. Better housing and improved standards of living have reduced the incidence of tuberculosis.

Medical science has made quantum changes since the turn of the century: Sulfonamides, antibiotics, chemotherapy, transplants and grafts, rehabilitation technology, lasers, CAT-Scanners are on a list that is virtually endless. All of these advances have reduced premature mortality and have contributed along with the environmental changes to an increased life expectancy for the total U.S. population from approximately fifty years in 1900 to almost seventy years in the late 1970s. As the discussion of health indicators in chapter 2 shows, we still have much to do to improve the length and quality of life, especially for our ethnic people of color as well as other minority groups.

Most of these environmental, immunological, and medical technological advances have been brought about by a relatively small group of public health and medical scientists. Very little conscious involvement, much less active participation, by the general public has thus far been required to bring about these changes in host, agent, and environmental relationships that have changed our life and death patterns. The increase in acute and chronic noninfectious conditions as leading causes of death, because of their complex and still incompletely understood etiologies, presents a new challenge to epidemiologists to learn more about their determinants so that we can intervene effectively in their prevention and control. For reasons we shall discuss later, the prevention and control of these noninfectious conditions is much more difficult than was the case with the acute and chronic infectious diseases.

Because of their chronic nature, many of the leading causes of death are responsible for considerable disability before they ultimately bring about death. Indeed the death rate from these acute and chronic noninfectious conditions is only the tip of the iceberg in terms of their prevalence in the total population. Some measurements and uses of disability data is discussed in the health indicators portion of chapter 2. We believe the most important challenge to modern epidemiology is to develop effective and economical measures especially for primary prevention of these and other acute and chronic noninfectious conditions that disable and kill our population.

THE CHALLENGE OF PREVENTION

The concepts of primary, secondary, and tertiary prevention were introduced in chapters 1 and 2. Here we shall discuss them at greater length and provide detailed examples. Primary prevention, as can be seen in table 9.3, is divided into health promotion and specific prevention.

TABLE 9.3 *Levels of Prevention and Illustrative Actions*

Primary Prevention		Secondary Prevention		Tertiary Prevention
Health Promotion	Specific Protection	Early Diagnosis and Prompt Treatment	Disability Limitation	Rehabilitation
Health education	Use of specific immunizations	Case finding of infected individuals	Adequate treatment to arrest the disease process and to prevent complications and sequelae	Provision of hospital and community facilities for rehabilitation.
Development of a lifestyle compatible with promotion of optimal level of functioning re: nutrition, exercise, sleep, recreation, relaxation, and nonuse of alcohol, tobacco, and drugs	Chlorination and fluoridation of water	Screening surveys: i.e., diabetes		Professional education re: appropriate use of rehabilitation and how and when to make referrals
	Protection against occupational hazards	Multiphasic examinations	Professional education regarding the need for treatment and early referral to appropriate rehabilitation facilities	
Health hazard appraisal	Protection against accidents: seat belts, vehicle safety, highway engineering	Education directed to early detection of disease by individuals		Public education to promote focus on people's abilities instead of their disabilities
Healthy personality development	Use of specific dietary supplements	Development of diagnostic and treatment facilities	Provision of community economic, social, cultural, and vocational support systems during acute process	Adequate support networks during entire rehabilitation process
Marriage counseling	Protection from carcinogens	Professional education		Vocational rehabilitation services
Development of a healthy social environment	Avoidance of allergens	Regular physical examinations		Sheltered workshops

TABLE 9.3 (*Continued*)

Primary Prevention		Secondary Prevention		Tertiary Prevention
Health Promotion	*Specific Protection*	*Early Diagnosis and Prompt Treatment*	*Disability Limitation*	*Rehabilitation*
Promotion of a sanitary and safe environment: air, food, home, school, water, work	Case finding and treatment to prevent spread of disease	Regular dental examination	Regular dental care	Education of industry regarding employment of the handicapped
Personal hygiene	Health education directed to specific protection			
	Genetic counseling			

Source: Modified from H. R. Leavell, and E. G. Clark, *Preventive Medicine for the Doctor in his Community: An Epidemiological Approach*, 3rd. ed. (New York: McGraw-Hill Book Co., 1965), pp. 19–28.

Health promotion is generalized and geared to improving peoples' functioning level in general rather than to ward off or treat any specific disease or condition. Much of the focus of the holistic health practitioners and self-help groups is on health promotion. Leading the list under health promotion is health education, which is discussed at length in chapter 10. Suffice it to say here, then, that one of the most, if not the most, important contribution community health nurses, as well as all professionals interested in health, can make to clients' optimal level of functioning (OLOF) is to teach them how to care for themselves and how to use available facilities and resources appropriately. Health education and other health promotional efforts are increasingly important as we learn more about the influence of lifestyle and health habits on all facets of our lives. General personal hygiene, promotion of a sanitary and safe physical environment, and a sound psycho-social milieu are other health promotion measures.

Because of their general nature, health promotional activities are very hard to justify on the basis of cost-benefit relationships (see chapter 11). Expensive longitudinal cohort studies arc needed to prove their value in promoting peoples' health as a means of preventing, reducing, or forestalling the development of disabling or lethal diseases or conditions, much less that they have a positive effect on peoples' OLOF. Monies for such studies are difficult to obtain initially and even harder to keep at a high enough level over time to finance the studies to their conclusion. Politicians who appropriate monies want results within their term of office to use in their next campaign. This phenomenon makes obtaining governmental funding of twenty-year studies very difficult. These kinds of data, however, must be gathered and their results made known so that we can develop and market effective health promotional activities. Now that's a challenge!

Specific primary protection measures are geared toward the prevention of particular diseases or conditions and are easier to sell. Some of the broad categories of specific primary preventive measures are listed in table 9.3. These include specific immunizations, chlorination and fluoridation of water, genetic counseling and other specific health education, and protection from occupational hazards, carcinogens, and other environmental hazards. Because these measures are specific and fairly well proven as effective, we have had much more success in getting programs for their use funded. Specific primary protection measures for four diseases and conditions are given in table 9.4 as illustrations.

Secondary prevention is also divided into two sections: (1) early diagnosis and prompt treatment and (2) disability limitation. Most of the resources spent for medical care in the United States are expended on

TABLE 9.4 *Protection Measures for Specific Diseases and Conditions*

	Acute, Infectious Disease: Infectious Hepatitis	
Primary Prevention	*Secondary Prevention*	*Tertiary Prevention*
Environmental sanitation, especially of water, sewerage.	Provide for adequate, early treatment.	Case teaching re: levels of damage; avoidance of stressors, toxins, re-exposure; carrier state.
Toilet cleanliness; handwashing facilities available and used.	Encourage development of better, early differential diagnostic tests for infectious hepatitis.	Adequate convalescent care as long as indicated.
Assertiveness toward those who do not use adequate measures.	Treatment directed to relief of symptoms, minimizing damage.	Vocational retraining for those whose occupational conditions were causal or would be detrimental to
Isolation from known cases, especially by high-risk persons.	Careful observation of general health of close contacts through duration of incubation period.	themselves or others.
Regulation of food preparation and handling.	General public education re: care of sick and indications for professional care when symptoms persist, worsen, etc. Danger signs.	
Mandatory paid sickleave for ill foodhandlers.		
Screen all blood donors for virus; test all blood for virus; avoid unnecessary transfusions.	During high-risk times (outbreak) or for high-risk groups, education for signs, symptoms, management, complications, etc.	
Teach proper sterilization technique for injections	Professional education to update knowledge of conditions, transmission, prevention, and treatment.	
Safe handling of blood-contaminated instruments and equipment.	Adequate acute care to manage symptoms, prevent worsening, secondary infections.	
Regular testing of health workers involved with patient interiors (surgery, anesthesia staff); exclusion of carriers.		
Contacts: –Hyper-immune gamma globulin as passive immunization.		

TABLE 9.4 *(Continued)*

Acute Infectious Hepatitis (Continued)

Primary Prevention	*Secondary Prevention*	*Tertiary Prevention*
–Maximize general good hygiene. –Identify source and route of infection; correction, education, etc., as indicated. –Reduce stress, exposure to other diseases.		

Chronic, Infectious Disease: Tuberculosis

Primary Prevention	*Secondary Prevention*	*Tertiary Prevention*
General hygienic practices to raise levels of resistance. Personal sanitation re: saliva—coughing, spitting, tissue disposal, etc. Assertiveness toward those not practicing such. Screening tests of those involved in intimate contact with public or high-risk groups: beauty operators, dentists, school teachers, child care attendants, etc. BCG immunizations to high-risk populations (not general practice in United States but frequent in other countries). Inspection and vaccination of dairy herds for bovine tuberculosis. Pasteurization of milk; careful handling and certifications of raw milk and its products. Programs to prevent overcrowding and inadequate nutrition in risk populations.	Annual physical exams to include screening test for tuberculosis. Regular testing appropriate to risk at lowest level of hazard to client (e.g., skin test is preferable to X-ray unless already positive; high-risk people should be more often than low-risk people). Community screening programs in high-risk populations. Intensive case-finding services to contacts, especially children. Education of cases re: isolation techniques when active, self-care, medication regimes, followup care. Education of professionals re: populations at risk, new therapies. Inclusion of screening as automatic part of all intake procedures for hospitals, group living arrangements, community health agencies and penal institutions.	Long-term followup, checkups, medication monitoring. Modification of lifestyle to permit optimal functioning within limits of physical state. Diminish exposure to other lung hazards: pollutants especially smoking, dust, asbestos, silicates, other lung infections. Regular repeat screening even after completion of therapy.

TABLE 9.4 *(Continued)*

Adequate housing.	Counseling to avoid inappropriate invalidism.	
Isolation from contact cases until they are no longer infectious.		
Prophylactic chemotherapy to newly converted positive skin tests in the absence of positive sputums, especially children and other high-risk individuals.		

Acute, Noninfectious Condition: Auto Accidents

Primary Prevention	Secondary Prevention	Tertiary Prevention
Seat belt use on all trips by all occupants; passive restraints, such as air bags.	CB radios for early reporting by truckers and motorists.	Development/utilization of rehabilitation programs: physical, occupational, vocational, speech, or whatever therapy is needed.
Driver's education programs.	Emergency Medical Services for treatment at the scene.	
Public education re: drinking, drugs, fatigue, various diseases and their impact on driving; mechanical failures; emergency actions.	Professional specialization in EMS. Public education in first aid.	Education of industry on employability of handicapped; of professionals to raise awareness of needs for/uses of rehab services; of community on services available for rehab and how to get at them with or without professional aid.
Maintain safe speed for conditions.	Training as paramedics for all ambulance drivers, police, fire personnel. In some areas funeral vehicles are still used as ambulances; their drivers also need training.	
Spot checks of vehicles for safety equipment: lights, horn, tires, brakes, etc.		Development of community services for handicapped: e.g., Goodwill Industries, vocational rehabilitation, job retraining through the schools for people who must change work as a result of injuries.
Law enforcement: suspension and revocation of licenses for drunk or reckless driving before any accident occurs.	Develop and upgrade trauma centers. Insure trained personnel quickly available in all emergency rooms.	
Defensive driving courses; brush-up courses for drivers.	Acute care services available after emergency dealt with.	Financial assistance: (a) during rehab and job retraining; (b) aid to totally disabled for those who cannot be retrained to return to work; (c) partial support for those whose rehab does not make them totally self-supporting but still able to work.
Mandatory retesting for drivers: knowledge of laws; adequate vision.	Teaching care to case/ family/attendant: home care acute and chronic. aid in preventing disability and complications between professional visits.	

TABLE 9.4 *(Continued)*

Primary Prevention	Auto Accidents *(Continued)* Secondary Prevention	Tertiary Prevention
	Teaching self-care: of a hand wound, for example; how to care for wound, when and where to have stitches removed, how to recognize infection, what to do for infection, how much to use wounded part now, tomorrow, next week, next month.	Remedial driver education for repeated offenders; revocation of licenses on those who refuse. Penalty insurance rates for repeaters. Standards of inspection for "rehabilitated" vehicles that have been damaged.

Primary Prevention	*Chronic, Noninfectious Condition: Hypertension* Secondary Prevention	Tertiary Prevention
Lower sodium intake for all: infants, children, adults, high-risk groups, etc. Improve regular involvement of all age groups in participatory sports, exercise, or other strenuous activities. Teach pro-heart nutrition at all age levels: eliminate from all schools foods that are high salt, high fat, high starch, the basic junk foods; institute programs of consumer education at supermarkets. Reduce (eliminate?) tobacco smoking: prevent it in children and youth; stop-smoking programs; support groups against backsliding; assertive behavior by non-smokers; push for laws restricting smoking in public.	Public education about need for at least annual BP screening and to insist on adequate treatment for control of elevation. Screening services at convenient locations at minimal cost to test all populations for BP elevations with reliable interpretation, advice, and followup. Professional education on need to detect and control BP in excess of 140/90; all health workers should be able to screen in their work sites: pharmacists and dentists as well as nurses and physicians. Physician education on diagnosis of hypertension, nondrug and drug therapies, contraindications, and adverse effects of drugs used to treat hyper-	Establish programs for comprehensive treatment of hypertension through multiple approaches, especially incorporating lifestyle changes for permanent control of high BP. Continuing public education on need to control BP as a primary preventive for stroke, heart attack, and congestive heart disease. Professional education in all of above plus common causes of "patient non-compliance," including unacceptable drug side effects, inadequate education programs, failure to adapt teaching to client lifestyle, lack of followup of detected high BP. Continued monitoring of

TABLE 9.4 *(Continued)*

Obesity management at all ages. Stress control programs: relaxation in work settings; hotlines for harried housewives; TV tips on ways to relax. Institute screening programs to test for hypertension precursors including high blood cholesterol and triglycerides; renal disease; diabetes; pregnancy, birth control pills; excess salt intake; genetic history; obesity; lack of exercise; high stress levels.	tension, on need to teach clients to manage their own treatment, and on community resources, especially the CHN, for work with clients who have hypertension.	known hypertensive persons to insure their continuance with adequate treatment to control their hypertension. This is necessitated by people's tendency to stop taking their medications because they "feel fine" and/or because their blood pressure has been controlled as a result of the medication although this control may not continue without the medication.

secondary prevention. The rise of chronic noninfectious diseases and conditions has provided impetus for the development of the current emphasis on primary care that focuses on early diagnosis and prompt treatment. To be sure, these are essential efforts when the diseases and conditions cannot be totally prevented. In table 9.3 we list some of the general kinds of measures employed for early diagnosis and prompt treatment. These cluster around efforts to develop and promote the utilization of regular medical and dental care including screening examinations as well as professional education for these activities and the provision of needed and appropriate treatment facilities. Table 9.4 contains specific early diagnosis and prompt treatment measures for the four diseases and conditions listed.

Until relatively recently, concern for limiting disabilities from diseases and conditions did not have the priority it must have today and in the future. Most of the acute infectious diseases that ravaged the population before the days of immunizations and specific pharmaceuticals to treat them were relatively short in their duration. The majority of people who had them either recovered fairly quickly or died. Because of treatment limitations, both chemical and technological, people who developed chronic noninfectious diseases or conditions often did not survive nearly as long as people with these same maladies do today. Our life expectancy has only recently reached the biblically promised three-score and ten and most people died before they developed any of the chronic noninfectious conditions for which the probability of incidence increases with age. Manmade environmental hazards have increased in quantum leaps since World War II, thereby exposing more people to the as yet not clearly understood effects of food additives, radiation, dyes, pesticides, and pollution, to name only a few. Even with our modern technology and pharmacology, we still cannot cure many of the chronic and acute noninfectious conditions that are increasing in our population. Therefore we must place increased emphasis on preventing or delaying the disabilities that so often follow or accompany all kinds of diseases and conditions. Table 9.4 gives examples of disability-limiting measures for four specific diseases and conditions.

Tertiary prevention focuses on rehabilitation with the objective of helping people attain and maintain their OLOF regardless of the disabilities present. Rehabilitation can be thought of as a process of capitalizing on and developing abilities, whatever they may be, as well as learning to cope with disabilities. The increasing numbers of peoples who are disabled as a result of trauma and chronic noninfectious diseases and conditions necessitates increasing emphasis on rehabilitation. Many people with disabilities can be restored at least to personal independence in caring for themselves. Many others can be returned to gainful employment thereby increasing their own self-esteem as well as contributing to the economy. Community health nurses who work for visiting nurse associations, home health agencies, coordinated home care programs, and an increasing number of official agencies are finding themselves more involved in rehabilitation activities.

THE CHALLENGE OF PREVENTING NONINFECTIOUS DISEASES AND CONDITIONS

Much progress has been made in the United States to overcome the scourges of acute infectious diseases. A good deal of this progress has been the result of activities that have:

1. *Created environmental barriers to the spread of disease*—for example, construction of safe water supplies and effective sewage disposal plants;
2. *Increased host immunity or resistance to invading organisms* such as specific immunizations for measles, diphtheria, and polio or in the use of

general immunizing agents such as immune serum globulin for the prevention of hepatitis;

3. *Destruction of the vector that carries the disease* from host to host, such as measures to kill the female anopheline mosquito, which is the vector for malaria, or the World Health Organization's current massive plan to eliminate the tsetse fly, which is the vector of trypanosomiasis or African sleeping sickness;

4. *Development of treatment methods* such as antibiotics and chemotherapeutics to treat more adequately infectious diseases, such as gonorrhea and tuberculosis, that have proven harder to prevent than others.

For the most part this progress has been brought about by the efforts of public health workers and agencies with minimal involvement of the general public beyond that of fiscal support. Perhaps that is why we have had such success in dealing with infectious disease control—that is, we have provided general health promotion and environmental sanitation for the public or have offered them specific protection such as immunizations that required only minimal participation on their part (Hilbert 1977:354).

The task confronting epidemiologists and other public health workers in the late twentieth century is much more complex. We are faced with the challenge of developing, implementing, and evaluating primary preventive measures for the noninfectious diseases and conditions that are increasing as disablers and killers of our population. We stress the need for primary prevention of these conditions because as advanced as our technology and pharmacology are, we still can neither cure most of them nor rehabilitate their victims adequately. The human and economic toll they take each year defies calculation. Traditionally public health has been charged with the responsibility to prevent disease, and we must not lose sight of that responsibility; it is our raison d'etre (Terris 1976:1155).

Research and epidemiological investigations are increasing our data bank on the etiology and natural history of many chronic noninfectious diseases and conditions. Mauser and Bahn (1974:310–12) point out some of the problems encountered in etiologic investigations of chronic diseases.

Absence of a Known Agent. Unlike infectious diseases many chronic, noninfectious diseases have no known etiologic agent; hypertension is an example. We do not really know what causes elevated blood pressure although many factors such as obesity, smoking, lack of exercise, family history, high sodium intake, and stress are often associated with its manifestation. Often diagnostic tests lack sufficient specificity to enable us to distinguish between diseased and nondiseased persons; arthritis is an example.

Multifactorial Etiology.   Some chronic diseases have many factors that are operative. The example of hypertension given above is an illustration. Another is the greatly increased risk of lung cancer in people who both smoke and are exposed to asbestos. Women who smoke and take oral contraceptives increase their risk of hypertension geometrically rather than arithmetically.

Long Latent Period.   A long period of time often elapses between pertinent antecedent events and the development of manifest disease. For example, a friend is claustrophobic but can not figure out why. Parental questioning reveals that as a charming child the only way the nursery school teacher could cope with her was to periodically lock her in the coat closet. The chronic fear remains although the etiology has long since been forgotten.

Indefinite Onset.   Many chronic conditions have insidious onsets that go unnoticed for periods of time. Hypertension is often asymptomatic for a long time, which thus accounts for peoples' surprise when they are told their blood pressure is elevated. Their almost inevitable response is "But I've been feeling fine." Most of us have aches and pains periodically so that the actual onset of one of the arthritides is hard to pinpoint. This inability to determine time of onset makes antecedent events hard to identify.

Differential Effect of Factors on Incidence and Course of Disease.   A factor that influences the incidence of a chronic disease in one way may influence the course of that same disease differently. Smoking, for example, is more closely associated with sudden death in coronary heart disease than with other forms of the disease.

PROTECTION MEASURES

In spite of the problems with determining the natural history of acute and chronic noninfectious conditions and diseases, protection measures can be implemented that parallel those listed in the previous section as contributing to the decrease in infectious diseases. The following are some examples of protection measures for acute and chronic noninfectious diseases and conditions.

Environmental Barriers to the Spread of Disease.   Some experts attribute the etiology of 60-80 percent of all cancer to environmental contaminants (Hilbert 1977:355). Cleaning up our environment and removing the chemical contaminants could go a long way toward decreasing the incidence of cancer. Recent moves to establish smoking and nonsmoking sections in planes and other public areas is another environmental barrier to the spread of known disease-causing agents.

Increase Host Immunity or Resistance to Disease. Breslow et al. (1972:353) have found that the following of a number of basic health habits is significantly related to increased life expectancy and better health. These habits are:

Eat three regular meals a day rather than snacks;

Have breakfast every day;

Have moderate exercise (long walks, bike riding, swimming, gardening) two or three times a week;

Sleep seven or eight hours each night;

Don't smoke;

Keep weight moderate;

Keep alcohol use moderate; no alcohol is even better.

These are health promotion activities except for the admonitions against smoking and alcohol use, which are specific preventives for lung cancer, emphysema and other obstructive lung disease, cirrhosis, and cardiovascular diseases—all of which are in the top ten killers of our population.

Destruction of Vehicles that Carry Disease. Terris (1976:1157) suggests some concrete actions that can be taken to eliminate some of the vehicles of noninfectious diseases and conditions. One major approach is through laws that, he suggests, would prohibit all advertising for cigarettes and alcohol and forbid smoking in public places. Another legal move would be to require that only unsaturated fats be used in commercial baking and that all labels be required to list the amount and degree of saturation of fats in all packaged foods. Another major approach, which should be coupled with the passage of these laws, is to provide economic incentives for compliance. Taxes on alcohol and tobacco should be increased to the point where these products are prohibitively expensive to buy. At the same time support should be given to farmers raising the crops needed to make these products so that they can turn to less lethal crops. Taxes should also be levied on food stuffs that are high in saturated fats. Subsidies could be applied to make the cost of food low in saturated fats more attractive to consumers. Farmers could also be given assistance to change cattle feeds to produce beef that is low in saturated fats. These suggestions are examples of how politics and economics can be made to work for primary prevention (see chapter 11).

Develop Treatment Methods.   Again we must point out that the majority—
the vast majority, in fact—of our health care resources is expended on
treatment of noninfectious diseases with little change in overall disability
and mortality rates. To be sure treatment is needed and developments
must continue; however, if we make nothing else in this chapter clear, it is
our conviction that primary prevention measures for the noninfectious
diseases and conditions must be given far greater emphasis than is currently the case if we ever hope to reduce the disability and mortality they
cause.

Much of the environmental cleanup and removal of disease-causing
chemicals and waste products can be carried out, as was the construction
of water and sewage treatment facilities in the past, with only minimal
public involvement beyond that of providing public or private funding.
To some extent community health professionals can help to bring about
the kinds of legal and economic incentives and disincentives Terris (1976)
suggests to remove the vehicles of toxic substances from the market.
Tremendous resistance will be encountered from those sectors of society
whose vested interests are threatened by these actions. This opposition
cannot be overcome without public understanding and participation. Absolutely the same is true of efforts to increase host resistance to noninfectious diseases and conditions through changes in our way of living.

The greatest potential for attaining and maintaining our own OLOF
lies in what we do to and for ourselves. No longer can we rely on others to
protect us or to provide us with quick and easy preventive measures such
as immunizations. Every one of the factors Breslow has identified (see
above) are do-it-yourself factors. We must learn self-reliance ourselves
and then teach it to our clients. We must serve as role models of positive
health promotional behaviors. We must change our lifestyles and help
our clients to change theirs, too. This type of teaching is the hardest part
of the role that we as community health nurses must play. We must be
prepared to teach and teach and teach again. A fantastic amount of data
are at our fingertips to back up what we teach. We must use it to help
clients understand what needs to be done and how to do it.

We have already heard the hue and cry when seat belts were mandated by law for all new cars. The seat belts are there now, but are they
used? Air bags have proven to be effective in preventing terrible injuries.
When will they be installed? Air bags have the advantage of working
automatically on impact and so do not depend on our conscious use of
them. Tobacco is clearly linked to lung cancer, cardiovascular disease,
emphysema, and a host of other diseases. How many people still smoke?
How many of *us* still smoke? These questions point to only a few examples of public reactions so far to efforts to help them help themselves. The

problem is not that we lack the information in many areas, it's that we have not yet learned how to make the information available to the public in such a way that they take on the responsibilities for promoting their own OLOF. To do so is the greatest challenge facing epidemiology and community health nursing in the late twentieth century.

SUMMARY

The case example that begins this chapter is an illustration of an epidemiological investigation of an acute infectious disease. The example is used to demonstrate the relationship between the three major actors in epidemiology; the host, the agent, and the environment. Epidemiology is an applied science that uses eclectic research methods to study the distribution of diseases and conditions and their determinants in the total population. This total population orientation separates epidemiology from clinical or case medicine and nursing, which focus on individuals or small groups of clients. Some of the uses of epidemiology as a major community health tool are discussed.

Diseases and conditions are classified on the basis of two factors, etiology and duration, into four groups: acute infectious, chronic infectious, acute noninfectious, and chronic noninfectious. Primary, secondary, and tertiary preventive measures are discussed generally and specifically for each of the four classifications of diseases and conditions.

Because chronic noninfectious diseases and conditions now account for seven of the ten leading causes of death in the U.S. population, considerable time is spent discussing these conditions. Although pharmacological and technological advances in the treatment of chronic diseases have made quantum progress since World War II, the real hope for reducing their effects lies in preventing or at least forestalling their incidence. Some of the limitations in the study of noninfectious diseases are discussed and some concrete suggestions for their prevention, which parallel measures that have been successful in reducing the incidence of infectious diseases, are given.

The greatest challenge presented to epidemiology and to community health nurses in the prevention of noninfectious diseases is to learn how to motivate the public to apply what is already known about lifestyle changes and their relationship to the development of noninfectious diseases to their own lives. As in the past, environmental safety and protection can be undertaken with minimal public involvement. Professionals can provide specific protection and treatment as needed. However, the real primary prevention must come through people's own control of their lifestyles in such areas as alcohol and tobacco use, obesity, exercise, nutrition, and rest. Community health nurses have a vital role to play in the health education that must take place if people are to learn how and why positive lifestyle changes can help them attain and maintain their optimal level of functioning.

GLOSSARY

Carrier   A healthy person who harbors and excretes an infectious agent often for long periods of time. Typhoid Mary is an example.

Case Studies   A detailed, intensive, factual description of individuals, groups of individuals, institutions, communities, whole societies, or even incidents, situations, inanimate objects, or animals.

Cohort Studies   A set of study subjects who are grouped together according to certain characteristics and observed longitudinally. Cohort studies are essentially repeated cross-sectional studies that involve the same subjects.

Demography   The study of mankind collectively, especially of their geographical distribution and physical environment.

Direct Contact   The term applied when an infection is spread more or less directly from person to person. It does not necessarily mean actual bodily contact but does indicate a rather close association.

Epidemic   The occurrence in a community of a group of illnesses of similar nature, clearly in excess of normal expectation.

Experimental Studies   Studies in which all elements of the research are under control of the investigator. They are often conducted in specialized research settings.

Fomites   Intimate personal objects such as drinking glasses, toys, and so forth.

Herd Immunity   Resistance of a group to the invasion and spread of an infectious agent based on a high proportion of individuals in the group being immune already.

Immunity: Acquired   Host immunity developed to a pathogen as a result of contact with the disease agent; for example, measles in humans.

Immunity: Active   Host immunity developed in response to an infecting agent or a vaccine and characterized by the presence of host-produced antibody.

Immunity: Natural   Species-determined inherent resistance to disease agent; for example, human immunity to the virus causing cat leukemia.

Immunity: Passive   Immunity derived from antibody produced by another host that is acquired naturally by an infant from the mother or artificially through the administration of an antibody-containing preparation, such as immune serum globulin as a prophylaxis for hepatitis.

Incidence   The number of new cases of a disease or condition within a specified time period.

Indirect Contact   The spread of a causative agent of a disease by such conveyers as milk and other foods, water, air, contaminated hands, and inanimate objects.

Intervention Studies   The conditions for the study are consciously manipulated or controlled. The researcher actually interferes with nature.

Life Expectancy   The average number of years a newborn can be expected to live.

Multiple Causation A situation in which many variables may be related to a single effect through a direct-indirect mechanism in which A is causally related to B, B to C, C to D, and so on until finally maybe R plays an important part in the development of the disease.

Natural Experiment A research situation in which the setting is studied just as it is without any modification or control over the environment.

Natural History of a Disease A comprehensive report on the disease: the nature of the agent, its source and distribution, its reservoirs and modes of transmission, and its impact on susceptible hosts. When many people speak of the epidemiology of a disease, they are referring to its natural history.

Prevalence The number of cases of a specific disease or condition at a given time in the population at that same time.

Probability Sampling A formal plan for selecting individuals for study in which, for every member of the population under study, the probability of being included in the sample is known and is the same.

Risk The probability that an event, in this case the occurrence of a disease or condition, will happen to a given person or group. For example, people who smoke have a greater risk of lung cancer than do people who do not smoke.

Risk Factors Factors whose presence is associated with increased likelihood that a disease or condition will develop. Obesity, high salt intake, and lack of exercise are risk factors for the development of hypertension.

Sensitivity Here used to refer to diagnostic tests that are sensitive if they detect a very high percentage of the people tested who have the disease or conditions tested for. Sensitivity deals with *true positives*—that is, accurately designating those people who do have the disease or condition.

Specificity Here used to refer to diagnostic tests that are specific if they determine that a high percentage of the people *without* the disease or condition being tested for are indeed free of the disease or condition. Specificity deals with *true negatives*—that is, accurately designating those people who do not have the disease or condition.

Vector An insect that plays a role in the transmission of an infectious agent from host to host. The female anopheline mosquito and the organisms causing malaria are examples.

Vehicle An inanimate object, such as clothing, food, water, soil, or other substances, by which the infectious or other disease-producing agent is transported to the host.

APPENDIX: FORMULAS FOR COMPUTING RATES USED IN VITAL STATISTICS

Name of Rate	How Computed
Annual Death Rate	Deaths from all causes in a calendar year × 1,000 ÷ population of July 1
Annual Age-Specific Rate	Deaths from all causes for given age group in year × 1,000 ÷ population for given age group, July 1

Appendix: Formulas for Computing Rates Used in Vital Statistics

Name of Rate	How Computed
Annual Death Rate from Specific Cause	Deaths from specific cause in year × 100,000 ÷ population of July 1
Annual Case Incidence Rate of a Specific Disease	New cases of specific disease in year × 1,000 ÷ population of July 1
Annual Birth Rate	Live births in year × 1,000 ÷ population of July 1
Case Fatality Rate	Deaths from specific disease in given period × 100 ÷ cases of specific disease in given period
Incidence Rate	Number of new cases of a specified disease occurring in a defined population during a specified time period × 1,000 ÷ estimated population a midpoint of the specified time period
Infant mortality Rate	Deaths under one year of age in year × 1,000 ÷ live births in year
Maternal Mortality Rate	Maternal deaths in year × 1,000 (or 10,000) ÷ live births in year
Neonatal Mortality Rate	Deaths under one month of age in year × 1,000 (or 10,000) ÷ live births in year
Point Prevalence	Number of cases of a specified disease existing in a defined population at a specified point of time × 1,000 estimated population at the same point in time
Prevalence Rate	All cases of specific disease at given time × 1,000 ÷ population at given time
Stillbirth Rate	Stillbirths in year × 100 (or 1,000) ÷ total births in year

REFERENCES

BAKER, D. J. P. *Practical Epidemiology.* London: Churchill Livingston, 1973.

BECKER, MARSHALL H. "The Health Belief Model and Personal Health Behavior." *The Health Education Monograph* 2 (Winter 1974):4.

BENENSON, ABRAM S., ed. *Control of Communicable Diseases in Man,* 12th ed. Washington, D.C.: American Public Health Association, 1975.

BRESLOW, LESTER. "A Quantitative Approach to the World Health Organization Definition of Health: Physical, Mental and Social Well-Being." *International Journal of Epidemiology* 1 (April 1972):347–55.

FOX, JOHN P., HALL, CARRIE E., and ELVEBACK, LILA A. *Epidemiology in Man and Disease.* New York: Macmillan Co., 1970.

HILBERT, MORTON. "Prevention." *American Journal of Public Health* 67 (April 1977):353–56.

KASL, STANISLAV. "Issues in Patient Adherence to Health Care Regimens." *Journal of Human Stress* 1 (September 1975):5–12.

LALONDE, MARC. "Beyond a New Perspective." *American Journal of Public Health* 67 (April 1977):357–60.

———. *A New Perspective on the Health of Canadians: A Working Document.* Ottawa: Government of Canada, April 1974.

LEAVELL, HUGH R., and CLARK, E. GURNEY. *Preventive Medicine for the Doctor in his Community: An Epidemiologic Approach,* 3rd ed. New York: McGraw-Hill Book Co., 1965.

MMWR: Morbidity and Mortality Weekly Report. Atlanta: Center for Disease Control, U.S. Public Health Service, published weekly.

MACMAHAN, BRIAN, and PUGH, THOMAS F. *Epidemiology: Principles and Methods.* Boston: Little, Brown and Co., 1970.

MAUSER, JUDITH S., and BAHN, ANITA K. *Epidemiology: An Introductory Text.* Philadelphia: W. B. Saunders Co., 1974.

MILIO, NANCY. "A Framework for Prevention: Changing Health-Damaging to Health-Generating Life Patterns." *American Journal of Public Health* 66 (May 1976):435–39.

PEACOCK, PETER B., GELMAN, ANNA C., and LUTINS, THEODORE A. "An Annotated Bibliography for Preventive Health Care Strategies for Health Maintenance Organizations." *Preventive Medicine* 4 (1975):328–72.

———. "Preventive Health Care Strategies for Health Maintenance Organizations." *Preventive Medicine* 4 (1975):183–225.

PENDER, NOLA J. "A Conceptual Model for Preventive Health Behavior." *Nursing Outlook* 23 (June 1975):385–90.

PESZNECKER, BETTY L., and McNEIL, JO. "Relationship among Health Habits, Social Assets, Psychologic Well-Being, Life Change, and Alterations in Health Status." *Nursing Research* 24 (November–December 1975):442–47.

"Profile of American Health." *Public Health Reports* 89 (November–December 1974):504–23.

ROGERS, RONALD E. "A Protection Motivation Theory of Fear Appeals and Attitude Change." The Journal of Psychology 91 (1975):93–114.

ROUCHÉ, BERTON. *Eleven Blue Men and Other Narratives of Medical Detection.* New York: Berkeley Medallion Books, 1955.

———. *The Incurable Wound and Further Narratives of Medical Detection.* New York: Berkeley Books, 1954.

SOMERS, ANNE R., ed. *Promoting Health: Consumer Health Education and National Policy.* Germantown, Pa.: Aspen Systems Corporation, 1976.

TERRIS, MILTON. "Approaches to an Epidemiology of Health." *American Journal of Public Health* 65 (October 1975):1037–45.

———. "The Epidemiology Revolution, National Health Insurance, and the Role of Health Departments." *American Journal of Public Health* 66 (December 1976):1155–64.

WYATT, H.V. "Investigating an Epidemic: A Seven-Part Simulation Used in Teaching." International Journal of Epidemiology 6 (1977):173–76.

10. Aspects of Health Education in Community Nursing

Ruth P. Fleshman

INTRODUCTION

During the early years of the Haight-Ashbury Free Medical Clinic, hepatitis was a major and recurrent health problem encountered by many of the young people who came to us for help. As a volunteer nurse, I began to notice that different physicians explained the disease and advised the clients about it in contradictory terms. Some presumed anyone with jaundice was using illicit needles. Some advised a low fat diet, others a high carbohydrate one. Some clients were told to adopt isolation techniques for droplet-borne organisms, others for fecal ones. The length of time clients were told they might be contagious also varied with which physician they saw. Such confusion suggested that even physicians' knowledge might not be the best on this subject. Thus I set out to see whether I could organize information into a handout sheet to reduce the inconsistencies and increase our reliability. I started with medical texts and then moved to journals since hepatitis research was ongoing and information constantly changed. I found these sources also were contradictory and that there were enormous areas of ignorance.

Luckily a research unit at the county hospital was working on hepatitis and I interviewed the medical director who flatly stated that if our clients wanted "to know more about their disease, they'd better get something other than hep!" Thus, even someone at the forefront of medical research admitted he couldn't be much help. The fact that our desire to answer questions and give advice outstripped the knowledge base available to anyone soon became clear. For example, apparently the common practice of giving gamma globulin to people exposed to hepatitis was only a part of the helping syndrome, since studies showed that even under ideal conditions, those given the injections had no lower rates of subsequent illness than those who had gotten no serum at all. Knowledge at the level of care delivery was not even consistent about which form of hepatitis might be the right one to try gamma globulin on.

My first three tries at writing out the information for our clients resulted in dry-as-dust, textbookish prose that bored everyone to death, including me. At last I realized that I was writing as if for an outside observer, for the professional, not the patient or potential patient. Finally, by turning the material inside out in a way, I was able to translate it into something that could be useful to someone who might have or might be getting hepatitis. It was quite a different thing to describe the external view of the course of hepatitis than to explain what if *felt* like and how to tell from the inside what was happening. I realized that this approach was one of the differences between medical textbooks and what needed to be a part of health education. I wondered whether this difference might also be one of the reasons why health professionals are often able to resist applying their knowledge to their own lives, as with smoking or lack of exercise: Textbook knowledge is remote, abstract, exterior while educational material needs to be personal, interior, specific. Medical texts are for observers; health education is for participants. In addition, bridges had to be constructed between explanation and application. Many pamphlets simply present recipes for what to do without giving any logic as to why or the risks of not doing so. The texts, on the other hand, present research findings, lab tests, epidemiologic information, and treatment procedures without explaining what people can do in everyday life to manage the illness in themselves or a family member.

Even with the new handout sheet, I soon realized that other approaches were needed. People would take the pamphlet home and return the next night to ask me questions about the material they had read. When I answered with information consistent with the handout, they seemed reassured. I thought their reaction was peculiar since they knew I had written it. But it seemed important for some to *hear* as well as read material. (Some couldn't relate to written information at all and needed to have the content talked over with them before they could absorb it.) To some extent, the material needed to be repeated or presented in a different set of words for people to deal with it successfully.

There was a great deal of satisfaction for me in having acquired a high level of knowledge even about a single subject such as hepatitis. However, by entering into exchanges with people concerned about the impact of this disease on their lives, I soon learned there were other areas of real impact that played an important role with this disease alone. One was the problem of fecally contaminated water, which was eventually to lead me to study more than I cared to know about water purification and the disposal of human wastes, including how to dig a proper privy in the country. The other big area of immediate concern to the people we served was nutrition: "Since you say diet is so important in preventing or curing hep, tell me how I can do it on a vegetarian diet?" With this subject, books were no help, since they didn't deal with some of the unusual diets people were following, and I had to turn to our clients to learn from them. I learned that I was uncomfortable with some of the claims made by followers of the Macrobiotic Diet or the Ehret Mucusless Diet, but I lacked the scientific knowledge to refute them even to my own satisfaction, let alone the clients'. So I turned to nutritionists who also had to do a fair deal of reading to analyze the precise problems with these diets. (This experience turned out to be educative for some of them too, since it made them realize the gap between their scientific beliefs and the dietary practices of various groups of young adults in our own community!)

By this time I was hopelessly entwined in the health-related information this population of young adults was asking for: nutrition led me to pregnancy problems among pure vegetarians, which led to the issue of home deliveries as a preferred practice. Nutrition also led to problems of low-cost food in the city, food conspiracies (neighborhood pooling to buy food wholesale and distribute it directly), and other forms of collective action. These issues in turn put me into contact with groups focused around health topics, such as the Berkeley Women's Health Collective, which has spent years refining its own knowledge about nutrition to produce a sensible and sound pamphlet about the subject. This pamphlet became a basic part of the material distributed to the young adults who were soon my community client group. It's far better suited to their style and level of knowledge than some of the simple-minded Basic Foods for Healthy Bodies things that had been a standard part of the old public health library.

The numbers of other topics I felt impelled to study have led some of my nurse-colleagues to wonder just what my specialty is. A nutritionist keeps asking, "If diet is so important to these people, why don't you just hire a nutritionist and be done with it?" Others wonder about our getting the aid of dentists, sanitarians, veterinarians (even pets have health problems!), or dermatologists. And I keep asking back what can they teach besides their specialty? I am not an "expert" on pregnancy and delivery, nor on diets, nor rural sanitation, nor community organization, nor even health education. I'm a community health nurse. I've learned about one group of people, tried to answer their questions, worked with some of them in advancing their knowledge and my own as well. I've gotten to know a lot about young adults and their eagerness to learn about themselves. I've become convinced that other community nurses have a vital contribution to make in this way with whoever their clients are: the elderly, a neighborhood, some particular ethnic group, some group with health deficits or handicaps, whoever goes to make up the clients they serve.

CLIENT-PROFESSIONAL COMMUNICATION

One issue of great concern is the trouble health professionals of all kinds have in sharing their information with their clients, patients, and with laypeople in general in terms they can understand. Until twenty or thirty years ago, the health professional could get away with doing things *to* the passive patient; the less interference the better. Great value was placed on patients' being cooperative—that is, docile. But now we've reached the stage where too much depends on the patients' active participation. The cost of hospitalization being what it is, patients can no longer sit passively in bed having things done to them. Home care and ambulatory services are the most feasible way to deal with many of the chronic illnesses. With the old, short, and dramatic infectious diseases, patients either recovered or died. But we have none of the sort of magic tricks that used to be enough. Cure has been replaced by maintenance. Prevention is no longer managed only by inoculations; education is the only primary prevention for many chronic diseases.

The health field's complexity is tremendous. Knowledge has expanded explosively and technical information is increasing faster than we can use it. There is an expanding variety of professionals involved in health care. Their specialized knowledge is pulling away from general lay knowledge at an increasing rate. It has never been more important, then, for clients to become fully informed members of the health team.

Professional Obstacles to Teaching

One problem in educating clients is the baffling unwillingness we occasionally meet in colleagues to accept the idea that knowledge should be shared. Sometimes they simply don't want to take the time or effort needed to translate the expert knowledge they have taken years to acquire into a form that would be digestible for clients who are not medically trained. Others believe that clients can't possibly understand *without* all that background, so there would be no point in trying; it would only confuse them! Some seem to consider clients to be slightly dim and incapable of complex thinking. Whatever information is shared is often phrased in Basic English or pared-down logic. The game plan here seems to be "If you're so smart, how come you're sick?" We all tend to think this way at times without checking whether clients are indeed dumb, simply ignorant, or the victims of events beyond the control of any of us. This is never more clear than when one of our own becomes a patient!

There is an entirely different set of problems presented for us by colleagues whose idea of professional practice does not invest other members of the team or the client with the same autonomy as they hold for themselves. For many reasons, it isn't possible for such workers to share—or permit others to share—the special information we might consider essential for client care. Some seem to fear that giving away even a part of one's professional bag of tricks would lessen the ability to go on being a health worker. Others seem to subscribe to the "a little knowledge is a dangerous thing" school of thought. The greatest obstacles for nurses trying to give needed information to clients are the professionals who believe that the whole health care enterprise rests in their hands and no decisions can be made in their absence. My impression is that hospital nurses are more plagued than community nurses with this problem since they exist in a stringently hierarchical situation where power and authority are apparently vested along professional lines. But it would be a disservice to any of us committed to the notion of a fully informed client to presume that everyone shares our belief. The first step in the nursing assessment of such a situation may well need to be the identification of barriers to client teaching and the development of strategies to change them.

Many nurses tend to identify physicians as the only authoritarian obstacles they need to deal with. This view is most true for those physicians educated along the traditional lines that suggested their responsibilities are onerous yet sacrosanct. The experience of New York's nurses in the early seventies found them successfully challenging their medical colleagues' view that nurses were incapable of independent judgments. By refusing to make *any* for twenty-four hours, the nurses more than adequately proved their point; they rousted physicians from sleep to check thermometer readings, *ad lib* and *prn* orders, reported unsorted observations of postoperative patients until their case was clearly demonstrated.

However, it is never wise to assume that even one's coprofessionals are in ideological agreement. For example, in my own experience I have observed many other nurses ducking the responsibility for independent decision making by referring thoroughly trivial matters to the physician even when agency policy does not demand it. Where have you ever seen it written, for instance, that patients may not be told their temperatures? And many of us are only too willing to feed back to physicians their notion that really important things, like teaching or other preparations for discharge, hang upon their written orders. Some of my coworkers in the free clinic have expressed great discomfort at watching me in rap sessions with clients, and one even admitted she feared that this would next be expected of her and that she couldn't stand the notion of being found unable to carry it off. I'm sure all of us know many times when we duck questions about what we are doing—not so much for fear of giving away some precious secret—but because we don't know what is really the basis for our actions and hate to let that be known. The importance of maintaining a mask of expertise may well operate in many refusals to give information.

During the planning stage of a hypertension screening program, we found the physicians on the planning team were aghast that we intended to give each client a copy of the blood pressure readings. Knowing this information, one said, would upset the clients too much until they could get to a physician for reassurance or treatment. We suggested that the concealment of such information behind guarded phrases would probably be even more anxiety-producing: "Your pressure *seems* to be up a little today—uh, er—maybe you should check with your doctor—soon—carefully!" Our colleagues agreed there was merit on both sides but accepted our firm decision to do it our way. Clients made many comments that they had never had blood pressure explained to them before; they had generally been dismissed with a cheery "Oh, it's just fine," and no notion of the numbers involved. No one had any problems from knowing normal or elevated readings, and those with the latter may well have sought medical care more promptly for being given the bases on which we made our suggestions that they needed to do so. The experience of the project finally convinced the particular physicians involved that maybe the idea hadn't been so bad after all!

Another barrier to communicating information is a problem common to all health professionals: our special language. It is, perhaps, harder to be unaware of this language in community health than in institutional services, but we all have a shorthand jargon that we use within our field that makes it easy to talk about very complex topics with a minimum of words: prognosis, syndrome, tachycardia, metastatic. But it's really a foreign language to the general population, a fact we tend to forget. If those workers who do take time to explain what's going on use this insider's speech, what they have to say is little better than telling nothing at all. Without translation, a jargon often conceals more than it reveals.

Often, however, we do not take into account the rise in the general level of education. In the 1940s, for instance, we could safely assume that a bare majority of the populace had graduated from high school. Few went on to higher education and generally the cream of that crop went to medical school, the most prestigious profession. Medicine, for most people, was an awesome mystery. This situation has changed, however. Expanding knowledge has bred new and equally mysterious disciplines and professions. Other careers besides medicine are open to bright men and women. There has also been an increased lay awareness of general health matters as well as wider availability of specific information. Look through general circulation publications; there's almost always some health-related column or article. People are interested and concerned.

The information explosion extends also to increased circulation of unreliable, misinformed, or outright false information about topics related to health and illness. Examples can be found in the wide number of nutrition books that appeal to wide numbers of people. Potentially harmful practices are advocated by authors who appear to base their doctrines on large doses of religious fervor and alienation from scientific authority. Another fascinating theme can be found in the kind of paranoia printed by small publishers with their own axes to grind. For example, I once came across a pamphlet stating that aspirin is a poison, a plot by organized medicine to get us to introduce a foreign substance into our bodies; that they don't know how it works; that aspirin causes chromosomal breaks; that it's derived from petrochemicals, which we all know cause air pollution and cancer; and that we should all go back to the natural remedy in willowbark tea. Such statements are all confirmable in a way. We *don't* know how aspirin works; it *is* derived from petrochemicals; more children are poisoned yearly by aspirin than any other single substance; it *does* cause chromosomal breaks (though the consequences are not yet determined). It is directly related to the chemical found in willowbark tea (salicin) but with a much *lower* toxicity potential than the so-called natural form.

The health questions written to Doctor Columns, the sorts of health books being written, bought, and read in increasing numbers, and the fact that diet books, for instance, actually make best-seller lists all suggest that people want to know more. Our free press permits anything short of libel to be printed, whether true or not, which thus makes it even more important that health professionals engage in sharing reliable, scientific information. The need for this information is borne out to us whenever we see people seeking medical help for problems that would have been preventable with the earlier application of accurate information—that is, when a little reliable knowledge put into action could make the difference between illness and absence of illness.

TEACHING HEALTH INFORMATION

HEALTH EDUCATION IN SCHOOLS

Those of us professionally involved with health often wonder why more people haven't gotten the basics of health information that we take so much for granted. Formal education is a part of childhood, and many people assume that children are taught all about health in school. But teachers have little or no content in health science as part of their preparation, unless they are planning to teach it as a distinct subject, so their information is probably little better than the average layperson's. Of course, science and biology teachers often incorporate material applicable to humans into their course outlines, but they usually have different objectives than trying to teach healthful living. Most school districts employ nurses either directly or indirectly. The presence of such a knowledgeable resource would seem a natural fit. But so few school nurses are able to make health education in the classroom a regular part of their job that it is still considered an innovative direction for school nursing.

You might expect that health educators would be involved in educational programs geared for individuals or groups. But, like teachers, they are often taught more of the process of teaching than of health improvement and more how to organize groups and libraries and bulletin boards and health campaigns than actually to transmit reliable health information to a population. Because the function of health education often has low visibility and is periodically cut from budgets as a mere frill item, many health educators use their other skills in following more remunerative trends—into community organizing, program development and evaluation, health care administration, wherever the budget goes this year.

How then does health education get done in the formal learning setting? Much often depends on teachers' individual concerns or on crisis campaigns centered on some particular health topic. An example of the latter is the big push against venereal diseases since communities became aware of the epidemic scope of the diseases among young people. The topic has been pounded by all the media to the point that many adolescents are bored to revulsion with any further attempts to add to their knowledge about VD. It often turns out they still lack sufficient information to detect risks and symptoms but are so turned off by the campaign approach that they block input on the topic. With such issues, teachers often use individual concerns to introduce special health topics. In one health class, the teacher introduced discussions of death after three violent deaths had occurred in a local high school. Death and dying are topics often too hot to handle for a lot of people, and even one attempt to deal with it in school should be applauded since adolescent suicide is a major health problem given very little attention in school or out.

There are generally two approaches to teaching health in schools. One way is to incorporate it into the general flow of the curriculum and thus utilize the teacher's skills and ease with the students. Many schools include specific topics in their curriculum master plans as mandated by legislators. These often include smoking, drugs and alcohol, dental care, and exercise. School districts often prepare a detailed health curriculum plan with many more subjects included, but closer scrutiny often shows room to doubt the degree to which it's actually carried out. Teachers who know little or nothing about a subject can hardly be expected to make it fascinating or even particularly clear and useful.

To counteract the problem, health topics are often set apart in special classes, where "experts" are brought in to deal with important topics that are beyond the scope of the regular teachers. This second method is often used in districts that do permit sex education, since this is another hot topic for teachers, parents, and school boards. (One district instructed its nurse to teach about VD prevention but to be sure she didn't include anything about sex, since the parents had created an uproar the last time that topic was introduced!) By separating a subject into a special unit, it is never put together with the rest of the curriculum nor for that matter with the thinking of the students, even when the school nurse is used as the hired gun. It is obviously different from the rest of the teaching process and easily kept apart in students' minds from their ongoing store of knowledge.

In many schools, nurses are not yet recognized as experts in an area of knowledge important to the education of the students—and faculty as well. These nurses are often relegated to first aid procedures and paper shuffling. However, a few are beginning to prove that nurses not only have an area of expertise, but also a wide array of properly academic courses incorporating learning theories, psychology, growth and development, and normal behavior. Strategies can be developed to create a health education curriculum drawing on teachers' expertise in methods and nurses' knowledge of health content. If classroom teaching is not always possible, a consultative role can still permit nurses to make their special contribution.

HEALTH EDUCATION FOR ADULTS

In looking for books to suggest as references in this chapter, we became aware that most listings under health education were clearly intended for school programs. A few were directed to the somewhat different area of patient teaching, to which we'll turn in a while. But almost nowhere could we find significant efforts directed toward people after they leave the school system. This lack may reflect the educational philosophy that holds that learning ends upon leaving school. This philosophy has never been true, but now more attempts are being made to change its operation, in adult schools, night programs, and alternative schools—free universities, self-help health groups, and so on. Otherwise, the information adults receive generally comes from mass media sources. These may be ads for health products which give flat-out advice on solving problems with some over-the-counter drug. Advertising techniques are also being applied to health campaigns: Learn Cancer's Seven Danger Signals; There's a Name for People Who Don't Use Seat Belts—Stupid; Warning: The Surgeon General Has Determined That Cigarette Smoking is Dangerous to Your Health. At best, media campaigns are designed only to present single-shot themes, to raise consciousness of health concerns, to transmit only the simplest message. Tying messages to an agency address or phone number does offer followup information, but also requires that further action will have to be taken by people interested in the topic.

Generally, material aimed for a mass audience is geared to a wide range of people and no one in particular. Such an approach may be compared to a shotgun blast that is hoped to hit something by the spray of a wide enough blast. Looking at mass media health information reveals a number of deficits. Much of it is geared toward some insultingly low estimate of the audience's intelligence. Health material is often presented from an authoritarian stance that condescends to the level of understanding and often comes across as "doctor knows best." Many times it gives specific directions for action without explaining the rationale for doing so or the consequences of not doing so. On the other hand, some materials stray so far into the theoretical bases for action that they never explain how the information can be applied in real life. This approach can be seen in the supertechnical kinds of articles generally prepared for professionals that are occasionally put into general circulation without considering just how useful they will be. Since wide circulation health information is often expensive to make up, large numbers are generally done at once to last awhile. Thus they often become dated both in terms of the rapidly expanding knowledge base and in shifts of basic problems and assumptions. These latter can be seen in prose that reflects racist or sexist slants to which we have only recently become sensitized. Many materials also reflect a presumption of unlimited resources (flush toilets require at least three gallons of water for each action; nonreturnable containers are still the general rule). Most health materials assume medical coverage for everything and everyone, give little or no self-help directives, and do not relate at all to people with alternative views of health care.

CONSUMER HEALTH EDUCATION

Within the past few years another aspect of health education has increased in importance and must be considered here even though it may seem quite different from what has been discussed so far. This form is directed to helping consumers of health services learn how to use those services, to evaluate the quality of the service they receive, and to participate in the improvement of services that do not meet their needs. A general theme of many community organizing activities has been the stipulation that a large portion, often a majority of the advisory or governing boards, must be comprised of community members—that is, laypeople, nonprofessionals, or whatever people call them to make sure they're not providers with a vested interest in the particular service. There have been some fascinating projects in community control of decision making, although a few of these have foundered in feuds and power grabbing.

For the most part, laypeople, elected to boards with professionals, are overwhelmed by the apparent expertise of the pros, and often go along for months until they begin to understand what's *really* going on. Then, just about the time they get a firm grip on how to make the board move in their direction, their term of office expires, and a new election brings fresh layfolks in to have to learn all over again. In projects centered around health services, it seems especially important that lay board members be given short, intensive seminars on their rights and responsibilities, how to see through professional jargon, how to ask questions over and over until the answers make sense, and how to counter all those things professionals do to cool out the outsiders. This sort of action may not always be seen as a nursing role, but there is certainly no reason why nurses could not work in this area. And lots of reasons why *community* nurses should.

Any nurse sooner or later encounters a client who is getting short shrift from the care system. What each of us does about such situations is partly related to how each of us sees the whole world, our profession and its relation to other members of the health team, the role of clients, and even how well we get along with the particular one in trouble. Clearly, we do have opportunities to teach clients how to get around some of the apparent obstacles and also how to make the most effective fuss per square inch to get things changed. Sometimes our action may be nothing more than reinforcing a client's notion to write a complaining letter about some upsetting event, or providing the really appropriate name and address to write to (with carbons on up the hierarchy!), or maybe actually addressing the envelope, or . . . , or . . . , or . . . .

At other times a single client may not be able to make effective and enduring changes in the system. For example, recurrent problems in service delivery may continue to impede client progress until basic policies are changed, and thus appropriate action may be as an advocate, if you see that as part of your role. (We've talked a bit elsewhere about some of the hazards involved in this very exciting line of work!) Some nursing groups have actually made patient care a major issue in contract negotiations and subsequent strikes.

However, there are times when clients are quite able to speak for themselves and indeed must do so. An appropriate nursing action at such a stage might well be to facilitate the formation of a client group, if nothing more, than by arranging a meeting room and providing support services. Further action is also possible if we know of other clients with similar interests and concerns and put them into contact. In taking such action, a helpful point to remember is, of course, that we are consumers too, even though we have another piece of identity as a professional. However, we are not always able to look at our own system through the same eyes as nonprofessionals, and there are even times when we are part of the problem! No matter how pure our intentions, there are still occasions when we nurses are seen only in our role as part of the service system that is causing trouble.

We discuss other specific courses of action in other parts of this book: Advocacy is briefly defined in chapter 1; the questions Terry and Bello ask in chapter 6 could be answered by client advocacy, and the advocate role is exemplified in chapter 14. Discussing health insurance with clients is an important act of consumer education by nurses as is suggested in chapter 12.

As discussed in chapter 22, the whole legislative process provides many chances for nursing input, starting with the initial public hearings at which many of us testify to help legislators better understand the problems consumers face in trying to use our system. Lawmakers seldom have adequate information about health care unless someone, often a lobbyist, provides it for them. Laws made only to reflect special interests often benefit only those interests and there are very few consumer lobbyists. Even after laws are written, there are opportunities for amendments and discussion in the legislature. After passage, the law must be transformed into operational regulations that determine how it really works; thus there is yet another chance to push for the consumer viewpoint, either directly from consumer groups or as one speaking for them. If nothing else, we can work on ways to help consumers become more assertive in behalf of their own interests. We can do so by clarifying with them how the care system impinges on their interests or, if it is more appropriate, by conducting assertiveness training sessions.

ILLNESS TEACHING

Just as many people tend to use the words *health care* to refer to services extended to the ill without any thought for positive or maximal health, so too, many who speak of health education actually limit their meaning to the processes of teaching clients and families about the management of disease. Aspects of prevention may, of course, be included when early warning symptoms are learned about or when information about complications is given.

Shorter and more expensive hospital stays as well as the increase of chronic illnesses have made clear the greater need for information as the basis for self-management of illness. All nurses, inside hospitals and out, must be prepared to participate in sharing this kind of information. Thus, much before students move into community nursing, they presumably have already begun to acquire skills in the kind of one-to-one teaching that most often characterizes this form of education. Community nurses do find more instances of illnesses managed at home and also need to be prepared for that kind of teaching.

Illness brings a new consciousness to the afflicted persons as what was before only abstract becomes very real and personal. Thus clients may well be more highly receptive to teaching than at any other time. However, we may first need to assess each client's understanding of his or her particular condition and take steps to be sure this understanding is consonant both with our own knowledge and with the medical status assigned by the other health workers. Misunderstanding medical jargon is common and nurses can well serve as translators to advance a client's knowledge. At other times a client may not have yet absorbed the full impact of the shift from well to sick role. For example, in rehabilitation units therapy cannot proceed beyond passive exercises until new trauma victims accept their status and cease to wait for miraculous recovery of function. Some diagnoses, such as VD or tuberculosis, are individually or culturally loaded with shameful connotations that must be overcome before control measures can be instituted. These examples are areas in which any teacher must try to implement one of the maxims of learning theory: Begin where the learner is.

As in any other teaching-learning transaction, it is important to be thoroughly aware of who the clients are—not only from the viewpoint of what their illnesses are about, but also their individual characteristics and the backgrounds they draw on for their ways of coping with illness. Individual differences are, of course, vital in working with clients. But their characteristics that may be attributed to membership in various groups also influence what approaches need to be used. For example, when one student investigated the health services available for pregnant, black adolescents it soon became glaringly obvious that though all the services took into account the pregnant part and many dealt well with the special factors of race, none (count them, *none!*) was geared to the fact that these were adolescents: younger than the "usual" pregnant client, with all the turmoil, role uncertainty, emotional liability, and on and on, that are part of the adolescent life period under any circumstances.

No matter what the particulars of the condition involved, we should think through the kinds of knowledge clients will need to manage their illnesses in the circumstances they are in. When I did home care, my favorite suggestion to hospital nurses trying to plan a discharge was "Figure what you'd have to have if this patient were coming home to your apartment." Homes don't have a handy Central Supply Service, autoclaves, or all those special therapists. Whatever is special will have to be acquired ahead of need or done without. Planning ahead also extends to procedures that will have to be carried out at home. Watching someone else administer insulin or irrigate a colostomy is quite one thing; doing it is something else. In the hospital, or at home, clients need a chance to practice under supervision before being turned loose. Often it is only after practice that problems become clear and clients find there are questions they need to ask. In these instances—as in so many others—giving clients a phone number they can use for unexpected need can give them a sense of security even if they never have occasion to call it.

MODELS FOR HEALTH EDUCATION

Traditional diagrams used to analyze the process of health education are often laid out in a linear fashion (figure 10.1). Most omit acknowledging the point where we here begin, the professional perspective (box A)—that

10.1   *Traditional Planning Model for Health Education*

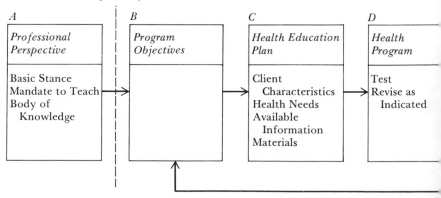

is, with the basic assumption of a body of knowledge, a scientific stance, an obligation, and a mission that gives you the right to set up your objectives (B) from which flows your plan (C) for health education. At this point you are required to take into account the characteristics of your client population and the sorts of materials or resources available to you. From these you create a tentative program (D) that you test and revise as needed before implementing it on a full scale (E). Because you have nicely built in measurable behavioral objectives, your evaluation (F) follows implementation, which is the feedback link in the process. This process model may do very well in certain education situations, but it is not constructed to achieve high levels of client agreement and involvement or even as high a degree of knowledge acquisition or behavior change as the professional would hope.

The rising demand among consumers to participate in more services of all kinds has brought growing criticism of the delivery and content of medical care and health education based on such a model. For an example, the nurses in a Commune Health Education Project worked with young adults in alternative lifestyles for four years. Having come from experience in free clinics, we knew better than to take on the "problem" of illicit drug use since our clients were far more knowledgeable than we. We did, however, attempt to try out some of the materials being used for drug abuse prevention, since many other health workers were eager to know how we were dealing with this "problem." We first eliminated the obviously false, dumb, and scary things and then tried several items on our clientele. The written materials got scant attention and were quickly dismissed if one or more inaccurate portions were found. Several of the films were eloquently voted against when the viewers simply got up and walked away. A few films provoked peals of laughter and only one or two engaged enough attention to stir arguments from the viewers. Thus we came to the conclusion that the available materials on drug use and abuse were inappropriate for our young adult clients who saw no need to be

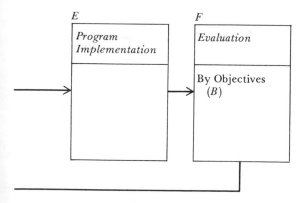

preached at to change their drug behavior. They had all had wide experience in and around drugs and had reached their own decisions on how to manage drugs, either by nonuse, controlled use, or transfer to licit drugs such as alcohol or legal herbal materials. The drug education materials seemed almost universally to be aimed at some very young or sheltered audience with no contact with drug usage who were to be deterred from experimentation. Whether or not this expectation is realistic is not important here; the point is that such an approach cannot be used with an audience already into or past the drug use scene. Their notion of an ideal informational presentation would be one that would give authoritative answers to the positive and negative questions they have about effects of common drugs. Such an approach does not exist, however, since no presentation can adequately balance the usual detrimental effects against the reported pleasant or beneficial effects without being accused of advocating something.

THE CLIENT-CENTERED MODEL FOR HEALTH EDUCATION

A variety of similar situations have led us to propose a model for client-centered health education (figure 10.2). In this model the basic assumption (A) is the client population with all its characteristics, lifestyle, position in time and space, language, and health concerns. As health workers, again carrying the professional perspective, knowledge, and mission (B), we propose to work with the client group in the area of our expertise: health. If the offer is accepted—and at times it may *not* be, if the clients have no health concerns or have some other system that deals adequately with their wants—the joint communication process leads to an identification of the health problem (C). Instead of deciding for a client what is *needed*, in this first stage we focus on finding out what is *wanted*. For example, in one of the early consumer-controlled clinics, the health workers were firmly convinced that contraception was the major health problem. The community, however, stated firmly that it wanted a program on cockroach control. In spite of the professionals' view that cockroaches were not a health problem nor even a very significant pest problem, the fact soon became clear that a control program was what the community wanted. So, the health professionals did the cockroach control program, after which the clients were willing to listen to what the professionals wanted to talk about. Of course, they made clear that this was the professionals' turn, but the willingness to do what the community wanted gave the professionals credibility and legitimacy. It proved they were not simply mouthing phrases about concern for community interests while ramming unwanted services down the collective throat.

Once a problem is identified, the community-professional team then

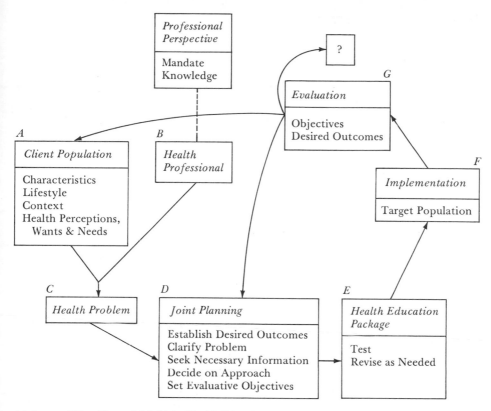

Client-Centered Model for Health Education

works toward a joint plan (D). On the basis of the identified problem, the team defines the desired outcome. For example, resolution of the VD problem can entail two quite different outcomes: Is the program designed to keep people from getting VD or is it meant to get them to seek treatment for it? China, with its puritanical morality and very little extramarital intercourse, has reportedly wiped out VD. The authoritarian structure of the country, combined with sufficient penicillin production, makes giving treatment to an entire population possible. Our nation, however, may have enough penicillin, but it does not have the morality, authority, or a situated population to use such an approach to VD control. In our country, to consider abstinence as a serious means of VD control seem to ignore social reality. The use by police order of therapeutic doses of penicillin on all prostitutes picked up on sweeps through one city's streets has formed the basis for a lawsuit charging, among other things, the use of medicine as a form of punishment. Another factor is travel, which is considered nearly a constitutional right by most of our citizens and often brings them into contact with a variety of exotic communicable diseases, including VD. Elimination of VD from a population would last only so long as sexual activity was limited to members of the guaranteed disease-free group.

Once outcome is clearly decided, the next step in the joint planning process is to seek the needed input, whether material or information. This step may be the first point where the decision is made for education. Many people have proposed solving the problems of the poor directly by giving them the money to buy the solutions. Clients with clear medical emergencies need direct and expert life-saving interventions. However, many chronic conditions require large inputs of education for prevention and maintenance, especially directed to the population at risk. Development of vastly improved surgical or chemical techniques would make far less impact on control of cervical cancer than would wider and more regular use of the Pap smear screening method.

The next stage in planning is to decide how to present the material, based on predictions of what works best with the material to be presented and how it will be received by the clients. The commune project noted, for example, that presenting materials in a slick, finished movie production puts the audience into a passive relation to the material, since movies are considered entertainment. Put a television tape before them and it is quite a different relation. This generation of young adults had grown up with TV sets in every home and felt free to argue with a television set and comment to one another about what was being presented. Discussion afterwards is much easier to get going than with a film. Of course, health video is not the same polished field that health films have become, and while learning can occur in both instances, of course, we found that commune dwellers were less able to adopt material from professionally produced, mass-audience films than from less slick, more tailor-made productions that made up in sincerity what they lacked in polish.

A natural tendency at this point in planning is to rush out and start doing. But without some notion of deciding beforehand how you'll know whether what you're doing is actually working or how well, you can end up with an inordinate effort for very little health return. Thus at this point evaluative objectives need to be set up. Transforming outcomes into measurable objectives not only provides a basis for deciding whether or not the project reached its goals but may also identify activities that are on target or those that are wandering afield. Contributions toward the outcome of decreasing VD, for instance, can be an increase in knowledge about symptoms and resources to treat VD, increased usage of screening and treatment facilities, or lowering the number of positive VD tests in a target population. Each is measured in quite different ways and would likely reflect entirely different project activities.

The interaction of all the steps of this stage will end up in the production of a health education package (E). By this time, all the participants are thoroughly immersed in the topic, have become increasingly expert in it, and often have moved closer to a shared perspective on the problem. Thus, the next crucial step is that the package be tried out on some audience that has not undergone this learning experience. Testing it will almost inevitably turn up areas that need revision to avoid omitting hugely significant information or harping needlessly at something the audience already knows or has long since picked up. Failure to test the material is one reason why single-shot health education experiences as students are often unsatisfying. It's only after presenting the material that you figure out what it was that was needed to make the performance more successful.

Although revisions may be continuous—knowledge does continue advancing, after all, and should be incorporated—the program is at last ready for implementation(F). It may be the launching of a pamphlet or book, the distribution of posters, showing a film or slide show, or arranging to present a videotape on the local cable or commercial TV station. It may also include the incorporation of health teaching in the regular activities of the professional at work. Although this latter is more often a side effect of the process, the health worker can become more aware of the importance of sharing information and more skilled in doing so.

Evaluation (G) is essentially testing the final package against the objectives set up during the planning stage, assessing the effectiveness of the outcome against the expectations, and reaching a decision about the quality of the whole process. At least three possible consequences flow from the evaluation. First, sometimes programs don't actually work out, either because of unforeseen circumstances or changed events or because the problem is bigger or more resistant than expected. For whatever reason, the problem remains and the approach must be revised. This consequence feeds back to the planning stage (D). Second, all may go along successfully, with the planned package answering the need. Such an outcome demonstrates the credibility of the health education enterprise and gives momentum to further joint participation in another planning cycle dealing with yet another problem. Third, evaluation may lead the project in a whole different direction, which also makes planning an ongoing process.

Problems of any kind are seldom so self-limited that solution does not create new problems or reveal others that had been lurking behind the greater urgency of the one at hand. Even the total success of a VD treatment campaign, as encouraging as that would be, could well reveal another problem that had not been clearly visible before. Such an emerging problem might be our growing awareness of repeaters—that is, individuals who, in spite of knowledge, screening, and treatment, continue to appear with positive tests. Clearly, some portion of the population at risk will not be kept disease-free. New approaches, then, become indicated if the old ones fail to accomplish the desired outcomes. These may involve teaching more about prophylaxis, exploring individual behavior change possibilities, or encouraging the development of immunizations against VD. The result may be the decision that the costs involved outweigh the benefits that would result. Ways to contain the problem may be devised while the bulk of your energies are put into health areas more accessible to change.

PRINCIPLES FOR CLIENT-CENTERED HEALTH EDUCATION

WANT TO KNOW VERSUS NEED TO KNOW

It is not always easy to find out what sorts of health information your clients want to know. Openly asking them to tell you often results in prolonged silence or stumbling attempts to answer what they think you want them to answer. Presenting a list of possible topics can be a little more helpful although in my experience I have met two extremes in using this approach: One group replied "everything" to a three-page, single-spaced list, while another group nodded a lot at the introduction but failed to vote for any items at all on a posterboard list. Often, by prior sifting of likely health problems, a nurse can present a list of choices for clients to rank in terms of their interest in learning about each one. Providing blank spaces for write-ins may result in some unexpected suggestions. A report back on the voting prepares the clients and encourages them to think ahead about a topic and, it can be hoped, prepare questions they will be interested in asking. Methods of increasing client involvement is one of the skills we as nurses can bring to health information planning discussions.

There is a flaw in the client-focused process, however, which comes up when certain health problems are clearly present and have bad effects on a population who refuse repeatedly to show interest in learning about them. This dilemma is difficult for nurses to manage and one where logical models get the heave-ho. For example, a colleague working with a high school group asked them to rate VD as a possible topic for discussion. She was met with a chorus of groans and looks of exasperation. Accepting that verdict and the voting they had done on her poll, she proceeded with topics they had shown interest in. Before the semester was over, however, she had managed to lead into the topic of VD several times without going into the full-blown pitch. Finally some of the class could stand it no longer and began asking questions that clearly indicated that in spite of their scorn for still more VD material, their knowledge had great gaps. They had finally become aware of these and were now willing to have them filled. This process, however, took time and planning that could not have occurred had our colleague been scheduled only for an annual nurse's lecture on VD.

A similar event occurred while several of us were having a VD rap group in the free clinic waiting room. A woman entered after signing in and hesitated before sitting down. "Come on in," I said, "we're just rapping about VD." Loftily, she replied, "I know all I need to know about VD." "Great," I said, "then you know that 85 percent of the women with positive clap tests have no symptoms at all?" She looked up from the book she had just opened and replied in a sobered voice, "Maybe I better have a clap test tonight."

As is well known in VD control circles, the moment educational programs are dropped, the VD rate begins to climb. But on the receiving end, there is a point when persistent hammering on the topic produces deafness to any more. The suggestion here is that it is not quantity of material alone that will result in behavior change, but that variation is needed in the approach to reach portions of the potential audience at levels or from directions that most directly appeal to their particular interests. Variety can be introduced in many ways: the use of different media, styles of presentation, or locations. Within a presentation, variations can be introduced: in timing, uses of different media, and changes in emotional tone. The advertising industry has gone through a number of studies showing the impact of changing the emotional character in selling. Humorous ads upped sales and every agency began grinding out funny commercials. Then sales levelled off. But shifting to the new theme and tone in nature-picture settings once again boosted sales. The conclusion, to no teacher's surprise, was that it was not so much one style over another but the mere fact of changing style that led people to pay attention long enough for the pitch to be heard.

Learner Motivation. If there were simple recipes for increasing learner motivation, public schools surely wouldn't be facing the dilemmas they are now. However, there are some factors in this area that we can take into account to improve the appeal of health information to the clients we serve.

A person, who is not a hypochondriac, tends to take his or her body for granted until it begins to misbehave. Then the body becomes a matter of vital interest and almost overwhelming concern. A person with a fresh heart condition or a family member with one suddenly becomes aware of all things cardiac: articles in the paper about someone age forty-six dying of a heart attack, a movie star under observation for a heart flutter, historical figures with heart trouble. These items leap out of the paper where before they had no personal meaning. Often people will seek out library books on their diagnoses, and thus become instant experts on the varieties of treatment used for their ailments. These examples illustrate one of the reasons it's so much easier to teach people about their illnesses and how to manage them than it is to persuade people to take preventive actions to avoid problems before they occur. Curing an existent illness is much more relevant to them than preventing a potential one. An important factor in learner motivation, then, is to try to personalize health teaching to a client's perceived needs. An adolescent is less interested in learning about childhood growth and development than are new parents. Contraceptive teaching is often most effective as part of the counseling that goes on at the time of an abortion; its personal applicability is clear at last then.

Some professionals rely heavily on the use of fear and threats to teach about health. "If you don't immunize your child, he'll surely get whooping cough and die," "If you drink raw milk, you'll get undulant fever, salmonella, and tuberculosis," "If you smoke marijuana, you'll become a heroin addict, impotent, and a welfare bum." The whole drug experimentation pattern of our youth is colored by defiance of this style of teaching, which has begun to spill into other areas. Now many young people are doubting the reliability of all medical authority and are asking questions where few have raised them before. People are also beginning to challenge the degree of risk actually involved in a variety of medical situations. One of the reasons for low consumer interest in measles immunizations may well be that most people do not consider that disease to be serious enough to want to eliminate it. Smallpox, on the other hand, is essentially an obsolete disease now because there was worldwide agreement about the degree of risk for human life. Thus we must be frank about the risks entailed in the various proposals we make to prevent or cure diseases. Just as promising a child "this little needle won't hurt at all!" is unfair so is failing to discuss the various risks that follow both treatment and nontreatment of a particular condition. At first clients may be totally freaked by so much information; indeed many professionals have refused to share such knowledge because they are certain it is far too upsetting to be dealt with. However, as our clients gradually become aware that there are no unmixed blessings, they will be able to make their own choices based on more complete data. And these can't help but be better decisions even if more painfully made.

Client Decision Making.   Many health workers believe their mission is to force people to avoid illness. Listening to many of us, one might think we have become obsessive about health. Since health concerns are the focus of our occupation, we act as if all our clients should be as eager to receive as we are to give advice. We are often surprised by the fact that when people are asked to list their top twenty concerns, health seldom ranks above sixteen or seventeen. But then, how many health professionals hand out advice they don't take themselves—on smoking, overweight, lack of exercise, or overwork?

The classic parental injunction to children—Do as I say and not as I do—is often used by many professionals to project a controlling, parental image into their relations with clients. One prenatal pamphlet even urges women to "Follow the orders (note the authoritarian trip there!) you are given; your doctor knows what is best for you."

Others of us, moving toward greater consumer participation, have tried simply to provide decision-making input for clients when their decisions affect only themselves and when there is time to go through the learning process. Like any principle, this one also cannot be the sole basis for operation. There are times when I don't want to have my head bothered with the factors involved in deciding what needs doing. For example, the only decision making I need to participate in for the repair of my car is whether or not I can afford to have it done or accept the consequences of leaving it undone. So too in life-saving circumstances, I prefer to have well-trained, superbly disciplined trauma workers in whom I have more or less blind faith. However, there are a lot of other times when I would resent having someone else usurp my right to make my own decisions—and my own mistakes. When there are alternatives, in matters that affect my health, I want to be an informed participant in the decision making that goes on. The same prerogative should be granted each client within the scope of his or her ability to participate.

There are times when the client's final decision does not match the one we would have advocated, but if the client makes it on the basis of the best information we can provide, we must accept it. The consequences, after all, are also the client's to bear. Women who want home deliveries often change their minds as they learn more about pregnancy and labor. Some do not, preferring to accept any of the possible risks since they believe what they gain far outweighs the dangers. Most health workers are very uncomfortable with this decision, and some even believe they must somehow force women to accept hospitalization "for their own good."

GETTING INFORMATION ACROSS

There are limits to the amount of material a person can absorb at any one time. Totally new information is always harder to understand than information that has been heard before. Thus, some basic notions in health education are to limit the input and repeat its content more than once. The ability to absorb is limited by emotional overlay; times of both great emotional stress and total stasis are inappropriate for information input. Mild levels of anxiety are considered optimal in learning, which may explain a lot of what happens to students.

Absorption is also inhibited if input does not correspond with the level of unmet needs facing the client. The leader of a women's self-help group identified the group's primary objective as state and federal political action to improve the status of women. Older women clients in the group, however, were immobilized by their failures to get jobs to supply money for food and rent. Health education would also be wide of the mark if it promoted better dental health through flossing when the client is suffering from acute appendicitis.

If professionals are to get health care past the sew-'em-up-and-turn-'em-loose kind of treatment, it is important to incorporate information at more than the minimal survival level. A newly diagnosed diabetic must have information and practice in the entire set of activities needed for self-care at home. The most dramatic procedure, for laymen, is the self-injection of insulin. But equally vital are the management of diet, urine testing processes, followup medical appointments, and the various screening procedures diabetics must become aware of, such as checking feet for unperceived wounds. Education can be geared at a procedure level that gets the technicalities across without the client understanding the principles involved. It can also be conducted at such a theoretical level that diabetic clients could pass an exam on endocrinology without ever figuring how to operationalize such knowledge for their own survival. Balancing acts are perhaps one major characteristic of health education at its best.

Health information must be useful to those who receive it. They have to be able to apply it to their own situations. The principles involved must be translatable into action terms. Few people are interested in facts or theories as ends in themselves. Not even too many are interested in facts that merely explain events—it isn't too helpful to know that the reason you feel ucky is you have a parainfluenzal infection unless you are also told what steps to take to become more comfortable. It may sometimes be reassuring to have a label to sort out the bulk of what you're experiencing into categories—"that is part of the ailment," and "that's just normal background discomfort," or maybe "that's part of something else we'd better investigate more thoroughly." But generally most people want health information linked to directions for what to do.

Directions must be within the range of possibilities for the client. A round-the-world cruise is therapeutic only for the wealthy; high meat diets are not appropriate to vegetarians; do-it-yourself surgery is still not generally possible. In addition, the action must *seem* possible to the clients; it must conform to their self-image. A young woman recently told me she rejected one hospital's procedure at time of delivery that every woman in labor had intravenous solutions started at the time of entry into the labor room. For her, IV tubes were indicative of "someone who is very, very sick" and she simply could not accept that as the attribute of a healthy delivery. She went to a good deal of effort and expense to find a situation that offered the kind of care she could accept.

To exemplify my favorite image of turning health information inside out to fit the client's point of view, I find a helpful exercise for nurses who must teach self-injection to diabetics is to give themselves a subcutaneous injection in the thigh. It does teach humility to learn that your own hand shakes like a leaf when it's *you* you're about to puncture! The exercise should also suggest that just as there is a real difference in giving someone else injections, so too, the information clients need to take care of their own health problems is quite different from that needed by health workers on the job.

Health professionals often have trouble remembering that their special language is not that of the rest of the world. In some areas, medical jargon helps make hot topics cool enough to be managed by health workers, who are only human. Death, sex, bodily functions, and emotional problems are only four subjects that we clothe with special distancing language that fends off their personal impact. Some people cannot comfortably discuss such topics in lay terms, and thus teaching everyone a cool language may be necessary before getting on with it. However, this approach can turn the discussion into a language class and get no further. One group of slow-learning high school students resisted learning medical terms for sex anatomy and the nurse finally asked them to teach her their terms for the various parts. She then used those in her discussions. Whenever she found they lacked the concept for certain body parts—usually those inside—she taught them medical names even while pairing them, whenever possible, with common terms, such as uterus-womb. The terms used depended on the level of comfort both for her and the students. Clients are quick to detect condescending uses of their own language and resent it even more than the use of technical terms. Probably a crucial factor is that the educator be at ease with the client's language as well as the content before trying to discuss it. Teacher discomfort is probably one of the major reasons for failure of sex education classes in the schoolroom.

Clients also speak a variety of languages and dialects. English may be very different in the United States or in Great Britain, let alone in places where it is not the native tongue. There are regional differences in all languages, including our own. Although language is not the only way we communicate, it can give clues that a given client group does not necessarily share our cultural assumptions. When we find ourselves puzzled by what's going on, it's generally wise to pull back and question our own assumptions. It's important to learn how the language and worldview of the client can best be incorporated into the attempt to translate medical-ese into people-ese. When you go into a strange situation or begin with a totally new group of clients, there's really nothing wrong with admitting you're a stranger here yourself. Asking clients to teach you what's going on with them so you can then try to do your job better is a far more helpful tactic than sailing in with the assumption that you already know everything you need to. That's sometimes hard to do when you're still new on the job, but putting yourself into a one-down position is easier to take than being put there by someone else. Besides, clients who have a part in decision making about what they are to learn become more committed to the whole process than those who just have to put up with what's handed to them.

Health information is directed to a real audience, and we must identify who they are before trying to present health materials. Many expensive productions attempt to reach everyone and end up speaking to no one. In addition there is a tendency, especially for a novice, to try to speak not only to the client audience but also to the hidden audience of coprofessionals—a bit of trying not to offend some ghost of instructor-past. When outside health workers asked permission of our commune project to attend one of our sessions to see our wares, they made clear that they were not considering these in relation to their own health but rather in an instrumental fashion: Did we have any new tools they could use for their clients? What magic formula did we have that they could lift? For us, presenting health information when the audience was split between consumers of the information and those who would utilize it for the benefit of others was clearly impossible. It was disconcerting to be in the middle of a presentation and have part of the audience turn to each other and begin commenting on the materials being used: "Yes, we have *that* in the department," or "We never had much luck getting them to use that film in the school," and other unrelated remarks.

Learning Enough to Teach It.   However you arrive at the subject of any education presentation, you need to consider two aspects: the method and the content. Teacher training manuals and journals are filled with age-graded projects for imparting knowledge about various health topics. The content, however, is presumed to come from an "expert" in the field who, in the school situation, is often the nurse. We already have a lot of useful information about health as well as special knowledge about where to seek even more, but we often take for granted our knowledge of references and other basic resources. We can also take some questions directly to local health workers in the field under consideration. In a VD program, for example, there are always epidemiologists and VD health educators to provide scientific and human interest information, as well as suggestions for reliable references. To simply relay textbook information is not particularly helpful to clients. You need to internalize and understand it thoroughly before you can turn it around for someone else's use. Trying a presentation out a few times on individuals or small groups soon begins to make clear what it is they want to know, hence what you need to go back and look up.

Admitting to clients that there are things we don't know is often very difficult. A much thornier problem is being unaware that you don't know. We all have the desire to be helpful, and some half-remembered line of advice may seem just the ticket. Sometimes, though, it's the wrong half that gets remembered. For example, an office nurse, very sympathetic to my report of nausea after taking tetracycline, explained that it was obviously due to having taken the medicine on an empty stomach, which usually makes anybody nauseated. My own knowledge told me that she was wrong, that food would interfere with the drug's absorption, and that my problem was an allergic response. But even knowing this, I had no way of dealing with her calm certainty. In fact, I had to go back to my books just to be sure of myself. If we were all less threatened by disagreement or questioning, such false advising would not have to go unchallenged. I'm not sure how to alter this but perhaps we all need to be sensitive to the slightly too-persistent "But are you *sure?*" or other clues that there is disagreement with what we say.

Variety Shows.   In the opening example of this chapter, I mentioned that some people absorbed spoken words better than printed ones. This situation can occur for a number of reasons. In this instance it was simply one of the differences in learning styles to be found in any group of people. However, there are also times when the spoken word must be used because the clients are unable to read. This is, of course, true with little children but also may occur with immigrants who may or may not even be able to read their own first language. Individuals with forms of symbolic aphasia may also be unable to read written materials.

Restriction to the use of words limits the effectiveness of many presentations. The vividness of graphics makes them a helpful supplement to printed material, and in some instances they may be even more effective. The use of a range of sensory and intellectual appeals can increase the interest and attention given to various health presentations. There comes a point, of course, when the use of multimedia becomes too much and either overwhelms the topic or is perceived as serving another purpose. An example can probably be recalled by any of you about what went on when a classroom was darkened for movies: holding hands, sleeping, whispering, and a lot of things other than paying attention to the film!

Education Is Anywhere.   Opportunities for health education occur wherever a group gathers with a concern for health. Elderly members of a senior recreation facility are avid for general information about the use of vitamins, exercise, sleep problems (both too much and not enough), and how to get medical care. Parents belonging to a local church group want very much to discuss child-rearing problems. The waiting room of the free clinic has been an exceptionally good place to start rap groups on food, contraception, crabs, or whatever topic is of interest to whomever is there.

In spite of many attempts to innovate within health facilities, a surprising number of health workers feel constraints against moving out into other kinds of locations. For instance, when I used the example of the home visits Chicago's Black Panthers made to test slum residents for tuberculosis and their use of the results as a basis for politicization, a pharmacy student scoffed at the idea, and said he couldn't see us becoming door-to-door salesmen for health. At first I agreed; but on second thought, I began to wonder why not? Moving onto the client's turf may change some of the rules under which we operate but certainly gives us a chance to rethink the values of our services as well as demonstrate our commitment to delivering such services to our clients. For example, a community pharmacy is a health facility, but the notion of nurses working there surprises many. But this location has proved a valuable place for nurses to be available to provide reliable health information and to perform a variety of health screening and monitoring functions. The sort of casual locations mentioned in our later community case study (chapter 14) demonstrate ways that community nurses may carry expert knowledge to people where they are.

Problems that tend to prevent nurses from seizing these opportunities include our frequent failure to identify ourselves as the appropriate persons to teach about health and illness as well as the failure of agencies to so define us and hence pay us to engage in such activities as a part of our jobs. Another problem is the difficulty a lot of us have in taking the initiative to begin a health education exchange. The clinic waiting room, for instance, feels like client territory and many of us are hesitant to invade it for the first time. By utilizing what is for many waiting clients wasted time, we can offer them the chance to ask questions about health or at least be presented with packaged health education material in what seems a valuable way to advance their levels of functioning.

There is also an interesting aspect of nursing that often operates either to prevent us from expanding into new areas of operation or justifies continuing to work in old ways with no attempt to assess their effectiveness.

This notion is that no matter how much you do, there's always more of the same to be done: more families to visit, more parent groups to organize, more unimmunized to reach. Breaking out of this pattern is often very difficult, even for something as clearly related to health as the kind of education we've been talking about in this chapter. On the other hand, there are the very realistic complaints raised by members of the health team when some worker selects all the goody tasks and leaves the dull stuff to the others. For example, the head nurse of a college health service complained, rightfully too, that one new nurse spent all her time teaching clients or doing group counseling with no time left over for such dull but essential chores as washing speculums or setting up rooms for an afternoon clinic. Having less-skilled workers available to take care of that sort of thing would be nice, but that thought is no help when budget realities put only nurses on the scene. It may be that the head nurse viewed health education as less valuable than did the new nurse; the latter obviously did not consider clinic management as legitimate a nursing task as did her immediate supervisor. Perhaps compromise would have lowered tensions on this job.

SUMMARY

Clients make health decisions on the basis of information available to them. Nurses (and other health workers) can improve the reliability and extent of this information base by sharing what we know and engaging in health education exchanges with clients at every opportunity. Formal education in schools, continuing education for adults, education for consumers of health services, and illness-focused patient teaching are four varieties of experiences nurses may use. A model for participatory, client-focused health programs is proposed and discussed. Selected principles that affect health learning are included.

REFERENCES

ALLEN, ROBERT E., and HOLYOAK, OWEN J. "Evaluation of the Conceptual Approach to Teaching Health Education: A Second Look." *The Journal of School Health* 43 (1973):293–94.

BAKER, M. H., ed. "Personal Health Practices and the Health Belief Model." *Health Education Monographs* 2 (1974):324–473.

BANTA, JAMES E. "Effecting Changes In Health Behavior in Developing Countries." *Archives of Environmental Health* 18 (1969):265–68.

BLAYNESY, KEITH. "Consumer Health Knowledge: Problems and a Comprehensive Proposal." *Alabama Journal of Medical Sciences* 9 (1972):403–09.

BOOTH, ALAN, and BABCHUK, NICHOLAS. "Seeking Health Care from New Resources." *Journal of Health and Social Behavior* 13 (1972):90–99.

CADY, RUTH. "Oh Where, Oh Where Should Health Educators Be?" *American Journal of Public Health* 62 (1972):79–81.

CONANT, RICHARD K., DELUCE, A. J., and LEVIN, LOWELL S. "Health Education—A Bridge to the Community." *American Journal of Public Health* 62 (1972):1239–44.

DALLAS, JAMES LEE. "Health Education: Enabler for a Higher Quality of Life." *Health Services Reports* 87 (1972):910–18.

DOWLING, IMELDA. "The Nurse's Role in a Community Health Education Program—Part I." *The World of Irish Nursing* 2 (1973):159–63.

FELDMAN, JACOB J. *The Dissemination of Health Information.* Chicago: Aldine Publishing Co., 1966.

KIESLER, CHARLES A., COLLINS, BARRY E., and MILLER, NORMAN. *Attitude Change.* New York: John Wiley & Sons, 1969.

KLEINSCHMIDT, H. E., and ZIMAND, SAVEL. *Public Health Education: Its Tools and Procedures.* New York: Macmillan Co., 1953.

MACQUEEN, IAN A. G. "Organization of Health Education." *Community Health* 4 (1973):239–43.

MEANS, RICHARD K. "Health Education: What, Why, and How." *The Journal of School Health* 39 (1969):209–16.

MOSS, BERNICE, SOUTHWORTH, WARREN H., and REICHERT, JOHN LESTER, eds. *Health Education,* 5th ed. Washington, D.C.: National Educational Association of the United States, 1961.

NEWELL, ALLEN, and SIMON, HERBERT A. *Human Problem Solving.* Englewood Cliffs, N.J.: Prentice-Hall, 1972.

PAUL, BENJAMIN D., ed. *Health, Culture, & Community: Case Studies of Public Reactions to Health Programs.* New York: Russell Sage Foundation, 1955.

POHL, MARGARET L. *Teaching Function of the Nursing Practitioner.* Dubuque, Ia.: Wm. C. Brown Co., 1968.

REDMAN, BARBARA KLUG. *The Process of Patient Teaching in Nursing,* 2nd ed. Saint Louis: C. V. Mosby Co., 1972.

RUDDICK-BRACKEN, HUGH. "The District Nurse as Health Educator." *Nursing Times* 69 (1973):1187–89.

RYAN, THOMAS ARTHUR. *Intentional Behavior: An Approach to Human Motivation.* New York: Ronald Press, 1970.

SANFORD, TERRY. "Educating the Public about Health: The Role of Formal Education." *Journal of Medical Education* (January 1975):3–10.

SIMONDS, S. K. "Health Education as Social Policy." *Health Education Monographs* 2, suppl. 1 (1974): 1–10.

SOMERS, ANNE R., ed. Promoting Health: Consumer Education and National Policy. Germantown, Md.: Aspen Systems Corp., 1976.

YACENDA, JOHN A. "Turning-On High Schoolers (About Health)." *The Journal of School Health* 42 (1972):597–99.

YARROW, A. "The Use of Mass Media in Health Education." *Community Health* 4 (1973):244–48.

11. Politics and Economics: How Things Really Work

Sarah Ellen Archer

INTRODUCTION

This chapter focuses on some of the major concepts in politics and economics and relates these concepts to health care delivery in general and to nurses specifically. Although much progress is being made, many nurses still don't know enough about either politics or economics except on an intuitive level. The reason is partially due to an absence of content about politics and economics in most baccalaureate nursing curricula. Nurses still tend to avoid involvement with them, in part feeling that politics is "dirty" and economics, since it uses mathematics, is difficult. Chapter 22 and 23 illustrate a variety of kinds of involvement with politics. The discussion in chapter 21 of community health nurses in administration illustrates the essential nature of our knowing a great deal about economics.

As this chapter's title indicates, we believe that politics and economics have great bearing on how things really work. If nurses want much voice in what goes on, we had jolly well better learn something about both subjects. We hope that this chapter will whet your appetite for further study since it is only a beginning. Knowing more, hopefully you will then feel more confident and so be more willing to develop and use political and economic skills.

Although this chapter is neatly divided into two parts—politics and

277

economics—be not confused that the separation occurs any place other than on paper. Politics and economics are two sides of the same coin. Economics, as we shall see later, seeks to explain how, why, and to whom questions relating to the distribution of resources. Politics deals with the means by which the people and organizations making allocative decisions gain and wield the power and prerogatives to do so. In short, politics determines who gets to play the decision-making games and economics defines the stakes and the bidding. For example, health care agencies' budgets are statements of priorities in terms of how much and to what ends resources will be spent during a given period of time. The budget can be viewed as a statement of the economic policy of the organization. Our advice to persons seeking employment in an organization is to read the organization's statement of philosophy and objectives and then to look at the budget. If there seems to be a discrepancy between what the organization says it is doing in its philosophy and objectives and the manner in which its budget reflects its allocation of resources, believe the budget.

In the face of inevitably limited resources, politics enters the budgetary process the minute there is more than one alternative for spending an organization's resources or more than one group or subgroup whose interests must be addressed. In the power struggles that ensue, agency administrators, relying on their responsibilities to their board of directors and the public, seek to exert ultimate authority. Physicians seek to have their wishes met on the basis of their expertise and responsibilities for patient care. Support disciplines such as nursing, pharmacy, dietary, and social service seek to have their budgets increased. Community people may demand or oppose an expansion of services or facilities. What follows is a struggle to force acceptance of one group's priorities at the expense of other groups' priorities. Thus the group that wins has the greatest power and so can exert the most influence on the allocation of resources to itself and therefore to others.

The process is often a fierce battle for power since seldom will all of the participants see their goals met due to limitations in the amount of resources available. The core struggle is to retain control or if a group is out of power, to gain access to the ranks of decisionmakers. These realities lead to tradeoffs, shifting coalitions, lobbying, name calling, ulcers, and hypertension. With the rise in nurses' assertiveness level that is in turn bringing about drastic revisions of the doctor-nurse game, the balance of power is shifting and new power centers are developing (Alberti 1977; Everly 1976; Pogrebin 1975; Thomstad, Cunningham, and Kaplan 1975).

One of the biggest stumbling blocks in negotiations during nurses' strikes is not salary or fringe benefit increases, but rather nurses' de-

mands for a greater voice in decisions on the numbers and levels of preparation of nurses assigned to special service units in the hospitals. Thus the
issue becomes one of power not money since the nurses are demanding
inclusion in decision making as legitimate on the basis of their professional responsibility for the quality of patient care. Apparently hospital
administrators and some physicians see this demand as a threat to their
autonomy and therefore as far more ominous than mere economic and
general welfare issues.

Systems theory, as discussed in chapter 3, reminds us that no subsystem's exertion of power in any arena and particularly in the allocation
of resources should be absolute. Some balance must be maintained for
even though subsystems compete for resources, they remain interdependent within the parent system. For this reason subsystems should not
seek to wipe each other out since such actions would seriously weaken the
entire system. This reality is often easier said than remembered in battles
over resources. This subsystem interdependence is increasingly important
in health care as more and more specialized disciplines are needed to
provide clients with comprehensive high-quality care.

Our discussion starts with politics and then turns to more specific
economic considerations. This information is presented to help community nurses become more effective advocates, coordinators, deliverers
of services, facilitators, organizers, and planners.

POLITICS

INTRODUCTION AND DEFINITIONS

Why, you may ask, does a community nursing text have a chapter partially devoted to politics? The answer is that if we really stop and think
honestly, we are about where Milio was when she began the "Moms and
Tots Center" in Detroit; she later noted, "My naivete at the time about
the politics of living, the use of power, the force of vested interests, was
immense" (1971:22). In chapter 3, we discussed an exchange model as a
basic concept for community nurses. Politics is an integral and essential
part of virtually every exchange or transaction that takes place in a community, regardless of the kind of community it is. Politics is equally important in one-to-one or small group interactions. An understanding of
the political realities—power, the necessity for decision making, vested interest groups, and "the politics of living" generally—that shape the situations in which or in spite of which we and our clients must act can help us
work with clients.

First, community nurses must decide what we believe in and state these beliefs to ourselves, our clients, and our colleagues. Do we really believe in equal opportunity for all people, that health promotion and teaching, a safe clean environment, and access to medical care are rights, that aged people in our society are entitled to dignified and humane treatment, and that the quality of all our lives can be improved if these things come to pass? These are ideological statements—that is, statements of normative beliefs and values. Adherence to these beliefs places us in direct conflict with other interest groups whose convictions are differently based. an interest group's ideologies are important since they shape the precursor or overriding goals that influence all other goals, objectives, plans for change, and evaluations of their outcome—in short, the way the group looks at the world.

Can we as community nurses develop an ideology upon which we can agree? Doing so would be a highly political process. Once agreed upon, these beliefs should be clearly stated and then stood by even in the face of conflict. This issue is one of the most critical facing all of nursing (Shaefer 1973:887–89). Benveniste states this necessity in more general terms:

> It is evident that fragmented professions cannot hope to accomplish political acts as long as they behave as if they were not involved politically and as long as they sharply limit the domain of their professional norms and values . . . . If all or part of the profession shares even a minimum set of values, it should find out what those values are and defend them [Benveniste 1972:21].

Lest there be any doubts, the reference here is not to partisan politics, although many of the major health-related issues, such as National Health Insurance, have been made "political footballs" by the major parties. Politics in our use of the term is much like Novack's definition:

> Politics is the art of creating actions by entire communities.Politics is the art of shaping many disparate social elements into societal, not private action. It is the art of directing societies [Novack 1973:9]

In this definition, politics is seen as a means of organizing communities so that they can act. The process is also called the articulation of collective interests. The political process helps draw disparate groups together into coalitions. Collective actions are often more effective and safer than individual ones; we have learned this from such groups as the Welfare Rights, United Farmworkers, and National Organization for Women. Often, groups seeking societal rather than private goals are born in and must live with conflict. To survive, much less accomplish anything, a group must be reasonably large, have a centralized organization, and stand up for what it believes, even if doing so means a fight (Gamson 1974:35–41). Nursing faces both internal and external forces with which it must come to grips if it is to survive. An increasing number of nursing speciality groups are developing, each of which addresses the particular interests of its constituents. While such organizations as those for operating room nurses, public health nurses, pediatric nurse practitioners, and emergency room nurses are of great benefit for their members, they also serve to divide nursing still further. Thus the political process can also bring about division and even polarization within groups. Knowing something about the forces in the arena and some strategies for coping may help (Deloughery and Gebbie 1975; Lawrence 1976; Perlman 1976; Powell 1976).

POWER

Power has been variously defined but most definitions deal with the ability of a person, group, or organization to cause or constrain others' actions. Power is sought by individual persons and aggregates both as a tool to influence others' behavior and as an end in itself; hence the comment "she's on a power trip." Power can be applied or used by individuals and groups to attain their ends; power can also be withheld from people, thereby keeping them in a helpless or at least one-down position. The rallying cry "Power to the People" sought to galvanize people who felt powerless in the face of "the establishment" and to bring them together for both safety and strength. Students, ethnic groups, welfare clients, all kinds of powerless persons found brief brushes with power under this banner. Although there was a brief response to the pressure of the organized groups, long-lasting change in the power distribution within the establishment has not followed. Our society has not really become more responsive to the needs of these kinds of groups and so we shall see another slogan and another wave of group effort seeking to share the power pie (Alinsky 1972; Altshuler 1970; Hawley and Wirt 1968; Kahn 1970; Scholnick 1969; Walzer 1971).

Weber linked his three types of authority—rational, traditional, and charismatic—to the kind of claim each made to legitimacy. Rational authority depends for its power on proof that what it does is based in law, thereby giving it legitimacy: The nursing director has authority because the organization's laws give it to the person in this position. Traditional authority rests on long-term customs; custom is often cited as the reason behind policies: "We've always done it that way." Little wonder that traditions are often an impediment to change. On the other hand, many laws are made to formalize what has been happening for some time. New state laws drafted to conform to the Surpreme Court's ruling on abortion are an example. Charismatic authority is vested in a person and is based on the person's exemplary characteristics (Weber 1970:35–44). Some of the early leaders in the free clinic movement were charismatic.

May defines and characterizes five kinds of power: exploitive—power from or in spite of others; manipulative—power over others; competitive—power against others; nutrient—power for others; and integrative—power with others (1972:105–13). I believe that community nurses must be prepared to understand and use all five kinds of power depending on the need and circumstances. We need to know what kind of power we are using at any given time—that is, we need to be aware that we are manipulating a situation, rather than doing so on an intuitive basis. I believe that any use of power—short of violence and criminal behavior—is justifiable in helping clients attain and maintain their optimum level of functioning; in fact using power to this end is my responsibility.

The first three of May's kinds of power—exploitive, manipulative, and competitive—are those types most often associated with "dirty" politics. As we shall see in the discussion of interest groups, exploitation, manipulation, and competition are three tactics of prime importance in getting things done. In trying to get things done for your clients, you too will undoubtedly have to use any or all of these techniques. For example, you have a client, a woman with two small children, whose husband is in jail. She is eligible for welfare, food stamps, and medical care for herself and the children, but she's getting the bureaucratic run-around from the welfare department. You have much more power in this situation than she does since you are a worker and not a client. So you call the welfare department and raise the roof. If you know someone in the department, you may call and ask for her help—and thus use manipulative power. Another use of manipulative power was the coaching we gave clients seeking abortions before the laws were changed. We knew the only way to obtain a therapeutic abortion was for the woman to say that her physical or mental health was endangered by the pregnancy. Since these statements had to be supported by a physician or psychiatrist, we advised our clients on how to obtain their support. Often, this coaching and the ensuing discussion precipitated real opportunity for crisis counseling—nutrient power—since suicide was a common thought among these women but one which they never dared talk about openly before. Like most other theoretical phenomena, the kinds of power we are discussing are not discrete entities, but rather overlap one another.

We use competitive power in client-centered community nursing by offering the information we believe to be most soundly grounded on the scientific evidence currently available. This responsibility is bound to put what we say into direct conflict and therefore in competition with many of the latest health fads. Diets are a marvelous example. Our responsibility is to counsel clients about the danger of many of the fad diets and to encourage them toward adequate nutrition. We are also in a position to help clients profit from competition among others. The health insurance chapter is included so that we can help clients read and understand the various competing insurance policies they are offered and select the one which best fits their needs.

Power for others or nutrient power is the kind nurses most often use with clients. Nutrient power involves working for, doing for, caring for clients; it is essential for many of the roles we have defined for community nurses. While the use of this kind of power on clients' behalf is essential, it must also be used appropriately. Too much nutrient power or doing things for clients can lead to a loss of their independence. Data on the leading causes of death and disability are making increasingly clear that if people are to attain and maintain their optimal level of functioning, they must be taught how to and encouraged to become increasingly responsible for developing and following sound rather than destructive lifestyles.

Integrative power means sharing our decision making, planning, and evaluating with our clients. It is the philosophical base that leads us to use the term "client" rather than "patient." Commitment to the use of integrative power will often place us in positions where we must use the other kinds of power as well. While working in the advocate, facilitator, and organizer roles, we may be called upon to use all kinds of power.

Finally, one of the ways to acquire power is to act as though you had power. Nurses long accepted the outside dictum that we cannot strike to force consideration of our various demands. In spite of that and even of legislation that forbade such actions, nurses chose to organize strikes. These have become more common since the late sixties. By taking power into our hands to strike, nurses have gained added power to do it again in the future, so that threats of strike also have power.

INTEREST GROUPS

We all belong to many groups. As Americans, we tend to be "joiners," and belong to groups on the basis of our sex, age, occupation, religion, location, and on and on. Many of the groups to which we belong have views and beliefs that are in conflict with the ideologies of other groups to which we belong. Decisions as to whom to follow on a given issue may be the result of careful consideration of the issue and our feelings about it or may be simply a matter of going along with the group to which we are most loyal. Loyalty as used here may mean an emotional commitment to an ideology or simply adopting a group's position due to necessity, such as keeping a job. Thus we must engage in the fine art of compromise within ourselves to determine where our multiple loyalties dictate that we give our support on any given issue. This situation is, in microcosm, what happens within interest groups on a larger scale.

Interest groups are aggregates of people or organizations drawn together by some commonality. They are the special interest communities discussed in chapter 2. Their purpose is to advance the cause in which they believe and which is stated in their ideology. The American Nurses' Association (ANA) is a special interest group that has as its purpose the advancement of the nursing profession. On behalf of the advancement of Nursing the ANA has, like many interest groups, a pressure group component that seeks to influence public opinion and government decisons to favor nursing. Many other professional orgainzations in the health care field serve the same function for their profession. The most powerful of these is the American Medical Association, although the American Public Health Association is gaining clout.

Both special interest groups and political parties seek to influence policies and to fill offices. However, the focus of special interest groups is more narrow than that of political parties. Thus, special interest groups tend to be more narrowly defined and appeal to a somewhat more selective populace, while political parties must appeal, or try to appeal, to many strata of voters and so tend to have more general statements of belief. They cannot afford to be as specialized or specific as can interest groups. To be able to judge the nature of interest groups, we need to know what their beliefs are and how they go about making them operational (Monsen and Cannon 1964; Dahl 1961). Interest groups may and do use all of the kinds of power discussed previously in pursuit of their causes.

One of the major reasons for the existence of special groups is to facilitate interest articulation—that is, that the group speaks with one concerted voice for the interests of its members. Group pressure has great value, particularly in a society as complex as ours. Government is too large and fragmented and the parties are too broadly focused to satisfy most groups, which thus have lobbyists and special branches to press their claims.

The constituencies of most interest groups are very widespread. Nurses are located all over the country, but they must speak with a united voice in their state capitols and in Washington, D.C. Hence we have state nurses' associations that are affiliated with the national group. The same process holds true for farmers, veterans, teachers, and a variety of others whose needs must be expressed. Of course, all interest groups have internal conflicts that are resolved through compromise—or through fractionation, if compromise won't work. To some extent, the development of specialty nursing groups is an example to nurses in various practice areas to develop their own organizations that will be responsive to their special needs. Many nurses hold memberships in the American Nurses' Association and its state affiliates as well as in one of the specialty organizations. The organizations all belong to a federation of which ANA is also a member. The possibility of schism from ANA is most likely, at this writing, because of nurse-administrators' dissatisfaction with ANA's posture on some economic and general welfare issues. These kinds of internal divisions serve to reduce a group's effectiveness in speaking for all of its constituents.

Cater and Lee (1972) define an interest group they call the "subgovernment of health." It is composed of certain political executives—that is, persons appointed to high-level positions by elected officials; career bureaucrats, such as civil servants and Commissioned Corps Officers who serve in the HEW; key congressional committeepersons like Edward Kennedy, the late Hubert Humphrey, and Warren Magnuson who have carved out empires as health advocates; interest group professionals who, like those from the American Medical Association, seek governmental protection for their group while opposing any governmental interference; and the public interest elites, such as the Naders and Mendelsons, who do research and prepare information for use by the other groups.

We must be aware of our own special interests, for they influence the way we view many of the issues confronting us. We emphasize this point to sensitize us to the fact that nurses, like everybody else, have biases. We must constantly ask ourselves whether the manner in which we are reacting to an issue, a situation, and, especially, to a client is based on what's really going on or is due to our special interests.

By the same token, we must be aware of a group's ideological position before we use the information they make available to us, much less decide to adopt their stance. In short, know your source's bias. In chapter 12 the background of the major sources of information used for the chapter is listed because knowing something of an author's background allows readers to judge statements accordingly. In collecting data for a community analysis, we suggest that you obtain information from many sources and consider the inherent points of view each may reflect. The Chamber of Commerce's information can hardly be expected to describe the problem areas of the town at length. Police department information deals with only a fraction of the area's residents. On the other hand, if you are searching for data on heart disease, an excellent source of information is the Heart Association. We must learn to know the groups in our communities and use them effectively and efficiently. People and groups without some kinds of vested interests are rather spineless and dull. The more we know about our own interests and those of the individuals and groups around us, the more able we are to interpret and use appropriately the information from these sources.

DECISION MAKING

Decision making is an essential and ubiquitous part of living. We cannot escape, although we can put off, making decisions. Sometimes if we refuse or procrastinate too long, other people will do our deciding for us, an approach some people seem to enjoy. Another "nonstrategy" is to wait until only one possible alternative is left and then do that. We call this decision by default. It really involves a kind of backhanded decision in that the defaulter decides to wait it out until the realities of the situation at hand make only one choice really possible. This kind of decision making gives rise to crisis management in which there is no long- or even short-range planning and needs are addressed only when they become crises. By this time options are limited by the nature of the situation and the decisionmakers must simply react to the realities of the situation rather than participate in shaping them. Having recognized that these are some of the ways not to deal with decisions, we shall now look at some tactics for weighing and selecting alternatives for action.

The moment we have more than one alternative, or more than one opinion on a given alternative is voiced, we have a situation that requires choice. Decision making, then, involves nothing more complex than picking one or more alternatives and ruling out the others. In most situations, since more will need to be done than we can possibly do, we have to set priorities, which thus requires that we select and rank some courses of action and completely rule out others—a decision-making process. A review of the planning process discussed in chapter 3 can make this look at some specific decision-making strategies more useful to you.

Normative Strategy.   Normative decision making focuses on what "should" be. Many decisions are made with little debate simply on the basis that such-and-such is the "right" decision and the one, therefore, that should be made. The process seems very simple, but it is not really. When life was simple and right and wrong were crystal clear, at least in some people's minds, normative decisions were easier to make, we are told. "Situational ethics" apparently evolved to help in considering what was really happening as well as what "should be." Our society has become much more complex, however, and the people who make it up much more heterogeneous, thus making normative decision making, based on long-standing doctrine, more difficult. We now have situations where one person's norm is another's anathema. This is the arena for compromise or conflict.

Compromise.   People try, at least to some extent, to resolve without violence differences of opinion over what should and should not be done.

The American form of government has survived in great measure due to the ability of people and groups to reconcile their differences through compromise. Nobody gets all that he or she wants, but nobody loses all that he or she wants either. One miserable failure in our ability to compromise was the Civil War. While compromise generally helps avoid violence, it also results in the passage of programs and budgets that are watered-down versions of the original proposals. Congressional compromise on Medicaid reimbursement for abortion is an example. In this situation, as in most compromises, no side gets all that it wants but by the same token, no side completely loses out, either. The real potential for compromise to bring about an equitable resolution of a situation is when all of the protagonists can agree at the principle level on what should be done. In this case selecting implementation strategies is less difficult. Thus if the Right to Life groups and the pro-abortion groups could agree on the principle that the decision to have or not to have an abortion is the prerogative of the woman involved, how and by whom the abortion should be paid for would become a much more simple decision. Agreement on this principle is not possible at present, and so the compromises that are negotiated are less than satisfactory for many people, particularly the poor and minority women who are directly affected by a decision in which they have had no voice. We chose the abortion example because it is controversial and extremely emotion fraught. It represents the kind of compromise that is simultaneously the most difficult to make and the most important to make. Unimportant issues aren't worth fussing over. The art, of course, is to be able to separate the important from the unimportant and act accordingly. Many decisionmakers have trouble doing that, too.

Tradeoff.   This strategy is a form of exchange and goes something like this: "I'll vote for the school bond issue you're interested in if you'll sign my petition for campaign spending reform." This example is a variation on "I'll scratch your back if you'll scratch mine." However, in many situations, tradeoff is a more realistic solution than compromise, particularly when a decision comes down to a vote; half a vote is useless. Compromise may have gone into the statement of the issue on which the vote is taken, but the only alternatives on a vote are yes, no, or abstain. The tradeoff is a mechanism by which things are accomplished. If I offer you my support on an issue and you accept it, then you owe me support on an issue in which I'm interested. Until such time as you "pay me back," the exchange is incomplete and you are in my debt. When I "collect," I complete the transaction. If I really want something done, I may delay introducing the idea until I have most of the people in the voting group in my debt for things I've done for them. Then I can "collect" my debts and get my proposal adopted. This type of process is precisely the way many persons, interest groups, political bodies, and nations reach decisions that result in policies (Lindblom 1968).

Games: In game theory, games are described as ". . . the structured group of activities that coexist in a particular territorial system . . ." (Long 1968:229). Players (decisionmakers) have goals that are interrelated and often in conflict with others' goals. Interest groups as well as persons, political jurisdictions, or agencies can be players. There are some rules by which the players are supposed to abide; generally the rules specify how each player's resources are to be used. Each player tries to figure out strategies—that is, plans of action to fit every contingency ahead of time. Payoffs are the outcomes of the game, and their value must be estimated in terms of the costs and benefits for each player. If the payoff is worth the gamble or risk of a given strategy, a player may decide to take the risk; if the payoff is not worth the risk involved, a player may pass or may leave the game. Card games and chess are microcosmic examples of games played in politics, business, and diplomacy. Win-win games are those where all players gain. Developing fieldwork placements for students is a situation where a win-win game can be played. In the course of negotiating with the agency, faculty should be prepared to offer the agency something in return for the time and effort agency staff spend with students. Such offerings could be in-service programs, clinical appointments at the school, or other kinds of benefits for the agency. In this situation everyone wins: The students are placed for fieldwork, the faculty members get some exposure to the real agency world, and the agency staff has the opportunity to participate in in-service education or learn more about the academic setting. Zero-sum games are those where the winner's gains are made at the expense of the other players; an election is a zero-sum game since the winner gets the whole office and the loser(s) lose the whole office (Shubik 1964; Smith 1968). Berne's writings have made people aware of games as part of the decision-making processes we all use (1964; Levin and Berne 1973).

Decision Matrix.   There is always or almost always more than one way to meet an objective. As we noted in the planning process discussion in chapter 3, decisions must be made among alternatives. Here we present a technique for making these decisions as objectively and rationally as possible. This technique uses the decision matrix, a grid that crossmatches the variables to be weighed in the decision-making process and to be used in selecting from among possible alternatives.

Our problem is to determine how best to make influenza immunizations available to high-risk population groups since an epidemic of influenza is spreading. The objectives of the program are to immunize 80 percent of the known population at high risk during a ten-day period commencing in three days. These objectives are clearly stated in measurable terms.

A model of a decision matrix is presented in table 11.1. The criteria, which appear on the vertical axis of the matrix, for evaluating the feasibility of any alternatives for meeting the objectives are fairly clear. The first two deal with the agency's capacity to meet the objectives in terms of its own resources of personnel and funding. In this kind of emergency situation, personnel can be made available from other programs and activities, at least up to a point. Funding is the same way. We do not here consider material such as the vaccine since that is being supplied from a central source in sufficient quantity to meet the 80 percent objective. Time is obviously a crucial factor since we have a ten-day limit for the program to be of value in preventing an epidemic. Despite the emergency situation the alternative chosen must be acceptable to the people or they will not participate. The alternative must also be technologically feasible. Finally, we must reach the target population (see table 11.1).

The alternatives considered are door-to-door campaign, immunizing regular clinic and hospital admission clients, and conducting special pro-

TABLE 11.1 *Decision Matrix: Influenza Immunization Program Alternatives*

| | | Alternatives | |
| | | | |
Criteria	Door-to-door campaign	Regular clinics and hospital admissions	Special programs in many locations
Sufficient personnel	0	2	1
Adequate funding	0	2	1
Sufficient time	0	0	2
Acceptable to the people	1	1	1
Technologically feasible	1	2	2
Reaches target population	2	0	1
TOTAL*	4	7	8

Scoring: 0 = not feasible or satisfactory
1 = moderately satisfactory or feasible
2 = quite feasible or satisfactory

*Total equals the number of points each alternative receives for each criterion.

grams in many locations convenient for the target population. These alternatives are placed on the horizontal axis of table 11.1. A simple threepoint scoring key (not feasible, moderately feasible, and quite feasible) is used to rank the alternatives according to the predefined criteria. Once the alternatives are ranked, the score for each alternative in terms of each criterion is entered in the appropriate box on the matrix. The scores are added up and the alternative with the highest score—in this case special programs in many locations—is the alternative of choice.

This process is all very neat and tidy, but there are some problems inherent in the use of such quantitative decision-making tools. Probably the most glaring one is that some of the criteria used to evaluate alternatives are more important than others. The more important criteria can be weighted or given additional scores according to their relative value. For example, in table 11.2 we have repeated the process we went through in the previous table, but this time we use weighted criteria. Reaching the target population is weighted highest (4) since it is the reason for the program. Time is weighted 3 since it is limited and cannot be extended. Personnel, funding, and technological feasibility are weighted 2 since they can be expanded through release of resources allocated elsewhere because of the high priority and limited time nature of this program. Acceptability

TABLE 11.2 *Decision Matrix: Influenza Immunization Program Alternatives Using Weighted Criteria*

Criteria	Weight	Door-to-door campaign	Regular clinics and hospital admissions	Special programs in many locations
		Alternatives		
Sufficient personnel	2	$2 \times 0 = 0$	4	2
Adequate funding	2	$2 \times 0 = 0$	4	2
Sufficient time	3	$3 \times 0 = 0$	0	6
Acceptable to the people	1	$1 \times 1 = 1$	1	1
Technologically feasible	2	$2 \times 1 = 2$	4	4
Reaches target population	4	$4 \times 2 = 8$	0	4
TOTAL*		11	13	21

Scoring: 0 = not feasible or satisfactory
1 = moderately feasible or satisfactory
2 = quite feasible or satisfactory

*Total equals the sum of the score times the weight for each alternative on each criterion.

to the people is weighted lowest (1), on the assumption that with enough public education regarding the importance of high-risk groups being immunized, the program will be acceptable. Such weighting essentially cancels out acceptability as a criterion in making this decision. Special programs in many locations is the alternative of choice using the weighted criteria method. Its margin of choice is greater in table 11.2 than in table 11.1.

Another problem with decision matrices is one that plagues all quantitative decision-making tools. Since we are dealing with people's lives we must consider those whose needs cannot be met by the alternate we have selected via quantitative methods. This consideration is qualitative. High-risk people confined to their homes and in institutions cannot come to special programs even if they are held nearby. These people will have to be sought out and immunized wherever they are, even though the 80 percent objective is attained without them. Economists and epidemiologists will have difficulty seeing the value of this added effort. The former's questions will stem from cost-benefit considerations, the latter's from herd immunity ones (see figure 11.2 and chapter 9). Our commitment to protect all those we can is based on a system of values that is more concerned with people's lives than with dollar values or probabilities and is thus the critical difference between people's decisions and those made by computers.

TYPES OF PARTICIPATION

There are many types of participation in decision making. Increasing the participation of consumers is needed in such programs as comprehensive health planning, where it is mandated by law. The demand for increased consumer participation is being heard more and more. Consumers are organizing into a variety of interest groups and seek input into all kinds and levels of decision making. We will discuss three models of participation.

In the first model, the consumer is given the opportunity to vote for or against a given course of action. This model represents a forced or polarized choice. The school bond issue on the ballot is an example. People can vote for or against the bonds. They may have had little or no voice in the decision that more schools are needed, how better to use existing facilities, where to locate the new ones, and so forth, but they can choose to support or reject the final decision. Of course, having this choice is better than no participation at all, but this model does not permit the greatest consumer input.

The second type of model allows consumers to participate in selecting one among several alternatives presented to them. Although they have no voice in selecting these alternatives, the choice is greater than a simple yes or no vote. We can assume that whoever selected the alternatives from which choice is permitted has made sure that all the alternatives are feasible and are acceptable to whatever group made the decisions. An example is presenting a list of extended care facilities to a family and permitting them to make their choice from it. If those preparing the list are experts in assessing the quality of such facilities, this kind of choice can be beneficial, since it protects the family against choosing a facility that does not meet minimum standards. Unfortunately, such lists are not always prepared with this objective in mind nor are they based solely on quality of care (Mendelson 1974). Interest groups may influence the choices offered the public, and these interests may not be readily apparent.

Some forced choice votes are genuinely seeking decisions from voters. "Do you or do you not want annexation to the municipal water district?" Often the presenting body appears only to be going through the motions on the assumption that the voters will *have* to come down on the "right" side of the issue. Health facility and school bond issues are often presented in this manner, which is proving to be politically naive. Presenters are finding that they must come up with contingency plans when opposition develops and voters come down on the "wrong" side. Multiple choices are more carefully thought through regarding the probable consequences of each alternative and whether these are acceptable to those in authority.

The third model is the most participatory and truly democratic. In small groups such as families, classes, and some planning groups, all those involved can sit down together and go through the decision-making process from start to finish. Communities are generally too large to make this model feasible, although the "town meeting" is still held in some places. If everyone cannot sit together to go through the process, representative forms of participation are the next possible approach.

Representation is always somewhat questionable since, when the chips are down, each represents herself and her own interests. If, however, representatives selected by and accountable to groups can be involved from the start in the planning or decison-making process, participation is improved. Representatives should be sought from all known interest groups. Publicity in the media can help others be aware of what's going to happen and decide whether they or their group want to participate. Meetings must be planned and held at times and places in which the people who need or want to participate can attend. For example, scheduling meetings in the evening or on Saturdays allows working people to attend without having to take time off—often at a loss in pay—to attend. Selecting locations that are easily accessible for both people who use public transportation as well as for those who drive private cars can also increase participation. Many problems with the outcomes of plans or decisions can be anticipated and either dealt with or eliminated by having broad representation from the outset, particularly when the decision group involves representatives from those having potential veto power over what is planned or decided. These representatives should have sufficient authority from their organizations both to make decisions at the meetings and to insure that these decisions will be supported by the organization later. The overriding principles here are that broadest representation possible be obtained and that the people representing the organizations have decision-making authority.

Once a decision-making group is constituted it can begin the planning process described in chapter 3. In participatory planning, as many people as possible are given a voice in setting objectives, establishing evaluation criteria, deciding among alternatives, discussing how and when to implement the plan, and evaluating the outcome. Along the way input can be increased by well-publicized public hearings that are open meetings any person or group can attend. They can hear what's happening and voice their opinions. Special priority should be given to the inclusion of the people who will be affected by the decisions made.

This kind of decision making is more process than product oriented; it takes much more time than decisions made by "experts" without input from others. However, it is more likely to produce plans and policies that will succeed through the cooperation of those affected.

POLITICAL SYSTEMS MODEL

In chapter 3, we presented a discussion of general systems theory and defined a number of terms. We also introduced an open systems model we applied to a family of four; this model illustrated the exchanges that occurred between the family system and its environment. In this chapter we apply the same open systems model to a community, in this case a decision-making body (figure 11.1).

The inputs include vested interest groups' opinions of what "ought to be," which is often a statement of the group's ideology. In this kind of open system in cities, interest groups seeking to influence decision-making bodies would include labor unions, parents' and teachers' groups, business organizations, neighborhood councils, ethnic groups, and a variety of others. The number of groups, the extent of their participation, and the coalitions they form will vary with the issues under consideration. Data from assessment of the situation are derived by the process described in chapter 3, "The Assessment Step in the Planning Process." Previous procedures are actions the group has already taken or precedents set by other groups, the courts, and legislation. Consideration of its

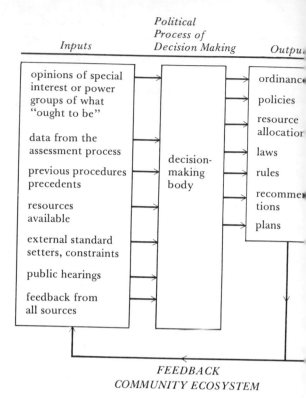

	Political Process of	
Inputs	*Decision Making*	*Outpu*

decision-making body

opinions of special interest or power groups of what "ought to be"

data from the assessment process

previous procedures precedents

resources available

external standard setters, constraints

public hearings

feedback from all sources

ordinanc

policies

resource allocatior

laws

rules

recommen tions

plans

FEEDBACK
COMMUNITY ECOSYSTEM

11.1   *Open Systems Model of a Community*

own previous decisions is part of feedback. Resources available is an input since these are generally limited and so choices have to be made about their use. External standards and constraints include guidelines such as those for implementing programs funded from other sources and regulations like those with Medicare and Medicaid services. Public hearings allow people who might not otherwise have the opportunity to voice their opinions on matters to be considered by the planning or decision-making body. Public hearings are also a forum for feedback from consumers and other sectors. Feedback from as many sources as possible, as indicated in figure 11.1, is essential if decisions are to be relevant and repeated mistakes are to be avoided.

We have briefly described the decision-making process in this chapter. As we noted, much of this process is an attempt to resolve conflicting and competing inputs. Once this is accomplished, the selection of alternatives, formulation and implementation of plans, and evaluation of the outcomes and their consequences follows more or less the type of planning process discussed in chapter 3.

The outputs of the system or decision-making body include rules,

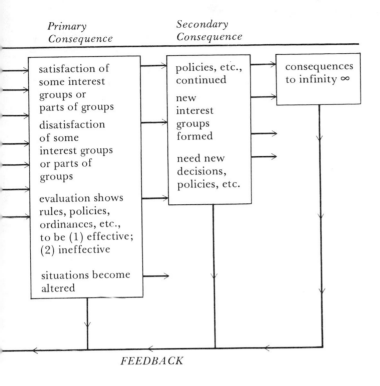

	Primary Consequence	Secondary Consequence

satisfaction of some interest groups or parts of groups

disatisfaction of some interest groups or parts of groups

evaluation shows rules, policies, ordinances, etc., to be (1) effective; (2) ineffective

situations become altered

policies, etc., continued

new interest groups formed

need new decisions, policies, etc.

consequences to infinity ∞

FEEDBACK

recommendations, policies, and the like. All of these outputs imply actions to be carried out or constraints to be followed. The decision-making body may have the power to enforce its decisions, it may rely on other organizations or systems in the environment to do so, or it may depend on voluntary compliance to its authority. Whatever the case, there will be a range of reactions to the decision from various interest groups. The implementation of the decisions may prove ineffective or effective in terms of predefined criteria. Over time, situations will change and necessitate new assessment and decisions based on new developments. All of these primary consequences will provide feedback for the decision-making body's subsequent deliberations. Secondary consequences can include the formation of new vested interest groups to support or refute policies or seek attention to new needs, the need for new policies, and the continuation of older ones. Again, feedback from increasing numbers of sources and quarters will return to become inputs. These kinds of consequences, their consequences, and feedback from them will continue indefinitely.

The process illustrated in this model is a complex and highly political one. Not all groups' interests can be served no matter how worthy they are or how well supported they may be. Resources are always limited, although they can be borrowed, stretched, reallocated, or priorities completely reordered. The fact remains that sooner or later decisions must be made. In open systems such as most of our institutions and decision-making bodies, the political processes described will and should occur. We believe the best decisions are those that include the greatest input possible from the largest possible number of people and groups.

ECONOMICS

INTRODUCTION

Economics (or political economy, as it has traditionally been called) deals with the alternatives and their consequences of the ways systems allocate or distribute limited resources. These include money, labor, land, and other natural resources. Economics is based on assumptions that include the following: All resources—land, labor, capital goods, and services—are scarce—that is, their supplies are limited. Supplies may temporarily be increased but not indefinitely because of the finite nature of all materials as well as competition for them by other systems.

The struggle to develop and enact a National Health Insurance or National Health Service illustrates both scarcity of and competition for resources. Bills proposing a National Health Service as well as bills proposing various types of insurance coverage, each with a different price tag, are introduced each time the issue of comprehensive access to health and medical care services is brought up. Both National Health Service and National Health Insurance are discussed in chapter 12. All these bills and proposals are supported or opposed to varying degrees by interest groups or subsystems within the health care delivery system: physicians, hospitals, drug companies, insurance companies, as well as by consumer groups and the national administration. This internal competition is brought on at least in part by each group's realization that there are not enough resources available to support all of the proposed programs. Only a part of the total national budget will go to National Health Insurance and each group, naturally, wants the supported program to be theirs. Furthermore, the whole health care delivery system will have to compete with the Departments of Defense, Labor, Commerce, Interior, and all the rest for any allocation at all, since the resources of the federal government are also limited.

A relatively recent and interesting group of entrants into the fray over legislation for federal level comprehensive health and medical care programs is industry, labor, and other portions of the private sector that see increasing amounts of the Gross National Product (GNP) being devoured by health and medical care costs. These costs to industry and commerce are passed along to consumers and, along with the spiralling expenses for health, medical, and dental care, whether paid for out-of-pocket or through third-party payers, are contributing to U.S. inflation. As the rest of this chapter will show, resources used for one purpose are not available to be used for any other purpose. Thus, business, industry, and labor are realizing that what the American people spend on health and medical care cannot be spent on other goods and services. Within the context of this competition for scarce resources, the political tradeoffs, games, and compromises discussed earlier in this chapter take place. Health and medical care may not be the only political game in town, but with growth to the second largest industry in the country and consumption of resources approaching 10 percent of the GNP, the political and economic impacts of health and medical care decisions are attracting increasing numbers of players.

In allocating scarce resources, a system must select from among several alternatives. Each alternative has a set of consequences that must be considered. There are costs and benefits involved in each alternative and its consequences. These costs and benefits can and should be analyzed to understand the relative effects various patterns of resource allocation will have on the extent to which a given system attains its goals. The budget of a community health agency exemplifies a set of given resources. The range of services offered is determined by the administrator's choice of which health care activities to support. The fact is possible, if unlikely, that more money could be obtained, but if it were, the amount would be limited and the selection of services would depend on the same decision-making process. The relative costs and benefits of each type of client service must be weighed against each other. For example, a home visit is very expensive and much of what is done during it can be done over the phone or through clinic services. However, some families cannot come to clinics, do not have telephones, do not read English and thus to be reached, must be visited in their homes. Initial visits that involve home assessments and extensive psycho-social history taking as well as visits where the community health nurse wishes to observe family members' interactions are most effectively done in the home.

Clinic services are generally less expensive per client served than are home visits. There are services that are given most effectively in the clinic, such as prenatal workups and services requiring X-ray or other extensive examinations. These are considerations of alternative uses of resources and their consequences, and they are critical to an agency's overall success in meeting its objectives.

The decision to allocate resources for one purpose precludes the use of these resources for any other purpose. This preclusion is called the opportunity cost and the other uses to which the resources might have been put but were not are called foregone or lost opportunities. Returning to our example in the community health agency, once resources are spent on home visits, they are not available for use in paying for clinic services or anything else. Consideration of opportunity costs is of critical importance in making resource allocation decisions.

ECONOMICS, NURSES, AND SALARIES

Peoples' efforts to avoid calamity and chaos attributable to the unpredictability of human nature are traced by Heilbroner through three developmental stages: tradition, authoritarian rule, and the "market system" (1972:17–18). Woman's traditional role has been caretaker of the sick and injured within the family. As this care became the responsibility of institutions more than families, nursing shifted to hospitals. These were generally religious or military organizations, under heavy authoritarian control. Secularization of hospitals did little to alter their traditional and authoritarian aspects. Women were trained in an apprentice model in local hospitals and generally continued to work there for extremely low wages or simply in return for room and board. Students "paid" for their training like any other apprentice—they worked for it. This pattern has only recently been altered in the United States and still continues in many other countries.

National examinations for individual licensure, teamed with the general mobility of the American population, permitted nurses to move about and learn that nursing skills are a scarce commodity for which the market will pay. Nurses are no longer bound to the institution where they are trained. This independence has made nurses notoriously mobile as Pape has shown (1964). Should institutional licensure be implemented, it could mean a return of this dependence on institutions. By making institutions rather than the individual professional responsible for quality control, hospitals and other health care facilities can return to training apprentices to fit the work situation in each institution. We must be aware that the development of institutional licensure will curtail not only our mobility potential, but also, and more importantly, will strip us of our individual R.N. licenses. A result will be a return to nurses' dependent role vis-à-vis the institution.

Moving nursing education from hospitals to institutions of higher education has placed nursing among the occupations for which advanced education is expected. Nurses are now more on a par with other health care professionals. We have increased self-esteem that together with impetus from the women's movement is moving nursing out of its traditional forms and lessening the hold of authoritarian institutions on us. We are now more willing to bargain in the market place for what is our due and for what we believe in. Nurses have realized not only that we have skills that are valuable and scarce commodities on the market but also that there is strength in collective action. Safeguarding individual professional licensure is essential to nurses' ability to influence the health care system.

Galbraith observes that industrialization has resulted in the loss of the servant class and threatens the entire field of personal services. The search for surrogates for the persons who historically provided personal services has resulted in the development of the paid homemaker, a women's trade. Unpleasant tasks must still be done and one way to persuade people to do them is to endow these workers with what Galbraith calls, "Convenient Social Virtue." Ascribing special merit to this work has long been used to obtain the services of nurses, custodial personnel, and other kinds of hospital workers. The general community views such social status as a partial substitute for adequate pay (Galbraith 1973:30–34). Status and social prestige are also applied to a variety of public employees such as college teachers, community health workers, clergy, and so on. As we all know, however, status is a heady thing but you can't eat it. Psychic dollars don't pay the rent.

We have heard people say, "It must be rewarding to be a nurse"—but they don't mean monetarily rewarding—or "I couldn't do it but I sure give credit to you girls who can be nurses." Outsiders still look at occupations such as ours through the rosy glow of convenient social virtue. Many inside the field are suggesting that nursing is instead exploitative and are beginning to demand remuneration comparable to that of other workers. The organization of domestic workers, the increased dollar value attached by insurance companies to disabled housewives, college teachers' demands for collective bargaining, and the nurses' strikes are all examples of insiders redefining the relation of their jobs to the market (Werther and Lockhart 1976).

Economic Terms

There are a wide variety of writers holding forth on all manner of economic specialties. In general, however, they share a special language that, like our medical jargon, makes sense to them and excludes outsiders. We include a selection of their terms with examples from our own field to illustrate their applicability to our own interests. The list is in no way complete but represents a sample of the terms most crucial to our understanding of the economic forces that impinge on our profession.

Capital.   Labor, land, and capital are the three basic resources or inputs with which the market works. Labor and land are primary inputs since they are not produced by the economy. Capital, shorthand for capital goods, is the output of market subsystems and is used as input by other subsystems of the economy. Capital includes buildings, machinery, and supplies. For many years the government has provided funds to hospitals and other care facilities for capital expenditures; part of the reimbursements that institutions receive from Medicare and Medicaid must be used for amortization of debts for capital expenditures. Presumably this arrangement will continue under whatever scheme of National Health Insurance is enacted.

Supply and Demand. Supply is the amount of goods or services that producers are willing to sell; the supply schedule or curve is the relationship between the market price offered and the supply of goods willingly sold. Demand is the amount of goods and services that consumers will buy. Demand is not what consumers *want* to buy, it is the amount they *do* buy. The demand schedule or curve is the relationship between the market price for goods and the quantity of these goods demanded. In Adam Smith's vision of the free market, it regulated itself on the basis of competition among many buyers and many sellers, no one of whom was sufficiently large to influence either the supply or demand for any good or service. This lovely theory has never worked except perhaps in true barter economies. It certainly does not work now (Keynes 1964; Galbraith 1973; Samuelson 1976).

The Law of Downward Sloping Demand says that with other things being equal, when the price of a good increases, the demand for that good decreases. The supply curve tends to rise since sellers increase their production in their anxiety to sell more goods at the higher price. The equilibrium price is believed to be the only price that is stable or in balance, since it is the point at which the amount of goods supplied is equal to the amount of goods demanded. Competitive equilibrium is the point at which the supply and demand curves intersect. This happy relationship occurs when all other things are equal; unfortunately, in the U.S. economy all other things are far from being equal.

Despite the ideology that characterizes the U.S. economy as purely capitalistic and the Soviet economy as purely communistic, in reality there are no pure economies. Every nation has a mixture of public and private enterprise. Our major businesses are selective about what parts of the free enterprise system they endorse. They seldom bite any feeding hand, even if it is a governmental subsidy or a system of price supports. Private medicine in the United States has been quite willing to permit government interference with health care as long as government confined its activities to caring for the very poor payment risks—seamen, native Americans, and the impoverished.

Elasticity of Demand.   This term describes the extent to which the quantity of a good or service changes its market price. Thus an increase in quantity of a good is likely to depress the price per unit. Producers may therefore receive less revenue when their production is high than when it is lower. The concern in measuring elasticity is with the total dollar revenues that consumers pay providers. This dollar revenue is the product of the price per unit times the total quantity purchased. Elasticity of demand is stated in percentage changes and takes three forms.

Elastic Demand.   A decrease in the price of a good or service increases the demand for it; the resulting increase in quantity purchased causes an increase in the total dollar revenues. Conversely, if the price increases, there is a decrease in the quantities purchased and the total dollar revenues fall. Commodities that are prone to elasticity of demand are luxury items such as jewelry.

Unitary Elasticity of Demand.   A price reduction of a given percent results in an equal percentage increase in quantity demanded so that the total dollar revenue remains unchanged—that is, price and demand vary in a one-to-one inverse ratio.

Inelasticity of Demand.   A cut in price causes no change or only a very small increase in demand and thus revenues decrease. With inelastic demand the converse is also true—that is, if price increases, total revenues increase since people continue to buy. Physician services and hospital care are considered commodities for which demand is fairly inelastic, since people buy these services when they need them with little concern for price. We know this statement is not entirely true except in theory; many put off seeking medical care because they cannot afford the costs.

Cost as a Barrier to Buying Services.   Cost is often a deterrent to people in making a choice to purchase goods or services. This phenomenon also works when they consider buying health care services. In some instances such procrastination pays off since some conditions clear up without medical intervention. Unfortunately, this situation is not always the case and people must seek care for conditions that do not just go away. When care is finally sought, the person is often so ill that cost is secondary to the need for immediate treatment—the client will worry about the bills later. Postponing care because of the cost all too often results in long-term or irreparable damage to the client's level of functioning. It may also result in a higher bill since longer or costlier care may be needed than would have been necessary earlier. Thus, postponing medical care as a means to save money may be like jumping over a nickel to get at a penny. We may need to explain this possibility to some clients and encourage them to seek care promptly, not only to decrease long-run financial costs but also to avoid or reduce long-term incapacities.

The effect of cost as a barrier to use of services varies with the kind of services needed. Demand for life-sustaining service is least affected by cost; demand for preventive services is most subject to cost as a barrier. Demand for services to alleviate minor ailments falls somewhere in between. Health insurance reduces the economic barrier to the use of health services, as we shall see in the next chapter (Bailey 1969:10.10–10.15). Before closing this discussion, we should note that because of the incidence of chronic illness, primary preventive services are increasingly essential, because they are precisely the ones most often foregone because of their cost.

Contrived Demand.   The creation of contrived or artificial demand is an objective of advertising. We are encouraged to buy large automobiles, to travel, to consume one brand of aspirin instead of another. Contrived demand induces us to buy things we neither need nor really want. The sales pitch often involves blatant appeals to status consciousness or being "in." Community nurses should be aware that food and dental and medical care budget items are often the first ones cut when clients must make sacrifices to keep up appearances.

Costs.   There are many kinds of costs. Some are particularly important to community nurses and are discussed here:

Fixed costs are the set, unchanging costs of running a system and producing outputs. They include rent, wages, and utilities and are the components of overhead. Fixed costs are the same for each unit of output the system produces. If the fixed costs for a day's hospitalization add up to $100, then each patient's charges will begin with $100 per day. One problem facing hospitals and other kinds of health care facilities is that their fixed costs remain the same whether or not their services are being used—that is, the fixed costs of maintaining an empty hospital bed add up to $100 per day just as they do for an occupied bed.

Variable costs are the cost of goods and services over and above the components of fixed costs—that is, everything else comprising the total cost. In a hospital, variable costs include x-ray services, laboratory work, medications, special treatments such as physical therapy, and so forth.

Total cost is the sum of fixed and variable costs. The total cost to the client of a hospital stay is composed of the fixed costs that are the same for everyone plus the variable costs, which are different for each client. Clients should be advised to obtain itemized bills following hospitalization so that they can see exactly what the fixed and variable costs of their hospital stay were. Occasionally mistakes in billing can be picked up by careful study of itemized bills. Also an itemized bill is essential when seeking explanation of reimbursements from insurance carriers, since only with an itemized bill can the client compare what a policy states it will cover and what the insurance company actually did pay for.

Average cost per unit of service is calculated by dividing the total cost of running the agency by the number of units of service provided. These data are among the more important cost accounting calculations used by administrators as a basis for making program decisions.

Let us say that we are running a home nursing program. Our agency's unit of service is the nurse's visit to a client's home for the purpose of giving nursing care. We want to know what the average cost per visit is. We would divide the total cost—that is, the sum of the fixed or overhead costs and the variable costs for the special services—by the total number of nursing home care visits. If the program's expenditures are $40,000 per year and the staff made a total of 1875 visits, the average cost per visit would be: $40,000 ÷ 1875, or $21.33 per visit.

The average cost per visit is an extremely important figure since it is the basic figure for determining how much to bill clients or third-party payers per unit of service—that is, per nurse's visit to a client's home to give nursing care. You will notice that the program's entire expenditures are used as the basis for determining the unit cost of a home visit. Often the mistake is made of counting only direct nursing service costs—salaries, transport, supplies, and the like—in determining unit cost. Since indirect costs such as administration, maintenance, utilities, and other expenses must be paid for out of generated revenues regardless of their sources, these indirect costs must be included in determining costs per unit of service. Budgets should be made up in such a way that all of nursing service's indirect as well as direct costs can be broken out and tabulated rather than being all lumped together in a single line item. Nurse-administrators like all other department or bureau managers must be alert to be sure that each subsystem of the organization is appropriately accounting all of its direct and indirect costs (see chapter 21).

In many instances home visits are only one of the agency's services or there may be more than one level of nursing personnel giving service. In such circumstances calculations of average cost per visit are far more difficult and reference should be made to such publications as "How to Determine Nursing Expenditures in Small Health Agencies" for assistance (Anthony and Herzlinger 1975; Borst and Montant 1977; Sweeny 1977).

The increased emphasis on cost accounting and cost-benefit analysis makes essential that these data be available to administrators, governing bodies, and ultimately to the public that is showing an increasing concern with how tax monies and donations are being allocated. Both as citizens and as employees, nurses should be aware of the influence of costs over an agency's budget and the extent of services it can provide, as well as the problems of adequate reimbursement.

Consumer Price Index.   The costs of medical care and hospitalization have contributed to the rising cost of living and the inflationary spiral. The costs of these services continue to rise at a faster rate than most other items in the Consumer Price Index (CPI). CPI is a measure of the current price of goods and services relative to their costs in a baseline period (see table 12.2). For example, if a particular prescription such as insulin cost $1.00 in the baseline period and now costs $1.50, it has increased in cost by 50 percent in the interval between the baseline and the present. CPI figures for a number of goods and services enable us to see how the relative increases in the prices of food, medical care, and other consumer items compare.

The Law of Diminishing Returns.   This law states that in a system that has both fixed and variable inputs, increasing the variable inputs relative to the fixed inputs will increase the output *up to a certain point.* Beyond that point no matter how much the variable inputs are increased, without an increase in the fixed inputs, the output will decrease. For example, our agency has a prenatal clinic; its output is the number of clients examined. The clinic facility has three counseling rooms and three examining rooms; these are fixed input. The variable input is the number of staff who can be assigned to the clinic. Assuming that client demand is greater than the amount of prenatal services currently available and that we want to increase the output of the prenatal clinic by seeing more women, we would look at the present and potential staffing patterns. There are four nurses assigned to the clinic to do prenatal teaching, return visit examinations, and assist the physician with initial or complicated examinations. Increasing the number of nurses from four to six can be expected to increase the clinic's output since with six nurses and six rooms we can assume that all of the rooms will be in use. This increase of staff relative to the fixed inputs of the six clinic rooms can be expected to increase the numbers of clients examined. But can we expect a continued increase in output if we add a seventh nurse? That the seventh nurse will increase the output as much as the fifth and sixth nurses did is doubtful; adding a seventh and an eighth nurse will not produce an output sufficient to justify the added cost for these personnel; we have thus reached the point of diminishing returns for additional investment of personnel.

Marginality.   Regardless of the context in which it is used in economics, marginal means something extra or additional. For example, I recently bought a new car and in the process of bargaining with the sales manager, I indicated that most firms' profit margin was approximately $100 per vehicle. This profit margin is the markup or added price over and above the actual cost of the good or service that enables the firm to make a profit. Marginal cost is the amount by which the total cost increases for each additional unit of output. Since fixed costs are the same for each unit of production and variable costs grow unitarily with total costs, which are the sum of the fixed and the variable costs, the marginal cost is computed by subtracting the total cost of producing two units of output from the cost of producing three units. For example, if the total cost of producing two batches of pills is $45 and the total cost of producing three batches is $50, then the marginal cost is $5, or the difference between total costs. Marginal cost is higher for initial units of service and then begins to decrease, although this decrease never reaches zero. Because of the Law of Diminishing Returns marginal cost eventually begins to increase again.

An example of marginality that has occurred in recent public health practice in the United States is the shift in TB control from the use of mass mini-screening X-rays to tuberculin skin testing in many areas of the country. The reason for this shift, besides the desire to reduce the dosage of radiation, was the realization that the cost of finding each case of tuberculosis revealed by mini-screening was prohibitive. In most of the United States the rate of tuberculosis is now so low that there is little likelihood of finding cases through mass X-ray screening. In many areas TB control people have turned to tuberculin skin testing of young children to determine their exposure to TB, as well as a search for index cases through followup. This approach has resulted in a much lower cost per case found than with X-rays. X-ray is now generally reserved for high-risk populations such as prisoners and hospital admissions. We used to talk about eradication of tuberculosis; now we speak of control since the cost of eradication is so high. Figure 11.2 illustrates the relative costs of programs with 25, 50, 75, and 90 percent eradication goals. Beyond 75 percent or so the costs of finding each additional case become prohibitive, and invoking concepts like herd immunity and probability become necessary to determine where marginal costs for each additional case found become too great.

Utility. We infer utility, the ability of a good or service to satisfy a want or desire, from the strength of demand for that good or service. Marginal utility is that amount of satisfaction which each added unit of a good or service gives the consumer. The utility or satisfaction derived from three cocktails may be greater for the individual consumer than that derived

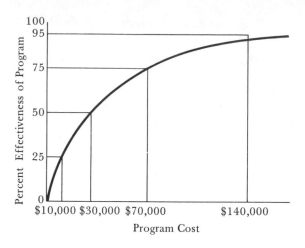

11.2   *Cost-Effectiveness Ratio of a Disease Eradication Program*

from two cocktails. The increased satisfaction from the third drink is marginal utility. If satisfaction peaks with four drinks, the marginal utility of subsequent cocktails will decrease since the peak has been passed. In economics this process is called decreasing marginal utility; clinically it is called inebriation or overdose. Utilization of health care services is often used as an index of the degree of consumer demand for these services. Heavy utilization is, therefore, justification for continuation and expansion of these services.

Cost-Benefit Analysis. Cost-benefit analysis is used to determine the relative value of alternative patterns of resource allocation in planning or in evaluating ongoing programs and their consequences. It is based on the ratio of dollar value of the costs or inputs of the system and the dollar value of the system's outputs, or the benefits the system produces. Costs are considered in dollar terms so that everything has a common denominator. Placing dollar value often brings economists and non-economists into disagreement. Economists can measure the value of any and all things including human life in dollar terms. For example, the dollar value of a white, college-educated male is greater than the dollar value of a white male who failed to complete high school. This evaluation is made by estimating the amount of income and therefore taxes each will have to pay and consequently their relative potential for supporting the economy; in other words, their relative efficiency in repaying the public resources invested in their care. Given limited services and supplies, the economist would argue that since the potential for return on the investment made is greater with the college-educated persons, they should have priority for the scarce services. This dollar value rationale makes investments in services for the aged seem frivolous. Obviously, persons who consider themselves to be humanists find such calculations odious as a basis for determining priorities among people. As with most arguments based on such contrary values, both sides make some telling points, and effective ways of analyzing and dealing with situations probably need to combine aspects of both arguments. Economists might be less quantification-oriented in terms of returns on the dollars invested, and humanists might be more concerned with efficiency as well as with matters of fairness.

Cost-benefit analysis is not only concerned about the effects of alternative patterns of resource allocation on the internal workings of the system, but also about the social or external effects of the various courses of action. Two important issues must be considered in any cost-benefit analysis. The first, efficiency, is concerned with getting the maximum output for each unit of input, according to marginal costs discussed above. Efficient use of personnel, for example, means that each category of personnel should do the things that they alone are best able to do. Thus, registered nurses who are the most highly trained and skilled can most efficiently do client teaching or family and home assessments, while licensed vocational or practical nurses are best prepared to give bedside care in the home situation under the supervision of the registered nurse, and homemakers are skilled in such activities as meal preparation, light cleaning, marketing, escorting clients, and so forth. From a dollar point of view, for a registered nurse to do homemaker tasks is inefficient, unless there is client teaching involved in so doing.

The second issue to be considered in cost-benefit analysis is that of equity. In seeking to determine the equity of a situation, we are interested in who pays the costs of the services given and who receives the benefits. If the payers and the receivers are the same people, then we have a situation that is equitable. Inequities exist when the persons who pay for services are not the recipients of the services. For example, taxpayers are bearing the costs of government-subsidized care through Medicaid programs. But taxpayers rarely receive Medicaid, and its recipients generally pay minimal taxes.

In doing cost-benefit analysis, we must consider all the alternative direct and indirect costs and direct and indirect benefits of the programs under study. Some *direct costs* such as out-of-pocket payments and third-party payments for health care services are fairly obvious. Less obvious direct costs are transportation to and from facilities, the burden placed on the client's family due to illness and loss or interruption of income, the loss to an employer by the client's absence, and that part of the institution's cost for providing care that is not covered by fees. *Indirect costs* include time lost on the job or in school by members of the client's family who must transport and care for the client, loss of taxes by the government, and other opportunity costs that are incurred by the family and client as a result of illness. *Direct benefits* of health care services include restoration of a level of functioning enabling the client to return to work or school with a minimum number of days lost or residual disability, the number of years added to the client's lifespan, the effect on the quality of life of the client, the family, the employer, and the community by restoration of the client's ability to function productively as a person and a worker. *Indirect benefits* of health care services include the employment of providers of services, the reduction of client's loss of economic and social status, and the effects on the community of a family group whose attitude toward life is better than it might otherwise have been. These are the kinds of cost and benefit considerations that must be studied in deciding among potential programs that are competing for scarce resources.

Bailey (1969 9.21–9.35) suggests that the following questions be asked in doing any cost-benefit study to be sure that the issues of efficiency and equity are considered: Which groups of people receive these benefits? How much benefit is required by a person being treated? How much return is there to the government in terms of taxes? Over what time periods do these benefits accrue? What kinds of services can maximize these benefits? What is the form of the cost; what is its magnitude and time span? Who shares in the costs—the person or family and taxpayers, or certain income groups of taxpayers? Do the groups receiving the services also bear the costs?

Taxes. The principle of taxation in a free society is the decision of citizens or their legislators on how and from whom resources will be collected and how these resources will be made available for public goods and services. In the 1970s U.S. voters directly influenced some taxes through referenda dealing with tax increases for such projects as rapid transit and construction or the acquisition of land to be used for open space.

Taxes are classified in three ways: proportional, progressive, and regressive. Proportional taxation takes the same proportion of income from everyone regardless of the size of that income; an income tax of 10 percent for everyone is a proportional tax. A progressive tax takes a larger fraction of income from the rich than from the poor; federal personal income tax is a progressive tax since the more money people make, the more taxes they are expected to pay. Discussion of deductions and loopholes is beyond the scope of this chapter. *In principle,* however, federal income tax is an example of progressive taxation that if properly collected, results in redistribution of wealth from the rich to the poor. Regressive taxes take a greater fraction of income from the poor than they do from the rich—that is, the rate of taxation decreases as the amount of the person's base for taxation increases. The property tax, highly criticized for many reasons, is a regressive tax. Two families own homes of equal value. The property tax on each home is $855. Family A's annual income is $15,000 and family B's is $5,000. The property tax is 5.7 percent of family A's total income and is 17.1 percent of family B's. That's why property taxes are regressive. Regressive taxes such as property, sales, and excise taxes are particularly devastating to persons with fixed incomes such as those on social security, disability, pension, and welfare. Many older people who paid off their homes long before they retired are now being forced to sell them because their retirement income does not increase fast enough for them to meet the spiraling costs of property taxes.

SUMMARY

Community nurses are involved in political and economic matters constantly in working with clients, whether individuals, families, groups, populations, or communities. In this chapter we have presented an orientation to how things really work, in our experience, by discussing some key aspects of politics and economics.

In the politics section we discussed what politics is and is not in our context. We then went on to talk about power; interest groups; decision-making strategies including compromise, games, tradeoffs, and decision matrices; and three types of consumer participation. The section on politics ended with a discussion of an open systems model of a community, patterned after the systems model developed in chapter 3.

The economics portion begins with an overview of the place that nursing occupies in the market system and some background on how we got there. Key economic concepts are defined and examples relevant to community nursing are given. These include: supply and demand, cost-benefit analysis, opportunity costs, marginality, and costs in general.

Neither of these discussions is exhaustive. They are meant, instead, to provide a baseline of information on which community nurses can build through their own experience and study.

REFERENCES

ALBERTI, ROBERT E., ed. *Assertiveness: Innovations, Applications, Issues*. San Luis Obispo, Calif.: Impact Publishers, 1977.

ALINSKY, SAUL D. *Rules for Radicals*. New York: Vintage Books, 1972.

ALTSHULER, ALAN A. *Community Control: The Black Demand for Participation in Large American Cities*. Indianapolis: Pegasus, A Division of Bobbs-Merrill Co., 1970.

ANTHONY, R.N., and HERZLINGER, R.E. *Management Control in Nonprofit Organizations.* Howewood, Ill.: Richard W. Irwin Publishing Co., 1975.

BAILEY, RICHARD M. "Economics and Planning." In Henrik Blum, ed., *Health Planning 1969.* Berkeley: University of California, School of Public Health, 1969.

————. "The Microeconomics of Health." In Henrik Blum, ed., *Health Planning 1969.* Berkeley: University of California, School of Public Health, 1969.

BENVENISTE, GUY. *The Politics of Expertise.* Berkeley: The Glendessary Press, 1972.

BERNE, ERIC. *Games People Play.* New York: Ballantine Books, 1964.

BORST, D., and MONTANT, P.J. Managing Nonprofit Organizations. New York: AMACOM, A Division of the American Management Association, 1977.

CATER, DOUGLASS, and LEE, PHILIP R., eds. *Politics of Health.* New York: MED-COM, 1972.

CLAUS, KAREN E., and BAILEY, JUNE T. *Power and Influence in Health Care: A New Approach to Leadership.* St. Louis: C.V. Mosby Co., 1977.

CONANT, RALPH W. *The Politics of Community Health.* Washington, D.C.: Public Affairs Press, 1968.

DAHL, ROBERT A. *Who Governs? Democracy and Power in an American City.* New Haven, Conn.: Yale University Press, 1961.

DELOUGHERY, GRACE L., and GEBBIE, KRISTINE M. Political Dynamics: Impact on Nurses and Nursing. St. Louis: C.V. Mosby Co., 1975.

EASTON, ALLAN. *Complex Managerial Decisions Involving Multiple Objectives.* New York: John Wiley and Sons, 1973.

EVERLY, G.S., and FALCOINE, R.L. "Perceived Dimensions of Job Satisfaction for Staff Registered Nurses." Nursing Research 25 (1976):346–48.

FERGUSON, MARION. *How to Determine Nursing Expenditures in Small Health Agencies: A Procedure Using Work Units.* Washington D.C.: U.S. Department of Health, Education and Welfare, Division of Nursing Publication No. 902, revised, 1966.

GALBRAITH, JOHN KENNETH. *Economics and the Public Purpose.* Boston: Houghton Mifflin Co., 1973.

GAMSON, WILLIAM A. "Violence and Political Power: The Meek Don't Make It." *Psychology Today* 8 (1974):35–41.

HAWLEY, WILLIS D., and WIRT, FREDERICK M., eds. *The Search for Community Power.* Englewood Cliffs, N.J.: Prentice-Hall, 1968.

HEILBRONER, ROBERT L. *The Worldly Philosophers: The Lives, Times and Ideas of Great Economic Thinkers,* 4th ed. New York: Simon and Schuster, 1972.

KAHN, SI. *How People Get Power: Organizing Oppressed Communities for Action.* New York: McGraw-Hill Book Co., 1970.

KEYNES, JOHN MAYNARD. *The General Theory of Employment, Interest, and Money.* New York: Harcourt, Brace and World, 1964.

LAWRENCE, JOHN C. "Confronting Nurses' Political Apathy." *Nursing Forum* 15 (Fall 1976): 363–71.

LEKACHMAN, ROBERT. *Economists at Bay: Why the Experts Will Never Solve Your Problems.* New York: McGraw-Hill Paperbacks, 1976.

LEVIN, PAMELA, and BERNE, ERIC. "Games Nurses Play." *American Journal of Nursing* 73 (1973):483–87.

LINDBLOM, CHARLES E. *The Policy-Making Process.* Englewood Cliffs, N.J.: Prentice-Hall, 1968.

LONG, NORTON E. "The Local Community as an Ecology of Games." In Willis D. Hawley and Frederick M. Wirt, eds., *The Search for Community Power.* Englewood Cliffs, N.J.: Prentice-Hall, 1968.

MARX, KARL. *Capital (Das Kapital).* Chicago: Encyclopedia Britannica, The Great Books, vol. 50, 1952.

MARX, KARL, and ENGELS, FRIEDRICH. *The Communist Manifesto,* 1848. Chicago: Encyclopedia Britannica, The Great Books, vol. 50, 1952.

MAY, ROLLO. *Power and Innocence: A Search for the Sources of Violence.* New York: W.W. Norton & Co., 1972.

MEADOWS, DONELLA H., et al. *The Limits of Growth: A Report for the Club of Rome's Project on the Predicament of Mankind.* New York: Universe Books, 1972.

MENDELSON, MARY ADELAIDE. *Tender Loving Greed: How the Incredibly Lucrative Nursing Home "Industry" Is Exploiting America's Old People and Defrauding Us All.* New York: Alfred A. Knopf, 1974.

MILIO, NANCY. *9226 Kercheval: The Store Front That Did Not Burn.* Ann Arbor: University of Michigan Press, 1971.

MONSEN, JOSEPH R., JR., and CANNON, MARK W. *The Makers of Public Policy: American Power Groups and Their Ideologies.* New York: McGraw-Hill Book Co., 1964.

NOVACK, MICHAEL. "Politics as Drama." *The Center Magazine* 3 (Summer 1969):9.

PAPE, RUTH H. (FLESHMAN). "Touristry: A Type of Occupational Mobility." *Social Problems* 11 (1964):336–44.

PERLMAN, JANIS. "Grassrooting the System." *Social Policy* 7 (1976) :4–20.

POGREBIN, LETTY COTTIN. *Getting Yours: How to Make the System Work for the Working Woman.* New York: David McKay Company, 1975.

PIORE, NORA. "Rationalizing the Mix of Public and Private Expenditures in Health." In John B. McKinlay, ed., *Economic Aspects of Health Care,* a Milbank Resource Book. New York: Prodist, 1973.

POWELL, DIANE J. "Nursing and Politics: The Struggles Outside Nursing's Body Politic." *Nursing Forum* 15 (Fall 1976) : 341–62.

REDMAN, ERIC. *The Dance of Legislation.* New York: Simon and Schuster, 1973.

SAMUELSON, PAUL A. *Economics,* 9th ed. New York: McGraw-Hill Book Co., 1973.

SCHAEFER, MARGUERITE J. "The Political and Economic Scene in the Future of Nursing." *American Journal of Public Health* 63 (October 1973): 887–89.

SCHOLNICK, JEROME H. *The Politics of Protest.* New York: Ballantine Books, 1969.

SHUBIK, MARTIN, ed. *Game Theory and Related Approaches to Social Behavior.* New York: John Wiley and Sons, 1964.

SILVERMAN, MILTON, and LEE, PHILIP R. *Pills, Profits, and Politics.* Berkeley and Los Angeles: University of California Press, 1974.

SMITH, ADAM. *Inquiry into the Nature and Causes of the Wealth of Nations.* Chicago: Encyclopedia Britannica, The Great Books, vol. 39, 1952.

SMITH, PAUL A. "The Games of Community Politics." In Willis D. Hawley and Frederick M. Wirt, eds., *The Search for Community Power.* Englewood Cliffs, N. J.: Prentice-Hall, 1968.

STIMSON, DAVID H. "Health Agency Decision-Making: An Operations Research Perspective." In Mary F. Arnold, L. Vaughn Blankenship, and John M. Hess, eds., *Administering Health Systems: Issues and Perspectives.* Chicago: Aldine-Atherton, 1971.

STRICKLAND, STEPHEN P. *Politics, Science and Dread Disease: A Short History of United States Medical Research Policy.* Cambridge, Mass.: Harvard University Press, 1972.

SWEENY, A., and WISNER J., JR. *Budgeting Fundamentals for Non-financial Executives and Managers.* New York: McGraw-Hill Paperbacks, 1977.

THOMAS, JOHN M., and BENNIS, WARREN G., eds. *Management of Change and Conflict.* Baltimore, Md.: Penguin Books, 1972.

THOMSTAD, BEATRICE CUNNINGHAM, and KAPLAN, BARBARA H. "Changing the Rules of the Doctor-Nurse Game." *Nursing Outlook* 23 (1975) : 422–27.

WALZER, MICHAEL. *Political Action: A Practical Guide to Movement Politics*. Chicago: Quadrangle Books, 1971.

WEBER, MAX. "Authority and Legitimacy." In Eric A. Nordlinger, ed., Politics and Society: Studies in Comparative Political Sociology. Englewood Cliffs, N. J.: Prentice-Hall, 1970.

WERTHER, WILLIAM B., and LOCKHART, CAROL A. *Labor Relations in the Health Professions: The Basis of Power, the Means of Change*. Boston: Little, Brown and Co., 1976.

ZINN, CHARLES J. *How Our Laws Are Made*. Washington, D.C.: U.S. Government Printing Office, Stock Number 5271–0304, 1972.

12. Health Insurance: How the United States Pays for Health Care

Sarah Ellen Archer

INTRODUCTION

Health care is a right in the United States and no one can be refused care because of their inability to pay. Fact or myth?

People who cannot afford private medical care can always be covered under Medicaid or some other public program. Fact or myth?

People in the United States no longer have to pay from their own pockets for health care since everyone has adequate health insurance coverage. Fact or myth?

Everyone has access to primary, secondary, and tertiary preventive health services, all of which are covered by health insurance. Fact or myth?

Requiring people to pay most of the costs for initial visits to the doctor or days in the hospital reduces the utilization of these services and results in cost containment. Requiring people to pay 20 percent or more of the total cost of all insurance covered services also reduces utilization and helps contain medical care costs. Fact or myth?

One of the greatest strengths of the medical care system in the United States is that it is pluralistic and many faceted. Coordination between the many components of the system is so good that all clients are assured of continuity of care as they move from one part of the system to another. Fact or myth?

313

All kinds of health care providers and consumers are actively involved in groups such as Professional Standards Review Organizations, which are concerned with the development of standards as a means of assuring quality of care. Fact or myth?

Generally people either are able to read and understand their health insurance policies themselves or have others such as insurance agents, physicians, or attorneys to interpret what their coverage means to them. Fact or myth?

As community health nurses, we must have information to be able to make our own decisions about whether these statements about the health care delivery system in the United States are fact or myth. The purpose of this chapter is to provide you with much of the needed information. Other chapters also address many of these same issues from a variety of points of view. Be alert for them as you read. We will come back to these statements in the section at the end of the chapter dealing with national health programs.

As you read this chapter loaded with statistics and definitions, you will repeatedly ask yourself, why do I have to know all this stuff? Here are a few reasons. One of your clients phones shortly after her husband's discharge from the hospital following surgery. They have just received the hospital's bill that indicates they owe several hundred dollars over and above what their health insurance paid. They are upset since they thought their health insurance would cover all expenses; they certainly were not expecting these expenses; in fact, they are already short of money because the family breadwinner has not yet been able to return to work. Another family is angry because a condition the mother has had for a long time is not covered by their new health insurance policy and so they will have to pay all of the costs for her treatment for that preexisting condition. Still another client can't understand why expenses involved in an illness that started a week after the family signed up for health insurance coverage were not paid by the insurance and so they got the whole bill.

Since community nurses are part of the health care establishment and often the closest one to whom clients can turn, we are often asked—many times angrily—why clients' health insurance didn't cover all their medical expenses and what they're supposed to do about it. They often don't realize that virtually no health insurance covers all expenses. A common question is, "Why didn't somebody tell me this before now?! What's the point of having insurance if you still have to pay?"

We hope this chapter will provide community nurses with background information on health insurance, which in turn will help us answer some of our clients' questions about their health insurance *before* they get into the kinds of situations we've just described. Our purpose is not to convert community nurses into insurance agents, nor are we planning to invade insurance sales territory or inflame clients against the industry. There is no doubt in our minds, however, that there is a direct connection between clients' optimum level of functioning and the kind and amount of health insurance protection they have to help them with the overwhelming costs of medical care.

INSURANCE COUNSELING

INSURANCE AGENTS

We are often told that an insurance policy is only as good as the agent who sold the policy to the individual or family. This rather sweeping statement is one that, I think, has validity. Much of the following section about the need for us as community health nurses to become involved in insurance counseling could be eliminated if more people had ethical insurance agents from responsible insurance companies and if the people knew how to use these agents appropriately. Insurance agents should be selected with the same care that one uses in picking a physician or an attorney. The best place to start is through your friends and business associates who can direct you to a local agent with whom they are satisfied. An agent who has been in business in the local area and is well established is likely to remain and to be there when you or your clients need his or her services for the filing of a claim or for additional insurance coverage.

An important aspect is that the client and the insurance agent establish a rapport in which they can work together comfortably. The client has a right to ask about the agent's training and experience. Is the agent a Chartered Life Underwriter? If so, this status indicates considerable training in insurance, including individual life and health insurance, life insurance law, group insurance, pension planning, income, gift, and estate taxation, and accounting and finance. In addition, we can assume that a Chartered Life Underwriter subscribes to the Code of Ethics that appears below.

When purchasing insurance of any kind, especially health insurance, the client must understand at least three things: the kinds of coverages available, the costs of each or combinations of these coverages, and what kinds and levels of coverage are needed to insure appropriately the person and his or her family. Time should be taken to gain this understanding and a good insurance agent should not only welcome these kinds of questions, but be able to supply answers in terms the client can understand. It behooves the agent to take this kind of time with the client for several

---

CODE OF ETHICS

Preamble: The position of the Life Underwriter is unique in that he is the liaison between his client and his company. As a life insurance advisor he owes a high professional duty toward his client, while, at the same time, he also occupies a position of trust and loyalty to his company. Only by observing the highest ethical balance can he avoid any conflict between these two obligations.
Therefore:

I Believe it to be my Responsibility:

To hold my business in high esteem and strive to maintain its prestige.

To keep the needs of my clients always uppermost.

To respect my client's confidence and hold in trust personal information.

To render continuous service to my clients and their beneficiaries.

To employ every proper and legitimate means to persuade my clients to protect insurable obligations; but to rigidly adhere to the observance of the highest standards of business and professional conduct.

To present accurately, honestly and completely every fact essential to my client's decisions.

To perfect my skill and to add to my knowledge through continuous thought and study.

To conduct my business on such a high plane that others emulating my example may help the standards of our vocation.

To keep myself informed with respect to insurance laws and regulations and to observe them in both letter and spirit.

To respect the prerogatives and cooperate with all others whose services are constructively related to ours in meeting the needs of our clients.

Source: American Society of Chartered Life Underwriters.

---

reasons. First, missunderstanding about the coverage in the policy purchased most often results in very dissatisfied customers when claim payments do not meet their expectations. This dissatisfaction will be vented on the insurance agent who not only sold the policy but is the one who handles claims and any problems around them. Thus the insurance agent benefits in the long run by being absolutely sure that insured customers

understand what a policy does and does *not* cover. Secondly, ethical insurance people like any other professionals take pride in helping people
and in having satisfied customers. Thirdly, the better the customers
understand that insurance premiums are directly related to the amount of
coverage a policy provides, the more likely they are to buy adequate
coverage for their financial and risk situations. Patient explanation can
result in the purchase of more realistic coverage rather than the cheapest
the customer can get. This explanation job pays off for the insurance
agent not only in fewer headaches later but also in higher payment for the
agent. Top insurance companies now require the applicant to sign a
statement that enumerates the limitations of the policy and indicates that
the applicant understands what these limitations are. The professional insurance agent, therefore, can be a very helpful person to have around.

COMMUNITY HEALTH NURSES AS INSURANCE COUNSELORS

Not everyone, unfortunately, has an ethical insurance agent to help
with health insurance problems and needs, particularly in the case of
mail-order insurance where the company is in another state and has no
local agents to work with clients. One should be very careful about this
kind of insurance. Again, unfortunately, the very people who most need
insurance help because their incomes are precarious or because their
health problems are great or both, are the very people to whom mail-
order insurance with its celebrity endorsers and fancy format, is most appealing. Even though an insurance agent may be available to the client,
for a variety of reasons the agent and the client may not be able to communicate. In still other situations, the client may seek validation and advice from the community health nurse about health insurance. In all of
these circumstances the community health nurse needs to be able to help
the clients understand their insurance or know what questions to ask and
of whom to ask them. If we don't provide this help, often no one else will
either.

Attorneys are a possible source of interpretation of insurance policies'
coverage except that their fees tend to put them outside of the reach of
many clients community health nurses see. Local bar associations are increasingly offering a short legal consultation, usually half an hour, for a
set fee that is often as little as $15 or $20. During this consultation period,
questions of a limited nature can be handled, such as those surrounding
many insurance policies, or referral can be made to an appropriate
source of legal help if that is indeed warranted. Many unions, fraternal,
and professional organizations offer group legal services as part of their
membership benefits and thus also become a source of legal assistance at
low cost. Generally physicians hate filling out insurance forms, much less

talking about them, and hospital accounting office personnel are usually too busy to help very much. Most of the population not receiving public assistance has only limited contact with social workers, so this source of information is not widely utilized. Thus, who is there to talk with most clients about health insurance, other than the community nurse— at least for many of our clients?

The next logical question is: "Why can't clients learn to understand their own health insurance?" They can, of course, but often they need some help; try reading your own or someone else's health insurance policy and we feel sure that you'll see why many people need help with the terms and the style. There is little doubt that some people are refused health insurance protection for reasons they do not know or cannot understand. Many more have what they think is adequate coverage only to find that there somewhere in the fine print is a clause, which no one explained to them, that invalidates their claims. We are all admonished not to sign anything without reading it carefully first, but most people are not likely to get through the dense prose of an insurance policy without despair. Besides, like much else related to health and health care, people seldom think about health insurance coverage except when they buy a new policy, have to pay premiums, or need to collect on its benefits. By the time they have to file a claim, it's too late to do anything about changing the policy's coverage, at least for that episode of illness.

Explanation of health insurance protection and alternatives open to our clients is thus another example of our roles as health educators and client-advocates. For all of the reasons above, we feel that part of our responsibility as community nurses is to make sure that our clients understand their health insurance protection. We recommend that the type, amount, and conditions of clients' health insurance coverage be included as a regular part of every nursing history. As the joke goes, "I have health insurance. If a camel bites me on the arm I get $25, provided that I am pregnant at the time." We and our clients need to know the specifics of health insurance policies covering us.

HEALTH INSURANCE INFORMATION

Types of Health Insurance

The vast majority of the civilian noninstitutional population of the United States has one or more types of health insurance. The numbers of people with coverage increased greatly during World War II when wage freezes made fringe benefits, including health insurance, a major target for collective bargaining. The proportion of the population with some form of coverage has grown ever since.

The six types of health insurance are:

Hospital Expense Insurance. This insurance provides protection for part of the costs of hospitalization resulting from illness or injury of the insured client.

Surgical Expense Insurance. Policies of this type help pay doctor's operating fees. The amount of the benefits paid each client is generally based on a schedule that states the maximum amount for each kind of surgical procedure that the policy will pay.

Regular Medical Expense Insurance. This kind of health insurance provides benefits toward the payment of physician's fees for nonsurgical care in the hospital, outpatient department, or home. Some of these policies also cover diagnostic X-rays and laboratory costs.

Major Medical Expense Insurance. More commonly known as catastrophic illness insurance, this coverage includes almost any kind of health care prescribed by a physician. These policies help cover expenses for care in and out of the hospital, special duty nurses, X-rays, prescriptions, medical appliances, nursing home care, ambulatory psychiatric care, and a variety of other expenses. Maximum benefits go as high as $1 million or may have no limit. After the initial deductible is paid, these policies reimburse up to 75 or 80 percent of the covered expenses; the policyholder as coinsurer pays the remainder.

Loss of Income Protection. The oldest kind of health insurance coverage in the United States, this type is designed to provide wage earners with regular cash payments during the period of time that their regular income is interrupted due to illness or injury. Short-term policies have a maximum benefit period of two years. Long-term income protection policies provide benefits for more than two years.

Dental Expense Insurance. This coverage is the newest kind of health insurance and helps pay for the costs of normal dental care as well as dental care needed as a result of accidents. Its coverage includes endodontics, orthodontics, bridge and denture work, fillings, extractions, and oral examinations including X-rays and cleaning. Dental insurance is an increasingly popular target in labor negotiations concerning fringe benefits.

HEALTH INSURANCE STATISTICS

The number of civilian, noninstitutionalized people in the United States with some form of private—that is, nongovernmental—health insurance in 1975 reached almost 178 million or eight out of ten as shown in table 12.1. This figure includes 165.4 million people under sixty-five years of age or nine out of ten. Six out of ten or 12.6 million people over sixty-five years of age have private health insurance policies as supplements to Medicare (Health Insurance Institute 1977:21–22). These figures do not address the adequacy of the health insurance coverage people have, however. A congressional study released early in 1977 indicated that 101 million persons in the United States, or nearly half of the population, have no or inadequate health insurance coverage. The report estimated that 40 million persons with projected family income for 1978 of under $10,000 either have no health care insurance, are not eligible for Medicaid, or have individual health insurance policies with "generally very poor" coverage. Payment for uninsured medical expenses was also estimated to consume more than 15 percent of the total income of 5.6 million families with incomes under $10,000 (*San Francisco Chronicle-Examiner,* January 30, 1977:A–15). The consumption of an excess of 15 percent of a family's income for medical care is significant and illustrates the regressive nature of the tremendously high medical care costs in this country: 15 percent of a $10,000 income is $1500; for a family whose income is $25,000 per year, $1500 is only 6 percent. The fact that the same amount, $1500, hits lower-income families harder by taking a larger proportion of their total income than is the case with higher-income families is what is meant by regressive costs. This situation once again illustrates the need for people to understand the extent of health insurance coverage they have bought or the need to have an adequate level of health insurance protection *before* they are ill and in need of costly medical treatment. As it is, Hilbert estimates that the average citizen works one month out of every year to help pay the nation's medical care bills (1977:355).

Hospital expense, surgical expense, and regular medical expense insurance are considered to be "basic protection." Hospital expense insurance in 1975 continued to be the leading kind of coverage, with 178 million or approximately 83 percent of the population having some kind of coverage. In the same year, 169 million or approximately 80 percent had some surgical expense coverage, and 162 million or about 75 percent had some regular medical expense coverage (Health Insurance Institute 1977:24–27). Other kinds of health insurance coverage are much less prevalent.

Major medical insurance to help pay for large, unpredictable expenses was carried in 1975 by 92 million Americans or approximately 43 percent of the population. An additional 55 million people carried "catastrophic" insurance, which are high-benefit hospital insurance plans (Health Insurance Institute 1977: 27–29). A survey done in 1975 by the Health Insurance Association of America of member companies insuring over 69 million people under group major medical policies showed:

TABLE 12.1 *Number of Persons with Health Insurance Protection by Type of Coverage in the United States*

End of year	Hospital expense	Surgical expense	Regular medical expense	Major medical expense	Disability Income Short-term	Disability Income Long-term	Dental expense
1940	12,312	5,350	3,000	—	N.A.	N.A.	—
1945	32,068	12,890	4,713	—	N.A.	N.A.	—
1950	76,639	54,156	21,589	—	37,793	*	—
1955	101,400	85,681	53,038	5,241	39,513	*	—
1960	122,500	111,525	83,172	25,371	42,436	*	N.A.
1961	125,825	116,376	90,393	32,334	43,055	*	N.A.
1962	129,407	119,766	94,717	37,130	45,002	*	N.A.
1963	133,472	124,105	100,095	42,003	44,246	3,029	N.A.
1964	136,304	127,092	106,007	47,338	45,092	3,363	N.A.
1965	138,671	130,530	109,560	53,020	46,927	4,514	N.A.
1966	142,369	133,995	113,986	57,881	49,931	5,068	N.A.
1967	146,409	138,898	119,913	63,428	51,975	6,778	4,639
1968	151,947	143,625	126,233	68,171	55,636	7,836	5,939
1969	155,025	147,774	131,792	73,752	57,770	9,282	8,929
1970	158,847	151,440	138,658	77,061	58,089	10,966	12,979
1971	161,849	153,093	139,399	80,252	59,280	12,284	16,347
1972	164,098	154,687	140,873	83,668	61,548	14,538	19,089
1973	168,455	162,644	151,680	87,839	64,168	17,011	22,476
1974	173,140	166,434	158,170	91,044	65,282	17,799	33,297
1975:							
Under 65	165,357	158,518	152,157	90,125	N.A.	18,396	N.A.
65 and over	12,623	10,377	9,697	2,041	N.A.	—	N.A.
Total	177,980	168,895	161,854	92,166	62,971	18,396	35,252
1976.							
Under 65	164,027	156,852	152,867	91,278	N.A.	17,779	N.A.
65 and over	12,554	10,580	10,227	1,913	N.A.	—	N.A.
Total	176,581	167,432	163,094	93,191	60,840	17,779	43,939

*Included in "Short-term," with the possibility of some duplication of disability income coverage for these years.

N.A.—Not available.

Note: Data are revised. For 1975 and later, data include the number of persons covered in Puerto Rico and other U.S. territories and possessions. The data refer to the net total of people protected, i.e., duplication among persons protected by more than one kind of insuring organization or more than one insurance company policy providing the same type of coverage has been eliminated. The "Hospital expense," "Surgical expense," "Regular medical expense" and "Dental expense" categories represent coverage provided by insurance companies, Blue Cross-Blue Shield and medical society-approved plans, and other plans. The "Major medical expense" category represents insurance companies only. The "Disability income" category represents insurance companies, formal paid sick leave plans and coverage through employee organization.

Sources: Health Insurance Association of America, Blue Cross Association, National Association of Blue Shield Plans and the U.S. Department of Health, Education and Welfare.

Reprinted with permission from *Source Book of Health Insurance Data, 1977–78* (New York: Health Insurance Institute, 1978), p. 21.

98 percent of the persons insured had maximum benefit levels of at least $10,000;

89 percent had maximum benefits of $20,000 or more;

67 percent had $50,000 or more;

39 percent had benefit levels of $250,000 or more, or benefits of an unlimited amount;

24 percent had some maximum out-of-pocket limit beyond which they paid nothing for the remainder of the costs of their care (Health Insurance Institute 1977:38).

These data show a considerable increase since 1966 in the percentage of insureds with maximum benefits in excess of $20,000. Also since 1966 the benefit ratios, or the proportion of the total of covered expenses paid under these policies, has increased from 80 percent to over 90 percent (Health Insurance Institute 1977:38). The increases in major medical benefits are reflective of the industry's attempts to protect insureds from financial disaster as a result of incredibly high medical expenses.

Disability insurance or loss of income protection insurance was carried by 80 million people or approximately 38 percent of the population during 1975. Sixty-three million or 79 percent of the people with income protection had short-term policies whose benefits are payable for up to two years. The remainder carried long-term policies with benefits payable for longer periods such as five or ten years depending on the stipulations of the individual policy. A study of a sample of new disability income protection policies during 1971 and 1972 showed that most policies were bought by people under forty years of age. Men preferred noncancellable policies whose annual premium was around $200 and whose monthly benefits ranged from $150 to $249 (Health Insurance Institute 1977:29).

Dental insurance is the type of health insurance carried by the smallest number of persons, 35 million or 16 percent of the population. For those fortunate enough to have this kind of insurance, coverage is usually for X-rays and cleaning as well as restorations, dentures, root canals, oral surgery, and orthodontics (Health Insurance Institute 1977:34). Any of you who have had any kind of extensive dental work done, can understand why the cost of such care is making dental insurance one of the most popular fringe benefits in labor negotiations.

Medical insurance for the aged under the Social Security Act, or Medicare, became law on July 1, 1966. The program has two parts: Part A, compulsory hospitalization insurance, is financed by contributions from employees and employers; Part B, supplementary medical insurance, is financed by the monthly premiums shared equally by those who buy this coverage and by the federal government. Part B is voluntary and is designed to help pay for physicians' services and some medical services and supplies not covered by Part A. Part B covers 80 percent of medical-surgical charges after payment of the $60 deductible. In 1975, 97.4 percent of all the aged enrolled in compulsory Part A also carried elective Part B of Medicare insurance. The 1972 Social SecurityAmendments increased the eligibility for Medicare coverage under Part A to some aged persons such as aliens and some federal civil service employees and annuity holders upon their payment of a monthly premium. This premium is based on the full cost of hospital care for this high-risk age group, and in 1976 was $45 per month. These people, like those enrolled in compulsory Part A coverage, have always had the option of voluntarily participating in Part B (Health Insurance Institute 1977:40–41).

Private insurance policies held by persons sixty-five years of age and older provide supplementary benefits for Medicare. These benefits are most usually in the form of a stated dollar allowance for the person while hospitalized and may also include nursing home and private duty nursing care (Health Insurance Institute 1974:41–42). In a recently conducted study we found that a number of older people carried *more* than one private insurance policy as a supplement for Medicare. In most instances this double insurance coverage does not pay off since insurance companies will not duplicate payments already made by another insurance company under another policy. The purpose of these supplementary policies is to cover the expenses that Parts A and B of Medicare do not cover. Unless there is written assurance *in the policy itself* that its benefits will be paid regardless of other insurance payments received for the same illness or injury, the payments received will not exceed the actual expenses incurred. Many clients, particularly older ones who fear catastrophic illness most, have several supplemental policies. For example, a case history given before the Senate Special Committee on Aging's hearings on private health insurance supplements to Medicare disclosed that a 76-year-old woman had 13 different health and life insurance policies whose $9000 annual premiums totaled 68 percent of her income. Many of the policies duplicated existing coverage. This woman had "stacked" her policies, but as a result of the investigation, the unnecessary policies were cancelled *(San Francisco Chronicle,* May 17, 1978, p. 4).

Finding this kind of situation, the community health nurse should advise the clients to read their policies carefully for assurances of their payment regardless of other payments. In the absence of such statements, the supplemental policy with the broadest complementary coverage to Medicare should be kept and the rest dropped since they are a waste of premium money. If the client has a reliable insurance agent, he or she should discuss the entire insurance package with the agent and seek advice (see the previous section on insurance agents).

Almost all insurance company plans as well as insurance from other insuring organizations such as Health Maintenance Organizations (HMO) and employing agencies offer protection not only for the primary insured person—usually the worker—but also, at added cost, to dependents. Dependents generally include the primary insured's spouse and unmarried children. Of the 178 million persons with some type of health insurance protection in 1975, 73 million (41 percent) were primary insureds and 105 million (59 percent) were dependents (Health Insurance Institute 1977:35).

In 1975, premiums paid to all private insuring organizations in the United States totaled $38.8 billion or the equivalent of 3.59 percent of our total disposable personal income—that is, the amount of money we have left to spend as we please after taxes and depreciation costs. This increase is more than 0.2 of 1 percent from the 3.36 proportion of personal disposable income so spent in 1974. Of the $21.8 billion that was paid to private insurance companies in 1975, the remaining $5.1 billion went to organizations such as Blue Cross–Blue Shield, 76 percent of $16.7 billion was for group insurance premiums, and the remaining $5.1 billion went for individual and family insurance premiums (Health Insurance Institute 1977:48–52). The private insuring organizations in 1975 paid out $31.7 billion in health insurance benefits, which represented a 16 percent increase over 1974. This increase is due mainly to rising costs of medical care, expansion of benefits, and rising utilization (Health Insurance Institute 1977:43). The difference between what the private insuring organizations took in in premiums, $38.8 billion, and what they paid out in benefits, $31.7 billion, is $7.1 billion or approximately 18 percent, which was used to maintain the insurance industry during 1975.

Data are hard to get on the ratio of administrative and overhead costs and actual benefits paid to clients for federal and state-administered health insurance programs. A mid-1974 report by the state auditor general on some prepaid health plans in California that enrolled Medi-Cal clients (California's name for Title XVIII, medicaid) showed that in some instances overhead, administration, and profits were taking 52 cents of every Medi-Cal dollar. He recommended a 25 percent ceiling for such costs in all prepaid health plans that enrolled Medi-Cal patients (*San Francisco Chronicle*, June 23, 1974: Section B, 3; see also Mendelson 1974). This example is but one of the numerous criticisms that have been levelled at the cost of the red tape involved and the financial slippages possible in publicly administered programs for health care. The 25 percent ceiling proposed would be a vast improvement and would compare favorably with the 18 percent overhead and administrative costs claimed by the private health insurance industry (see above). Controlling the costs of running the system will be a major challenge for whatever scheme of National Health Insurance is enacted.

MEDICAL COSTS AND HEALTH INSURANCE

It's no news to anyone that the costs of medical care are going up. In fact they are rising faster than most other items on the Consumer Price Index. The Index lists food, apparel, housing, transportation, medical care, personal care, reading and recreation, and other goods and services, as shown in table 12.2, which compares the Consumer Price Index (CPI) for September 1977 with that of September 1976. The increase in medical care on the CPI is exceeded only by the increase in the costs of fuel and

TABLE 12.2 *Comparison of the Average National Consumer Price Index for September 1976 and September, 1977 (1967 = 100)*

Group	September 1976	September 1977	Difference
All Items	172.6	184.0	+11.4
Food	181.6	194.5	+12.9
Housing	179.5	192.7	+13.2
Shelter	181.5	194.7	+13.2
Rent	146.2	155.3	+ 9.1
Homeownership	194.4	209.1	+14.7
Fuel and utilities	185.1	205.5	+20.4
Fuel oil and coal	250.8	285.1	+34.3
Gas and electricity	192.2	218.0	+25.8
Household furnishings and operation	170.2	178.9	+ 8.7
Apparel and upkeep	150.2	156.2	+ 4.0
Men's and boys'	150.1	155.8	+ 5.7
Women's and girls'	145.0	148.6	+ 3.6
Footwear	152.3	158.1	+ 5.8
Transportation	169.5	178.5	+ 9.0
Private	168.6	177.9	+ 9.3
Public	176.9	184.1	+ 7.2
Health and recreation	165.3	176.1	+10.8
Medical care	187.9	206.3	+18.4
Personal care	162.8	172.8	+10.0
Reading and recreation	152.8	159.8	+ 7.0
Other goods and services	153.9	160.6	+ 6.7

Source: U.S. Department of Labor, Washington, D.C.

utilities, especially fuel oil and coal. In absolute terms, medical care is fourth behind fuel oil and coal, gas and electricity, and homeownership (U.S. Department of Labor). The rise in individual medical care items that go into the medical care category in the CPI since 1967 is shown in table 12.3. Hospital costs continue to be the fastest rising item with physicians' and dentists' fees second and third, respectively. The average cost of one hospital day's stay in 1970 was $81.01; in 1974, $127.70; and in 1975, $151.20, for an increase of 86.6 percent between 1970 and 1975 and 18.4 percent between 1974 and 1975. The average length of hospital stay decreased from 8.2 days in 1970 to 7.7 days in 1975. The savings that might have been brought about by this shortened length of stay were obliterated by the rising costs per day with the result that in spite of the shortened average length of stay, the cost of the average patient stay in the hospital increased by 75.3 percent from 1970 to 1975 (Health Insurance Institute 1977:5). In January 1978 in a TV documentary on medical care costs, the estimate was made that the increase was currently running *$1 million per hour!* (NBC, "Medicine in America: Life, Death, and Dollars," January 3, 1978).

Helpful though public and private insurance benefits are to those who have coverage, the American people continue to pay a considerable portion of the costs out of their own pockets. As noted, we paid a total of $38.8 billion in premiums to all private insuring organizations, which represents an increase of $13.1 billion since 1972. Total national health

TABLE 12.3 *Consumer Price Index for Medical Care Items*

Year	All Medical Care Items	Physicians' Fees	Dentists' Fees	Optometric Examinations and Eyeglasses	Semiprivate Hospital Room Rates	Prescriptions and Drugs
1950	53.7	55.2	63.9	73.5	30.3	88.5
1960	79.1	77.0	82.1	85.1	57.3	104.5
1967*	100.0	100.0	100.0	100.0	100.0	100.0
1968	106.1	105.6	105.5	103.2	113.6	100.2
1969	113.4	112.9	112.9	107.6	128.8	101.3
1970	120.6	121.4	119.4	113.5	145.4	103.6
1971	128.4	129.8	127.0	120.3	163.1	105.4
1972	132.5	133.8	132.3	124.9	173.9	105.6
1973	137.7	138.2	136.4	129.5	182.1	105.9
1974	150.5	150.9	146.8	138.6	201.5	109.6
1975	168.6	169.4	161.9	149.6	236.1	118.8

*1967 = 100.0 percent and is the baseline price against which the other prices are compared.

Source: U.S. Department of Labor, Washington, D.C.

expenditures reached $118.5 billion in fiscal 1975, which is an average of $547 per person in the United States. In 1975 health expenditures represented 8.3 percent of the country's Gross National Product (GNP) (Health Insurance Institute 1977:55; 1974:51). The NBC documentary cited 1977 expenditures at $181 billion, approaching 10 percent of our GNP ("Medicine in America: Life, Death, and Dollars," January 3, 1978). Of this $118.5 billion, $103.2 billion is classified as personal health care spending. This category excludes all expenditures for medical research, medical facilities construction, administrative costs, public health activities such as disease prevention and control, some philanthropic organizations' expenses, and the net cost of health insurance—that is, the difference between premiums collected and benefits paid. For persons under sixty-five years of age in 1975, private health insurance paid for 35 percent, government paid for 29 percent, philanthropy paid for 2 percent, and the remaining 34 percent of personal health care expenses were paid for personally and directly by the consumer. Thus direct payments out-of-pocket still account for over one-third of personal health care expenditures. When we add the almost 30 percent the government pays for personal health expenses—all of it derived from our taxes—the proportion of our income paid for these services increases. Again note, that these out-of-pocket and tax expenses borne directly by the people do not include health insurance premiums (Health Insurance Institute 1977:55–57).

COMMENT

By this time, you are no doubt asking yourselves, why carry on about all these statistics and cost information? The fact is that the tremendously rapid increase in health and medical care costs is driving our national inflation up at a rate second only to the influence of the surge in the cost of energy. Cost containment in the medical industry is rivaling quality of care as the prime concern. Obviously the two are absolutely interdependent in the medical care system, and increasingly, questions are being asked about whether we can *afford* to provide the quality of care we are *technologically capable* of providing. If access to quality medical care is a right, then can we deny everyone the maximum access to all care regardless of the cost? If the persons involved cannot pay and their insurance does not cover all the costs, then who pays? Should the public bear the financial burden for self-induced conditions such as lung cancer in heavy smokers of cigarettes or accidents occurring while driving under the influence of drugs or alcohol? In the face of increasingly limited resources for medical care, who gets the care and who doesn't?

All of these are terribly complex questions that are inextricably bound up in conflicting values and ideologies. The dollar figures only reflect these dilemmas although we are very close to being in a Catch-22 situation. People are clamoring for better and more accessible care facilities; practitioners want the latest equipment and supplies; industry and business are increasingly rumbling over the proportion of disposable personal income going into medical care and so not available for the purchase of their goods and services; third-party payers, both government and private insurance carriers, continue what seems to some of us an insane practice of "reasonable and customary fee" reimbursement, a practice that almost amounts to a blank check. As community health nurses, we must strive to understand the issues involved ourselves and then to work with our clients who at best are confused and frustrated and at worse are angry and bankrupted. This understanding is not easy; important things rarely are.

MEDICAL INFORMATION BUREAU

The Medical Information Bureau (MIB) is a clearinghouse and data storage and retrieval facility for medical and nonmedical underwriting information for its 700 member insurance companies located in the United States and Canada. MIB is an unincorporated, nonprofit trade association. Each of its member insurance companies must sign a pledge to abide by the MIB's rules. All of its members qualify as life insurance companies under the Internal Revenue Code of the United States. MIB participant companies must report to MIB all significant personal medical and nonmedical information they obtain on preliminary and completed formal applications for insurance. The applicants' data are coded and filed and then released by MIB to member companies on request when they are considering an application for insurance by a particular person (Swarts 1977:48–49). Thus MIB can be likened to a nationwide credit organization for insurance companies that compiles and shares information with other member companies to whom the person in question may apply for insurance. Persons judged to be substandard risks can be identified through information supplied from the MIB, and the member company can decide whether to issue a policy to the applicant. The purpose of the MIB is to protect the insurance industry—and ultimately all who are insured—from the costs that substandard risk persons are more likely than other people to incur.

Much seems to have happened to the MIB since I first wrote about it several years ago. At that time the now-retired Executive Director J.C. Wilberding was very helpful in supplying information as a basis for the material contained in the first edition of *Community Health Nursing*. In preparing this revision, I again wrote to the MIB asking for information, and William B. Swarts, III, Associate General Counsel, provided the information upon which much of this update draws. We would not go so far as to say the MIB is totally open to consumer scrutiny, but the implementation of the Fair Credit Reporting Act, P.L. 91–508 passed in October of 1970, has had its effect on MIB as it has on so many other organizations that gathered and used information about people without their prior knowledge and consent.

MIB became involved in the legislative process after the passage of the Fair Credit Reporting Act (FCRA) in 1970. As a result of hearings for the purpose of amending FCRA chaired by Senator William Proxmire in 1973, the MIB was criticized for three areas of its operation. These areas and the MIB's reported actions to meet them are described below.

First, applicants were not notified that information about them might be sent to MIB. In response, MIB reports that it has developed a "Pre-Notice Program" that involves an amendment of its General Rules to require that member companies provide each applicant with "pre-notice" information before completion of the application for insurance so that he or she knows: (a) of MIB's existence and operations; (b) of the possibility of a report being made to MIB; and (c) of the availability of disclosure and disputed accuracy procedures (Swarts 1977:50). Under this rule, no member company can give information to MIB or receive reports from MIB unless this "pre-notice" has been given to an applicant. Under the provisions of FCRA, consumers may request their records from an organization like MIB, review the reports and then if they feel that the information is inaccurate, begin "disputed accuracy proceedings" to correct the misinformation. MIB has had more than 18,000 disclosure requests since 1974. Of the 9,015 filed in 1976, 150 (less than 2 percent) are reported to have developed into disputed accuracy proceedings. As a result of these proceedings, 61 records were changed (Swarts 1977:50). Under the provisions of FCRA, any time people are denied credit or insurance on the basis of a report from an organization such as MIB, they must be told the reason and given the name and address of the organization. Consumers may then write the organization, in this case MIB, to request a copy of their record in a form they can understand rather than in company code. If they feel that the information is incorrect, incomplete, or obsolete, they may notify the consumer reporting agency of this fact. The organization must then reinvestigate the case and make whatever changes in its records warranted by the data revealed by the reinvestigation (Fair Credit Reporting Act, P.L. 91–508).

Second, sensitive nonmedical information such as "sexual deviation" and "social maladjustment" were included in the MIB records. Criticism has resulted in code changes and eliminations. Specifically "sexual deviation" and "social maladjustment" codes have been removed from the

MIB codes and eliminated from records in which they already were included. Other nonmedical codes such as "insurance hazard" and "age" have also been deleted.

Third, the rule enforcement mechanisms carried out by MIB on its member companies were inadequate. In response to this criticism, MIB expanded its Company Visit Program to enable members of the visiting team to do a site visit and audit on each insurance company at least once every two years. The typical company visit is described as including a review of compliance with MIB's security agreements and an audit of twenty carefully selected records. These records are chosen by the MIB visiting team and are reviewed against a set of specific criteria derived from MIB rules such as the giving of "pre-notice" to the insured that information given on the application and in subsequent documents will be sent to the MIB and the maintenance of security for the records (Swarts 1977:50–51).

As a result of MIB's appearance before the President's Privacy Protection Study Commission in 1976, the MIB's rules regarding consumer privacy and the confidentiality of information for both MIB and its member insurance companies have been tightened. Annual self-audits by member companies must be conducted and these reports sent to MIB. These self-audit data are used by MIB's on-site review teams and the Company Visiting Program has been stepped up to enable more field audits to be done. Careful monitoring of information coming from member companies is also done to identify companies that consistently report incomplete or inaccurate information. Greater attention is also being given to the security of MIB's data base and communication systems that have been automated. The MIB computer bank contains some 11 million individual records and receives about 9,000 new reports and 18,000 requests for checking information against the central file each day. About 500 member companies have computer terminals located in their offices that provide them with direct access to the MIB's computer files. Finally, MIB has further modified its nonmedical coding to separate pertinent nonmedical underwriting information from subjective lifestyle information contained in the same consumer report (Swarts 1977:51–52). These facts remind us that health insurance is big business.

How much clout does the MIB have over its member insurance companies? The short answer is plenty. Like any other financial industry that must rely on people's past history as a basis for deciding how much capital to risk on the person, the insurance industry must have some kind of central clearinghouse for information on consumers. This information is supplied by its member companies on the persons with whom these companies deal. This information is used to determine who are standard and who are substandard risks for insurance. Banks and other financial credit organizations have a similar system that results in a person's credit rating. MIB can be thought of as an organization that provides a person's insurability rating to insurance companies, as already noted. Swarts reports that MIB's activities are great money savers for member insurance companies. He reports that one company estimated that it saved $45 for every $1.00 it spent on MIB services (1977:52). We can assume that these savings to the insurance company resulted from decisions not to insure people whose MIB file information indicated that they were high risks and therefore could be expected to have many claims. Whatever the reason, such a savings ratio is very difficult to dispute and indicates a major reason for insurance company membership in MIB. In terms of the effectiveness of MIB's rules on the functioning of its member companies, the vice president of a large Midwestern insurance firm said in an interview that because the ultimate penalty for not abiding by the MIB rules is suspension from membership and because insurers simply cannot function effectively or efficiently without MIB membership, MIB's sanctions are remarkably effective.

The point of including this information about the Medical Information Bureau is to alert you to the fact of its existence and functions both for yourselves as potential insurance buyers and for work with clients. Under the provisions of the Fair Credit Reporting Act, a notification of the insurance company's intent to sent the information given them in the application process for insurance to the MIB and request information about the applicants from MIB must be given to applicants and their "informed consent" must be obtained before the process can be initiated. If you or one of your clients is turned down on the basis of the information obtained from MIB, the insurance company must tell you or the client this. Then you can follow or advise your client to follow the disclosure and disputed accuracy procedures already discussed. Have no doubts, the MIB's purpose is to protect the insurance industry by weeding out applicants who are judged to be substandard risks. By so doing the MIB helps to control the costs of all of our insurance premiums. However, that still leaves unanswered the question about what is to be done to protect substandard risk people, from the point of view of insurability, from the devastating costs of medical care that they are more likely than the rest of us standard risks to incur and for which they have no insurance coverage. Many of us are seeking the answer to this question through the promotion of a National Health Service, which is discussed later in this chapter. In the meantime, if you have questions for the Medical Information Bureau, you can contact them at their home office at 34 Mason Street, Greenwich, Connecticut 06930, telephone (203) 661-8344. MIB has been very cooperative in sending me information about the MIB; presumably, they will treat you the same way.

HEALTH INSURANCE TERMS

This section on health insurance terms is included to enable community nurses to help our clients better understand their health insurance protection. It also contains some examples of how we may be called upon to use the information in practice. The list is representative rather than exhaustive and includes terms that in my own experience and in investigation with other nurses I have found are not generally understood. These are important terms both for us and for our clients. The definitions are derived from many sources, the major ones being the Health Insurance Institute's 1977 *Source Book of Health Insurance Data* and *Introduce Yourself to Health Insurance* (1971), a programmed text for insurance agents; other sources are noted in the text. The terms are listed alphabetically for easy reference later.

Accumulation. Some policies provide for an increase in the amount of benefits provided as a reward for continuous renewal of the policy by the insured. In counseling clients who may wish to change their policies or companies, we should be alert for this kind of clause in the policy the client already has. The added benefits that accumulation may provide could make changing policies a costly transaction.

Adjustable Premium. This term refers to a policy payment whose amount the insurance company may modify under certain circumstances, such as high risk, that are specified in the policy. Clients' policies should be searched for these kinds of clauses, and the clients should be sure they understand what such clauses mean.

Aggregate Indemnity or Amount. Some policies specify the maximum dollar amount that can be collected either for any disability, a period of disability, or from the policy in total. For example, the aggregate indemnity for a major medical policy may be $50,000, which means that the insurance company will pay up to that amount but no more. When the aggregate limit is reached, the policy expires and protection ceases. A history of large claims reduces the client's insurability with any private insurance company.

Aggregate limits are used in certain noncancellable or guaranteed renewable policies and should be discussed with the agent. The amount of the aggregate indemnity contained in the policy should be evaluated against the probable costs of services covered by the policy during the period that the client plans to pay for it. These data may make the consideration of other alternatives to health insurance worthwhile.

Assigned Risk. This term refers to the means by which insurance companies offer insurance coverage to "bad risks"—that is persons who either because of their history or occupation are more likely to become ill or suffer injury than are other people. The most common kinds of insurance programs to have assigned risk requirements are workmen's compensation and automobile insurance. In the case of workmen's compensation, state laws require that each insurance company that writes workmen's compensation insurance in the state must take on its share of the "bad risks." The purpose of this assigned risk program is to provide insurance coverage for those who could not otherwise get it and at the same time distribute these so-called "bad risks" equitably among the insurance companies. Assigned risk programs are rare in the private health insurance arena, with the result that some people cannot obtain any kind of private health insurance coverage if they are labeled "bad risks." Examples may include people diagnosed as accident prone or those known to have been treated for alcoholism. About the only alternatives for these people are to save sufficient money to cover any possible health care bills or to become members of a group insurance plan through a place of employment, the government, or a prepaid health plan such as a health maintenance organization. Even these alternatives may not prove feasible for very high-risk persons to obtain health insurance protection.

Assignment. Assignment refers to the transfer of benefits from the insured person to some third party. Since insured persons must sign transfers, efforts must be made to be sure that they understand that they are signing away the benefits of their insurance to someone else. Some nursing homes and other long-term care facilities require that persons moving in assign their life insurance benefits to the facility. Clients should understand that by doing so the facility rather than themselves or their families will receive any forthcoming benefits.

Blanket Medical Expense. Under this provision in loss of income protection policies, the insured is entitled to collect benefits up to the maximum established in the policy for all types of medical expenses—whether the insured is hospitalized or not. To the extent that this coverage can be used for outpatient services, clients will no longer be required to pay for these services out-of-pocket nor be unnecessarily hospitalized for services that could be given on an ambulatory basis.

Cancellation. Cancellation occurs when the insurance company unilaterally terminates a client's insurance coverage regardless of the reason. With any record of cancellation, the client may have extreme difficulty in getting insurance coverage again. Therefore, if clients are in danger of having their insurance canceled—regardless of the reason—they need to know of the likelihood of subsequent problems in obtaining insurance. They may then decide to protest, to terminate the coverage themselves, or to wait it out.

Claim. This term refers to a demand the insured person makes to the insurance company for payment of benefits for losses or disabilities that are covered by the provisions of the insurance policy. When clients file claims, many companies require that they complete forms that ask for virtually the same information in terms of medical history questions as did the original application form for the insurance. Clients should be very careful to be sure to give the same information on their claim forms as they did on their original application. Most companies now include a photostatic copy of the completed application form as a part of the policy for future reference. Obviously the application should have been both complete and accurate in the first place.

Discrepancies between original and claim applications can cause insurance companies to raise questions about the client's misrepresenting original statements. Suspicion of misrepresentation is sufficient grounds for the insurance company to declare the client's claims invalid and to refuse to pay benefits. Here is another instance where clients must be fully informed about their health histories. Our failure to help clients really understand their health histories can lead to their being accused of misrepresentation when, through ignorance, they fill out applications incorrectly. As will be shown later, part of the insurance application the client signs often contains a release of information from all hospitals and physicians who have treated the client; this information is kept in a central data bank at the Medical Information Bureau and made available to other insurance companies requesting information on applicants before they are insured. Discrepancies between client's applications, claim forms, and histories from medical care sources are often assumed to be misrepresentations on the part of the client. These kinds of data in clients' files can make impossible their obtaining subsequent insurance coverage from other companies and may cause cancellation of what they now have. This potential for depriving a client of insurance coverage suggests that community nurses must contribute to clients' knowledge about their health as well as give direct assistance as needed with the completion of both application and claim forms. Clients should retain a photocopy of all forms they send to insurance companies. These documents should be kept with the policy for easy reference. Again, if the policy does not contain a copy of the original application form, a copy should be requested *before* it is needed for reference in filing a claim.

Clients should also be advised that the following are warning signals for insurance companies.

1. Claims filed very soon after the policy goes into force are often considered to be for preexisting conditions, except for claims resulting from accidents.
2. Discrepancies between statements on applications and claim forms are considered to be misrepresentations.
3. Claims not filed promptly are questioned.
4. Presence of indefinite diagnoses, such as "back injuries" or "mental disorders," are more likely to cause inquiries than are more specific diagnoses.
5. Claims for services in excess of the average durations listed in insurer's experience tables are checked.
6. Use of unapproved practitioners—that is, those not specifically stated in the policy—can result in denial of claim.
7. Infrequent medical treatment such as only once or twice a month while collecting disability can cause inquiry into the state of the client's disability (Gregg 1973:101–02).

To avoid delays or denials of benefits, clients should be counseled to seek help in filing a claim.

Coinsurance.   In this policy provision, also known as percentage participation, the insurance company and the insured person share in a specified ratio all the costs of covered medical expenses after the deductible is paid by the insured person. In most major medical policies, both private and governmental, the ratio of coinsurance is generally 70 to 80 percent of the specified expenses borne by the insurance company and the remaining 20 to 30 percent is paid by the insured. Clients should examine their health insurance policies so that they know what percentage of any bill for covered services they will be expected to pay.

Coordination of Benefits.   In instances where two or more insurance policies cover the same insured, the companies collaborate for the coordination of benefits. For example, in a client family both spouses work and are covered by the group policies at each one's place of employment as are their dependents. When one spouse files a claim, the two companies work together to coordinate the amount of payments. The first step is to determine which policy constitutes primary coverage. If the claimant is the wife then her policy will usually be considered the primary one and the claim is paid according to its provisions. The second company—that is, the company under whose policy the husband is insured and which also covers the wife—will pick up the portion of the claim payments not covered by the primary policy, under the conditions of that policy. In some cases payments may be shared by both companies up to the maximum of the broadest coverage of the two policies. Again, recall that unless written in the policy itself is a statement that the policy will pay allowable claims to the full extent regardless of other insurance payments for the same claim, we must assume that this coordination of payments will ensue. Unless this specific assurance is given, claim payments will not exceed the actual amount of the claim.

Deductible.   In most cases, the insured person must pay part of covered hospital and medical expenses before the benefits of the health insurance policy begin to be paid by the company. Deductibles are most common in major medical insurance plans. As with coinsurance, clients should understand the amount of deductible they must pay before their policy's benefits begin. This amount is clearly stated somewhere in the policy.

Both coinsurance and deductibles serve a gatekeeper function to prevent over- or indiscriminate use of health care services by policyholders. Since insured clients must pay all of the costs up to a given amount (deductible) and a stated percentage of all expenses beyond that amount (coinsurance) for covered services, the rationale is that they will not seek unnecessary or frivolous services since such use will increase their out-of-pocket expenses for health care services. Of the total amount of money paid in 1966 for medical care from all sources including both public and private health insurance payments, out-of-pocket expenses for health care services amounted to 51 percent; the share of the total health care expenses not covered by any kind of insurance and thus paid directly by clients in 1975 was 34 percent (Health Insurance Institute 1977:56). This 34 percent represents not only deductible and coinsurance costs but also those health care service costs that were not covered by policies held by persons and group insureds as well as those costs for health care services borne by the roughly 10 percent of the population that has no insurance.

Clearly, many people are deterred from using services when they must bear its entire cost or that part determined by deductible and coinsurance provisions. Without such financial barriers to early care, health care emphasizing prevention and early detection might reduce the number and amount of subsequent claims for severe illness and complications. This possibility would not only save money insurance companies otherwise pay in claims but also reduce interference with a client's abilities to function and lower the overall costs of health care services.

Elimination Period.   Also called the waiting period, this term refers to the

time between the beginning of an insured person's disability and the start
of payment of the policy's benefits. The longer the elimination period, the
lower generally are the premiums for the policy. Thus policies that have
immediate coverage are more expensive than policies whose benefits
begin at a later time. First-day sickness coverage, unless hospitalization is
involved, is generally not written, especially where the person has sick
leave with pay from a place of employment. The usual optimal coverage
is payment for the first day after an accident and for the seventh day of
sickness not involving hospitalization. Clients need to weigh the advantages of having insurance protection that begins on the first day of illness
against the higher premiums they would have to pay. Then they can
decide on the elimination period they want.

Exclusions.   These are the kinds of hazards, conditions, and health care
services for which a health insurance policy does *not* provide benefit payments. These exclusions are listed in the policy and should be examined
carefully to see what the policy does not cover. Dental, maternity, and
psychiatric services are among the most common exclusions, although for
higher premiums these services are increasingly available. Group plans
are also adding broader coverage in these areas for their members. Knowing what kinds of illness and accidents are prevalent in clients' occupations, age, sex, ethnic, or other group can serve as a basis for helping them
sort out which of the most commonly needed services are and are not included in the list of conditions for which the policy will pay benefits. Obviously, study of the exclusions is vital to making decisions about the adequacy of various kinds of health insurance coverage.

Experience Rating.   Premiums are set for a particular group's risks wholly
or partially on the basis of the insurance company's past losses and expenses incurred in the settlement of claims and other expenses involving
members of this group. For example, premiums for persons who engage
in certain hazardous kinds of activities such as motorcycle racing or flying
are relatively high because the rate of injuries resultant from these activities is greater than for people who engage in less hazardous ones. Experience rating is one of the reasons why premium costs differ among individual clients for much the same basic kind of health insurance protection.

Grace Period.   For a specified period of time after a premium payment is
due, the premium can be paid without penalty and the policy's protection
remains in force. The grace period protects clients from having their
health insurance protection canceled if the mails are slow or should they
forget to pay the premium, be away, or otherwise be unable to do so.
Clients should be cautioned about misusing the grace period. Marking

the premium's due-date on the calendar so it's not forgotten is one way; another is to investigate the possibility of having the premium, especially if it's due monthly, drawn directly from the client's bank account and paid to the company. Many insurance companies have forms that when filled out and signed by the insured, permit the bank to make premium payments automatically. Many business firms deduct their employee's health insurance premiums automatically from their paychecks. All of these alternatives reduce the possibility of forgetting to pay an insurance premium. Should clients forget, they should contact their health insurance agent as early in the grace period as possible and make necessary arrangements.

Group Insurance.   These are policies that cover a specified minimum number of people who have something in common, such as the same employer, profession, or labor union. Group policy underwriting sets premium rates on the basis of the characteristics of the group and so evidence of insurability is not required from each individual member as long as the group seeking insurance coverage meets the insurance company's minimum group size. Group premiums are generally lower than individual rates for comparable coverage. Group policies are tailored to the group's needs. If the group is large enough and well enough organized, it can bring pressure on the insurer to make changes in benefits and procedures. For example, if Medicare subscribers were sufficiently organized they could demand that Blue Cross and other fiscal intermediaries present them with itemized bills that enumerate precisely what the bill covers and how much each item costs. Some hospitals and insurance companies do not want people to know this information, or at least so it appears. Another area in which group pressure needs to be brought is that of decreasing the time lapse between filing for reimbursement under Medicare and the time at which the subscriber gets that reimbursement.

Some group policies, where the group is well organized and vocal, often have very broad coverage and excellent and prompt service when claims are filed. Group insurance is noncancelable as long as the persons stay in the group and pay their share of the premiums; the insurance company cannot cancel a group member's policy no matter how much the person has to use it. Entire group policies can and are canceled by the company at the renewal period if claim experience has been very bad and the group refuses to pay increased premiums to cover these incurred expenses. Again, cancellation can only occur at renewal time and not in the interval between. Many group policies have a conversion right clause that enables members leaving the group to convert their group coverage to individual guaranteed renewable coverage through the same company without having to supply proof of insurability through a physical examination. This provision is an advantage for the person who might not be able to qualify for individual coverage any other way. Like all private health insurance, group insurance rarely covers all expenses or offers protection against all conditions. Group coverage does not duplicate or replace coverage offered under workmen's compensation. If clients have the option for either individual or group health insurance coverage, the group plan is generally more to their advantage.

Guaranteed Renewable.   This provision gives the insured the right to keep the policy in force by prompt payment of premiums up to a specific age, generally sixty-five, or for life, depending on the period stated in the policy. For the duration of the policy, the insurance company has no right to unilaterally make any changes in the individual policy's provisions. The insurance company may increase the premiums for all such policyholders as a class should it wish to. Clients should be advised to seek this kind of policy although it often carries a somewhat higher premium; it may more than pay for itself in the long run. Care should be taken to note any limiting clauses such as aggregate indemnity, discussed earlier.

Health Maintenance Organization (HMO).   These organizations provide a wide range of comprehensive health care services for a specified group of enrollees for a fixed, periodic, and usually prepaid payment. HMOs have a variety of sponsors—governments, medical schools, private organizations, labor unions, consumer groups, and insurance companies. Emphasis is placed on preventive care, early detection and treatment of dysfunctions, and ambulatory care. HMOs are one of the leading proposals for the organization of National Health Insurance. The Kaiser-Permanente Plan is suggested as a model.

Indemnity.   This term refers to the benefits paid by an insurance company to a policyholder for all or part of losses insured under the policy. The insured is indemnified or protected against the losses covered in the conditions of the policy. Double indemnity is a policy provision usually associated with death that doubles designated benefits if death results from certan kinds of accidents. Standard life insurance policies are incontestable for any reason after they have been in force for two years so that even suicide or misrepresentation of medical information does not invalidate the double indemnity clause. If a misrepresentation of age has occurred, benefits will be adjusted to the appropriate age.

Limited Policies.   These policies cover only certain specified diseases or accidents. In buying these policies, clients should be careful that they know specifically what the policy covers and that this coverage is adequate to their needs.

Mail-Order Insurance.   Many insurance companies offer insurance protection by mail, and many people complete these applications and send in their premiums. In some instances all may be well and good; however, as noted earlier, many people cannot understand many of the insurance terms contained in the advertisements for these policies and fail to understand the significance of some of the questions on the application. For example, if the client fails to complete the health history section of the application adequately, the insurance company can refuse to pay subsequent claims based on the lack of this information in the policy application. Although some people do not put down their complete health histories in hopes that their past experiences will not be found out and they will have insurance coverage should they become ill, the previous section on the Medical Information Bureau should demolish this hope. Other people do not know enough about their health histories to complete accurately and adequately health insurance applications—another reason for health professionals to be sure clients know and understand exactly what their health conditions are. In either case the insurance company can refuse to pay claims for illness on the basis of inaccurate or fraudulent applications. Clients are probably better off dealing face-to-face with an insurance agent rather than trying to complete their own application for a mail-order policy.

Many mail-order insurance companies seek "third-party endorsement" in which the insurance company persuades an organization such as a fraternal order or labor union to endorse a policy it will offer the organization's members. Such an arrangement may be an opportunity for organization members to obtain health insurance at a lower rate; often this isn't the case and insurance coverage is not forthcoming. Enough problems occurred with mail-order insurance that the Unauthorized Insurers Service of Process Act was passed. This act subjects all mail-order insurance companies to the authority of the insurance commissioner in every state where they solicit for policy applications. If fraudulent practices occur, these mail-order companies can be taken into the state's courts by the insurance commissioner (Gregg 1973:19–34).

Should you be asked about the value of mail-order insurance policies by clients or indeed receive solicitations, yourself, you would be wise to inquire from the state insurance commissioner about the reputation of the mail-order insurance company; to check with the organization, if one is present, that is endorsing the proposed policies for its members; to ask a local insurance agent about the proposed policy. Anyone who decides to file an application for mail-order insurance should be sure that all of the terms used are understood and all of the information asked for is given.

Recently an advertisement for hospital confinement indemnity coverage endorsed by a national celebrity appeared in our Sunday newspaper. It promised that no one could be turned down and that the policy once issued was noncancelable. It listed several alternate plans with different benefits and premiums. The company's home office was listed as being in another state, so I called our State Division of Insurance—in your state it may be called the Commissioner's office—to ask about the reliability of the company and the provisions of the policy. The man with whom I talked indicated that the company was licensed in our state and so met the minimum standards under our laws. He would not advise me pro or con on the specific policy but suggested that I contact a local insurance agent or two and compare relative benefits and premium costs before making a decision about buying the policy. He also indicated that because there was no agent or middle person in mail-order insurance, the cost of premiums might be much lower than would be the case where an agent was involved. He suggested, however, that the lower rate might be a false savings when it came time to file a claim (see the section on insurance agents). I also contacted the Better Business Bureau, which could not be of much help because it had not received any comments, pro or con, on the company or the policy in question.

We believe that comparison shopping is as valid when buying insurance as it is when buying an automobile or any other major purchase. Insurance companies are beginning to suggest, as part of their own television and other media advertising, that people compare benefits and premiums before they buy insurance. Comparative shopping should be done especially with mail-order insurance. In such cases, it is particularly critical since often no one in the potential buyer's area can give advice on specific mail-order policies until they have been used by someone who can report on application, information-gathering, and claim-filing procedures. If you or your clients are already insured by the time negative reports begin to reach the Better Business Bureau, then this information will be too late.

Never is skepticism more warranted than when one is considering insurance advertising in general. We must ask ourselves, how, logically, can the companies promise so much to so many for so low a premium? We can reasonably assume that for policies where the advertisement assures us "no one will be turned down," many high-risk people who cannot obtain health or life insurance coverage elsewhere will subscribe and therefore the claim rate will be higher. Sooner or later, either premium raises or more stringent criteria for persons who are substandard risks or both will be necessary. Knowing, as we do, that at least 18 percent of all monies taken in by insurance companies will be used for running the company, how can they promise, as some do, to return all of the money one has paid in if no claims are filed? Such a promise would seem to mean that the company is assured of making at least 18 percent interest on its investments to break even. My own doubts about the realities of this situation lead us to caution buyers to beware.

Mutual Company. This type of insurance company is owned and controlled by policyholders. Management of the mutual company is in the hands of a board of directors or trustees chosen by the policyowners. Blue Cross and Mutual of Omaha are examples of mutual companies. Blue Cross is controlled by hospitals and doctors and was founded to help them collect their bills. Since Blue Cross is run by the hospitals—it was founded by the American Hospital Association in the early 1930s—we can assume that Blue Cross' primary interest is in serving the hospitals' interests rather than the subscribers' (Michelfelder 1960:59–72). This fact is still true and nursing homes have been added to hospitals as primary loyalties for Blue Cross, especially since it became fiscal intermediary for the government's Medicare and Medicaid programs. Because of the relatively free hand that the government has given Blue Cross, it has few outside regulations imposed on it, and its self-regulation costs the taxpayers a great deal of money (Mendelson 1974).

Applications for insurance from many mutual insurance companies contain proxy clauses. In signing the applications, clients also sign a proxy statement and so give up their right to vote for officers. Mutual companies are really nonprofit cooperatives, but signing the proxy deprives the policyowner of a voice in the running of the company (Gregg 1973:70–71). Many people do not realize this fact; others do not care. The point is that such mutual companies as Blue Cross and Blue Shield, commonly called the Blues, are extremely powerful in the total health insurance business because of the numbers of persons and groups they insure and because of their position as fiscal intermediaries for Title XVIII and XIX of the 1965 Social Security Amendments, Medicare and Medicaid. As such, they are in a prime position to exert considerable influence on National Health Insurance. As mutual companies, the Blues are potentially more open to consumer control than are other companies or the federal government's bureaucracies. Therefore, we and our clients must be aware that signing away our legal voice as policyholders in such mutual companies as the Blues to unknown proxies is the loss of one more potential force in bringing about change in the health care delivery system. Proxies may be revoked at any time and voted in person or assigned to another who would vote in line with our preferences.

National Association of Insurance Commissioners. This organization was founded in 1871 and is composed of all state insurance commissioners, directors, and superintendents. Its major purpose is to propose and encourage state legislatures to pass uniform procedures for insurance regulation. Although it has no legal authority, the organization's existence and regulatory effect on the insurance industry has been a major factor in the insurance industry's contention that federal regulatory legislation is not necessary. The late 1970s will see more concern with consumer protection and an increased emphasis on public involvement in the activities of regulating bodies such as this one.

Noncancelable. See *Guaranteed Renewable* and *Aggregate Indemnity.*

Optional Renewable Policies. These are policies that may be renewed at the option of the insurance company. Clients should be aware that the final decision to renew—that is, continue—the client's insurance protection is the company's.

Preexisting Condition. This term refers to a physical condition, injury, or sickness the person had prior to the issuance of a health insurance policy. Some preexisting conditions may be covered at additional premium costs; others may be subject to rider or exclusion from reimbursement under the policy. For example, some policies that cover expenses associated with childbirth indicate that the client cannot claim benefits for maternity services until the policy has been in force for ten months. This clause means that the policy will only cover expenses incurred for a pregnancy that began after the policy was in force. Some major companies are now writing coverage for preexisting conditions that applies after the policy has been in effect for a period of time, usually six months. Many of these policies are for limited benefits such as supplemental to Medicare. We must be sure to counsel our clients to complete the medical portions of health insurance applications accurately and completely since the company will check with sources of medical information such as the Medical Information Bureau and will find out about clients' preexisting conditions especially if they have been treated for such conditions under the coverage of another insurance policy.

Most applications for health insurance contain a medical authorization statement the applicant must sign; it permits hospitals and doctors whom the client has seen within a given period of time to release information about the client's health history contained in their records. Many individual health insurance application procedures also require a physical examination as proof of insurability. At this time conditions might be found that the insurance policy may not cover since they already existed at the time the policy was issued.

Prepaid Group Insurance Plan. These plans offer specified handling of health care services rather than reimbursement. Payment, from either the insured persons or their employers, is made at regular intervals in advance of need to use the service. The first such plan was developed in 1929 among Dallas school teachers. The Kaiser Plan is another example and is the model for health maintenance organizations. Many plans involve their own facilities and personnel in the delivery of services; others contract for the services to be performed for their subscribers.

Probationary Period. This period is the number of days specified in the policy that must elapse between issuance of the policy and the time when coverage of sickness begins. It is also called the "incubation period" and is designed to preclude claims for sickness contracted prior to the time the policy went into force. Since this period varies with different policies and companies, clients should be sure to note how long it is and that it is useless to file a claim for sickness that developed during the probationary period.

Prorating. This practice reduces the amount of benefits payable to the insured persons for various reasons: because they have changed to more hazardous occupations since a particular insurance policy was issued or because the benefits paid to them by all of the insurance policies they carry exceed expenses for the present claim or exceed their average income. This process obviates the advantage for clients of carrying duplicate policies since total benefits will not exceed expenses. We have found that older people tend to carry more than one private policy as a supplement to their Medicare coverage. Unless there is written proof from the companies that all policies will pay regardless of the total amount of benefits the client receives, we should advise our clients that they are wasting their money paying premiums on duplicate policies. As noted frequently in this section, the communications network among the insurance companies is excellent and electronic; trying to beat it rarely pays off.

Recurring Disability Clause. This clause is a provision in the policy that states the period of time during which the recurrence of a condition is considered a continuation of a prior period of disability or hospitalization. Note should be taken of this clause since deductible and coinsurance payments by the insured are often based on each *new* episode of illness. Thus if the condition recurs within the time stated in this clause, the client does not have to treat it as a new episode and therefore may not have to pay the second round of deductible or coinsurance costs. Awareness of the length of time stipulated in the recurring disability clause provides the community nurse with another incentive to persuade clients not to put off seeking additional treatment when the fact first becomes apparent that convalescence is not progressing well or additional services are needed. However, some policies may limit the benefits for a single episode of illness and if these have already run out, the best approach may be to wait out the specified time before the benefits can be received. Then clients can again seek care with a fresh extent of coverage; the community nurse's role here would be to marshal resources as much as possible to wait out the necessary time.

Rider. Riders legally modify the protection offered by a policy. They may expand or decrease its benefits or add or exclude certain conditions of the policy's coverage. Preexisting conditions are subject to a rider that is usually exclusionary. Riders are specifically stated in the policy. Filing claims for conditions that are "ridered out" is useless. Often clients are not aware of these rider clauses and cannot understand why their insurance does not cover everything. Again the community nurse may be in the best position to explain the meaning of riders to clients as well as to help them find other kinds of insurance coverage where their conditions will be covered even if premiums are prorated higher. See *Group Insurance.*

Risk. Risk is a basic concept that underlies the whole insurance business. Technically it means the probability or degree of chance that a given event will occur—the odds. In epidemiology we are concerned with defining and studying the population at risk—that is, those for whom the probability of a given event is higher than the rest of the population. The risk of cancer of the lung is higher for smokers than nonsmokers, and their premiums may be prorated accordingly. Sophisticated tools have been developed to aid the insurance industry in calculating various risks.

Schedule of Allowable Charges. Insurance companies set up their own schedules of allowable charges for procedures, lengths of hospital stay, approximate costs of equipment and personnel, and other predictable expenses. They base the amount they will pay for conditions and procedures on these calculations. Generally the amount is 80 percent of the estimated cost less the deductible and coinsurance portions paid by the insured. This approach seems perfectly reasonable assuming that the schedule is adjusted periodically to take cost increases into account. The problem comes when the insured gets the bill and finds that the physician, surgeon, or anesthesiologist has charged a "reasonable and customary fee" that exceeds the amount the insurance company has on its schedule of allowable charges. If the client has good major medical supplemental coverage, these excess fees may be covered up to the limits of the provisions of the supplemental policy. Often superspecialists charge super fees that can be two or three times those charged by other physicians and surgeons and that far exceed any kind of insurance coverage most of us can afford. The excess of fees over and above what any or all of the client's insurance policies will pay become an out-of-pocket expense. The practice of "reasonable and customary fees" is one factor in the excessive and rapidly rising cost of medical care in this country and is closely guarded by the medical profession that believes that the practice of charging "reasonable and customary fees" is its prerogative. Two of the many ways that have been suggested to bring about cost-containment in the medical care industry is for the federal government to introduce specific reimbursement schedules. One is to set a national reimbursement schedule based on a fixed rate per stay per diagnosis. The second is establishment and mandatory acceptance of reimbursement fees for provider services that will be payment in full (Berman 1977:56). While these fees for both providers and institutions could be based on geographic differences and other variables, once set for an area, they would be the maximum that could be charged to either third-party payers or consumers as out-of-pocket expenses.

In the absence of such rational systemwide solutions to inflationary and unreasonable fees, we must find ways to deal with the reasonable and customary fee business on an individual basis. We must advise and encourage our clients to be blunt about asking fees *beforehand* so that they are not dumbfounded when the bill arrives. Another question that needs to be asked is what relationship the fee quoted has to the local standard for insurance reimbursement. Many physicians may not be able to answer this question but its asking would get us all thinking more clearly about costs. The answers clients get to these kinds of questions can make them more aware of the personal dollar drain they are about to incur and help them in making decisions about limiting the physician's activities they are willing to pay for. Finally, consumers must demand itemized bills so that they can see in detail what each service, lab test, office or hospital visit, medication, and piece of equipment they have been charged for actually costs. The malpractice scare in many areas has given rise to the practice of "defensive medicine," which results in unnecessary tests and consultations being ordered, not because the client needs them, but rather to protect the provider. Consumers and providers *must* become acutely aware of the cost of every item they request or prescribe if the inflationary spiral of medical care expenditures under the present system in the United States is ever to be understood, much less contained.

Senior Citizen Policies. These policies for persons sixty-five and over are usually supplementary to Medicare benefits. In working with older clients whose fears about devastating medical expenses are both considerable and realistic, we should advise that they seek adequate but not unnecessary or "stacked" supplemental coverage.

Substandard Health Insurance.   Individual policies may be issued to persons whose health status prevents them from meeting the requirements for standard health insurance policies. Some of these substandard policies require higher premiums because of greater risk; others pay lower benefits for a specific loss than do standard policies for the same amount of premium. Still other substandard policies may be written with certain conditions under rider, which thus releases the company from paying benefits for losses sustained as a result of ridered conditions. While these policies are far from ideal from the client's point of view, they may be the only kind that some of our clients can obtain. In discussing this fact with our clients, we may point out that these substandard policies at least cover some conditions and so are better protection than no health insurance at all.

Trial Application Procedure.   This technique is used to protect the applicant from some of the adverse consequences of being denied health insurance such as listing with the Medical Information Bureau should the client prove to be a substandard risk or not insurable for any other reason. If there is a possibility of rejection following accurate and complete filling out of the health insurance application, the applicant should instruct the agent to print "TRIAL APPLICATION—MAKE NO RECORD UNLESS ACCEPTED" across the top of the application form. The applicant then gives the agent a $10 or $20 deposit instead of the total and usually a substantial amount of the advance premium with the understanding that should the policy be rejected, the deposit will be returned or if the policy is accepted, the remainder of the advance premium will be paid immediately (Gregg 1973:59–60).

Unallocated Benefit.   This term refers to the total amount of reimbursement up to a maximum amount for the costs of all extra miscellaneous hospital services. Specification is not made for how much will be paid for each treatment or dressing, only the total amount for all such expenses is given.

The Uniform Individual Accident and Sickness Policy Provisions Law.   This law was drawn up by the National Association of Insurance Commissioners and adopted during the 1950s by all states. It establishes model provisions that are required to be in every policy issued or authorized in the states. The law sets up the format, wording, and procedures policies must follow. Thus reading policies regardless of the company's home state becomes easier since all conform to the law's model (Dickerson 1968:632–47).

Waiting Period. The time between the beginning of the insured's disability and the start of the policy's benefits is called the waiting period. See also *Elimination Period.*

Waiver. This agreement that appears in the policy releases the company from liability for certain disabilities or conditions that the policy would ordinarily cover. Waivers are often placed on preexisting conditions for which the client cannot collect benefits under the provisions of the policy. See *Preexisting Conditions* and *Rider.*

Waiver of Premium. This provision written into some policies, exempts clients from paying premiums for a stipulated interval during the period in which they are disabled. Applicants should ask about this feature in the process of applying for insurance since during a period of disability every possible savings is helpful.

Our intent in including this section on health insurance terms is to make community nurses more comfortable in helping clients read and understand their policies as well as to be alert to some of the problems clients encounter with health insurance. Well-known terms such as beneficiary and the like have purposely been left out in order to concentrate on terms that our experience has shown nurses and clients are far less likely to be familiar with. We suggest you go over your own family's health insurance policy with these terms as guides; I would bet you are likely to find things that you didn't know were there and might want to have changed. If you know someone in the health insurance field to whom you can talk, make a list of questions and go ask them. All this will help you understand your own health insurance coverage as well as better prepare you to cope with clients' questions about health insurance.

Evaluating Health Insurance Coverage

In evaluating your own or clients' health insurance coverage, some major questions should be asked:

1. What conditions and services are covered?
2. What conditions and services are excluded or ridered out?
3. Is this coverage adequate for you or your client? How important are the exclusions or riders in terms of the actual risks you or your client faces?

4. What percentage of the cost of covered services does the insurance pay? Is this level of coverage realistic in terms of the kinds of expenses that can be expected?

5. Do the insurance companies pay hospitals and providers directly or are you or your client required to pay the bills first and then file a claim with the insurance companies? If the insureds have to pay and then wait for the company to reimburse them, how long is that waiting time, based on other peoples' experience with this kind of coverage?

6. How much is the deductible?

7. How much is the coinsurance?

8. At what point in an illness or hospitalization does the insurance coverage begin to pay?

9. Are there supplemental policies available that will help to pay what the basic coverage does not?

10. Are the total benefits from the basic policy plus the supplemental policies reasonable in relation to current health care costs as well as to your own or your client's financial and risk statuses?

11. Do you or does your client understand these questions and how to find the answers?

NATIONAL HEALTH PROGRAMS

INTRODUCTION

An optimally functioning or healthy population is a vital—perhaps *the* most vital—national resource. This realization is one of the factors underlying modern nations' development of national health programs for the delivery of personal health care services. There are two basic types of national health programs: national health insurance (NHI) and national health service (NHS). Most nations that have national health programs have chosen one or a combination of these two approaches. In many instances, historically, one has evolved into the other with the most common sequence being national health insurance programs developing into a national health service (American Public Health Association, January 1978). This country has followed a pattern of national health insurance, with Medicare and Medicaid being examples. The United States has also developed national health service-type programs, with the Veterans' Administration's and the military's health and medical services being examples. The Congress is currently considering a number of national health program proposals. The majority are variations on the national health insurance theme. A bill to create a national health service was introduced in 1977 (H.R. 6894, May 1977).

A major difference between NHI and NHS has to do with the status of the service providers and institutions. Under NHI, as with the present health insurance programs in the United States, the government purchases medical and health services from the private sector: hospitals and individual or groups of providers. An insurance company, such as Blue Cross, may serve as the fiscal intermediary or middleman, between the government and the providers. We see this model in Medicare and Medicaid. In an NHS system, the government owns the health and medical care facilities. Providers are salaried employees remunerated on the basis of their preparation and responsibilities. The Veterans' Administration, as noted, is an example. Table 12.4 lays out the major differences between NHI and NHS. This table is based on the generally accepted definitions of NHI and NHS.

As noted earlier, many proposals for a variety of national health programs have been put before the Congress. Because of the monumental size of the task of selecting one and because of the violent disagreements among the many vested interest groups that will be directly affected by whatever national health program is enacted, the process will continue to be drawn out. After all, thirty years elapsed between the passage of the original Social Security Law in 1935 and the enactment of Medicare in 1965, and some people think even that was too soon. Since whatever measures are passed effect us directly, both as providers of health care services and as potential consumers of these services, we must keep up with what is being proposed and the actions being taken on these proposals. The intricacies of the present proposals for national health programs that are before Congress or about to be introduced are not in-

TABLE 12.4 *Major Differences Between National Health Insurance and National Health Service*

Characteristic	NHI	NHS
Scope of services	Varying scope based on coverage purchased	Comprehensive services
Population served	Defined groups, not necessarily universal	The entire population
How services are provided	Via contractual agreements with independent providers	Via NHS's own personnel and facilities
Financing	Insurance contributions with government subsidies	General tax revenues

cluded here because they will change before the printer's ink is dry. Therefore, each of us must keep up with the process through our daily media as well as contacting our local congressperson's office and asking that we be kept informed directly of progress toward a national health program. Our major professional organizations, the American Public Health Association, the American Nurses' Association, and the National League for Nursing, are all actively involved in lobbying and testimony for various proposals. Bear in mind that these groups, like all others, have vested interests in one or another proposal. This is perfectly legitimate and, indeed, necessary. Learn what these organizational biases are so that you can judge what the organization espouses accordingly. As always, a good rule of thumb is to have as many sources of information as possible so that you can get many points of view and then make your own decision. Whatever that decision is, make it known to your legislator to try to influence his or her voting. In short, be informed and actively involved in the process of developing a national health program for us all. (See chapters 9, 11, and 22.) As this book goes to press, the prospects of National Health Insurance or a National Health Service of any kind seem further away than ever. The congressional leaders who have been trying to devise a compromise bill in cooperation with the administration and the administration are in open and bitter disagreement about fundamental issues. This rift, plus the inflationary spiral in the United States, unfavorable balance of payments, and plummeting value of the U.S. dollar in world money markets, are vastly important issues, both nationally and politically, and may preclude serious attention to health insurance matters for some time to come.

HISTORY OF NATIONAL HEALTH PROGRAMS

The earliest recorded instance of any kind of insurance, based like all insurance on the concept of sharing large and often unexpected expenses from a pool of resources, is the ancient Greek funeral societies. Medieval craft guilds set up welfare funds for use by sick and needy members. In the United States the Marine Hospital Service began in 1798. The federal government compelled ship owners to contribute a stipulated amount per month per seaman in their employ for a sickness fund. The government then built facilities and hired providers to care for the seamen. This program was the beginning of the U.S. Public Health Service.

The state of Prussia experimented with national social security legislation in 1854. This legislation included broad coverage compulsory health insurance and soon added workmen's compensation and old-age pensions. By 1911 France and Britain had similar national coverage. During and following World War II many other countries developed national health insurance plans and in 1948 the British Health Service was founded, building on a long history of governmental involvement in social programs. Canada has developed a national health program that has many strengths, particularly in the area of primary prevention (Lalonde 1974, 1977).

The United States is one of the few industrial countries in the world that does not have a comprehensive national health insurance program. The Social Security Act of 1935 contained many social programs but did not include health insurance. Private health insurance developed and grew rapidly following World War II until reaching its present status. Many people feel that the Medicare and Medicaid amendments to the Social Security Act passed in 1965 are the first parts of what will become a comprehensive national health program in this country. We shall see. In the meantime, we should bear in mind that nationally controlled and administered health insurance programs are not new—either in this country or elsewhere in the world. I recommend that readers seek additional information about national health programs since we will all soon be intimately involved in one (Borrow 1963; Corning 1969; Fishbein 1947; Redman 1973; Social Security Administration 1976).

ISSUES A NATIONAL PROGRAM MUST ADDRESS— OR MYTHS REVISITED

Rather than labor through the specifics of the various national health program (NHP) proposals, let us instead consider the statements that appear in the introduction to this chapter. They raise many of the salient issues that any NHP must address if it is to improve our health status or our abilities to function optimally. As the discussion of health indicators in chapter 2 and the information about spiralling costs in this chapter make eminently clear, improvement is badly needed. The purpose in going back to our opening statements is to help us to focus on these issues because they are essential criteria to use in comparing and analyzing the many NHP proposals about which we will hear a great deal during the next few years. Whatever NHP we eventually have will not spring full grown from anyone's head but rather will evolve slowly, and probably falteringly, into an organized and integrated system that addresses the following pertinent principles.

Health care is a right and no one can be refused care because of their inability to pay for it. At present in the United States we pay lip service to this idea but do not practice it. Whatever NHP this country develops, it must provide care for us all since the ability of the people to function well is any nation's greatest natural resource. Because resources are and will remain scarce, priority decisions on the distribution of health care will have to be made. There are more humane ways of making these allocations than the present practice that gives higher priority to ability to pay than to need for care. These decisions are not easy ones, and at present much work is needed in the areas of values and ethics to help us make the hard decisions about who gets what and how much, when there are more needs to be met than resources available can accommodate. The ability to pay should not be the major basis for making these choices as is now so often the case.

People who cannot afford private medical care can always be covered under Medicaid or some other public program. At present the people who are hardest hit by the costs of medical care are those whose incomes are too much for them to be eligible for public assistance programs and yet too little to permit them to pay for anything like adequate insurance coverage much less the additional out-of-pocket expenses. These are the people who have no choice but to put off needed care until they either get over the condition by themselves or become so ill that they have no choice but to go for services regardless of the costs. In fact, the costs are often higher under these circumstances since the people are more ill when they come and take longer to regain their former state as a result of having postponed treatment. Whatever NHP we have must provide for universal coverage so that no one is excluded because of income or any other variable such as geographic location.

Everyone has access to primary, secondary, and tertiary preventive services, all of which are covered by health insurance. Part of the problem with primary preventive and, to a lesser degree, tertiary preventive services is that for the most part they are not covered by health insurance. Insurance companies are currently experimenting with coverage of ambulatory and preventive care and reimbursements for organized home care programs and nursing homes (Health Insurance Institute 1977:15). However, the fact remains that less than 1 percent of our $181 billion expenditures for health and medical care in the United States in 1977 was spent for primary prevention (NBC, "Medicine in America: Life, Death, and Dollars," January 3, 1978). As we saw in chapter 9 on epidemiology, greater emphasis on primary prevention, particularly of chronic noninfectious conditions, is essential if we are to make a significant impact on the population's leading causes of death and disability. Therefore, NHP must provide for comprehensive services including greatly increased emphasis on primary prevention. We have heard repeatedly that many providers are not terribly interested in primary prevention. Our experience has proven time and again that where there is money for research and the development of services, provider interest soon follows. We in community health are already there and we'd like to get paid for it.

Coinsurance, deductibles, and waiting periods reduce utilization of medical care services and so result in cost containment. The private insurance industry reports that numerous recent studies confirm that there is a direct relationship between these kinds of cost-sharing arrangements and a decrease in the utilization of medical services (Health Insurance Institute 1977:15). No doubt this is true. The crucial question in my mind every time I see this kind of report is what happens to those people who indeed do not use the services they need or at least think they need because of the cost barrier? We have already noted that many get over whatever it is that's interfering with their level of functioning without medical help; others do not. Again, recall the data in the epidemiology chapter and the imperative raised there about our need to work to help people develop lifestyles to prevent or at least forestall their occurrence. The cost-sharing arrangements presently in effect throughout most of our medical care system are a real deterrent to peoples' use of the few existing preventive services. Further, the insidious onset of so many of our chronic noninfectious killers and maimers makes early diagnosis and prompt treatment essential if life itself, much less abilities to function, are to continue. Since cost sharing does indeed reduce utilization, at least in the short run, what effect does this practice have on long-term and costly utilization brought about by people's failure to seek early diagnosis and treatment because of the cost barriers? Thus whatever NHP is enacted must provide incentives for people to seek services early so that conditions can be diagnosed and treated promptly when the prognosis is best.

One of the greatest strengths of the medical care system in the United States is that it is pluralistic and many faceted. Close reading of chapters 6 and 19 will give some idea of the difficulties of providing for continuity of care for clients. The medical care programs in the United States are increasingly often referred to as a nonsystem. Clients all-too-frequently fall into the cracks or chasms that exist between various kinds of services. NHP must draw all of the components of the medical care system into a coordinated network of services that is understandable to and usable by both consumers and providers. Whether all of the components and providers belong to or work for the government is not the critical point here. What is essential is the coordination of the components to make the whole system work effectively and efficiently. This is certainly not the case with our present chaos.

All kinds of health care providers and consumers are actively involved in groups such as Professional Standards Review Organizations (PSROs), which are concerned with the development of standards as a means of assuring quality of care. Presently there is very little involvement in PSROs by any group other than physicians. Change in this situation is in the wind but has not occurred yet. Many other disciplines, nursing included, have developed their own standard-making groups with little, if any, input from outside their own group. Regulatory and licensing boards are classic examples. Consumer involvement in all of these activities is an idea whose time is long overdue. Most standard-making organizations are a long way from the Health Systems Agencies that under P.L. 93–641 are required to have a majority of consumers on all of their boards, councils, and committees (National Health Planning and Resources Development Act of 1974). This requirement of a majority of consumers on all standard-making organizations is a model that any NHP should adopt.

People generally are either able to read and understand their health insurance policies themselves or have others to interpret what their coverage means. Our own and our clients' experiences probably already have shown us that this statement is not true at present. This whole chapter is aimed at helping us as community health nurses to be able to understand our own insurance needs and coverage and in turn to help our clients to the same understanding. We are no substitute for reliable professional insurance agents, but in their absence we are likely to be the ones called upon to answer questions and give counsel. If you've made it through the chapter this far, you already know that understanding our current insurance is no easy matter. Whatever NHP is enacted in the United States must be simple enough for us all to understand and use effectively and efficiently. If that were the case, this chapter would be much shorter—to everyone's relief.

Finally then, whatever national health program we ultimately have should uphold the philosophy that optimal level of functioning is everyone's right and that access to the means to enable us to meet this goal must be available to everyone without financial barriers. The system must emphasize primary preventive services as well as secondary and tertiary ones and must be coordinated so that people can understand it and do not get lost in it. Finally, consumers and all kinds of providers must have a voice in setting standards and other decisions about the national health program. Does this sound idealistic? It is meant to, for after all, idealistic is not synonymous with unrealistic or impossible unless we choose to make it so. We must be informed and actively involved in the process of bringing about an ideal national health program in the United States. We owe our clients and ourselves no less. Chapters 9, 11, 14, 21, 22, and 23 among others will assist you in this involvement.

SUMMARY

The purpose of this chapter is to orient community nurses to some of the basic terms and concepts in health insurance so that we can better assist our clients in their dealings with or attempts to obtain health insurance. Many insurance terms are defined and illustrations relevant to community nursing practice are given. Terms are given in alphabetical order to facilitate the use of this section of the chapter as an ongoing reference. The chapter concludes with a brief history of national health programs and a discussion of some of the critical issues that any sound national health program must address.

REFERENCES

American Public Health Association. "Resolutions and Position Papers." *American Journal of Public Health* 68 (February 1978):182–83.

BERMAN, RICHARD A. "National Health Insurance: Reintroduction of Federal Controls." *Hospital and Health Services Administration* 22 (Summer 1977):45–57.

BORROW, JAMES G. *AMA: Voice of American Medicine.* Baltimore, Md.: The Johns Hopkins Press, 1963.

BUREAU OF LABOR STATISTICS. *Consumer Price Index.* Washington, D.C.: U.S. Department of Labor, Bureau of Labor Statistics, Published monthly.

Changing Times, The Kiplinger Magazine. Published monthly by The Kiplinger Washington Editors, Inc., Editors Park, Md. 20782.

CORNING, PETER A. *The Evolution of Medicare . . . from Idea to Law.* Washington, D.C.: U.S. Department of Health, Education and Welfare, Social Security Administration, Office of Research and Statistics, Research Report No. 29, 1969.

"Criteria for Assessing National Health Service Proposals." The Nation's Health (January 1978).

DICKERSON, O.D. *Health Insurance,* 3rd ed. Homewood, Ill.: Richard D. Irwin, 1968. (One of the Irwin Series in Risk and Insurance.)

ENGLISH, CHARLES O. *Report on Examination of the Medical Information Bureau as of December 31, 1971.* Albany: Office of the Superintendent of Insurance, 1973.

FALK, I.S. "National Health Insurance for the United States." *Public Health Reports* 92 (September–October 1977):399–406.

FISHBEIN, MORRIS. A History of the American Medical Association, 1847–1947. Philadelphia: W.B. Saunders Co., 1947.

GOLDSTEIN, JOYCE. "What Price Health? The Crisis Behind Medical Inflation." Mimeo. Health Service Action, Washington, D.C., October 1977. (P.O. Box 6586, T Street Station, Washington, D.C. 20009.)

GREGG, JOHN E. *The Health Insurance Racket and How to Beat It.* Chicago: Henry Regnery Co., 1973.

HEALTH INSURANCE INSTITUTE. *Source Book of Health Insurance Data, 1973–1974,* 15th ed. New York: Health Insurance Institute, 1974.

————.Source Book of Health Insurance Data, 1976–1977. New York: Health Insurance Institute, 1977. (277 Park Avenue, New York, N.Y. 10017.)

H.R. 6894. *Health Services Act.* Washington, D.C.: House of Representatives, May 1977.

"Health Insurance Scene Shifts." Independent Journal (San Rafael, Calif.) July 26, 1977.

"Health Insurance Umbrella: Half of U.S. Unprotected." *San Francisco Sunday Examiner–Chronicle,* January 30, 1977, A–15.

HILBERT, MORTON S. "Prevention." *American Journal of Public Health* 67 (April 1977):353–56.

LALONDE, MARC A. *A New Perspective on the Health of Canadians: A Working Document.* Ottawa: Government of Canada, April 1974.

———. "Beyond a New Perspective: Fourth Annual Matthew B. Rosenhaus Lecture." *American Journal of Public Health* 67 (April 1977):357–60.

MCSWANE, DOUG R. "Role of Insurance Third-Party Payors in Cost Accountability for Health Services." In E. Gartly Jaco, ed., *Cost Accountability for Health Services in the United States: Proceedings of the 1976 National Health Forum.* San Antonio, Tex.:Trinity University, Center for Continuing Education in Health Administration, 1977.

MENDELSON, MARY ADELAIDE. *Tender Loving Greed.* New York: Alfred A. Knopf, 1974.

MICHELFELDER, WILLIAM. *It's Cheaper to Die: Doctors, Drugs, and the American Medical Association.* Derby, Conn.: Monarch Books, 1960.

NATIONAL ASSOCIATION OF INSURANCE COMMISSIONERS. "The Uniform Individual Accident and Sickness Policy Provisions Law." In Charles O. Dickerson, ed., *Health Insurance,* 3rd ed. Homewood, Ill.: Richard D. Irwin, 1968.

NATIONAL BROADCASTING COMPANY. "Medicine in America: Life, Death, and Dollars." Documentary, January 3, 1978.

NATIONAL LEAGUE FOR NURSING. "Goals for a National Health Insurance Program." New York: National League for Nursing, February 1974.

"One Woman's 13 Insurance Policies." San Francisco Chronicle, May 17, 1978, p. 4.

P.L. 88–581. *The Social Security Amendments of 1965.* (Particularly Title XVIII, "Medicare," and Title XIX, "Medicaid.") Washington, D.C.: U.S. Government Printing Office, 1965.

P.L. 91–508. *Fair Credit Reporting Act of 1970.*

P.L. 93–641. *The National Health Planning and Resources Development Act of 1974.*

REDMAN, ERIC. *The Dance of Legislation.* New York: Simon and Schuster, 1973.

ROSS, DONALD K. *A Public Citizen's Action Manual.* New York. Grossman Publishers, 1973.

SOCIAL SECURITY ADMINISTRATION. "Chronology of Health Insurance Proposals, 1915–1976." Washington, D.C.: Social Security Administration, DHEW Publication No. (SSA) 76–11700, July 1976.

SWARTS, WILLIAM B., III. "A Decade of Change at MIB." *CLU Journal* 31 (April 1977):48–53.

13. Quality Assurance Programs for Health Care Delivery Systems

Patricia Porter

INTRODUCTION

"NURSES ON WARPATH ABOUT POOR HOSPITAL CARE," shouts the newspaper headlines. Provocative as the headline is, it is not as startling as it would have been ten years ago. We are in an "age of accountability" for health care systems and their professionals. Official funding agencies and consumers alike are asking for accountability from health care providers in areas of accessibility, cost, and quality of health services provided. Nurses, as members of the delivery team, are being held accountable for their contribution or lack of contribution to safe, efficient, and cost-effective services.

What is meant by the term *accountability?* As the use of the word has increased, it has taken on a variety of meanings in different settings. In discussing the development of quality assurance programs, Froebe and Bain (1976:10) provide a comprehensive definition of the term: "Accountability means a measure of individual, group or institutional efficiency and productivity that is judged against a predetermined guide or standard by both the agent and the client." Passos' (1973:17) description of accountability more specifically relates to nursing. She sees accountability as the ". . . 'dues paying' aspect of the increasing emphasis in nursing on greater autonomy and independence for the nurse practitioner." Revi-

358

sions in Nurse Practice Acts in several states clearly delineate the expanded role functions and the concomitant responsibilities.

DEVELOPMENT OF QUALITY ASSURANCE

Traditionally, professionals have had the privilege and the responsibility of monitoring their own practice. Individual licensure has insured us of the privilege. Evidence that the two major health professions, medicine and nursing, have not policed ourselves adequately is apparent in the increased threat of malpractice suits and the growing unfavorable public image of the attitude toward these professions. Many doctors and nurses are also expressing concern over our failure to hold ourselves and our peers accountable for the quality of services we provide to the public. Consequently, agencies outside of the specific disciplines of medicine and nursing have entered the picture in an attempt to insure quality of services to the consumer. The enactment of Title 11 of the Public Law 93-603 was a direct assertion of authority by the federal government. Enacted in 1972, this legislation mandated the establishment of Professional Standards Review Organizations (PSROs) to review the quality of medical services to Medicare, Medicaid, and maternal-child health programs. Despite the ridiculous limitation of the law that allows for the exclusion of membership of all health professionals except physicians, the mandate has influenced evaluation procedures in hospitals. Prior to the enactment of P.L. 92-603, hospitals were already being required by the Joint Commission on Accreditation of Hospitals (JCAH) to develop a quality control system. A recommendation of JCAH was most responsible for moving nursing in hospitals toward the development of a quality control system. The JCAH standards for nursing services clearly delineate the responsibilities of nursing. Standard IV states:

> There shall be evidence established that the nursing services provide safe, efficient and therapeutically effective nursing care through the planning of each patient's care and the effective implementation of the plan [JCAH 1972:51].

The clarity of the JCAH's expectation of nursing leaves no room for doubt; nurses must plan, document, and evaluate the care we provide. Yet, the nursing literature reveals very few reports of evaluation studies related to the process and outcome of nursing care. How can nurses fight for the right to individual licensure when they are unable or unwilling to state what they contribute to health care and how they insure the quality of that nebulous product called "nursing care"?

The Council of Home Health Agencies and Community Health Services (CHHA-CHS) of the National League for Nursing and the American Public Health Association jointly accredit home health agencies and community nursing services. CHHA–CHS publishes the following criteria for insuring accountability at various levels within an agency seeking accreditation. On the organization and administration level, agencies are required to have ". . . a governing body accountable for the management of the agency" (CHHA–CHS 1976:3). On the program level the following criteria specifically address accountability:

> 6. Conferences of workers providing services to a patient/family are held [for evaluation, reevaluation, and planning of total care]. A professional nurse has the responsibility for coordinating the agency plan for patient care.
> 7. The agency has an established mechanism for ongoing review of the quality of services rendered by each discipline.
> 8. The agency has established procedures for program evaluation [CHHA–CHS 1976:11–12].

On the staff level criteria for personnel supervision and development through continuing education opportunities are clearly spelled out (CHHA–CHS 1976:14–17). Standards for facilities and personnel are also clearly delineated in "Conditions for Participation" under Medicare and Medicaid. State bodies issuing licenses to agencies and individual practitioners also have minimum specifications that must be met before a license to practice will be issued. Thus, we are again reminded that we live in the "age of accountability."

Schlotfeldt (1973) has written provocatively of the nursing profession's need to remain a viable social system. She has explored the discrepancies that exist in stated nursing philosophies, policies, and practices. She summarizes the problem in the following statement:

> A clearly conceptualized role for the professional known by the term 'nurse' stated in terms of outcomes to be attained has not yet been adequately communicated and generally accepted, either within or outside the profession. As a consequence, the role of the nurse is not yet fully and generally understood, and outcomes that are consequences of scientifically based, humane nursing practice are not generally recognized and valued [Schlotfeldt, 1973:786].

Avoiding feelings of shock and dismay on reading such words from one of the profession's leaders is difficult. How can nursing, as a profession, have existed these many years without the consequences of its practice being recognized and valued? Dismaying as reality often is, the time has come to deal with that reality and get on with the task of developing standards and assuring the performance of those standards.

APPROACHES TO EVALUATION

Historically, nursing care has been evaluated from the perspectives of structure and process. *Structure standards* have often been set by licensing and accrediting bodies and have focused on such areas as physical facilities, staff to patient ratio, and educational preparation of care providers. The existence of structure standards attempts to incur necessary components of care but does not guarantee the quality of these components. *Process standards* speak to the actions of care providers—that is, what they do in response to the identified needs of the patient. Recently much attention is being given to a third type: *outcome standards*. Knowing merely what is done to whom and under what circumstances is not sufficient; the survival of nursing as a distinct health profession may depend on what difference nursing care makes in the health status of the consumer and the community.

To illustrate the kinds of standards and audits that are being developed and utilized in community health nursing agencies, examples of the protocols or standards and the audit tools used to evaluate the nursing services are given under these protocols in the appendix, at the end of this chapter. These example standards and audit tools were developed by the nursing division of the Santa Cruz County Health Services Agency and are currently in use in that agency's well child programs. They illustrate the type of quality assurance tools described in the following discussion and can serve as models for the development of similar tools for other community health nursing services.

ESTABLISHING A QUALITY ASSURANCE PROGRAM

ROLE OF NURSING ADMINISTRATION

Nursing administrators' leadership and direction are crucial factors in the development and the success of quality assurance programs. The development and implementation of the necessary guidelines and procedures for quality assurance programs require a substantial financial investment on the part of a nursing services division. Nursing administrators must be committed to programs and support that commitment with adequate resources. This action often involves justification of such expenses to hospital administrators, agency directors, and various funding groups.

Therefore, nursing administrators must be clear in their own thinking as to the purpose of proposed programs to evaluate quality of care.

There can be several objectives for developing quality assurance programs, and the components of a given program will conform to its specific objectives. The nursing management group is in the position to decide what is needed and wanted from an evaluation of nursing care. A frequently stated objective relates to improving the quality of nursing care the agency provides clients. Other objectives include: (1) complying with external mandates such as those of the Joint Commission on Accreditation of Hospitals or the Council of Home Health Agencies and Community Health Services/American Public Health Association, (2) demonstrating cost-effectiveness, (3) selecting program priorities, and (4) determining staff development needs. It is often possible and desirable to design quality assurance programs to meet many objectives, but such programs are complex and require much planning and care in implementation. A quality assurance program containing structure, process, and outcome standards as well as controls for assuring the attainment of those standards facilitates the accomplishment of any or all of the objectives previously identified.

THE DEVELOPMENT OF STANDARDS

Once an administrative decision regarding the purpose and basic structure of a quality assurance program has been made, the next step is that of developing standards. Staff participation at this level of program development is essential. A first step is to provide information to staff on the basic objectives of the quality assurance program, the general plans for its development, the proposed time framework, and the projected level of participation of each staff member. Following an adequate period for discussion and understanding of the concept of the quality assurance program, the coordinator of the program can begin to implement the specific components of the program with appropriate staff members.

As mentioned before, *structure standards* are often determined by licensing and accrediting bodies, but they are also influenced by the philosophy of nursing adhered to in any institution. Staffing patterns, supervisory styles, and commitment to staff development are among the structure standards influenced by the agency's philosophy. In the developmental stages of an evaluation program, nursing administration must critically review the spoken or unspoken philosophy and relate it to the structure standards in existence. One cannot deny the tremendous impact these structure standards have on the process of care.

Process standards are not new to most nursing organizations. *Nursing process* refers to the activities of nurses as they deliver care. Although definitions of the nursing process may differ slightly, there is a general recognition of the inclusion of the components of the nursing process: assessment, planning, implementation, and evaluation. These components have been incorporated into ANA's standards of nursing practice (ANA 1973). The delineation of process standards is facilitated when the standards relate to the elements of the nursing process as it exists in any given client service situation.

There are excellent tools available for auditing the nursing process. One of the most comprehensive is Phaneuf's Nursing Audit (1972, 1976). The tool measures seven functions of professional nursing, which, according to Phaneuf, provide the foundation for the nursing process. These seven functions are:

Function I:	Application and Execution of Physician's Legal Orders
Function II:	Observation of Symptoms and Reactions
Function III:	Supervision of the Patient
Function IV:	Supervision of Those Participating in Care (Except the Physician)
Function V:	Reporting and Recording
Function VI:	Application and Execution of Nursing Procedures
Function VII:	Promotion of Physical and Emotional Health by Directing and Teaching [1976:60–71].

The nursing audit is a fifty-item instrument designed to measure a cycle of care. The audit is done on a closed record, following the discharge of the client from the service (Phaneuf and Wandelt 1974). The instrument has been used extensively in hospitals and community health agencies. The two tools that have been used in conjunction with the nursing audit are the Slater Nursing Competencies Rating Scale and the Quality Patient Scale (QualPaCS). The Slater Nursing Competencies Rating Scale measures competencies displayed by the nurse and the QualPaCS measures the care received by the client. Use of the QualPaCS involves measurement of care after it has occurred, whereas the Slater Scale can be used for on-the-spot ratings as well as in retrospect. The nurse's actions, therefore, can be evaluated against established standards of care (Wandelt and Phaneuf 1976).

Wandelt and Phaneuf (1976) suggest that the QualPaCS be used with the Slater Scale to provide a measurement of the quality of care received by the client. Derived from the Slater Scale, the wording of the QualPaCS is designed to describe the nurse's action as it was received by the client rather than as it was performed by the nurse. Ratings are done by a nurse who directly observes the care provided a client during a two-hour period. In reviewing the Nursing Audit, the Slater Scale and the QualPaCS, Wandelt and Phaneuf (1976:56) acknowledge, ". . . there are questions about the validity and about subjectivity of the rater." However, the three tools do represent a tremendous step toward uniform and systematic measurement of the nursing process.

The three tools described in the preceding paragraphs are meant to be representative of nursing audit tools that are available; there are many other tools that have proven effective in auditing nursing care. Krumme (1975) has provided a detailed description of the use of many instruments.

The utilization of *outcome standards* for measuring nursing care is a more recent development in nursing. Program evaluations, which have considered output, if not outcome, have been more common in public health agencies than in hospitals. The reason is likely due to the fact that many community health nursing programs serve identified needs of a specific population; for example, the provision of well child services to inexperienced parents. Due to the nature of funding for such programs at federal, state, and county levels, nursing administration has often been required to formulate program goals and then document the services related to the goals. Keeler (1972) points out that the accountability of community health nursing programs has often been limited to documenting resources spent on the program rather than what difference the services made. Although accountability for the distribution of funds will always be a major and realistic component of any evaluation program, there are other issues that must be addressed.

Now that agencies outside the health care systems and consumers of health care are beginning to look at what their health dollar is buying, there is a need to be specific about the results of nursing care. Zimmer (1974a:308) has defined a patient health/wellness outcome as ". . . an alteration in the health status of the patient that is the end result of care." There are many possible ways of approaching the development of outcome standards and the myriad leaves many groups defeated before they begin. A staff group assigned to develop outcome criteria will need direction from an expert as they decide on an approach.

Stevens (1975) has provided a taxonomy for the selection of client groups. The grouping criteria include: (1) disease, (2) like treatment, (3) like needs, (4) geographic criterion, (5) life stage, and (6) illness stage. Grouping according to specified criteria allows for the prediction of similar outcomes. The classification system needs to vary with the client population and the services provided, but some type of grouping is imperative.

Aside from the initial problem of deciding on a grouping for clients and/or problems, there are several other difficulties that can be anticipated in attempts to develop outcome criteria. One of the most difficult is that of describing outcomes that are specific enough to be measurable without producing a document of a size that would threaten our forests with extinction. Too detailed an audit tool often engenders some interesting but predictable feelings of "being controlled." Nurses express the feeling that individualized care is not possible when standards spell out every interaction and expected outcome of that interaction. Arguments then rage on as to whether standards should reflect a baseline of care or the optimally desired level. Obviously, the standards must portray safe and therapeutically effective care or else we are better off without them. At the other end of the spectrum are the professionals who advocate standards that reflect the highest possible level of care. The existence of unrealistic standards for a setting result in undue frustration on the part of staff and contribute to the failure of patient care evaluation systems. Given the many factors that influence an individual nurse's ability to provide for the identified needs of an individual client, a reasonable approach would seem to call for standards that fall somewhere between baseline and optimum.

Another difficulty encountered in developing outcome criteria that has been discussed by various authors (Bloch 1975; Zimmer 1974; Taylor 1974; Stevens 1975) is that of overlap between care given by the different disciplines and the difficulty in any attempt to define nursing-specific outcomes. Commenting on the role of the different health disciplines, Schlotfeldt clarifies the issue:

> That which differentiates the several types of health professionals in the essential, primary, enduring focuses of their practices—their stable roles, so to speak—and the outcomes each is expected to achieve. Conceptualizing the practice of each type of professional practitioner defines the jurisdiction (responsibility and accountability) of each and identifies the competencies requisite for execution of each role [Schlotfeldt 1973:769].

Acknowledging that both physicians and nurses are concerned with the health of people, Schlotfeldt continues her differentiation of roles by describing the *practice* focus of the physician and the *practice* focus of the nurse:

> The physician's *practice* focus, however, is on differentially diagnosing and treating pathologies through the selective application of medical science and the discriminating use of available medical strategies. The nurse's *practice* focus is on assessing peoples' health status, assets, and deviations from health, and on helping sick people to regain health and the well or near-well to maintain or attain health through the selective application of nursing science and the use of available nursing strategies [Schlotfeldt 1973:769].

We should not anticipate universal agreement with Schlotfeldt's delineation of the practice foci of nurses and physicians, and since both are dynamic professions, the practices will change. The point is that the differentiation is and will be possible to make. The differentiation is an important factor in the development of patient outcomes related to services delivered. Part of the difficulty in developing client care outcome is simply one of semantics. Bloch (1974) has contributed much toward the clarification of terms used in nursing. My own experience in working with groups attempting to develop outcome standards supports Bloch's preference for *health* as a referent for such terms as *need, problem,* and *assessment.* The use of *health* as a referent puts the focus where it belongs: on the client, not the provider. This view does not mean that we abandon the development of outcome standards that are related to care provided by specific disciplines. Many of the factors that require evaluation in health care—for example, cost effectiveness and preparation of personnel—are directly related to the establishment of outcomes related to services provided. As Taylor (1974) has pointed out, there must be an assumption that some outcomes are primarily attributable to nursing care and some are not and that each can be identified. Nursing practice can do nothing but gain from an exploration of the process of care and the end results of that care. Neither of the three standards, structure, process, or outcome, used alone will provide a comprehensive evaluation tool.

DOCUMENTATION OF NURSING PROCESS AND PATIENT CARE OUTCOMES

Once the task of developing standards of care is completed, the job of assuring provision of care that meets the standards begins. Again, staff involvement is crucial. Getting their input at this point is not usually difficult if they have shared in the development of standards. However, present in the input from staff are usually many misgivings about the ominous "quality control" and what it means. Peer review remains a tense issue for most professionals. Reporting on an experiment in peer review one group of investigators (Gold, et al. 1973) reported that one of the major problems was the reluctance of the staff to judge and be judged. Yet, as Froebe and Bain (1976) have suggested, if peer accountability is not present in nursing, then its professional status is lost. That statement would certainly apply to all health care professionals, but it is more crucial for nursing's survival at this point in history.

To implement a comprehensive system of audit, as complete and accurate a record as possible is necessary, for the reality is that financial resources do not allow for continuous, nonsubjective observation of nursing care. This statement does not mean that the giving of care will never be observed, but rather, that observation cannot become the major source of quality control information. Once standards are identified, we can include documentation of the nursing process and the outcome of the care in the client care record.

Weed (1971) has made a major contribution to care by devising a system of recording that reflects the process, including the decision making and the outcomes. The nursing process is easily documented utilizing Weed's format. Again, staff can be held back by semantics, unless someone makes an arbitrary decision on what terms will be used in labeling the components of the process. Utilizing terms that have similar meaning to all health care professionals—for example, "health," "client care outcomes," "assessment," rather than "nursing outcomes" and "medical impression"—would be advantageous to any system for auditing nursing care.

Earlier, the components of the nursing process were identified. In utilizing a problem-oriented format for documentation, the components of the process can be clearly delineated and audit is greatly facilitated.

ASSESSMENT

The assessment of the health status of a client involves, first of all, the collection of data. Weed (1971) refers to this first step as the gathering of a data base, which is hopefully a universal phenomenon in the helping professions. The specific data needed will vary with the client, the setting, and the services provided, but it must be standardized in relation to the designated criteria agreed upon by the entire team. Nothing is more exasperating or trust defeating than six health care "team" members' asking a client the same questions! Surely clients speculate that we never talk to each other. Once standardization of a data base occurs in a setting, each team member is then accountable for documenting the particular portion for which he or she is responsible. It is a simple matter to audit the absence or presence of these kinds of information on the record.

The collection of the data base is only the beginning point of the assessment. Once data are collected, the team members must make judgments and inferences to identify problems. The intellectual process involving the analysis and synthesis of data and the resultant conclusions is thus revealed. Reviewing this process is an excellent source of information for determining a health professional's level of functioning. Because the Weed System is so revealing, many professionals have resisted the system! Care must be taken in introducing this system to staff. A nurse's comment that "a client appears to be sleeping" is a long step from the assessment, "the illness allows the client to meet dependency needs." Although Benedikter (1973) advocates the avoidance of use of the audit tool as an evaluation tool for individual nurses since the overall objective of a quality assurance program is not usually evaluation of individuals, it is difficult to understand how that can be avoided. To fail to identify a practitioner who provides less than acceptable care constitutes professional negligence on the part of peers—threatening? yes; necessary? absolutely!

PLANNING

Following the identification and the documentation of the client's problems on the record, the persons involved, including the client, the next step is to develop treatment plans. Documentation of the identified problems allows for setting priorities. This step is crucial in any health care setting, for every team member and certainly the client has his or her own view of what is most important in any situation. The volumes written on clients' lack of "compliance" attest to the lack of mutual goal setting among and between providers and recipients of care. Knowledgeable health care consumers are no longer willing to passively sit back and allow professionals to "do what is best."

Treatment planning among providers avoids duplication of efforts and outright conflict. Duplication is expensive, and conflict in plans can be less than therapeutic for the recipient. On the positive side, treatment planning allows for a sharing of knowledge and experience among team members that facilitates the differentiation of roles and an appreciation of the contributions of the individual health disciplines.

As with the documentation of problems, the written treatment plan portrays the level of knowledge and skill of the team members. One member's adherence or lack of adherence to standards of care is immediately demonstrated to all members of the team. Having stated a treatment plan, the practitioner must be able to discuss the rationale for the plan. "Home visit monthly to provide support" won't fly as a treatment plan without a great deal more being said about "support" and the anticipated outcome of "support."

IMPLEMENTATION

Another aspect of the helping process in nursing is the "action" taken by the provider in response to identified needs. In multidisciplinary settings there is often thorough formulation of treatment plans, agreed upon by all, but implemented by no one! "But I thought you were going to do that," is a common expression heard when an irate client confronts two or more team members with perceived lack of action. Thus, designating the who's, and how's of the implementation phase is necessary. Ideally, the action should be taken by the team member best prepared to perform the task. The action taken is then documented in the record and can be measured against the predetermined process standards.

The client progress notes are the usual source for documentation of actions taken. Weed's format of recording subjective observations, objective observations, assessment, and plan (S.O.A.P.) frequently causes confusion as to where the "action taken" is to be recorded. This decision is one that can be made by an agency. There is nothing sacred about the S.O.A.P. format, and it can be modified, as long as the modification becomes standardized for the setting. Many procedures for recording include the action statement after the assessment, prior to the statement of the ongoing plan. The advantage to utilizing the S.O.A.P. format with the action statement is that the information upon which the action is based is readily available for retrieval when implementing quality control systems.

EVALUATION

Evaluation of the effectiveness of the services provided has been one of the least formalized and standardized aspects of the nursing process. Much of nursing's contribution has been intuitive and ill defined and, consequently, difficult to evaluate. A problem-oriented format for documentation permits the retrieval of information that indicates the action taken and the client's response to that action. Subjective and objective observations, documented in relation to an identified problem, clearly describe the status of the problem at any given time and make possible comparing actual outcomes with the predetermined outcome standards.

Various levels of problem resolution need to be identified if effective treatment planning and implementation are to occur. The effectiveness of the treatment plan as reflected in the outcome statements in the progress notes can be evaluated on an ongoing basis. Ongoing evaluation allows for the development of time frameworks for expected outcomes and encourages the development of new treatment plans if the expected outcomes do not occur within the projected time.

In addition to the ongoing evaluation of care that is essential for quality, terminal evaluation of outcomes is desirable. Large numbers of cases can be reviewed to determine overall levels of care for any particular group of clients. Problems can be identified and steps taken at an agency level to correct the difficulty. At this point, structure standards are often evaluated and changes made.

SUMMARY

The need for quality assurance programs for health care delivery systems has been demonstrated and approaches to developing programs have been outlined. The nursing process, with the identified components of assessment, planning, implementation, and evaluation, has been utilized as the basis for evaluation of client care within the framework standards for structure, process, and outcome. The identification of such standards and a means of documenting the implementation of the standards allows for the "holding accountable" of the health care provider. Examples of nursing standards or protocols and audit tools for well child and family planning programs are included to illustrate the development of a quality assurance program.

Appendix: Protocols and Audit Tools of Santa Cruz County Health Services Agency*

13.1   *Problem-Oriented Format for Evaluation of Child Health Services*

SANTA CRUZ COUNTY HEALTH SERVICES AGENCY
Evaluation — Child Health Services

Date Opened_____   Date Closed_____

Common Problems	Outcome Criteria	Met	Not Met	NA	Comments

Source: Adapted by the Santa Cruz County Health Services Agency, Santa Cruz, Calif., from Joyce Waterman Taylor, "Measuring Outcomes of Nursing Care," *Nursing Clinics of North America* 9 (June 1974): 305–315.

*All materials in this appendix are reprinted with permission of the Division of Nursing Services, Santa Cruz County Health Services Agency, Santa Cruz, California.

13.2   *Frequency Schedule for Well Child Health Services*

Screening Procedure	Under 2 Mos.	2-3 Mos.	4-5 Mos.	6-8 Mos.	9-11 Mos.	12-17 Mos.	18-23 Mos.	2 Years	3 Years	4-5 Years	6-8 Years	9-12 Years	13-16 Years
Initial or Interval Health History	×	×	×	×	×	×	×	×	×	×	×	×	×
Height and Weight	×	×	×	×	×	×	×	×	×	×	×	×	×
Head Circumference	×	×	×	×	×	×	×	×					
General Physical Examination	×	×	×	×	×	×	×	×	×	×	×	×	×
Dental Inspection				×	×	×	×	×	×	×	×	×	×
Developmental Appraisal	×	×	×	×	×	×	×	×	×	×			
Denver Developmental Screening Test				×		×		×		×			
Vision Screening Test	×	×	×	×	×	×	×	×	× or	×	×	×	×
Hearing Screening Test				×					× or	×			
Blood Pressure									× or	×	×	×	×
Hematocrit or Hemoglobin					×			×	×	×		×	×
Tuberculin Test					×				×		×		×
Urine: "dipstick"					×					×			×
Assessment of Nutritional Status	×	×	×	×	×	×	×	×	×	×	×	×	×
Assessment of Immunization Status		×	×	×	×	×	×	×	×	×	×	×	×
Administration of Immunizations Necessary to Make Status Current[1]		×	×[1]	×	×	×	×	×	×	×	×	×	×
Special Procedures as Appropriate					×					×	×	×	×

[1] Refer to Santa Cruz County Health Services Agency's Immunization Protocols for recommendations.

TABLE 13.1 *Child Health Services Protocol*

Philosophy

Santa Cruz County Health Services Agency is committed to activities directed toward maintaining and improving the health of children. To that end, child health care services are organized throughout the agency on an integrated and cooperative basis. Services are available for families who consider the Health Services Agency their primary source of care and for selected families in need of intensive public health nursing services. Health services for children include Child Health Nursing Conferences, Child Health and Disability Prevention Clinics, and Outpatient General Medical Clinics for ambulatory care.

OBJECTIVE I

To provide health services to eligible families requesting well child care from the Health Services Agency.

Activity	Problem	Standing Orders	Expected Outcome
Determination of eligibility for CHNC	Identifying Criteria	PHN/PHA visit family requesting service	Need for intensive public health nursing is identified and noted on CHNC record
		PHN performs interview and initial history taking	
		Families in need of intensive nursing care due to –language, cultural and/or financial barriers, –difficulty coping with parenting, –mental or social dysfunction, drug abuse and/or parental stress, are eligible for CHNC	
		PHN –performs physical inspection of child –explains purpose and limitations of CHNC.	Parents have accurate information about services available in CHNC. Majority of children

Activity	Problem	Standing Orders	Expected Outcome
Determination of eligibility for CHDP Clinics	Family is financially unable to secure a primary source of care	MediCal recipient up to age 12 and children from birth to age 6 whose family income is within 200% of poverty level are eligible for CHDP Clinic	Payment mechanism established. Appointment given for CHDP Clinic
Determination of eligibility for Outpatient Health Care Clinic	Family is without a primary source of care	MediCal recipients 12 years of age and older, & children of families who consider HSA their primary source of care are eligible for well child care through the Outpatient Clinic	Appointment into Outpatient Clinic

OBJECTIVE II

To identify and to notify the child's primary source of medical care that the family has intent to utilize the CHNC.

Activity	Problem	Standing Orders	Expected Outcome
PHN gives family requesting CHNC a letter of intent		Parent(s) and PHN sign appropriate section of letter. Family requests physician to acknowledge plan for care	Physician signs letter of intent. Completed original (white copy) is placed in CHNC record
	Physician determines child is not appropriate for CHNC due to medical problems	Refer back to physician for ongoing care. Continued family follow-up unless indicated otherwise	

TABLE 13.1 *(Continued)*

OBJECTIVE III

To determine the intervals that the physician requests the child enrolled in CHNC to return for continuation of primary care.

Activity	Problem	Standing Orders	Expected Outcome
Plan for continuing care		PHN follows recommendations of primary provider for periodic referral back for care	Physician is provider of primary medical care. CHNC is supplement to that care.
	Physician makes no recommendations.	PHN refers family back to primary provider no less than annually and as necessary, in the event of illness or suspected abnormality	
		Copy of CHNC record should accompany family for appointments with provider	

OBJECTIVE IV

To provide periodic evaluations of health status through performance of physical, dental and nutritional assessments integrated throughout with anticipatory and situational counseling.

Activity	Problem	Standing Orders	Expected Outcome
Scheduling for well-child clinic		Nursing staff: −appoints child into CHNC or CHDP clinics −encourages appointments for General Medical Clinic but allows drop-in if clinic load permits −schedules clinic visits for 20–30 minutes per	Child attends clinic as appointed

Child is/appears ill	—cancels appointment —refers parent/s to child's primary source of care as indicated. —reschedules visit.	Ambulatory care for illness is not available in well child clinics
Scheduling for return visits	Nursing Staff —refers to Frequency Schedule —appoints or instructs parent/s to call for return appointment according to schedule.	Child returns for continuing care according to schedule.
Recording	PHN —initiates or continues clinic record, CHNC record (MCH-20), or CHDP record as indicated —gives parent/s Child Health Supervision Record —records findings of each clinic visit —explains results of screening to parent/s —gives parent/s a written summary of the screening.	Findings are documented in the medical record of the Agency and in a record for the parent/s use
Certification for school entry	PHN in CHDP or General Medical Clinic	Certification of screening is signed by PHN and given to parent/s

TABLE 13.1 (*Continued*)

OBJECTIVE IV (*Continued*)

Activity	Problem	Standing Orders	Expected Outcome
		–performs screening to include screening evaluation of health status, developmental assessment, immunizations as needed, tuberculine testing, laboratory tests, and vision and hearing tests if not already done by school	
		–signs State certification form for school entry and gives to parent/s	
		–gives parent/s Agency's certification form with screening results listed (HSA-23a)	
		–explains results of screening to parent/s	
	Parent/s are not required to share *results* with school	PHN encourages parent/s to share results of screening with school	Parent understands advantages of sharing child's health status with the school
	Parent/s refuse any component or the entire screening exam	PHN –determines the reason for refusal if possible –instructs parent/s who refuse to sign the waiver component on the certification form	Reason for refusal is identified Parent/s are informed of the State requirements for school entry Follow-up referral is made as appropriate

		Record documents activities
Health history to include: –demographic data –details of pregnancy, birth, and neonatal period –illness history –hospitalization history –summary of growth and development –immunization history –family health history –nutrition history	–instructs parent/s who refuse the entire exam to notify the school in writing of their refusal –refers family for PHN follow-up as indicated PHN –takes initial history or reviews past history –elicits interval history at each clinic visit	Health history is documented in record
Unclothed physical examination to include skin, head, eyes, ears, nose, mouth, and throat, neck, chest, abdomen, genitalia, extremities, brachial and femoral pulses	PHN performs physical examination at each clinic visit	Results of physical examination are documented in record, signed by the PHN

Table 13.1 (*Continued*)

OBJECTIVE IV (*Continued*)

Activity	Problem	Standing Orders	Expected Outcome
	Health history and/or physical examination reveal a potentially handicapping condition not receiving diagnostic evaluation or treatment by a source of medical care	PHN in CHNC refers to child's primary source of medical care using Agency's routine referral form PHN in CHDP clinic –reviews all potential referrals with CHDP physician consultant before completion –uses CHDP referral and follow-up form –refers to child's usual source of care or assists family to secure such care PHN in General Medical Clinic –refers to clinic physician for consultation and/or evaluation of the child –refers to an appropriate source of medical care as indicated, using Agency's routine referral form	Child with any potentially handicapping condition is referred to an appropriate source of medical care for diagnosis and treatment if indicated Record signed by PHN documents findings and subsequent activities
Nutritional and growth assessment		PHA –measures height and weight at each clinic visit –measures head circumference at each visit until 12 months old	Child's growth is within normal limits

	PHN	
Underweight (less than third percentile by Harvard-Iowa growth charts)	PHN —determines nutritional status at each visit —performs situational and anticipatory counseling related to nutritional needs of child and family at each clinic visit	Parent/s have information appropriate to nutritional needs of family.
Low stature (less than third Percentile by Harvard-Iowa growth charts)	PHN refers to primary source of care for evaluation	Problem is identified and corrected if possible
Overweight as determined by:		
Height 25th percentile 50th percentile 75th percentile		
Weight 75th percentile 90th percentile 97th percentile		
No source of vitamin supplement in the diet	PHN —gives prescription for multivitamins with Fluoride 0.6cc daily for child under 12 months	Adequate vitamin intake is provided via supplement or diet

TABLE 13.1 (*Continued*)

OBJECTIVE IV (*Continued*)

Activity	Problem	Standing Orders	Expected Outcome
		–instructs parent/s in administration –gives Fluoride warning –encourages vitamin supplement for child over 12 months with questionable dietary intake Chewable vitamins for children are available without prescription	
Dental Screening	Gross abnormalities of soft and hard tissues of face and/or mouth, caries, malocclusions, infections, or other dental disease	PHN –performs oral health inspection including soft and hard tissues of face and mouth at each clinic visit –recommends regular dental care beginning when child is 3 years. PHN refers to primary source of medical or dental care	Results of dental screening are documented in record Parent/s select dental provider Diagnosis and treatment by appropriate provider are instituted.
	Prevention of dental caries	PHN counsels parent/s regarding oral hygiene and diet –advises Fluoride use –gives prescription as appropriate	Reduction of preventable dental caries in child.

statement

	Multi-Vitamins with Fluoride —birth through 12 months 0.6cc. p.o. daily Fluoride qtts —birth through 3 years 0.5 mg p.o. daily —3 years and over 1.0 mg p.o. daily Chewable Fluoride —child under 3 years 0.5 mg (½ tablet) p.o. daily —child over 3 years 1.0 mg p.o. daily			
Determination of blood pressure	PHA/PHN determines blood pressure when child is 3 years, if possible, and at annual visits thereafter PHN palpates femoral pulse at each visit	Brachial artery cuff blood pressure is elevated above 130/80 mm. Hg. in right arm of children less than 6 yrs. of age, or 140/90 mm. Hg. for children 6 yrs of age or older		Record documents finding
	PHN repeats evaluation of blood pressure when child is *at rest*. If elevation continues, refers to primary source of care for evaluation			Diagnosis and treatment if indicated by primary provider
	PHN refers to primary source of care	Femoral artery pulses are absent to palpation		Record documents findings

TABLE 13.1 *(Continued)*

OBJECTIVE V

To provide routine immunizations and TB skin tests.

Activity	Problem	Standing Orders	Expected Outcome
Routine immunizations DPT—initial series		PHN or other licensed nursing staff	Record signed by the nurse documents the immunization series and the sites
		—begins initial series when child is at least 2 months old	
		—gives 3 injections of DPT 0.5 cc IM using alternate lateral thigh muscles	
		—allows at least 4 weeks between immunizations and may give at 2 month intervals to correspond with Polio	
		—notes immunization and site on record	
	Child is under 10 pounds	Immunization is delayed until child is over 10 pounds	DPT is not given to child under 10 pounds
		PHN or other licensed nursing staff	Record signed by the nurse documents the booster immunization and the site
		—gives first booster DPT 0.5 cc IM at 12 months after last injection of initial series	
		—gives second booster DPT 0.5 cc IM at 5 yrs of age, before school entry	

Trivalent Oral Polio Vaccine—initial series		PHN or other licensed nursing staff —begins initial series when child is at least 2 months old —gives 3 doses of Oral Polio Vaccine qtts II p.o. —allows 2 months interval between doses		Record signed by the nurse documents the booster
		—gives first polio booster qtts II p.o. at 12 months after last dose of initial series. —gives 2nd polio booster qtts II p.o. at 5 years of age, before school entry		Record signed by the nurse documents the booster
Rubeola, Rubella, and Mumps Vaccine	History suggests child has had measles and/or mumps	PHN or other licensed nursing staff gives combined measles and mumps vaccine when child is over one year of age —gives combined measles only, if measles and mumps not available —gives injection in subcutaneous area	Immunization is given	Record signed by nursing staff documents immunization and the site
	History reveals allergy to eggs	Refer to the primary source of care for immunization or consult General Medical Clinic Physician		Allergic reaction to immunization is prevented in well-child clinics

TABLE 13.1 *(Continued)*

OBJECTIVE V *(Continued)*

Activity	Problem	Standing Orders	Expected Outcome
	Immunization reactions	Unless instructed otherwise by the primary source of care, the PHN –recommends Baby Aspirin (gr 1¼ [75 mgm] per tablet) for immunization reactions Under 6 months of age— –½ tablet q 4 hr. ×3 Six months to 1 year— –1 tablet, (gr 1¼) q 4 hr. × 3 One year to 6 years— –1 gr. per ten pounds of body weight q 4 hr. × 3 –advises parent/s not to exceed 3 doses urless instructed by physician –advises parent/s that liquids must be given to and retained by children receiving aspirin	Parent/s have information to recognize and cope with immunization reactions Plan for emergency care is implemented as necessary. Record documents activities
	Severe immunization reaction —immediate	PHN –brings emergency box to outlying clinic –notes location of emergency equipment at each clinic site	

Severe immunization reaction –delayed	–initiates emergency resuscitation measures according to HSA standing orders –notifies child's primary source of care	Prevention or minimization of severe immunization reactions.
–fever over 104 R (103 oral) for 12 hrs. or more. –extreme irritability with fever for a 24 hour period –convulsions secondary to fever	PHN –performs assessment of current status –refers to primary source of care if parent/s have not already done so –refers child back to primary source of care for further immunizations	Continuing care is given by primary source of medical care.
Child is out of step with routine immunizations	PHN or other licensed nursing staff refers to Immunization Protocols	Record signed by nurse documents immunizations status and plan for bringing the child up to date. Immunizations including the sites are documented in the record signed by the nurse
Tuberculin Testing	PHN or other licensed nursing staff	Record signed by nurse documents

Table 13.1 *(Continued)*

OBJECTIVE V *(Continued)*

Activity	Problem	Standing Orders	Expected Outcome
		—gives initial Tine Test when child is over 9 months old —gives Tine Test 2 months before Measles vaccination —gives yearly Tuberculin Test thereafter —gives standard intermediate P.P.D. 0.1 cc intradermally when cooperation of the child permits —advises parent/s to call in 48 hours if injection site reacts in any way whatsoever—if any doubt exists as to a reaction, the child must be seen and evaluated by nursing staff or physician	test, the site, and the results
	The tuberculin test is positive by the tine method, or greater than 5mm. in duration results from application of intermediate strength standardized P.P.D.	PHN refers child to primary source of care for follow-up	Diagnosis and treatment if indicated by primary care provider

OBJECTIVE VI

To perform selected health screening procedures such as Denver Developmental Tests, vis on and hearing screening, hematocrit, and urine screening as a part of the assessment process.

Activity	Problem	Standing Orders	Expected Outcome
Developmental assessment		PHA and/or PHN performs Denver Developmental Screening Test in home, office or clinic setting when child is 6 months, 12 months, 2 years, and 4 years of age or more frequently if indicated	Results of Denver Dev. Screening Test are documented in record
		PHN –interprets findings to parent/s –performs situational and anticipatory counseling related to development	Parent/s have information concerning the present and expected development of the child
	The developmental assessment reveals developmental delay not receiving diagnostic evaluation or treatment	PHN –repeats Denver –interprets findings to parent/s, taking care that no diagnostic term is used or inferred. –refers to the primary source of care for further evaluation	Record signed by the PHN documents activities. Diagnosis and treatment if indicated are given by the primary source of medical care
Vision Screening		PHN –performs inspection of external eye at each clinic visit	

TABLE 13.1 *(Continued)*

OBJECTIVE VI *(Continued)*

Activity	Problem	Standing Orders	Expected Outcome
		−evaluates for strabismus by means a cover test or Herschberg Test at each clinic visit until Snellen is used −evaluates retinal (red) reflex through undilated pupil on initial visit PHA −performs Snellen screening test when child is 3 or 4 years, as possible, and at each annual visit thereafter PHN interprets findings to family	
	Vision screening reveals any of the following abnormalities:	PHN refers to primary source of care for evaluation	Diagnosis and treatment if indicated are provided by child's primary source of care
	Persistent symptoms of visual discomfort or fatigue associated with use of the eyes		
	Suspicion or presence of strabismus		
	Absent or abnormal reflected retinal reflexes or fundus abnormalities		

	A visual acuity of 20/50 or worse (missing more than half the symbols on the 20/40 line or test) for children six years of age; 20/40 or worse (missing more than half the symbols on the 20/30 line or test) for children 6 years or age or over; of a difference of visual acuity between the eyes of two lines on the Snellen chart	PHA/PHN repeat Snellen. If child fails test again, PHN refers to primary source of care for consultation and/or referral to ophthalmologist	Unnecessary referrals are prevented. Record documents findings and referral
Hearing Screening		PHN performs hearing screening as part of the general examination, noting behavior in response to sound as well as speech and language development at each clinic visit for child under 4 years	Results of hearing screening are documented in record
		PHA performs individual pure-tone audiometric screening test at 1000, 2000, 3000, and 4000 Hz for child 3–4 years of age, as possible repeats test at age 5; on initial visit if over 5	

TABLE 13.1 (*Continued*)

OBJECTIVE VI (*Continued*)

Activity	Problem	Standing Orders	Expected Outcome
	Health history reveals positive finding which places child in high risk for hearing loss, delayed or abnormal speech development	PHN interprets findings to parent/s PHN schedules repeat audiometric screening test with audiologist regardless of outcome of initial test. If child fails repeat test, PHN refers to primary source of care for further evaluation	Children at high risk of hearing loss and with abnormal speech development are screened by audiologist. Medical record indicated reason for special screening and outcome
Urine Testing		PHN or other licensed nursing staff –performs test for presence of sugar, protein, and blood in the urine –uses the rapid test method known as "dipstick" –give initial test when the child is 9 months and at yearly intervals thereafter –attempts whenever possible to secure a clean catch, mid-stream urine specimen	Record documents test and results
	Urine "dipstick" reveals unexplained blood, 1+ sugar or 2+ protein	PHN –repeats test at the next voiding after careful instruction for clean catch specimen. –refers child to the primary	Avoid contaminated specimens if possible. Further evaluation is given by the pri-

Topic	Condition	Process	Outcome
		source of care, givirg results of both tests	mary source of care
Testing for anemia		PHN or laboratory staff administers standard microhematocrit measurement when child is 9 months old initially, and at 2 years, 4 years, and 9 years of age thereafter, or at any age after the initial test at the PHN's discretion	Record documents test and the results
	Hematocrit is below 35% but above 30% in the absence of other significant findings	PHN –performs nutritional assessment and dietary counseling –schedules child back in 6–8 weeks for repeat test	Hematocrit below 35 which is due to inadequate diet will improve
	Hematocrit remains below 35%	PHN requests consultation from child's primary source of care or HSA's pediatric consultant as appropriate	Further evaluation and/or referral is made as indicated Record documents assessment and plan
	The hematocrit is 30% or below, or hemoglobin is 10 grams or below	PHN refers to primary source of medical care for evaluation	Diagnosis and treatment if indicated are provided by primary source of care

TABLE 13.2 *Common Problems and Outcome Criteria in Clients Receiving*
        Child Health Services

Common Problems	Outcome Criteria
1. Family is financially unable to secure a primary source of care	payment mechanism established appointment given for CHDP clinic
2. Family is without a primary source of care	appointment into outpatient clinic
3. Physician determines child is not appropriate for CHNC due to medical problems	well child supervision is provided by PMD
4. Physician makes no recommendation for continuing care	child is seen by PMD no less than annually and as necessary in event of illness or suggested abnormality
5. Child in CHNC is ill	child is referred to private provider
6. CHDP—parents do not wish to share results of screening with school	parent has information regarding advantages of sharing child's health status with the school
7. Parent refuses a component of entire screening exam for school certification	parent has information regarding state require-ments for school entry
8. Health history and/or physical exam reveals a potentially handi-capping condition not receiving diagnostic evaluation or treatment by a source of medical care	referral is made to appropriate source of care
9. Child is underweight (less than 3rd percentile by Harvard-Iowa growth chart)	child is referred to primary source of care for evaluation treatment plan developed by provider is supported by PHN during ongoing well child supervision.

TABLE 13.2 *(Continued)*

Common Problems	Outcome Criteria
10. Low stature (less than 3rd percentile by Harvard-Iowa growth charts)	child is referred to primary source of care for evaluation
	treatment plan developed by provider is supported by PHN during ongoing well child supervision
11. Overweight (defined in protocol)	referred to primary source of care for evaluation
	treatment plan developed by provider is supported by PHN during ongoing well child supervision
12. No source of vitamin supplement in diet	adequate vitamin intake is provided via supplement in diet
13. Gross abnormality of soft and hard tissues of face and/or mouth, caries, malocclusions, infections and other dental diseases	referred to primary source of care
	parents and child have information necessary for carrying out treatment plan and for prevention of further dental disease
14. Brachial artery cuff B/P is elevated above 130/80 mm. hg. in "R" arm of child less than 6 years of age; 140/90 mm. Hg. for child 6 years of age or older	child is referred to primary source of care
15. Femoral artery pulses are absent to palpation	child referred to primary source of care
16. At 2 months of age, child is under 10 pounds	immunizations are delayed until child is over 10 pounds
17. History suggests child has had measles and/or mumps	immunizations are given
18. History reveals allergy to eggs	referred to primary source of care for immunizations

TABLE 13.2 *(Continued)*

Common Problems	Outcome Criteria
19. Immunization reaction	Parents have information to recognize and cope with immunization reaction
20. Severe immunization reaction— immediate	plan for emergency care is implemented
	child referred to primary source of care immediately and for ongoing immunization provision
21. Severe immunization reaction— delayed	parents have information necessary for taking appropriate action
	continuing provision of immunizations is done by primary source of care
22. Child is out of step with routine immunizations	immunization protocol is followed
	child's immunization status is brought up to date
23. Tuberculin skin test is positive by the Tine method or greater than 5mm in duration resulting from application of intermediate strength PPD.	child is referred to primary source of care
24. The developmental assessment reveals developmental delay not receiving diagnostic evaluation or treatment	DDST is repeated in 2 months
	parents have information regarding findings
	child is referred to primary source of care
25. Vision screening reveals: a. persistent symptoms of visual discomfort or fatigue associated with use of eyes b. suspicion or presence of strabismus	referred to primary source of care

TABLE 13.2 *(Continued)*

Common Problems	Outcome Criteria
c. absent or abnormal reflected retinal reflexes or fundus abnormalities	
d. visual acuity of 20/50 or worse for children 5 years of age, 20/40 or worse for children 6 years or older or a difference of visual acuity between eyes of 2 lines on Snellen chart	Snellen is repeated child is referred to ophthalmologist
26. Hearing screening test is failed (child does not respond in either ear to the screening level of 25 db at any one or more of the frequencies of 1000, 2000, 3000, or 4000 Hz.)	child is retested by audiologist if child fails, referral is made to primary source of care
27. Health history reveals positive findings which places child in high risk for hearing loss, delayed or abnormal speech development	child is retested by audiologist if child fails test, referral is made to primary source of care
28. Urine "dipstick" reveals unexplainable blood, 1+ sugar or 2+ protein	test is repeated using clean catch if findings positive on 2nd test, child is referred to primary source of care
29. Hematocrit is below 35% but above 30% in the absence of significant medical findings	nutritional assessment and diet counseling are provided test is repeated in 6–8 weeks hematocrit remains below 35%—referral is made to primary source of care
30. Hematocrit is 30% or below, or hemoglobin is 10 Gms or below	child is referred to primary source of care

TABLE 13.3 *Audit Tools for Measuring the Nursing Process: Child Health Services*

Objectives			
I.	To provide health services to eligible families requesting well child health care from the Health Services Agency.		
	1. Was a determination of eligibility for CHNC made by the PHN?	Yes	No	NA
	2. Did the PHN conduct an interview and gather standardized data base?	Yes	No	NA
	3. Was a physical inspection of the child done by PHN?	Yes	No	NA
	4. Was family given an explanation of services available in CHNC?	Yes	No	NA
	5. Was a determination for eligibility for CHDP made?	Yes	No	NA
	6. Was a determination of eligibility for Outpatient Health care clinics made?	Yes	No	NA
II.	To identify and to notify the child's primary source of medical care that the family has intent to utilize CHNC.		
	1. Did the PHN give family a letter of intent?	Yes	No	NA
III.	To determine the intervals that the physician requests the child enrolled in CHNC to return for continuation of primary care.		
	1. Did the PHN follow recommendations of primary provider for periodic referral back for care?	Yes	No	NA
IV.	To provide periodic evaluations of health status through performance of physical, dental, and nutritional assessments integrated throughout with anticipatory and situational counseling.		

TABLE 13.3 *(Continued)*

Objectives			
1. Were appointments made into CHNC, CHDP, and General Medical Clinic at intervals recommended in Child Health Services Protocols?	Yes	No	NA
2. Were parents given the Child Health Supervision Record with explanation of findings of each visit?	Yes	No	NA
3. If CHDP, were parents provided with a written summary of screening?	Yes	No	NA
4. If CHDP, was certification for school entry provided?	Yes	No	NA
5. Did the health history include:			
a. demographic data	Yes	No	NA
b. details of pregnancy	Yes	No	NA
c. history of birth	Yes	No	NA
d. history of neonatal period	Yes	No	NA
e. illness history	Yes	No	NA
f. hospitalization history	Yes	No	NA
g. summary of growth and development	Yes	No	NA
h. immunization history	Yes	No	NA
i. family health history	Yes	No	NA
j. nutritional history	Yes	No	NA

TABLE 13.3 *(Continued)*

Objectives			

6. Was interval history elicited at each
   clinic visit?   Yes   No   NA

7. Did the PHN perform physical examination
   at each clinic visit?   Yes   No   NA

8. Did the physical examination include:

   a. skin
                                                          Yes   No   NA

   b. head
                                                          Yes   No   NA

   c. eyes
                                                          Yes   No   NA

   d. ears
                                                          Yes   No   NA

   e. nose
                                                          Yes   No   NA

   f. mouth
                                                          Yes   No   NA

   g. throat
                                                          Yes   No   NA

   h. neck
                                                          Yes   No   NA

   i. chest
                                                          Yes   No   NA

   j. abdomen
                                                          Yes   No   NA

   k. genitalia
                                                          Yes   No   NA

   l. extremities
                                                          Yes   No   NA

   m. brachial and femoral pulses
                                                          Yes   No   NA

Table 13.3 *(Continued)*

Objectives			
9. Was measurement of height and weight taken at each clinic visit?	Yes	No	NA
10. Was head circumference measured at each visit until 12 months?	Yes	No	NA
11. Was a determination of nutritional status made at each visit?	Yes	No	NA
12. Was anticipatory and situational counseling relative to nutritional needs of child and family performed at each clinic visit?	Yes	No	NA
13. Did PHN perform oral health inspection including soft and hard tissues of face and mouth at each clinic visit?	Yes	No	NA
14. Did PHN counsel parents regarding oral hygiene and diet?	Yes	No	NA

V. To provide routine immunizations and tuberculin skin testing.

1. Was initial series begun at 2 months or later?	Yes	No	NA
2. Did child receive 3 injections of DPT, 0.5 cc IM?	Yes	No	NA
3. Did PHN allow at least 4 weeks between immunizations?	Yes	No	NA
4. Was first booster of DPT given at 12 months after last injection of initial series?	Yes	No	NA
5. Was 2nd booster of DPT given at 5 years of age?	Yes	No	NA
6. Was initial series of trivalent oral polio vaccine begun when child was 2 months of age or older?	Yes	No	NA
7. Were 3 doses of oral polio vaccine, gtts 2, p.o. given at 2 month intervals?	Yes	No	NA

TABLE 13.3 *(Continued)*

Objectives			
8. Was 1st oral polio booster, gtts 2, p.o. given at 12 months after last dose of initial series?	Yes	No	NA
9. Was 2nd polio booster, gtts 2, p.o. given at 5 years of age?	Yes	No	NA
10. Was combined measles and mumps vaccine given when child was 1 year or older?	Yes	No	NA
11. Was initial Tine test done when child was 9 months or older?	Yes	No	NA
12. Did child receive yearly tuberculin test thereafter?	Yes	No	NA

VI.   To perform selected health screening procedures such as Denver Developmental Screening Test, vision and hearing screening, hematocrit and urine screening, as a part of the assessment process.

1. Was DDST performed when child was:			
a. 12 months	Yes	No	NA
b. 2 years	Yes	No	NA
c. 4 years	Yes	No	NA
2. Were findings interpreted to parents?	Yes	No	NA
3. Was situational and anticipatory counseling related to development provided to parents?	Yes	No	NA
4. Did PHN perform inspection of external eye at each clinic visit?	Yes	No	NA
5. Was cover test utilized at each clinic visit?	Yes	No	NA

TABLE 13.3 *(Continued)*

Objectives			
6. Was retinal reflex evaluated on initial clinic visit? ·	Yes	No	NA
7. Was Snellen screening performed when child was 3–4 years of age and annually thereafter?	Yes	No	NA
8. Did PHN perform hearing screening at each clinic visit for child under 4 years of age?	Yes	No	NA
9. Was individual puretone audiometric screening test done for child 3–4 years of age?	Yes	No	NA
10. Was audiometric testing repeated at age 5?	Yes	No	NA
11. Were findings of hearing testing interpreted to parents?	Yes	No	NA
12. Was the child's urine tested for presence of sugar, protein, and blood at age 9 months?	Yes	No	NA
13. Was urine testing done at yearly intervals?	Yes	No	NA
14. Was the standard microhematocrit measurement administered when child was:			
a. 9 months	Yes	No	NA
b. 2 years	Yes	No	NA
c. 4 years	Yes	No	NA
d. 9 years	Yes	No	NA

Source: Adapted by the Santa Cruz County Health Services Agency, Santa Cruz, Calif., from Irene Ramey, "Setting Nursing Standards and Evaluating Care," *Journal of Nursing Administration,* May–June 1973.

REFERENCES

AMERICAN NURSES' ASSOCIATION, CONGRESS ON NURSING PRACTICE. *Standards of Nursing Practice.* Kansas City, Mo.: The Association, 1973.

BENEDIKTER, HELEN. *The Nursing Audit—A Necessity (How Shall It Be Done?)* New York: National League for Nursing, 1973.

BERG, H. "Nursing Audit and Outcome Criteria." *Nursing Clinics of North America* 9, no. 2 (1974):331–35.

BLOCH, DORIS. "Some Crucial Terms in Nursing: What Do They Really Mean?" *Nursing Outlook* 22 (November 1974):689–94.

COUNCIL OF HOME HEALTH AGENCIES and COMMUNITY HEALTH SERVICES. *Accreditation of Home Health Agencies and Community Nursing Services: Criteria and Guide for Preparing Reports.* New York: National League for Nursing, 1976.

DAUBERT, ELIZABETH A. "A System to Evaluate Home Health Care Services." *Nursing Outlook* 25 (March 1977):168–71.

FROEBE, DORIS J., and BAIN, R. JOYCE, *Quality Assurance Programs and Controls in Nursing.* St. Louis: C. V. Mosby Co., 1976.

GOLD, HAROLD, et al. "Peer Review: A Working Experiment." *Nursing Outlook* 21 (October 1973):634–36.

JOINT COMMISSION ON ACCREDITATION OF HOSPITALS, NURSING SERVICES. *An Accreditation Manual for Hospitals.* Chicago, 1971.

KEELER, JANE D. "The Process of Program Evaluation." *Nursing Outlook* 20 (May 1972):316–19.

KELLY, MARY E., and ROESSLER, LINDA M. "Development of Interdisciplinary Problem-Oriented Recording in a Public Health Nursing Agency." *Journal of Nursing Administration* VI (December 1976):24–31.

KRUMME, URSEL. "The Case for Criterion-Referenced Measurement." *Nursing Outlook* 23 (December 1975):764–70.

LEWIS, EDITH P. "Accountability: How, for What, and to Whom?" *Nursing Outlook* 20 (May 1972):315.

NATIONAL LEAGUE FOR NURSING. *Community Health Agency Evaluation.* New York: National League for Nursing, 1976.

PASSOS, JOYCE Y. "Accountability: Myth or Mandate?" *Journal of Nursing Administration* III (May–June 1973):16–23.

PHANEUF, MARIA C. *The Nursing Audit: Profile for Excellence.* New York: Appleton-Century-Crofts, 1972.

———. *The Nursing Audit,* 2nd ed. New York: Appleton-Century-Crofts, 1976.

PHANEUF, MARIA C., and WANDELT, MABEL A. "Quality Assurance in Nursing." *Nursing Forum* XII, no. 4 (1974):328–45.

PORTER, PATRICIA. "Protocols and Audits." Division of Nursing, Santa Cruz County Health Services Agency, Santa Cruz, Calif., 1976.

RAMEY, I. "Setting Nursing Standards and Evaluating Care." *Journal of Nursing Administration* 3 (April–May 1973):35–43.

SCHLOTFELDT, ROZELLA. "Planning for Progress." *Nursing Outlook* 21 (December 1973):766–70.

TAYLOR, JOYCE. "Measuring the Outcomes of Nursing Care." *Nursing Clinics of North America* 9 (June 1974):337–49.

STEVENS, BARBARA. *The Nurse as Executive.* Contemporary Publishing, 1975.

WEED, L. L. *Medical Records, Medical Education, and Patient Care.* Chicago: Year Book Publishers, 1971.

ZIMMER, MARIE. "Quality Assurance for Outcomes of Patient Care." *Nursing Clinics of North America* 9 (June 1974):305–15.

ZIMMER, MARIE, and ASSOCIATES. "Guidelines for Development of Outcome Criteria." *Nursing Clinics of North America* 9 (June 1974):317–21.

14. Community Health Nurses in Action: A Case Study

Ruth P. Fleshman
Sarah Ellen Archer

INTRODUCTION

Much of this book is written for nurses who are new to community nursing. We feel that an excellent way to illustrate many of the concepts and techniques that have been discussed thus far is to present a case study of community nurses in an actual work setting. This study describes work that we and our colleagues in community nursing have done and are still doing in a rural community. We first present the case study that describes the area being served and the process by which we community nurses gradually became involved in the community's ongoing concerns with health. We then pull out and discuss some of the principles and methods we used with a variety of client groups. Unlike other chapters, we refer here to our own participation in these events by using our names—try to forget that we are also the writers! It seemed the best way to clarify who did what without being too stilted. And because several sets of nurses were involved, we have had to come up with special terms for each. We hope you can keep straight which particular set we mean from the context.

Writing down all the information about a community even at a single moment in time is never possible. At best, a case study is like a single photograph that momentarily stops the whole flow of action coming from history and going on into the future. The community is never static and

403

so what is true today may become different tomorrow. For this reason we emphasize the *process* of what happened in a brief period in the past, while mentioning only some of the outcomes and forecasting some probable futures.

CASE STUDY

The coastal plain of Pomo County, like other north-coast areas, is separated from the central population and services by the coastal mountain range. Thus services are accessible to the coastal residents only over difficult roads. The population of twenty thousand is sparsely spread over an area served by 110 miles of winding, two-lane state roads. The only significant settlements in our target area are Charleston, Pomo, and Yerba Buena. Local maps are dotted with names of settlements, but these are sometimes no more than a barn with an old plaque indicating a lumber town stood there forty or sixty years ago. Other towns are little more than a cluster of decaying wood houses around a decrepit bar or a combined grocery–gas station–post office. Old school buildings are closed for lack of children; some are converted to tourist trade; others are used as private dwellings.

The coastal plain has been settled by whites since 1852, with lumbering, fishing, and sheep ranching the only current local significant sources of income. Within the last two decades the Pomo Coast began to develop a modest art enclave and, more recently, became one of the low-cost areas to which many alienated youth moved in their search for a rural utopia they could not find in San Francisco's Haight-Ashbury. They arrived to become uncomfortably associated with remnants of an older population composed of Scandinavian lumbering folk, Portuguese fishermen, long-time American rural people (some descended from unreconstructed exiles from the Civil War South), and a smattering of retired city people who had come to run the summer motels and live on pensions just adequate, at best, to the lower costs of Pomo.

Remnants of the indigenous Indian tribes live scattered throughout this county. A small cluster live in the Yerba Buena area. The agricultural central part of the county provides some work for Mexican-Americans; few are seen on the coast. Occasional Asians live along the coast, where some of the Chinese have lived for several generations and a few Japanese returned after their imprisonment during World War II. Although blacks are counted in the census data, there are disproportionately few in the coastal strip. Black families stationed at the small military base in the central county are reportedly advised to seek their recreation outside the local area.

Tourists envisioning sandy beaches, ocean swimming, and days of endless sunshine come from all over to California. Those who travel over the twisting road from the central freeways are shockingly disappointed. The heat from inland valleys collides with chilly ocean air and the coast is generally fog-shrouded most of each summer day. Temperatures are low enough that daytime wear requires at least a sweater and coats are always at hand. Although little actual rain falls in summer, the fog is thick enough to require windshield wipers. The chill Alaska current makes for occasional good salmon seasons, but no swimming is possible without wet suits to combat the cold. The fabled abalone diving grounds have been depleted by local and outside skindivers. Local fishermen rage while huge automated fishing factories from Japan and Russia sieve the offshore fishing territory. Lumbering has fallen more and more into the ownership of giant nationwide corporations, none of which is based nearby.

Labor unions are ineffective in rural areas in general, and Pomo workers have few aids in their battles against a high rate of unemployment. Rumor has it that workers are regularly laid off from the mills just before they would have qualified for state unemployment benefits. Moreover, getting on welfare roles is very difficult since the country itself is very poor and the conservative policy makers rank welfare services very low in their priorities. Applicants frequently complain they are endlessly barraged with bureaucratic harassment each time they try to seek service at the distant county seat.

Thus, the economic setbacks that began to be felt statewide in the early part of 1970 had little impact since the coast area had long been experiencing recession conditions; lumbering had been sharply curtailed and coastal small-boat fishing was apparently becoming a dying trade. The local Economic Opportunity Council project, never as militant as any urban project, had nevertheless stirred much county controversy by 1971 by organizing local volunteers to distribute food commodities during the last five months of 1970 to the coastal poor. The county government refused to participate in the food stamp program. The January 1971 food distribution served twenty-seven hundred who qualified to receive these packages often made up of white sugar, white flour, lard, much butter, some canned vegetables, occasionally canned lunch meat, powdered milk—whatever products the Department of Agriculture was stockpiling to help maintain farm subsidies. (Urban nurses who had assumed food stamps were universally available found the commodities both demeaning and unnutritious.) On the two days a month when commodities were distributed, the poor had to line up in front of the EOC warehouse beside the highway outside Charleston. The recipients always allowed the elderly and disabled to go through ahead of the younger poor. Some of the unemployed young men volunteered to act as proxies for persons too ill or old to leave their homes and thus collected and delivered their commodities. The local radio talk-shows those days focused on the outrageousness of able-bodied people taking free food paid for by the hardworking taxpayers. The fact that some of the men were long haired and bearded only added to the outrage since it identified them in the eyes of the callers as outsiders and voluntarily poor.

HEALTH CARE

The entire coastal plain was served by ten physicians in 1969 when this study began. There were two small hospitals in Charleston, as well as the office of the one public health nurse assigned to the coast from the head office, thirty tortuous miles across the mountains at the county seat. The distance to the nearest metropolitan area from Pomo is 155 miles, much of it along winding, hilly roads. Health care services were clearly inadequate to the area's needs (table 14.1).

Both of the small hospitals in Charleston were inadequate to serve the coastal area. One had been condemned as a fire hazard when its physician-owner refused to bring it up to code. The other was safe but too small, cold, and dreary. A bond issue had been approved by the local voters who pinned their hopes for better health care on the construction of a new facility. The people did not realize that the new hospital would be administered by exactly the same personnel they had so severely criticized in the campaign for the bond issue for inept management of the current facility.

Perhaps in reflection of the nationwide trend in rising expectations for health care, many residents had begun criticizing the adequacy of local health services. The old rural fatalism was being replaced in some by a desire to upgrade the quality of physician care as well as increase their numbers. Care was frequently unavailable, either because residents could not afford it, would not beg for it, or were rejected as unacceptable by the medical professionals. The last was the experience of many of the counterculture youth.

Ruth, a nurse researching communal youth, was working with some of those living in communes in Pomo County and eventually made contact with a local psychiatric social worker, Sue, who shared Ruth's concern for setting up some service geared to their young clients. Because they shared a common background of work in free clinics, the two professionals considered this model for delivering care to their clients. They decided against a free clinic since the social worker felt that the hostility of the local "straight" residents might well take the form of a fire bomb some rowdy Saturday night. Later, a group of timid but sympathetic

TABLE 14.1 *Medical Care Resources and Demographic Distributions*

Ratio of physicians to population:

Pomo Coast	1:2000±	(1970)
San Francisco	1:306	(1970)

Selected demographic distributions, U.S. Census, 1970:

Over age 65:

State	9.0 percent
Total County	11.1
Pomo	14.3
Charleston	11.8
Yerba Buena	9.7

Growth of County population 1960 to 1970: 0.1 percent

Distribution of population

   Vicinities of Pomo and Charleston: 26.3 percent of county total
   Coastal area: approximately 40 percent of county total

Leading causes of death for Pomo County 1969:

Circulatory diseases	280 deaths
Neoplasms, malignant	81
Respiratory system diseases	44
Digestive system diseases	35
Non-vehicular accidents	28
Motor vehicle traffic accidents	22
Certain diseases of early infancy	14
Neoplasms, benign	11
Suicide	10

---

health professionals volunteered their services and a telephone-tree referral system was tried. In this system callers seeking aid reach a publicized, central answering service. After the caller explains what is needed,
referral is made to another number where specific information and help
on the stated need can be arranged. This operation is like the volunteer
"switchboards" that have developed in many communities to provide information and referral services. This system proved too awkward in Pomo
County, and the two health professionals realized that a visible facility of
some kind was needed, especially if the transients who could not break
into such a closed system were to be served. Use of the referral system required prior knowledge of its availability, which meant that service would

not expand beyond those already in contact with it except by very slow word-of-mouth publicity. The nurse and social worker finally realized that many of the problems of providing a special service to the counter-culture youth in the area actually came back to the issue of the dislike by the resident power structure for this minority. By this time, a number of local youth activists had begun to work with the social worker around the problems they were meeting in trying to get health care. Out of all of these activities grew the decision to develop a health center where people could get acceptable health services.

FORMATION OF THE HEALTH CENTER OF THE POMO COAST

After many informal meetings among interested young people of the area, an executive board was constituted from those most involved in developing plans for service. When the fact that needs existed far beyond the young became clear, the board was expanded to include more than the youth who had begun the project and especially to involve some of the older people able to influence community attitudes. After more than a year of planning, community members and health professionals in 1971 established the Health Center of the Pomo Coast, a nonprofit corporation aiming to improve health care to all residents of the coastal plain.

Because the local physicians were immersed in their daily caseloads, volunteer services came mainly from other health workers (primarily nurses but also a local pharmacist, lab technicians, and excorpsmen) as well as laypeople. A number of the local nurses early expressed a desire to work toward remedying what they had long felt were glaring defects in care delivery. When the center opened, six nurses gave their time to staff it one day a week and to develop health educational programs geared to the needs and wants of the community. Examples of the latter included an evening seminar on nutrition that brought together various types of persons with widely divergent beliefs about food (vegetarian, herbal, macrobiotic, scientific, and so on) that was attended by ninety-three people. A series of meetings was held centering on natural childbirth with a somewhat similar format to explore the range of beliefs present in this highly unorthodox population.

Services at the health center, in the first stage, were health education, first aid, and referral as indicated to available medical and dental services. Space was donated by the local Presbyterian church. One community physician agreed to provide whatever medical supervision the nurses felt they needed. Several other physicians agreed to treat free any patients referred from the center if they could not pay for services. Supportive services, such as laboratory, were slow to develop. In general, the board refused to use the idea of "free" and spoke rather of the health center as a "low-cost center."

In the first few months of the center's once-a-week operation, there was concern about the extent to which demand would develop. If community response were great, the existing medical resources would be overwhelmed since the physicians were already working nearly as close to peak as they wished to. Members of the executive board engaged in continuing attempts to recruit professionals by touting the attractions of living in the area as well as trying to muster resources to subsidize them on their arrival. They were able to recruit a dentist and a general practitioner from New York. Also, a pediatrician from the interior valley was persuaded to begin a regular office day on the coast, which could be expanded if the demand was sufficient.

The Pomo Coast's isolation from centers of medical care and education created many problems in getting care and in upgrading the quality of available care. If such a deficiency made the residents more self-reliant, it also created health hazards not encountered where health resources are qualitatively and quantitatively greater. The nurses staffing the health center expressed a desire to provide high-quality service to their clients; yet their knowledge of nursing trends, professional roles, support possibilities, and care delivery skills was clearly restricted.

To assist the local nurses, Ruth, who was also on the faculty at a school of nursing in the metropolis, proposed a program to bring in nurses who had completed their master's degree in nursing. During a summer's residency experience in community nursing, these graduate students could work with the Pomo County nurses in the health center. Ruth's written proposal was submitted to the state health department and funded by them through special project funds (title 314d of the Comprehensive Health Planning Act of 1966, P.L. 89–749). The project was designed to serve multiple functions: provide advanced nursing input from a metropolitan health center campus, immerse the master's level nursing students in a community health system, and expand the coverage and services offered by the Pomo health center. In addition, the project was designed to test the extent to which nurses could function as primary care practitioners in an area where such services were viewed as the domain of physicians.

Even with the active support of state health officials in speeding the proposal, moving from idea to actual receipt of funds took nearly six months. The proposal had to be endorsed by the health center board and the school of nursing administration and had to be heard and approved by the state comprehensive health planning agency and after that by the local comprehensive health planning council for Pomo County. After approval in each of these steps, the proposal was sent to the state capitol for fiscal review. Since the funds had to be awarded out of a budget due to lapse by the end of June, there was some urgency to getting it processed but bureaucratic wheels take their own sweet time. A sympathetic official finally phoned notice of approval, but the project could not officially begin until the contract was actually in hand at the school of nursing's administrative office.

THE SUMMER RESIDENCY PROGRAM

After the bureaucratic intricacies of both the state department of public health and the university were unwound and the contract actually validated to everyone's satisfaction, four graduate students in nursing moved to Pomo County to begin a twelve-week residency program in community health nursing. Their coming had been publicized to the coastal communities by newspaper articles in the Pomo *Lighthouse* and over the Charleston radio station, both of which were exceedingly cooperative in using whatever materials were given them about the graduate students and their consulting faculty. The four nurses were selected to be as broadly representative of nursing clinical specialties as any four could be.

Sister Margaret, a member of a religious order, came from southern California, although she spent nine years of her childhood in Brazil and still speaks Portuguese. In the fifteen years of her nursing career, she had worked in a wide variety of specialties as a supervisor, including coronary and intensive care units, pediatrics, and psychiatry. Her master's program had been in community mental health.

Flora, during her five years of nursing, worked primarily with youth and young adults in clinic situations. The year before entering the master's program, she taught pediatric nursing at a midwest university where her husband was pursuing graduate studies in history. Her master's program in pediatrics had increased her abilities in working with children and expectant parents.

Mary was born and raised in the southern part of the state. After receiving her nursing degree there, she worked as a staff nurse at a major burn treatment center. Later she taught nurses in a general hospital for one-and-one-half years. Her main interest in expectant families in the community was reflected in both her community health nursing major and her work in the master's program with a nurse-run prenatal storefront clinic.

Joan came from the midwest and had received her nursing degree from a midwest university before coming west for graduate studies. She had most of her nursing experience in intensive care units and surgical recovery areas. Her master's degree focused on medical-surgical special-ization, thereby rounding out the clinical range of the group.

Three members of the graduate faculty of the school of nursing also participated in this program to provide the faculty consultation required for its definition as a clinical residency faculty program. Their areas of ex-pertise were in community health (Ruth), community mental health (Jane), and maternity nursing (Kit). (Sarah did not become a part of the community nursing faculty until after 1971 when she became involved in other Pomo projects of her own.)

The first major problem was to locate housing for the four nurses; because of the delay in funding, community members had not held the rental housing they had tentatively pledged. This problem was only the beginning of the impact of the precarious economic conditions encoun-tered during this summer program. Flora and Mary found a farmhouse ten miles inland that they were able to afford by sharing it with other health workers also involved in summer projects. Sister Margaret found a suitable apartment within the city of Charleston itself. Joan finally lo-cated a trailer in the fishing settlement near Charleston.

At their first joint meeting with the health center personnel, the new nurses realized that the center's six volunteer nurses were relying on the newcomers to work miracles when their leader presented a monumental list of projects they saw as outcomes of the summer's program. The new nurses (hereinafter called resident-nurses) listened through the entire list, but then gently suggested that their own particular goals and interests had led them to consider three community projects: prenatal classes, child rearing, and outreach to the elderly to assess their needs for medical and health care. In addition they intended to try to expand the hours and services of the health center itself. They proposed that each of them should work with one of the local nurses as a counterpart in areas of shared interests, as well as in the operations of the health center sessions. Because several local nurses were, or were planning to become, pregnant, interest in the prenatal project was high. Mild interest was expressed in the parenting classes, and none at all in the problems of the aged.

At the start of the summer, the clinic was moved from a Sunday school room it had shared with a class in the basement of the Presbyterian church to a huge, bare room in an abandoned schoolhouse leased to the EOC project by a local lumber-land development firm. This move came as a deterrent to the planned full-week clinic operation since the room was without heat or lights. It also required painting, wiring, plumbing work, carpentry, and a variety of other modifications before the various county inspectors would contemplate approval of gas and electricity. Each set of improvements only resulted in more demands by inspectors, and the summer ended before either utility was used. Community groups as well as the resident-nurses spent many hours making the needed modifications both to meet utility inspections and to attempt esthetic improvements in the barn-like room. Patient privacy was one of the nurses' major concerns, and two tiny closet-like rooms were converted with donated furniture and screens into examining and treatment rooms. Examinations would be unnecessarily painful when both client and nurse were shivering with cold, and at least these rooms faced the afternoon sun, if there was any.

SETTING UP SPECIFIC PROGRAMS

The first step taken by Sister Margaret and Joan in assessing care for the elderly was to contact various health professionals in the area. Their efforts ranged from visits to or other attempts to contact local practicing physicians, hospital and public health staffs, and former health care workers. A cold reception was found and was consistently accompanied by such statements as "you are not needed" and "our senior citizens are well taken care of." These comments suggested that the resident-nurses were considered redundant and/or that their presence constituted some kind of threat to other health care personnel. Attending meetings of the senior citizens club, going to church, and actually making home calls soon convinced the nurses, however, that the opinions of the health care people were not shared by the elderly. Three major categories of need were eventually identified: (1) patients attempting to carry out medical regimes with unclear understandings of instructions, (2) patients discharged from the hospital without instruction, supplies, or realistic plans for followup, and (3) persons without any medical surveillance and unwilling to seek it due to fears of the expense involved. Few of these persons saw the health center as a possible solution to their needs, partly because of its distance from their homes, but also because of its association with the youth of the community.

Information about a home nursing service that had reportedly failed for lack of need was uncovered during the summer. Contacts with local physicians revealed that few had even the vaguest awareness that such a service had existed. On the other hand, they seemed acutely aware of the need for such a program and were eager to refer patients who needed assistance through the health center. One physician attempted to define the resident-nurses' role as persuading the hospital to engage them for inservice staff education for discharge planning. This role was incompatible with the objectives of the program but may have contributed to later moves by the hospital staff for some in-service program. Another physician decided that the resident-nurses' appropriate function should be to assist him in liberalizing the patient admission policies of the local hospital.

Mary concentrated primarily on expectant parent education and

Lamaze psychoprophylactic preparation for childbirth. Although none of the local nurses' interest persisted, a local Lamaze instructor was found who agreed to continue working after the summer with the health center clientele and to barter goods in exchange for her services with people who hadn't the cash to pay for them. Although there was no obstetrician on the coast, one in the county seat inland reportedly planned to hire a nurse to conduct expectant parent classes even though the patients would have to travel across the mountains for the actual deliveries. The emphasis among alienated youth on home deliveries presented a major problem since only one physician was willing to provide even prenatal care for young women who expressed their intention to deliver at home. Even he refused to see these women after a few of them evidenced complications in their deliveries. Finding obstetrical care had not been worked out by the end of summer, and so several pregnant women had no medical followup available to them on terms they could accept.

Early in the summer, a newly arrived pediatrician invited Flora to co-lead a discussion group on child rearing. Parents in the community expressed polite interest but few attended and even the pediatrician lost interest after a few sessions. Two explanations for the low attendance were offered. First, the "hip" population, pursuing a primitive lifestyle, were more oriented to action and would not respond to intellectual discussion groups. Second, the more conventional local residents were suspicious of any newcomers and would hesitate to come until such a group proved itself over a period of many months. Indeed, longevity in the community was highly valued for individuals and organizations, and acceptance of both the nurses and the health center proceeded at a much slower rate than might have occurred in an urban setting.

A well-baby clinic was proposed for the health center in July. It was seen as an opportunity to develop a program to assist the attending physician and to develop nursing in such a clinic. If a stronger nursing identity in the clinic could evolve, it might be possible to then move toward some pediatric nurse-practitioner skills, an interest shared by both Flora and one of the local nurses. Lack of county funding and procedural details, however, blocked the opening of such a clinic at the time.

Almost every attempt at innovation originating either from the local health center volunteers or the resident-nurses seemed to meet with frustration. During the summer, the local volunteer nurses had more and more difficulty in meeting their commitments to the health center, and they gradually withdrew their services, thereby leaving the resident-nurses to perform staffing duties and to recruit new local volunteers. Their project objectives shifted toward documenting and demonstrating community need in the hope of involving other persons in the process so that what they were doing in the community would continue after their summer residency was over.

Clinic experiences made many client needs very evident to the resident-nurses. Needs for pregnancy and abortion counseling had been felt early in the health center's operation. On any given day as many as half of the clients served might request pregnancy testing and the consequent counseling regarding birth control, prenatal referral, or abortion services. The lack of antenatal services of any kind on the coastal strip necessitated referral to other cities: usually to the county seat for prenatal care and 155 miles to the metropolis for abortions. The entire nursing staff and lay volunteers interested in pregnancy and abortion counseling felt inadequately prepared to assist these clients in crisis. A one-day workshop was planned by the resident-nurses with resource persons from the school of nursing's graduate faculty to discuss abortion laws, counseling, the normal crisis of pregnancy, and nurses' roles in each. One result of this meeting was a planned counseling service for all women coming in for pregnancy testing or counseling. This service included referral where feasible for prenatal care, dissemination of available written information, counseling and referral for abortion, and, during the summer, a program of counseling and health education for expectant parents. Arrangements were made for three local volunteers to attend a planned parenthood training session on abortion and pregnancy counseling in the near future.

During the summer the clinic was open two half-days weekly for medical drop-in services and one half-day for Lamaze classes and pregnancy counseling. Clients were sent in by their physicians for dressing changes, catheter irrigations, and similar technical procedures. Many came in on their own for evaluation of various symptoms or problems: itching, rashes, infected wounds, sick children, persistent coughs. Where the explanation was clear—as for instance poison oak—the clinic staff advised helpful procedures. Appropriate referrals were arranged as indicated. Seventy clients were seen each month and approximately thirty-five to forty referrals were made for physician care.

The community's response to the health center was overwhelming to the medical resources of the area. The four physicians most supportive of the health center in the early stages soon began refusing to take any further referrals; they said they did not have time to take new patients. Another possible reason for their refusing center referrals was the failure of clients to keep the barter bargains they had made with the physicians for the care received. One of the nurses attempted to meet this challenge by urging expansion of counseling to include advising use of various standard (nonprescription) remedies. There was much hesitation by the others, and her attempts did not continue long enough to create a positive model for nonphysician care. Nurses as deliverers of primary care seemed possible only with longer and closer contact with local physicians and less conservatism among the nurses attempting this role. The two immediate steps toward alleviating care shortages considered by the local physicians and a consultant from Regional Medical Programs were (1) encouraging more physicians to move to the area to practice and (2) encouraging group medical practices. To this end, Sue, the director of the health center, recruited a new physician from New York. However, upon arrival he showed no eagerness to take over medical direction of the health center or even contribute toward its services.

COMMUNITY OUTREACH

In spite of the lack of interest in the pediatrician's parent classes, the nurses decided to try the community class method again since a number of the people in the inland area expressed informal interest in discussions on some kind of first aid self-help. Clearly, success was more likely if classes were developed around what the people wanted. After careful negotiations with the conservative grange hall directors, that site was used for an afternoon home nursing–first aid course. Attendance at the first session was fifteen (everyone invited in that small community came). Interest continued through the six weekly sessions, whose subjects included setting up a first aid kit; treatment of common home emergencies such as burns, cuts, sprains, and fractures; and childhood and other communicable diseases such as hepatitis. The importance of these sessions seemed twofold: the first was to share health information and experiences. The second was to make known the role of nurses living in the community and working with the health center in order to make that service real and legitimate in the eyes of the townspeople. More people brought their health problems to the center after the classes began. (None of the community residents attending these classes were among those felled by the subsequent hepatitis outbreak in that area!)

Late in the summer an opportunity for community outreach came from one of the clients at the center who invited Flora to come to the river to speak with some of the fifty to one hundred persons living along its edge. Diarrhea was a recurrent problem in the summer community camped by the river. Flora and her counterpart local nurse talked with twenty or so adolescents and young adults gathered on the beach. Soon the crowd tripled as they explored the causes and treatment of diarrhea. Overcrowding and indifference to minimal sanitation contributed to cyclic recontamination and the recurrence of diarrhea. Leadership in the group was diffuse and few mentioned any commitment to action. That the conditions leading to the problem would persist seemed likely. Counseling on a one-to-one basis provided some help with individual health problems for some and a few came in to the center as suggested. The nurses gathered river water and stool samples, which were sent to the state health department for analysis. (The water analysis was still pending by summer's end, but the samples showed no bacterial source of infection.) Consequently, no general treatment was instituted and individuals had to rely on private medical care for treatment.

The resident-nurses' regular practice of identifying themselves in even casual encounters as the summer nurses at the health center served as an opener for expression of many concerns about health problems that local residents had no one to ask about. Contacting community members outside the health center allowed all the participants to identify health needs, engage in on-the-spot health education, express concern and caring, and suggest appropriate ways to deal with matters requiring investigation or further work. Knowing about the nurses before actually meeting them made it easier for residents to accept this unusual kind of role. Sister Margaret's uniform was a bonus for recognition since it provided an entry with the older community members. She was regularly stopped coming out of mass to be told of elderly people needing home visits. Health issues were raised in a wide variety of settings: stores, living rooms, bars, restaurants, street corners, in short, wherever people gathered to talk. Their limited time in the community motivated the nurses to work more intensively on breaking through to local people than would be necessary for permanent nurses. What they accomplished did indicate how effective nurses can be who keep their nursing identity visible and operative even when "off duty."

During the summer, a young man came to stay at the farmhouse while he worked on a campaign to persuade local voters to approve a referendum permitting an out-of-state land developer to create a giant retirement community in a ranchland area of eastern Pomo County. The defeat of the referendum reflected not only ecological consciousness but a deep hostility to outsiders. This same theme operated in slowing the innovative processes attempted by the resident-nurses and the new physicians, who assumed health care standards were a purely professional issue. It was later the rallying point for the refusal of permits to a franchise recreation facility on the coast and was an impetus to the EOC's creating an indigenous homemaker service in the face of a possible arrival of a national proprietary enterprise. When Ann (see the update section later in the chapter) planned to regularize her home nursing service, this element was deliberately invoked to mobilize local support.

A student from another university was carrying out her own summer project testing all the water wells in the area around Mary and Flora's farmhouse. By summer's end she published her report that almost all of them were grossly contaminated with coliform organisms. Although such a report would ordinarily create a major furor and result in immediate correction, it was received by the local people with profound boredom. They dismissed it and commented that the water had been the same for forty years and they saw no reason to worry about it now. All the resident-nurses and their faculty and guests had noted that very soon after coming to visit they would be afflicted with diarrhea, which was given various earthy nicknames. Some also commented that minor skin abrasions would invariably become infected until they returned to the metropolitan water supply. The temporary process used was to wash only with hexaclorophene soap and drink as little unboiled water as possible. Even ice cubes were made from boiled water to keep cocktails moderately sanitary. The foolhardiness of the local residents was borne out the next fall; there was a major outbreak of hepatitis when one of the local merchants refused to isolate himself while still jaundiced. One of the local volunteer nurses was hired temporarily by the health department to work with the health officer attempting to introduce sanitary measures among the homes in the affected area. They noted that the counterculture youth in the area were not the ones most affected but the so-called straights, which thus suggested that their immunity was not as high as that of the youth who had had greater exposure to outside organisms. The physician also commented that he could no longer use the term "dirty hippy" since he found their homes were generally cleaner than were those of their straight neighbors.

During the summer residency program, the nursing faculty conducted weekly seminars for both local and resident-nurses, which, in addition to the pregnancy and abortion workshop, dealt with the community dynamics, interprofessional relations, problems of cross-clinical integration, and recruitment, retention, and in-service education for health center volunteers. One result of a seminar was the initiation of postclinic review sessions when all the nurses involved that day discussed client problems and their management as well as aspects of staff interactions. These sessions generated ideas of general interest which were then brought to meetings of the total nursing group. They also served to deal with interpersonal problems before these reached the conflict stage.

One gain was the developing contact with the county health officer. The EOC-funded program for family planning held one clinic a month in the health center office (despite the lack of heat and electricity), which gave both health department and EOC personnel a chance to become better acquainted with the health center volunteers. The public health nurse seemed to become very slightly less threatened by the resident-nurses. The EOC workers tried to aid the health center gain equipment and furnishings. Through the efforts of the school of nursing faculty, a grant was prepared for EOC requesting funding for an integrated venereal disease screening, treatment, and education program. However, national and state priorities being what they were, it was not funded. EOC staff continued attempts to find funds for a project to demonstrate the need for such a program.

As if the health center's circumstances had not been precarious enough all along, late in summer the one local nurse who had been most active in managing the health center announced that she would be moving with her community-organizer husband to another area and would no longer be able to spark the work of the center. Her withdrawal was a severe blow since she had knowledge of the community and access to local hospital personnel through her regular job there.

OUTCOMES

Based on events during the summer residency program, the following outcomes and recommendations were presented in the final report.

Health center services were expanded to include prenatal classes preparing for delivery, pregnancy testing, counseling and referral for either abortion or prenatal care, home visiting of community residents, especially the elderly, for sick care, and occasional office procedures as ordered. The overloading and subsequent loss of community physician care resources suggested a need to involve the newly recruited physician more directly or, failing that, to recruit additional physicians more specifically committed to the health center. This recommendation required some source of funding or, if at all feasible, an attempt to work out a fiscal relation with the health department.

The loss of the regular community volunteer nurses required the recruitment of more to provide the necessary minimum of service. This recommendation highlighted the need to increase the rewards of the work, possibly on a material level, at least for the support of the nurse assuming major responsibility for managing the clinic schedule.

In the demonstrated absence of an adequate level of medical care, means should be developed to permit nursing and lay volunteers to expand their roles legitimately into areas of direct care needed and wanted by clients but otherwise unavailable. This recommendation would require long and close contact with some enabling physician since both the timidity of nurses and the conservative bias of medical practitioners can only be overcome by trust developed over more than a three-month span. Several physicians indicated interest in such role expansion by the nurses but none could provide the financial backing necessary to attempt it. One inland pediatrician is reported to have hired a nurse to be trained for a pediatric practitioner role, but she had not appeared on the coast by summer's end.

In spite of attempts by the health center to establish a wide-ranging community service image, many of the older patients identified it as a service only for youth and especially those of the hip variety. In an area where those so identified constitute a despised minority, a service catering to them is not viewed as appropriate to straight people. Outreach services by the very respectable nurse-volunteers, continuing media information

appealing to problems of other than hip population, and public appearances at straight functions would be required for the survival of the clinic
and its development as a community-wide service.

One local nurse, who had expressed great personal interest in a community nurse-practitioner role in the spring, was unable to follow
through within the structure of her marital role. By year's end, she had
not only withdrawn from participation as a volunteer at the health center,
but she and her physician-husband had moved out of state, thus depriving the area of two professionals. Although causation is always complex
and peculiar to each situation, the likelihood of women still being dependent on their husbands' career movements should be considered when experimentation with new work roles for a basically female occupation is
being contemplated.

BASING NURSES IN A COMMUNITY

The acceptability and feasibility of nurses as community health
workers, even within the limited scope attempted that summer, can be
shown by the following actions. Local physicians were willing to make
referrals for home and health center nursing services. The local physicians strongly (but vainly) urged the nurses to initiate and participate in
action improving local hospital policies and in-service education programs for hospital nurses. The county health officer was willing to approve using nurses in setting up special well baby sessions and extended
nurse role within the health center. Local residents were willing to make
referrals to and accept services from the nurses. They were willing to attend evening community health education seminars and afternoon classes
in preparation for childbirth and in first aid and home nursing.

The strength of this acceptance, however, was never tested along
financial lines since services were free. In fact, whenever funding was discussed, other health professionals made clear that they were very willing
to tolerate and use free nursing services but unwilling to pay for them or
even arrange to work out funding possibilities. The evolution of an independent nurse-practitioner was a relatively new concept (in 1971 when
the residency was done) to many of the local physicians and seemed to
threaten most of the local nurses. None of the orthodox agencies responded positively to the new role, and considering other ways of supporting a nurse in such an area is clearly necessary. A fee-for-service approach may be possible if a nurse is found with the commitment to experiment with this notion.

Although the previous volunteer nurse staff underwent marked deple-
tion, the resident-nurses' efforts resulted in the recruitment of two
master's prepared nurses, one of whom had only recently moved to the
area and was known to one of the faculty (and instantly recruited). The

other was Flora, the pediatric specialist, who decided to experiment with her own interest in preschoolers and set up a child care center in conjunction with a group of local parents. She began negotiating with a group of pediatricians to be taught primary care skills and worked as volunteer coordinator of the health center services.

The impact of their residency on the other three nurses was profound. The experience provided them with a highly realistic appreciation of the complexities of attempting changes even in a relatively uncomplicated small-town health system. Joan and Mary, who both went into nursing education, have reported how the experience has influenced their teaching. Sister Margaret looks back on the summer as the single most important learning event in her education.

Becoming even temporary members of rural communities enabled the nurses to experience sharply the distinctions between urban and rural areas and their impact on health care in general and the operations of the health center in particular. The impact of the economic depression of the area was acute; funds for health concerns were clearly lacking. This fact was of little concern to those controlling the area's resources. The conflict between population sectors along age, ethnic, social, and philosophic lines was clear-cut and vital to the work of the nurses.

Although physician obstacles were frequently encountered in trying new approaches to the summer's work, the resident-nurses were most discouraged to find their fellow nurses as even more resistive to change or new ideas. Although they realized continuation of the health center would depend on recruiting new nursing staff, they simply could not carry out all the steps they knew would be required to involve other local nurses, such as locating and attending meetings of the county nurses' association, searching out license-holding nurses, and so on.

THUMBNAIL UPDATE, 1971–1978

After the summer nurses left, the health center had to decrease its services to one day a week with entirely new volunteer nurses from the community. A few new physicians settled in the area, including a board-certified obstetrician-gynecologist. Flora's preschool lasted two years under her direction and was taken over by one segment of the parent board she had established for policy direction. She worked a year as a pediatric nurse-practitioner, but the sponsoring pediatricians inland could not agree with her desire for a professional fee-for-service. She and her husband became a part of the Charleston business community and she no longer works in nursing.

The report submitted to the state following the summer residency was circulated to the local health department where it stirred a slight furor. A leaked copy of the internally added margin comments suggests that the presence of nurses in the community who were not controlled by official nursing was a territorial threat. Several notes mentioned that failures we encountered would never have occurred had we entered under the department's aegis. We predict, however, that the value of an agency-linked experience would not have outweighed its limitations on the resident-nurses' opportunities to stimulate and respond to community needs. It seems interesting that all the subsequent nursing innovations (see below) have come from outside nurses and not from bureaucratic ranks. Our experience with other large health institutions suggests that system maintenance procedures can evolve so fast that they leave no leftover energy for creative or reflective nursing innovation within the ranks.

In 1973, a small two-year private grant was made through Sue to fund nursing services in the health center. With purely volunteer staff, it had virtually collapsed but now interest was revived. After consulting Ruth, Sue began negotiating for backup services from the county health department and the EOC project. Helen, who had just completed her master's program with Ruth and Sarah, agreed to share the single salary with her friend, Suzanne, whose new master's degree was done in medical-surgical nursing. The excitement of developing an innovative service from scratch made up, at least for a while, for the low income. During the first year, they earned certificates in a family nurse-practitioner program and thus expanded both the number and extent of services offered. Their demonstration was successful enough to induce county officials to take both of them onto the payroll at full salaries. Their nurse-run clinic became an accepted part of the county health department, and special job categories were established that acknowledged the unusually high levels of their expertise.

While helping Helen try to locate housing when she first moved to Pomo, Ruth and Sarah stopped by to see Mrs. Place, an old friend of Ruth's ex-sister-in-law. Mrs. Place, the wife of one of Pomo's prominent artist-businessmen, was not an oldtimer in the area, but had lived there long enough to become a recognized social force. She was the leader of a socially prominent older women's club that had become concerned with the lack of health care and low-cost housing, especially for the elderly. They had begun to prepare a community survey to identify the extent and scope of concerns among local residents. Ruth and Sarah helped revise the survey form and eventually involved several groups of graduate students in carrying out this opinion poll and interviewing various significant figures in the coastal area about health problems. Data from these studies will eventually be used to formulate proposals for improved health care that local residents will take to the county board of supervisors and the Health Systems Agency.

Sarah introduced the concept of the 911 emergency telephone system (the single county-wide number for all emergency services: ambulance, fire, police, and so forth) to Mrs. Place and put her into contact with the local phone company official charged with installing this system. The value of such a service was clear to the women's group and they began urging local officials to move somewhat less reluctantly toward installing the system.

After the new obstetrician had been in Charleston about a year, he came to a childbirth workshop organized by members of the commune project of which Ruth was the director. There he mentioned his interest in hiring a maternity nurse-practitioner. Several months later he had interviewed several and hired Elaine, an older woman who had just completed the experimental MNP program and who just happened to be Ruth's ex-sister-in-law and Mrs. Place's old friend.

During one of the visits with Mrs. Place, she mentioned a local nurse who had been making home nursing visits and receiving no fees from those who could not afford to pay but who were covered by Medicare. Sarah began to make the contacts necessary for this nurse, Ann, to begin to qualify for reimbursement under Medicare provisions. Friends in the state health department suggested shortcuts and contacts to make this interminable process shorter.

Nothing remains in one place as time passes and many changes have occurred more recently. After being a part of the development and running of the clinic for four years, Helen began to be aware that she was repeating herself, going through routines without seeing anything new, and saying the same things over and over. In addition, the lack of social life for a young single woman in a rural area finally became a major problem as the reward of a stimulating job began to disappear. Thus a chance to combine an expanded practice with teaching led Helen away from the coast to an urban medical center with greater potential for professional and personal activities. Her post in the health clinic was taken by a newly graduated practitioner without a background of community health or the experience of pioneering this new role. Whether the remaining nurse, Suzanne, can share this spirit with her remains to be seen. Whatever else can be predicted, the fact is clear that the nurse clinic will change with new staff.

The same is true for the larger system around the clinic. The county health department has had a complete turnover of administration. Many more physicians have moved into the Pomo coast area, although most of them still prefer to work less than full time while they "find themselves." The nurse-practitioner role has proved a success as other communities ask for similar clinics in their own areas. The involvement of community residents, so important in getting the original health center going, has become nearly nonexistent now that the service is operating full time. Their original vision has been made real and they could be expected to turn energy into new areas. An interesting aspect is seeing how often professionals manage to ease out those who pioneer a program with more enthusiasm than credentials. Few of those now on the scene were part of the original work and often fail to understand the role played by the local founders and even the various outsiders, such as Ruth and Sarah.

DISCUSSION

We have included the detailed case study of the residency program in the summer of 1971 and the brief update from that time until the time we wrote this chapter to illustrate the variety of roles and functions available to community nurses working with all segments of communities. At various times we have worked with individuals, families, groups, other professionals, business, economic, political, and religious groups, agencies, governmental bodies, utility companies, and anyone else who didn't move fast enough to get away from us. We have learned that community nursing as we practiced it in Pomo County is a twenty-four-hour-a-day job, seven days a week—if you are going to sell a new role to the community in which you want to work. Every person we meet is a source of information about the community, a potential client, and a possible convert to supporting our efforts. We have used and continue to use every bit of the network we developed in the community through friends and relatives and have sought to expand this network through their friends and relatives.

There should be a conscious effort to make associations with community members and groups as diverse as possible. By doing so, we can obtain as many inputs as possible to aid in analyzing the system we want to work with. Furthermore, such diversity prevents people, including ourselves, from thinking that we are working with only one group. The original clinic almost failed in its outreach efforts—especially with the older straight members of the community—because of its heavy initial association with the young hip members of the area. Helen and Suzanne had to work hard to overcome this assumption, too. Although it did not occur in the Pomo situation, a supportive faction or group can become smothering in its support of your efforts and can sometimes neutralize innovative outreach by creating unseverable bonds of obligation to that one faction. Such support may be well-meaning but it can be the barrier that keeps you from reaching other clients who need your services and are either cut out by the supporting group or are reluctant to associate with any enterprise supported by "those people." Careful analysis of the community power structure and social system is essential very early in relations with the community. (See chapter 23.)

OBTAINING A DATA BASE

To begin planning rational health services one needs some notion of the characteristics of the population being served. The community we have discussed is a rural area, and the first difficulty encountered there was the lack of extensive statistical information. The most recent data available are from 1969–70, at which time there were neither pediatric nor obstetric specialists within the entire coastal area. Few figures are gathered for rural areas, and those that are tend to be underrepresentative of the actual numbers: people in the country are often hard to find, some have irregular mailing addresses, and a few have none at all. As a consequence even the U.S. Census misses many individuals and families. One student preparing a grant proposal was given the only figures available for her rural county: the total number of people and the number of square miles. Thus nurses involved in health services must be prepared to piece information together and even conduct their own surveys. The ideal situation would be to obtain the U.S. Census forms or, lacking those, to copy the format used by the Census Bureau for a Standard Metropolitan Statistical Area (SMSA). These forms and those used in the National Health Survey can provide valuable statistics in a form that can be compared with data from other areas. However, one reason rural areas do not have good statistics is the lack of staff time to gather them.

Information can also be gathered from a wide variety of secondary sources. Use of data collected by other groups or agencies avoids duplication of effort. However, we must be sure about at least two points in using others' data. The first and easier is to learn when the data were gathered. The second is to find why they were collected. Often an agency's philosophy and purpose for gathering information influences the questions they do or do not ask and how they look at the answers. For example the Chamber of Commerce and the local grange or farming organization may well seek and interpret data on available land and its potential use quite differently. We must use secondary data sources or else spend a great deal of time and energy collecting information and have too little left over for action. Our concern is that in using others' data, we be aware of their biases—as well as our own!

Local schools have data on the school-age population. Senior citizens' clubs or associations of retired persons may have data on the numbers of elderly. State employment offices are a valuable source of information about working-age people. Other health and social agencies can often give information on their clients. Problems arise because boundaries defining populations for different information sources are seldom comparable, and these limits must always be remembered. Government agents, such as tax assessors, voter registrars, and police, often have helpful data.

Other kinds of information can be gathered from influential figures in the community. These may or may not be official leaders, but they are often well known for having more than the usual understanding of what goes on. We must recall, however, that such people have biases that influence their own particular views of problems. Many are unaware of health issues that do not impinge on their own consciousness. One industrial leader, for example, maintained there were no drug problems in his community even though health workers repeatedly commented on both legal and illegal drug abuse as major unmet needs. Many men are also unaware of health problems since health is largely a concern of women, especially those with children. Local newspapers occasionally run feature articles about local problems and often have a view of issues. Long-term residents are often a good source of gossipy kinds of information about trends in the area although their biases must be identified and considered. Health practitioners of all kinds are obviously a valuable source of information about health problems although solo practitioners seldom keep statistical records. They also tend to have a foreshortened view of the adequacy of services. We repeatedly heard physicians tell us there was no service problem since they were working at full capacity and saw all patients who presented themselves. They were quite unaware of the community reservoir of unserved. Community nurses need to make a habit of subscribing to and carefully reading whatever local newspapers are available. Even want ads help increase awareness of community problems. Active membership in local organizations, church, and clubs is also important.

Sometimes possible survey data are gathered for some special purpose by other groups. These may be the local high school civics class, a social action club, a land developer, or perhaps some state official intent on tracking some other problem. Health departments at both county and state level maintain data on selected health indicators (which are actually measures of illness!). These include death rates from various causes, rates of selected diseases, maternal death rates, infant morbidity and mortality, fetal deaths. The county also maintains records on births, marriages, and divorces. The reliability of all these figures is somewhat variable. Not all births are registered, for example, when they occur outside hospitals. Reporting of various communicable diseases, even the major health problems, is notoriously low. Recorded causes of death may be more reliable in counties that have a physician as coroner than in those that do not.

Despite all the limitations, a county's statistical records can give valuable insights into the state of health services in the county as compared to a larger area. Comparison of selected statistics for Pomo County with those of the total state gives an appreciation of some of the problems encountered by people who live in an area lacking many medical services.

GAINING PROFESSIONAL ACCEPTANCE

All disciplines have professional territory and react when threats to this territory from outsiders are perceived. This professional territoriality is quite understandable especially when fees-for-service, and therefore basic economics, or decision-making rights and power issues are involved. Innovators should proceed with some degree of caution although not so much that nothing ever gets accomplished. The reality is that no single health care discipline can meet clients' needs and so we must learn to work together. Collaboration, coordination, consultation, and coercion are all ingredients in interdisciplinary relationships.

Our specific attempts to work with members of other health disciplines are paying off to different extents. Sue, the social worker, has been an essential ally throughout the eight years of the project in Pomo County. The local pharmacist has also been consistent in his support and good will. Physicians have come and gone; some, such as the four who have consistently provided backup for the health center, have been great. Others are growing more accustomed to the activities of the group of nurses, and there is generally far more acceptance now for many reasons: The nurses who have worked in Pomo have all been well prepared and experienced practitioners. We have been in the community long enough to be viewed with less suspicion. Through the health officer's work, relations with the health department have improved greatly. Since the beginning of the Pomo project the concept of expanded roles in nursing has developed and the resultant professional publicity has helped our cause.

Although physicians and other health care discipline members do not always understand what we are doing, they have not presented as many obstacles as encountered from other nurses in the community. It is curious and discouraging that members of our own health care discipline have been our greatest problem. Our experience in Pomo and elsewhere has led us to believe that there is danger for those of us who pursue innovative ideas and who seek to make the health care system responsive to client needs. Nurses engaged in such pursuits are likely to encounter as much and often more resistance and hostility from other nurses than we do from other groups, both professional and lay.

GAINING LEGITIMACY

Clients, whether they are individuals, families, or communities, are not willing to accept any of us immediately. First we must prove our good intentions, competence, and commitment to do what we say we will do—

in short, we first must pay our dues. This certainly has been our experience in Pomo County. Rural areas like urban ghettos have been promised much and, for the most part, given little. Having been burned already, such communities tend to be highly cautious in accepting outsiders who come in to "help" them.

Acquiring legitimacy can be helped in a variety of ways. Involving clients in the plans for health care programs, such as the health education presentations, rather than simply presenting them as accomplished facts, provides a chance to work together and learn greater respect for one another. Carrying out programs the client community wants gives evidence of our willingness to meet their needs rather than ours. Helping the Pomo women's club carry out its health surveys as well as discussing uses of the data gave them ammunition to take to the county authorities to obtain additional services tailored to the needs of the coast. The nurses who elected to live as well as work in Pomo County came to be better accepted because they lived there, although they were viewed as newcomers. Ruth and Sarah have not lived in Pomo but rather worked through members of the community such as Mrs. Place and Ann, rather than be visible as individuals.

Another way to gain legitimacy is to do something that is relatively easily and quickly accomplished. The first aid–home nursing classes are an example. Community people were asked what they wanted from a class and the material was organized immediately and the class begun. Supplying information about and contacts for the 911 emergency telephone number is another project that can be carried out without a great deal of time or an elaborate support system. Once they see that the community nurse will deliver, the probability of client cooperation and involvement goes up.

FINDING FINANCIAL SUPPORT

All community work takes a great deal of time and time is often our scarcest resource. The amount of time needed to get this kind of community project going is frustrating for creative/innovative people who want to see their ideas tried out at once. Our grant proposal took some six months to make its way through the convolutions of bureaucracy before there was any money to support the residency program. Six months is fairly fast for government projects; thus lead time must be planned for and proposals developed and submitted far enough in advance to get them through channels. Funding agencies generally require evidence of client support before they will even consider a proposal. By the time client groups are sold on a proposed program, they are ready to get on with it. Unless the client group itself can fund the program or can obtain funding locally, then all must wait for outside sources. Great skill and persistence are needed to avoid losing the client group at this point;

they too are frustrated by the lead time necessary to obtain financial support. We have done rather well in terms of obtaining support for the Pomo County project and have been extremely fortunate to find colleagues whose interest in trying innovative roles have outweighed their concern for material gain. Suzanne and Helen lived a year on one salary; Flora's income through her various community projects was far less than she could make in an urban setting. Ruth and Sarah have donated their time as part of their commitment to client service and have been able to add woman power to many efforts through arranging student field work. Such fortunate circumstances and dedicated people cannot always be found.

If programs are to survive they must have adequate financial support. Unless we are independently wealthy, we who have ideas for innovative programs must often turn to organizations for the fiscal base to implement them even on a modest scale. The price for this support may well be modification of our ideas. We may find ourselves in a dilemma. Do we hold out for the program that we and our clients conceived, which may well mean we get no place, or do we modify the program to conform to the requirements of our potential sources of financial support on the premise that a modified program is better than no program at all? This kind of decision is another source of frustration for innovative people.

The Pomo County community nursing effort has been going on for more than eight years; we expect that it will continue in some form for an indefinite period of time. Our roles have diminished recently although both of us continue to show interest and input whenever possible. The ultimate success, however, of this or any other community program requires that the people of the community be involved and preferably in charge of the program. Thus the summer residency project stressed the need for each resident-nurse to have a counterpart from the local community. The local nurses were expected to participate fully in the residency program and then continue to work in the health center and community projects after the resident-nurses left. When they ceased participating in the health center, and worse yet when the nurse who had been the mainstay of the entire program moved away, there was a frantic scramble to find other local nurses who could carry on the health center. Flora's decision to stay in the community and the continued availability of resources of the school of nursing were unusual occurrences. A program really succeeds when the local community can and does carry it on after outside people and funding have gone. Community assumption of responsibility is a slow process and involves careful planning.

When planning an innovative project, wanting it to come out successfully, just as envisioned and, best yet, to get credit for it is natural. Early in this kind of community nursing work, however, the decision must be made as to whose needs are to be met and who is to be primarily served: the client community or the outside innovator's ego. There must be some degree of mutual benefit, but the balance must be clearly established since it determines much of what is to be done and how it is accomplished. Although difficult to do, we must often be satisfied with only our own knowledge of how our intervention made some whole chain of events possible.

LOCAL POLITICS

If community nurses are going to change existent health services or create new kinds, we must become involved in political activities at all levels but especially on the local and county levels. The processes through which Sue and the executive board went to start the health center in the first place exemplify grassroots politics. So was the work our colleagues have done in running, or persuading others to run, for the community hospital board to add another voice in the policy decisions of that body. Some of this political involvement has been by individuals and others by coalitions, which tended to be more successful. (See chapter 22.)

The realization by coastal residents that they constitute 40 percent of the county's population but clearly did not receive 40 percent of the county services helped galvanize these usually private people into group action. The data from surveys on health needs and availability of services to meet them were collected with the aim of having hard facts to take to the board of supervisors to back the coast residents' demands.

Helen and Suzanne both engaged in a wide variety of community activities in working with all kinds of groups in careful and continuous management of their public relations. This approach has paid off not only by enabling them to build a large and satisfied clientele but also by enabling them to secure additional funding from the county for the clinic and their own salaries.

The kinds of political activities described in the case study take tremendous amounts of time and effort, but they do bear fruit.

EPIDEMIOLOGY IN ACTION

Rarely does the epidemiological process follow the order encountered in the hepatitis epidemic in Pomo. More usually we must proceed from an outbreak of the illness to a variety of tests to find its possible source or sources. To have such a recent study of water pollution in the exact area was fortuitous, especially since the health department didn't have to pay anything to have one done. Hepatitis was not an unknown disease to the young hip immigrants, as was well known to free clinic workers and the commune researchers. That the new youth population did not also get it during the epidemic may not have been solely a tribute to their cleanliness or their knowledge of the disease and its prevention. Many of them may have had sufficient levels of immunity either from frequent prior exposure or subclinical and clinical disease that might have provided individual immunity, an acquired immunity the less-travelled oldtime residents did not have. (See chapter 9.)

RESEARCH

Most of the jargon of research has been avoided in this case study. However, Ruth, Sarah, and the various graduate students brought a research stance to the project that enabled them to gain much information. The identification of nursing role possibilities, analysis of community resources and strengths, and surveys of citizen opinions on health issues, as well as the original commune project that was the opening wedge for community nursing experimentation were all formal research enterprises. This project's participants were constantly asking the basic field research question: "What's really going on here?" The general atmosphere was one of experimentation and innovation. (See chapter 8.)

SUMMARY

Starting with a description of the physical locale of Pomo, we have presented short elements of its history, climate, population, industries, economy, and pertinent social characteristics. Because we are, after all, health workers, the health care system and the lack of services there is of special concern to us. The development by community members of the local health center is traced, as is our graduate students' involvement in a special summer project there. The main portion of the chapter is devoted to the summer's experiences: the nurses' entry into the community, meeting their local counterparts, developing plans for programs, the attitudes of other health workers and the local people toward the nurses in the summer residency project. After describing the programs carried on in the health center and in the community, we assessed the outcomes of the summer. The seven years following the residency project were reviewed as additional community-oriented nurses moved into the area to expand the nursing role where needs were greatest.

Discussion of the case study focuses on the ways our theoretical framework is actually applied: involving clients in planning health services, founding plans on sound bases of information, the problems of achieving legitimacy in the eyes of clients as well as with other professionals. We also mention some of the often neglected issues involved in health services: financing, politics, epidemiology, and research. Even a small community presents a reality far too complex to be fully considered.

By showing the way some of the themes common in community health nursing may be observed and dealt with, we hope you have been stimulated to look to your own communities for similar eye-opening experiences.

We purposely selected a rural area for our case description and analysis. Most schools of nursing are in cities and so many students do not have an opportunity to experience rural community nursing as part of their basic preparation. We have found working in a rural area, such as along the Pomo Coast, to be fascinating and challenging. We hope at least a few of our readers will be intrigued enough to try it too. Should you do so, you will be helping solve one of the most serious problems facing our health care system—people who cannot obtain needed services because of maldistribution of health professionals.

15. The Community Nurse's Yellow Pages

Ruth P. Fleshman
Sarah Ellen Archer

INTRODUCTION

In this chapter we present a sampling of the kinds of information sources we have found useful in working with a variety of clients and in pursuing our own continuing education. The lists are by no means exhaustive, but we have tried to make them suggest the possible range available. Our point here is to acquaint you with the kinds of *questions to ask* and *places to look* to find the resources you need in your practice. Consult telephone directories for the resources that are readily available in your area. The national addresses we have included may be useful to you in obtaining information about what is or could be created in your locale.

The reason for this chapter is that community nurses often must help clients find what they need. We are generally the ones who deal with client problems that arise outside the hospital, and so we are most reliant on community resources. We may also be the first professionals to become aware of the need for such organizations as Parents Without Partners, Meals on Wheels, and the like. Another possibility is that we may have to serve as catalysts to help groups form within the community to meet their own needs. To do so, we need to know where and how to find information. Knowing that resources exist in a field of practice and knowing where to look for them are essential components of any professional's function. No one can remember them all. What we must know is where to begin to look when we need them. For example, unless you use statistical formulas all the time, you will not remember them. Thus you have to know where your notes from statistics class are, where stat books can be found, or what state consultant to call in.

There is so much new information in almost all fields that professionals find keeping up with developments, even in highly specialized areas, is becoming increasingly difficult. Many community nurses have neither time nor ready access to extensive library facilities, and so have to make every minute count. For this reason we include a brief discussion of the indexes and abstracting services we have found most helpful as well as some shortcuts we have used. In the near future there will be many changes in the way information is disseminated. We are told that books and magazines will cease to be a major source of information. Until that time, we hope that the material in this chapter will help you make the most of whatever time and energy you can devote to keeping up with what's happening.

SERVICE RESOURCES

We health workers tend to be monomaniacs about our topic and presume that anybody with health problems will beat down our doors to get the services our agencies provide. This notion fails to take into account at least two facts. First, we forget that we are only one layer in a complex structure of health resources. The resources available for dealing with problems range far beyond the one health agency where you work; they begin with mothers and work along through neighbors, friends, books, church, druggists, curanderos, newspaper columns, and on and on. Second, in most communities—and especially in urban areas—there are a wide number of other professionals dealing with various aspects of health problems. Sorting out all these workers is very confusing, but we can sift through until we help clients make the best possible match between their problems and whichever agency deals with it best. This is not to say that there aren't both geographic areas and health-related problems for which services are grossly inadequate. But many areas, especially urban ones, have plenty of services if we know where to look for them.

Therefore, we present here the beginnings of a list of kinds of agencies and types of resources that may well be available in your area. If not, we try to give you some leads on where you might get information about organizations that can help you find nearby resources or even start your own.

Your telephone book is the obvious place to begin. Start with the large headings in the yellow pages. Just browsing can give you an idea of unsuspected resources you may someday need. Abdominal supports; Acupuncture; Adoption agencies; Alcoholism; Ambulance services; Animal shelters; Artificial breasts, eyes, limbs, voice; Associations; Audiologists—and that's just the A's. Some communities are lucky enough to have social service directories, United Fund listings, newpapers that periodically run series on agencies in the area, and some even have full-dress information and referral services where anyone can call up and be given the name and phone number of an agency nearby that can either help with the need described or be of service in arranging help. All of these assisting services are great helps, but we must be sure they are up to date. One way is to keep them informed of changes in agencies of which we become aware—feedback again.

When you've been at this for a while, you'll find that you're developing your own form of resource file. It will be based on the experience your clients have with resources, your own contacts and development of friends in other agencies, and other sources. One of the most valuable exchanges we make goes like this, "I've got a family who needs marriage counseling; where's the best place to send young people?" "I sent a couple to family services; they've got a really great social worker, Helen Thomas, who's really good with them." Take note of these exchanges even when they're not pertinent to your present clients; chances are you'll soon be able to use them.

Almost every health problem has its own special interest support system. The national organizations we include generally have local chapters, although you may have to write for their addresses. Sometimes there is competition among various organizations dealing with a single health problem and you may find that one type will not mention as resources those organizations that compete with them. For instance, there are various approaches to drug abuse, alcoholism, preparation for childbirth, and each approach has its advocates. There is little chance that orthodox medicine will suggest the use of even slightly different services such as chiropractic, let alone some of the new-old alternative approaches such as herbalism, homeopathic medicine, or psychic healing. Psychiatry tends to forget that clergy have long carried out counseling services; even bartenders are beginning to receive training for dealing better with the kind of clients who make that choice for therapy.

Listing even a substantial portion of the national groups involved with major aspects of health care would be impossible, but we include a few examples of the range of services available in different categories. Information about local services can be requested. All of the age groups mentioned may be further served by organizations focusing on diseases that are disproportionately found among the particular age category.

MATERNITY SERVICES

American Society for Psychoprophylaxis in Obstetrics (Lamaze Method), 505 E. 79th Street, New York, NY 10021

International Childbirth Education Association, 208 Ditty Building, Bellevue, WA 98004

La Leche League International, 9616 Minneapolis Avenue, Franklin Park, IL 60131

Maternity Center Association, 48 E. 92nd Street, New York, NY 10028

SERVICES TO CHILDREN AND YOUTH

American Association for Maternal and Child Health, P.O. Box 965, Los Altos, CA 94022

Association for the Care of Children in Hospitals, P.O. Box H, Union WV 24983

Child Welfare League of America, Inc., 67 Irving Place, New York, NY 10003

Easter Seal Society for Crippled Children and Adults, 2023 W. Ogden Avenue, Chicago, IL 60612

National Aid to Retarded Citizens (formerly N.A.R. Children), 2709 E St. East, Arlington, TX 76011

National Association for Children with Learning Disabilities, 4156 Library Road, Pittsburgh, PA 13624

Play Schools Association, Inc., 111 E. 59th Street, New York, NY 10022

Shriners Hospital for Crippled Children, 323 N. Michigan Avenue, Chicago, IL 60601

United Cerebral Palsy Association, Inc., 66 E. 34th Street, New York, NY 10066

United States Government.

Child Health Affairs, Department of Health, Education and Welfare, 5600 Fishers Lane, Rockville, MD 20852

National Institute of Child Health and Human Development, NIH, 9000 Rockville Pike, Bethesda, MD 20014

SERVICES TO THE AGED

American Association of Homes for the Aging, 1050 17th St. NW, Washington, DC 20036

American Association of Retired Persons, 1909 K St. NW, Washington, DC 20006

National Association for Spanish Speaking Elderly, 3875 Wilshire Blvd., Suite 401, Los Angeles, CA 90005 (legislative work)

National Center on Black Aged, 1730 M Street NW, Suite 811, Washington, DC 20020 (education, information, consultation)

National Council on the Aging, 1828 L Street NW, Washington, DC 20036 (literature)

National Indian Council on Aging, P.O. Box 2088, Albuquerque, NM 87103 (advocacy, action, newsletter)

Pacific/Asian Coalition, 1760 The Alameda, Suite 210, San Jose, CA 95126 (general resource, clearinghouse, newsletter for aged)

SELECTED NATIONAL ORGANIZATIONS

The following national agencies usually offer services of various kinds at local levels. In addition to these, you may want to check life insurance companies, pharmaceutical firms, and many other health-connected industries that offer nutritional or health literature. Of course, you have to filter them for their own self-interest bias!

Alcoholics Anonymous, 468 Park Avenue S, New York, NY 10016

American Alliance for Health, Physical Education, and Recreation, National Council for School Nurses, 1201 16th St. NW, Washington, D.C. 20036

American Can Company, 1660 L St. NW, Washington, D.C. 20036 (Most food companies have divisions that provide information of a nutritional or health nature.)

American Cancer Society, 777 3rd Avenue, New York, NY 10017

American Diabetes Association, 1 W. 48th Street, New York, NY 10020

American Heart Association, 44 E. 23rd Street, New York, NY 10010

American Institute of Baking, 400 E. Ontario Street, Chicago, IL 60611

American Lung Association, 1740 Broadway, New York, NY 10019

American Medical Association, 535 N. Dearborn Avenue, Chicago, IL 60610

American National Red Cross, 17th and D Streets NW, Washington, DC 20006

American Optometric Association, Inc., 7000 Chippewa Street, St. Louis, MO 63119

American Parkinson Disease Association, 147 E. 50th Street, New York, NY 10022

Arthritis Foundation, 221 Park Avenue S, New York, NY 10003

Family Service Association of America, 44 E. 23rd Street, New York, NY 10010

Mental Health Materials Center, 419 Park Avenue S, New York, NY 10016

National Asthma Center, 875 Avenue of the Americas, New York, NY 10001

National Association for Mental Health, Inc., 1800 N. Kent Street, Rosslyn Station, Arlington, VA 22209

National Association for Sickle Cell Disease, Inc., 945 S. Western Avenue, Suite 206, Los Angeles, CA 90006

National Association for Visually Handicapped, 305 E. 24th Street, New York, NY 10010

National Cystic Fibrosis Research Foundation, 3379 Peachtree Road NE, Atlanta, GA 30326

National Dairy Council, 6300 River Road, Rosemont, IL 60018

National Epilepsy League, 6 N. Michigan Avenue, Chicago, IL 60602

National Fire Protection Association, Public Information Department, 470 Atlantic Avenue, Boston MA 02110

National Hemophilia Foundation, Room 903, 25 W. 39th Street, New York, NY 10018

National Medical Association, 1720 Massachusetts Avenue NW, Washington DC 20036

National Multiple Sclerosis Society, 205 E. 42nd Street, New York, NY 10017

National Organization for Women, Action Center, 425 13th Street, NW, Washington, DC 20004

National Research Council, Food and Nutrition Board, 2101 Constitution Avenue NW, Washington, DC 20037

National Science Foundation, 1800 G Street NW, Washington, DC 20019

Planned Parenthood, 810 7th Avenue, New York, NY 10019

Salvation Army, National Headquarters, 120 W. 14th Street, New York, NY 10011

Sex Information and Education Council of the U.S. (SIECUS), 137 N. Franklin Avenue, Hempstead, NY 11550

Shriners Hospital for Crippled Children, 323 N. Michigan Avenue, Chicago, IL 60601

United Cerebral Palsy Association, Inc., 66 E. 34th Street, New York, NY 10066

United Ostomy Association, 1111 Wilshire Boulevard, Los Angeles, CA 90017

United States Government.

U.S. Government Printing Office, Division of Public Documents, Washington, DC 20403

Department of Agriculture, Agriculture Research Service, Federal Center Building, Hyattsville, MD 20782

Department of Health, Education and Welfare, Public Health Service, National Institutes of Health, 9000 Rockville Pike, Bethesda, MD 20014 (National Institute on Aging; Allergy and Infectious Diseases;

Arthritis, Metabolism, and Digestive Diseases; Cancer; Child Health and Human Development; Dental Research; Environmental Health Sciences; Eye; General Medical Sciences; Heart and Lung; Neurological and Communicative Disorders and Stroke)

Health Agencies located at 5600 Fishers Lane, Rockville, MD 20852: Health Services Administration; Office of Quality Standards; Bureau of Community Health Service (Indian Health Service, Bureau of Medical Service, Bureau of Quality Assurance); Office of Health Legislation; Food and Drug Administration; Office of Long-Term Care; President's Council on Physical Fitness; Office of International Health; Policy Development and Planning; Population Affairs; Bureau of Health Planning and Resources Development; Mental Health Administration

Other health-related government offices:

Office of Human Development, Administration on Aging, 300 Independence Avenue SE, Washington, DC 20023

Equal Employment Opportunities Commission, 2401 E Street NW, Washington, DC 20506

Division of Research Grants, 9000 Rockville Pike, Bethesda, MD 20014

Social and Rehabilitation Service, 300 C Street SW, Washington, DC 20024

Library of Congress, Division for the Blind and Physically Handicapped, 1291 Taylor Street NW, Washington, DC 20011

National Library of Medicine, 9000 Rockville Pike, Bethesda, MD 20014

Department of Labor:

National Labor Relations Board (NLRB) 1717 Pennsylvania Avenue SW, Washington, DC 20006

National Transportation Safety Board, 800 Independence Avenue SW, Washington, DC 20003

Occupational Safety and Health Administration (OSHA) 200 Constitution Avenue NW, Washington, DC 20001

LISTINGS OF HEALTH SERVICES

Whether for you or your client, breaking into the health system without a name or phone number of the agency delivering service is very difficult. It's even hard to start if you don't know *where* in the phone book to begin. However, service delivery in all categories—diseases, age groups, special populations, whatever—is changing so constantly that any publication would be instantly out of date. Agencies that specialize in particular services try to keep rosters of the agencies they are liable to refer folks to, but no one has all the agencies. Local rosters are more likely to be up to date than statewide ones and certainly more so than national listings. Typically, you will be able to find lists, files, or looseleaf folders more or less updated in local social service agencies, family service agencies, information and referral centers (whether general or only for the aged), and in the social work office of major health agencies. For instance, the Family Service Association of America annually publishes a *Directory of Member Agencies* with names and addresses, state by state for the United States and Canada. The price was $7.50 in 1977 and can be ordered through the FSA, 44 E. 23rd Street, New York, NY 10010. Special topics are often covered in journals applicable to those topics. For example, a national journal, *American Annals of the Deaf,* publishes one of its regular issues as a directory of services for the deaf. This issue lists teachers of the deaf; associations concerned exclusively with the problems of the deaf and blind; and centers for the rehabilitation or training of the deaf. You can probably check a copy at some agency concerned with hearing problems or subscribe to the whole journal by writing its editor at Gallaudet College, Washington, DC 20002. The 1977 price was $6.

Many of the services for special populations or age groups can be learned about from those already involved with them. Programs for the aged, for instance, are supposed to be coordinated by the local Area Agency on Aging. However, since the agencies often have different names in various places, you may have trouble locating them in a directory, but persistence can finally pay off with the name and phone number of a person with information about services. Many areas maintain information and referral services or Hotlines for special topics, such as child abuse or sex information, which are also likely to maintain files of good referral sources.

Many public service groups start projects to publish city or county service rosters, work hard at it for a year or two, then give up on the difficulties of keeping the manuals updated. A few of the bigger ones are trying to use computer technology to turn out regular supplements, which may help somewhat. If updating depends on agency people inserting many new entries, however, the roster will turn out to be only as useful as those folks are compulsive about pasting new slips over old slips as services come and go, move, change staff, change fees, even change entry requirements. The end result generally is that the service workers develop their own particular set of referral sources that have proved helpful to them and generally ignore all the others. This approach helps keep the information flood under control, but often limits the services we all can offer clients. Sometimes, then, browsing through service directories, even obsolete ones, to see the range of approaches to care that could be available can pay off.

PROFESSIONAL RESOURCES

If we're not careful we'll drown in information. There's so much being written now that it's almost impossible to keep up on new things even in narrow specialty areas—much less a general field like ours. The eighteen thousand journals dealing with medicine and related fields are only a start since there are all those other fields—sociology and so on—that we need to know about. There is no way we can do it all. Right!

So we've got to be selective. Those of us in metropolitan areas with university libraries and medical centers have an overchoice. Those in rural areas whose only nearby resource is the local hospital or health department library often have a different kind of problem.

What we are doing in this section is suggesting journals and basic books on a variety of topics that you may want to buy. The books are either those we use or ones our colleagues in the specialty areas indicated they use and recommend. Before you buy any book, remember that the information in it is two to four years old—depending on how long it took the publisher and author to make arrangements. In some fields it's not smart to buy books at all since the field is developing so rapidly. Journals are better. Their lead time is usually somewhere between six and eighteen months. Paperbacked, as opposed to clothbound books, are about one or two years from writing to bookstore.

Find a local bookstore or library that has a current copy of *Books in Print* for both hard- and paperbound books. Identify publishers who produce a number of books in your fields of interest and get on their mailing lists for announcements of new books. Talk with your local librarian or bookstore salesperson. We've found they are almost always willing to help you find things and will even contact you when things you might be interested in turn up.

PERIODICALS

Subscribing to periodicals is less expensive than buying books, and as we have indicated, the lead time between writing and publication is generally shorter for journals than for books. Many journals deal with topics of interest to community nurses, but we cannot possibly subscribe to them all, much less read them. With this in mind, we asked Mary Heatherman and Margaret Hoff of the Learning Resources Information Center, School of Nursing, University of California, San Francisco, to help us select journals of most relevance to community nurses. They reviewed literature from a three-year period and found that approximately 60 percent of the articles applicable to community nursing and public health appeared in six journals. These six with their 1978 addresses and prices are:

Nursing Times, £ 11, Macmillan Journals, 4 Little Essex Street, London, WC2R, 3LF, England (Cost in U.S. currency will vary depending on exchange rate and cost of postage.)

Nursing Outlook, $14, American Journal of Nursing Company, 10 Columbus Circle, New York, NY 10019

Australian Nurses Journal, $16 (Australian), Royal Australian Nursing Federation, 132–136 Albert Road, South Melbourne, Victoria, Australia 3205 (Cost in U.S. currency will vary depending on exchange rate.)

American Journal of Nursing, $12, American Journal of Nursing Company, 10 Columbus Circle, New York, NY 10019

American Journal of Public Health, included in membership dues and sent automatically to American Association of Public Health members or available at $30.00 per year, Circulation Manager, *American Journal of Public Health,* 1015 Eighteenth Street NW, Washington, DC 20036

Gerontologist, $20, Gerontology Society, 1 Dupont Circle, Washington, DC 20036

(We find it interesting that so many articles related to community health are beginning to appear in publications from England and Australia. From other sources, we hear that there is a good deal of ferment as nursing moves into what for these countries is a newer field: the community.)

Other journals helpful to community nurses include:

Association of Rehabilitation Nurses Journal, $15, Association of Rehabilitation Nurses, 1701 Lake Avenue, Glenview, IL 60025

Canadian Journal of Public Health, $20 (U.S.), *CJPH,* 55 Paredale Avenue, Ottawa, Ontario, Canada K1Y 1 E 5

Canadian Nurse, $9 (U.S.), Canadian Nurses Association, 50 The Driveway, Ontario, Canada K2P 1 E 2

ICN—International Nursing Review, $12 (U.S.), I.N.R., Imprimeries Réunies S.A., 33, avenue de la Gare, CH–1001, Lausanne, Switzerland

Journal of Continuing Education in Nursing, $18, Charles Slack, 6900 Grove Road, Thorofare, NJ 08086

Journal of Gerontological Nursing, $10, Charles Slack, 6900 Grove Road, Thorofare, NJ 08086

Nursing Clinics of North America, $14, W.B. Saunders Co., Washington Square, Philadelphia, PA 19105

Nursing Digest, $12, 12 Lakeside Park, 607 North Avenue, Wakefield, MA 01880

Nursing Mirror (weekly), $49.40 (includes air postage), I.P.C. Specialist and Professional Press, Limited, 161–166 Fleet Street, London EC44 P4 AA England

Occupational Health Nursing, $16, Charles Slack, 6900 Grove Road, Thorofare, NJ 08086

Journals in disciplines other than nursing may also be of interest. We've found the following more helpful than a lot of others in the medical library:

Administrative Science Quarterly, $12, Cornell University Graduate School of Business and Public Administration, Ithaca, NY 14850

American Sociological Review, $15 to nonmembers, American Sociological Association, 1722 N Street NW, Washington, DC 20036, or *Journal of Health and Social Behavior,* $12 to nonmembers, (includes reprints from *ASR* of articles about title topics)

Gerontologist, $20, Gerontology Society, 1 Dupont Circle, Washington, DC 20036

Health Values: Achieving High Level Wellness, $10, Charles Slack, 6900 Grove Road, Thorofare, NJ 08086

Human Organization: Journal of Applied Anthropology, $10 for students ($17, regular), Society of Applied Anthropology, 1703 New Hampshire Avenue NW, Washington, DC 20009

Journal of the American Geriatrics Society, $21, American Geriatrics Society, 10 Columbus Circle, New York, NY 10019

Medical Care, $17 for students ($33, regular), J.B. Lippincott Co., E. Washington Square, Philadelphia, PA 19105

Preventive Medicine (quarterly), $46, Academic Press, Inc., 111 Fifth Avenue, New York, NY 10003

Psychology Today, $12, P.O. Box 2990, Boulder, CO 80302

Public Administration Review, $25, American Society for Public Administration, 1223 Connecticut Avenue NW, Washington, DC 20036

Society, $8.50, Rutgers University, New Brunswick, NJ 08903

Urban Health, $9.95, *Urban Health,* P.O. Box 42409, Atlanta, GA 30311

Besides these, there are journals devoted to any particular medical specialty you can think of as well as the sciences that contribute to all areas of practice: genetics, mental deficiency, nutrition, occupational therapy, physiology, psychiatry, surgery, tropical medicine, venereal diseases, veterinary medicine, and so forth. For whatever you need, there's a journal—and people writing articles—and other people trying valiantly to keep up. Good luck! Furthermore, subscribing to all of the magazines may not be necessary to have access to the content. Before subscribing, check with your local hospital, health department, school of nursing library, and even public library to see whether they receive any of the journals. Also inquire among your friends and colleagues for members of the American Public Health Association. Chances are that you can find other ways to be able to read articles of interest in the six journals of primary interest to community nursing (expect possibly those from overseas) rather than subscribing to them all yourself. Should you find that the journals simply are not available in your locale, you and a group of colleagues might want to coordinate your subscriptions and share them. That way each could subscribe to one journal but have access to them all.

If you plan to keep magazines, it often pays in the long run to have them bound; that way they're less likely to get lost or destroyed. If you prefer to make notes on pertinent articles and only keep the notes, then recycling the journals when you've finished with them is worthwhile. That way more nurses can have access to them. Your local hospital, health department, nurses' association, or library might be happy to get your copies. The journals themselves often print calls for copies to be sent to new schools of nursing or for other uses. Any of these uses make more sense then dumping your old journals when they become a storage problem.

Writing abstracts on articles is an easy way to keep the information handy. We have found that 5-X-8-inch cards are a happy compromise; they're big enough to write a fair amount and yet are reasonably compact. When doing abstracts, the important thing to know is that they are *not* outlines, reading notes, or strings of quotations. Abstracts are summary statements of the essential message or content of a publication, a specification of the underlying theme or theory used by the writer, and your evaluation of the material. Be sure to start with a complete citation of the material. There are a number of forms for recording reference information, and a wise approach may be to pick the one most closely related to your particular field. Manuals of style list various formats, and you should follow a particular one for all your citations. The listings of our references in this book, for example, follow the format of the University of Chicago *Manual of Style*. A complete citation will keep you from having to go back to the library unnecessarily to write a bibliography. After that the content should include the following:

1. Focus of the publication being abstracted;
2. Theory presented by the author;
3. Methodology of data collection, theory development, and so forth;
4. Findings;
5. Conclusions the author draws;
6. Pertinence of the publication to your frame of reference—that is its relation to community nursing.

Articles often contain particularly meaty quotations you may wish to use or other reading notes you may wish to keep. These should be kept separate from the abstract; the back of the card may be the best spot, along with the particular pages to be cited for each item. Once you practice for awhile, abstracting becomes easy. Perhaps you can convince your colleagues to follow suit; exchanging abstracts can save time and be an excellent way to share information! We simply cannot read all of everything that interests us!

PHARMACOLOGICAL REFERENCES FOR COMMUNITY NURSES

American Hospital Formulary Service, American Society of Hospital Pharmacists, 4630 Montgomery Avenue, Washington, DC 20014. The first year's price includes a complete set of the AHF monographs, binders, and supplement service for the current calendar year. Renewal subscriptions at considerably lower price keep the supplements coming. Contains complete information on drugs assembled by the professional society for use in hospitals and community pharmacies. Supplements update subscribers on new information, drugs, dosages, and effects. The most complete pharmacological resource available but quite expensive.

Handbook of Non-Prescription Drugs, American Pharmaceutical Association, Order Desk, 2215 Constitution Avenue NW, Washington, DC 20037. Lists nonprescription drugs by name in large categories (antacids, antitussives, cold medicines, and so forth) with discussion of their relative values, side effects, uses. New editions advertised in the *Journal of the American Pharmaceutical Association* since publication is irregular.

Physicians' Desk References (PDR), Medical Economics Company, Oradell, NJ 07649. Contains information compiled from package circulars in drugs available only on prescription. Publication financed by drug companies that purchase space for their drug product descriptions. Supplements mailed twice during year to update material. Considerably less costly than *AHFS* but contains less comprehensive and often more biased information.

BOOKS FOR THE GENERALIST'S PORTABLE LIBRARY

Nobody knows everything about anything. There are times when it's nice to be able to stop and look something up right on the spot. We work with one storage box that contains a set of books that have answered most of the questions that come up in the average client visit. Be sure to check for the lastest edition. The ones we're partial to are the following:

Boston Women's Health Book Collective, *Our Bodies, Ourselves: A Book by and for Women,* 2nd ed. revised and expanded (New York: Simon & Schuster)

Silver, Henry K. et al., *Handbook of Pediatrics* (Los Altos, Calif.: Lange Medical Publications)

Watt, Bernice, and Annabel, Merrill, *Composition of Foods* (Washington, D.C.: Department of Agriculture)

Benenson, Abram S., ed., *Control of Communicable Disease in Man* (Washington: American Public Health Association)

Physician's Desk Reference (PDR) (Oradell, N.J.: Medical Economics Co., published annually)

Griffenhagen, George B., ed., *Handbook of Non-Prescription Drugs* (Washington, D.C.: American Pharmaceutical Association)

Holvey, David N., ed., *The Merck Manual of Diagnosis and Therapy* (Rahway, N.J.: Merck, Sharp & Dohme)

Robinson, Corinne H., *Normal and Therapeutic Nutrition* (New York: Macmillan Co.)

Wagner, E. G., and J. N. Lanoix, *Excreta Disposal for Rural Areas and Small Communities* (Geneva: World Health Organization)

Hanks, T., *Solid Waste/Disease Relationships* (Cincinnati: United States Department of Health, Education, and Welfare, Solid Wastes Program)

Manual of Individual Water Supply Systems (Washington, D.C.: United States Department of Health, Education, and Welfare, Special Engineering Services Branch)

MAKING LIBRARY TIME COUNT

Even those of us in extremely rural areas have occasional access to libraries. There are many aids that make literature searches easier and much less time consuming. We mention some of them; inquire at your library to find which are available and whether your library offers others.

Indexes and abstracts make locating and acquiring information far easier than poring through volumes of journals. Before talking about specific kinds of indexes, we list some general idea aids to finding material in periodicals:

1. Define your topic clearly enough to be able to decide which index to use to locate pertinent material

2. Determine the proper date of index to consult. Generally the most recent issue should be consulted first; you can then work backward through other issues. If the material you want to locate relates to the occurrence of a specific event, such as the passage of a law or the development of a vaccine, look directly at the index volume for that time period and then work forward in time through the index's subsequent volumes.

3. If you have difficulty finding your topic in the index, consider alternative subject headings under which your topic may have been indexed. Use the indexes' cross references to help locate other useful headings. The Subject Headings List in *Index Medicus* and other indexes should prove useful.

4. Copy the complete citation when you find an article in the index that you think may be useful. It should include the name of the periodical, volume number, author, title, page on which the article appears, and the date of the journal issue. This information can save your having to come back to the index for missing information and help avoid the frustration of not being able to find what you want.

Indexes that are generally available and pertinent to community nursing include the following:

Cumulative Index to Nursing Literature. This index has been published quarterly by the Seventh Day Adventist Hospital Association since 1956 with annual cumulations. It includes English-language journals covering nursing and ancillary services. It also indexes the kind of lay publications your clients are liable to be reading. However, it is not tied into Medlars or the other computer retrieval systems. Sections on book reviews, pamphlets, films, filmstrips, recordings, and so on are provided. Indexing is done by author and subject.

Hospital Literature Index. Published by the American Hospital Association, Chicago, since 1955, this index provides quarterly author-subject listings of articles in periodicals about hospitals.

Index Medicus and Cumulated Index Medicus. Published by the U.S. National Library of Medicine. It appears monthly and is cumulated annually. It is a comprehensive index of the world's medical literature presented according to authors' names and some 8,000 headings. These headings are listed in *MeSH,* which accompanies the January issue of *Index Medicus* each year.

Index of the National Audiovisual Center. This index is prepared by the General Services Administration, National Archives and Records Services, National Audiovisual Center, Washington, DC 20409. The index lists the following:

Audiovisual materials for loan by federal agencies, listed by agency;
Audiovisual materials for loan or sale by federal agencies and nonfederal sources, listed by subject;
Audiovisual materials for loan by federal agencies, listed by subject;
Addresses of offices that distribute United States Government audiovisual materials;
Miscellaneous printed material;
United States Government audiovisual materials for loan by the National Audiovisual Center;
Audiovisual materials for sale by the National Audiovisual Center.

Many journal articles include an abstract written by the author. There are also regularly published journals made up entirely of abstracts within a particular field. Any of these can be useful to you in several ways. They may provide sufficient information to enable you to know whether or not an article or book is pertinent to the topic you are studying. Often the abstract will provide you with all the information you want and so you need go no further. Other abstracts will help you know which articles and books you should seek out and read in their entirety.

Sources of abstracts which may be useful to you include:

Excerpta Medica, a coordinated series of forty-one abstract journals in the field of medicine. Articles included are from some thirty-five hundred foreign and English-language journals. Books and conference proceedings are also indexed.

Nursing Research, a bimonthly journal published by the American Journal of Nursing Company. It includes abstracts of reports of studies related to nursing.

Psychological Abstracts, prepared by the American Psychological Association, Lancaster, Pa. This publication provides a bibliographical listing of new books and articles grouped by subject, with an abstract of each item.

Sociological Abstracts, a classified abstract journal covering a broad range of sociological articles. It is published nine times a year by the Eastern and Midwestern Sociological Societies.

International Nursing Index, a listing by subject and author prepared in cooperation with the United States National Library of Medicine. This index has been done since 1966 on a quarterly and annual basis and includes many of the journals that are not in *Index Medicus.* Sections on "publications of organizations and agencies," "nursing books," and "dissertations" are useful and tend not to replicate information available elsewhere. Help with headings and cross-references is found in the *Nursing Thesaurus,* which is revised each year and is part 2 of the first issue of *International Nursing Index.*

Readers' Guide to Periodical Literature, compiled and distributed several times each month by the H. W. Wilson Company. This index covers approximately two hundred nonprofessional journals. Listings are by subject and author. Most public libraries subscribe to this service.

Social Sciences and Humanities Index, formerly entitled International Periodicals Index. Published quarterly, it indexes scholarly journals in the humanities and social sciences by author and subject.

INFORMATION AND RETRIEVAL SERVICES

ERIC (Educational Resources Information Center), a network of clearinghouses supported by the National Institute for Education. Clearinghouses focus on a specific area of interest in the field of education, such as communication skills and education of the disadvantaged. A list of the clearinghouses and their specific functions can be obtained from the National Institute of Education, 4833 Rugby Avenue, Suite 503, Bethesda, MD 20014.

MEDLARS (Medical Literature Analysis and Retrieval System), a service begun in 1964 by the National Library of Medicine. MEDLARS provides individualized bibliographies called "demand searches" from materials in *Index Medicus*. To initiate a search, health professions submit written requests describing the details of the information wanted. Requests are processed by trained analysts and approximately three to four weeks are needed to complete a requested bibliography. Inquire at the medical school/medical center library, state health department, or state library system nearest you for the availability of this service and the specific procedures to be followed at that institution. If you cannot locate the MEDLARS nearest you, write the National Library of Medicine, Bethesda, MD 20014 for information and assistance.

MEDLINE, a retrieval service run through a typewriter-like device connected to the National Library of Medicine via telephone. This service retrieves material from approximately 60 percent of the material in *Index Medicus*. Again consult your nearest facilities for the availability of MEDLINE or write the National Library of Medicine.

LAYPERSON'S HEALTH INFORMATION RESOURCES

Professional journals aren't the only source of valuable health information for either our clients or ourselves. Health consciousness now extends to nearly every general interest publication and to the other media as well. We had the unsettling experience of learning from one of our elderly clients that the local radio station had broadcast something about breast cancer and blood pressure medicine. The same items began to appear on television and in weekly news magazines before we could finally track it down to *Lancet,* a highly respected British medical journal. The time taken by other health publications to move into interpreting this information was far too long for many anxious women already frightened by newspaper reports of breast cancer in nationally known women. Many ceased taking their antihypertensives without knowing the full risks entailed. Thus keeping up with health topics presented in mass media may add to our reading overload, but it also keeps us current on client inputs and gives us some lead time to check out the sources used for the presentations. In our society, health is generally a part of a woman's work (even now), so magazines geared to women's interests usually contain much general health information. If you are working with clients from some special population group, you may want to be aware of the contents of media geared to their special interests. This topic is discussed in chapter

10. A short time spent browsing at the magazine section in the local library should reveal a number of unsuspected sources of health information that you would do well to keep up on.

RESOURCES FROM ELECTRONIC MEDIA

Electronic technology is enabling us to get more information faster and from farther away than ever. The Medical Society of Fresno County, California, pioneered a system that adapted the Dial-A-Prayer technique—that is, they installed a cassette message system that allowed 150 different prerecorded messages to be played by request to a special operator. The system disseminates to clients information that has been prepared by local medical specialists. Selections include lung cancer, drug abuse, bee stings, and vasectomies.

Nurses in isolated areas have set up their own tape cassette circuits to exchange ideas over great distances. We have heard from a Maine nurse who corresponds this way with nurses having similar interest areas in New England, Texas, and Australia.

The use of half-inch videotape and small video recording systems has been gradually spreading. The combination of moving images and sound has an impact that is second only to personal contact. Many schools and hospitals have this equipment. Videotape has the advantage over film of being instantly available for playback. One group used this capability to improve communication between community residents and the local health professionals. They would tape one session of residents' comments about health care delivery problems, play it back to the care providers, record their responses, and then play the whole thing to the community groups to complete the feedback loop. However, far more could still be done in other areas of health information. Although the original equipment is fairly expensive, a modest investment in reels of tape, which can be reused almost indefinitely, could provide an excellent means of transmitting information.

SHORTCUTS

Just looking over the essential things we've just said you should do, we find ourselves getting very, very tired. But immediately a series of ways to cut down the energy flow occurred to us.

Speed Reading: If you don't already read at high speed, taking courses that will enable you to skim rapidly while you concentrate only on those materials you truly need to know would be worthwhile.

Specialize: The whole world is fascinating but there are limits to us all. Concentrating on a few areas will keep your reading time from engulfing your whole life.

Take Notes: Keep your reading cards filed in some order, preferably with some form of subject retrieval system (we use code words in the upper right corner so we can riffle through to find what we need).

Cooperate: If your classmates are in close contact, circulate copies of your notes so everyone doesn't have to read the whole batch of articles. Your work unit or local nurses' association can set up a share-the-note circuit.

Publicize: Make your own areas of specialty known and ask coworkers to shoot pertinent finds off to you; of course you'll do the same for them.

Learn to Say No: Realize that no matter how much you cover, there's always more produced than you can handle, so select with discrimination.

Have your eyes tested regularly.

Read Abstracts: The short summaries will tell you soon enough if the original article needs to be read or if the essence is enough.

Pick Experts' Heads: Books are, after all, only packaged experts. Go direct to the source and ask your own questions.

SUMMARY

This chapter contains many "bits and pieces" that we hope will be useful, especially to our rural colleagues whose access to information is complicated by distance. We all need all the help we can get in learning to cope with the overwhelming amount of printed material that threatens to bury us each month.

Difficult as the task of trying to keep up in our areas of interest and expertise is becoming, we must do it. As community nurses we are perhaps even more burdened by the knowledge explosion since we are far more generalized than most of our colleagues. If we are to continue to offer our clients the kinds of services they need and to which they are entitled, we must put forth the effort to keep abreast of what is happening. As professional people, continuing education is our individual responsibility. We have offered some resources and suggestions here that we hope will be helpful to all.

PART IV
Community Health Nurses' Roles

EDITORS' INTRODUCTION

In this section we have drawn upon the specialized areas of expertise that we and some of our colleagues, in community health nursing possess. In speaking from our own experiences, we seek to show you the realities of community health nursing as we have known them as indicators of the breadth of possibilities this field offers.

Chapter 16:   Nurse-Practitioners in Community Settings
Ruth Fleshman and Sarah Ellen Archer describe the continued expansion of many specialists' interests into the community. Community health nursing was the first expanded role. Recently we have been joined by clinical specialists and nurse-practitioners in moving beyond the usual hospital-based practice of nursing. The chapter describes six types of distinctive, although not mutually exclusive, practices that community health nurse-practitioners reported. Each of the six is built upon a community health nursing base: community/diagnostic or disease speciality; community/primary care; community/population; community/place; community/middle management; and community/systems focus. Each of these areas is described in relation to principle activities, clientele, focus, decision making, and sites of practice. The first four are classified as direct client service activities;

451

community/management is semidirect client service activities; and community/systems focus is an example of indirect client services.

Chapter 17:   Community Health Nurses and Community Mental Health
Key mental health concepts for use by community health nurses such as stress adaptation, systems assessment, and reciprocity are Carol Edgerton Mitchell's initial focus. She gives examples of primary, secondary, and tertiary prevention, many of which are drawn from her work in the prevention and treatment of alcoholism. The chapter begins with a description of some community mental health roles that community health nurses often fill and closes with a brief discussion of research and evaluation.

Chapter 18:   Community Nursing in Schools: Developing a Specialized Role
School nursing has long been an area of specialization in community health nursing. Dorothy S. Oda sheds some light on what school nursing is, what practices influence it, and what some issues and concerns that school nursing faces are. The description of what school nurses do focuses on health supervision, health counseling, and health education. This chapter concludes with a discussion of how to develop a specialized role in nursing and uses school nursing as an example.

Chapter 19:   Community Health Nurses as Discharge Planners
Suzanne Brodnax describes some of her joys and frustrations as a public health nurse working in a hospital as a discharge planner. In addition to discussing the vital role of discharge planner in assuring continuity of care between parts of the health care system, she gives a number of specific examples of her direct client services. The chapter repeatedly emphasizes the need for discharge planners to understand the system in which they work and the essential nature of attaining and maintaining sound working relationships with colleagues both inside the hospital and outside of it. A thorough and up-to-date knowledge of all kinds of community agencies and facilities is a must for discharge planners.

Chapter 20:   Community Health Nurses in Ethnic Communities of Color
Many of the clients community health nurses serve are ethnic people of color who differ economically, socially, and culturally from community health nurses who are predominantly white people from the middle class. Unless we learn to understand the values and aspirations of the ethnic people of color whom we serve, we cannot help them attain or maintain their optimal level of functioning. Teresa Bello and Ruth Terry, both of whom are ethnic people of color, have written this chapter to help us understand phenomena such as individual and institutional racism,

"blaming the victim syndrome," and some of the offensive tactics used, often unconsciously, by a majority people to oppress a minority people. Until we consciously come to grips with these behaviors, we cannot serve ethnic clients and communities of color effectively.

Chapter 21:   Community Health Nurses in Administration
Carol Dana Brancich and Patricia Porter focus on giving staff nurses in community health some insights into the whys and wherefores of nursing administration. They focus on the administrative functions of planning, organizing, directing and controlling with examples of participative management in each one. The division of labor between direct, semidirect, and indirect client service providers is stressed to show how these divisions facilitate the effective and efficient running of a health care agency.

Chapter 22:   Community Health Nurses' Involvement in Legislative Processes
Jean Moorhead describes the process she went through in initiating and facilitating the passage of a state law to enable minors to receive treatment for alcohol and other substance abuse without parental consent. Her message is that all of us can and must be more actively involved in legislation and that we, too, can have an effect. She discusses the paths an idea follows on both the state and federal levels from initial contact with a legislator's aides to the enactment of a law. Legislation, since we and other health providers are increasingly regulated by laws, is much too important to leave to the legislators!

Chapter 23:   Community Health Nurses and Community Organization
Teresa Bello describes her experiences as a member of the Board of Directors, East Los Angeles Health Task Force. She then relates her activities in the case study to the literature on community organization. Community organization is an increasingly important role for those of us who work with whole communities as our clients. A step-by-step guide for community organization is included to help community health nurses realize our potential to work with community members to identify problems and bring about changes.

16. Nurse-Practitioners in Community Settings

Ruth P. Fleshman
Sarah Ellen Archer

INTRODUCTION

A long view of nursing history suggests that we have made repeated attempts to upgrade our internal and external images to gain respectability and status. In the early part of this century, nurses united to secure independent status by fighting for individual licensure rather than have it vested in their training schools. We have played various semantic games, naming nursing a "profession" instead of a "calling," being "educated" rather than "trained." We have moved our schools out of hospitals into institutions of higher learning. Many nurses resist our organization's involvement in collective bargaining and issues of economic welfare as somehow beneath the dignity of a professional organization. Individual nurses gained rank, title, and higher income by moving up the administrative ranks. Despite all these maneuvers, there always seemed to be a nagging dissatisfaction.

At the end of the sixties, nursing was trying to invent still another way to become independent, autonomous, and fully professional. The chosen route then was clinical specialization, an attempt to adapt nursing practice to the diagnostic categories that reigned in medical practice. This direction was clearly appealing to nurses in the traditionally delineated clinical areas of medical-surgical nursing and maternal-child health nursing. These nurses could easily become specialized in pediatrics, chest diseases, or orthopedic nursing.

Psychiatric nursing moved less rapidly in this direction since it was more focused on different styles of treatment or the location where the care was given than on a patient load divided into diagnostic categories. The nurses' specialties did not vary if the clients were schizophrenic or manic; instead practice varied according to use of the different individual or group therapies and whether the clients were in psychiatric institutions or ambulatory agencies.

The ensuing debate in nursing education and service circles about the functions, roles, and needed preparation of such specialists tore community health nursing in a variety of directions. With higher education in nursing firmly focused on increasing specialization, nurses who championed community health nurses as generalists were in a lonely position. Those of us who could identify areas of diagnostic concentration could more easily work within agencies that concentrated on those areas: diabetes, abortion, family planning, heart disease, cancer, and so on. Local and national budget priorities continued to emphasize categorical items, in part because incidence figures for diseases are convincing bases for determining need. The concept of total health care, let alone preventive services, has not yet been satisfactorily operationalized.

Beginning in the late sixties the emphasis on accountability and cost-effectiveness made it even more unlikely that programs that could not produce quantitative accomplishments—that is, countable events to divide into the budget expenditures—would be able to stand up against programs that could. It's likely that the urge to meet these requirements was one factor that weakened the innovative stance community nurses have traditionally taken in working with their client populations. When budget departments demand quantity—numbers of home visits, time studies, actual face-to-face client contacts, numbers of injections given, active cases detected, contacts interviewed—little time and energy are left to develop administratively respectable measures of the quality of care delivered or illnesses prevented. Quality, as an issue both for life in general and of health care in particular, has not yet been satisfactorily addressed. However, unless qualitative measurements are included in the evaluation of care being delivered, we may well find ourselves pushed to see more clients in less time with nothing more than a deepening discontent to explain why such care is inadequate. Some nurses are beginning to wrestle with the need to produce objective standards of quality care and, eventually, some method of measuring it as respectably as cost-effectiveness measures quantity. (See chapter 13.)

EXPANDING AWARENESS OF COMMUNITY

One early manifestation of a growing interest in quality was centered on hospital episodes and focused on continuity of care. Nurses in acute care settings realized they needed to know more about where their patients came from and would return to after increasingly shorter stays. Many of us jokingly said at that point, "Everybody's suddenly discovered 'the community'!" But those of us who had been out there forever became aware that it was becoming very crowded. Community-consciousness has infiltrated everywhere now; health workers have become more aware that their clients have a significant existence outside agency walls. Many disciplines have now moved at least partially outside the walls. Despite radioisotopes, immunology, transplants, and the other wonders of medical technology, more health problems have begun to be linked to larger contexts. Disease causation, for instance, is found not only in microscopic organisms but in everyday stress, environmental pollution, and genetic inheritance. Medicine has proliferated specialties and only recently has there been any significant move to return to general or family practice. Nursing has resonated to the impulse to develop in-depth expertise in categories that match those in medical care.

All of nursing has experienced the sequelae of the development of specialty areas; new categories of workers arise to pick up the discarded portions of work that still need doing. Nursing itself has inherited physician tasks and has, in turn, ceded functions to social workers, rehabilitation specialists (Sister Kenny, famed for her work with polio victims, was basically a nurse), LVNs or LPNs, aides, dietary staff, and so on. The growing complexity of health care has also resulted in totally new occupations: inhalation therapists, kidney dialysis technicians, play therapists.

Another group, more recently recognized, has arisen from the movement to include representatives of the general populace or the consumer group. The public schools, the church, have all gone through the process of having their clients—students or parishioners—demand participation in institutional decision making. Health care, especially in its community aspects, has seen the same impulse both in the legislation requiring community participation on OEO projects and planning boards, as well as in the development of indigenous workers. The latters' functions have ranged from organization and agitation against recalcitrant health institutions to client advocacy for delivery of service. They have often served a mutual translation or "bridge" function: interpreting the institution's peculiarities to the client and explaining the client's linguistic or stylistic nature to those attempting to deliver health care.

Part of the present ferment in the health care system is related to the realization by clients who pay premiums for insurance that, so far, the return for their money is beyond their control. Clients have more say-so in HMOs such as the Kaiser-Permanente system. The contrast is striking between clients there and those in a nearby charitable teaching hospital, who are grateful, docile, and silent. Many Kaiser subscribers firmly assert their rights to demand care on terms they establish, both through their contract negotiator and in person at the time of a clinic visit. Knowing they have already paid for service makes them less tolerant of being kept waiting or of having decisions made without their understanding. Such client assertiveness in the decision making creates tensions in the previous homeostasis and it follows that "something's got to give." All professionals including nurses are beginning to feel this pressure. Further, we must all realize that if a national health program does indeed take the form of an insurance scheme, one of the likely consequences will be to make care delivery problems even more costly (see chapter 12).

The upward pressures from clients and the lateral pressures from other workers who have "discovered the community" are not the only forces impinging on community nurses (figure 16.1). Some elements of organized medicine seem threatened by nurses who assert their own professional goals. A number of individual physicians support us in our individual and collective moves toward increased expertise and autonomy. However, some have taken a reactionary posture by opposing legislative moves to expand nursing practice (such as nurse-midwifery and other primary care roles), by creating yet more categories of ancillary health workers who will still be physician-controlled (physician-assistants, physician-extenders, Medex, and so on), and by opposing nurses' efforts to control the collection of their own fees for service. For example, one medical society officer recently labeled as "childish" attempts by nurses

16.1   *Compression of Community Nursing by Outside Forces*

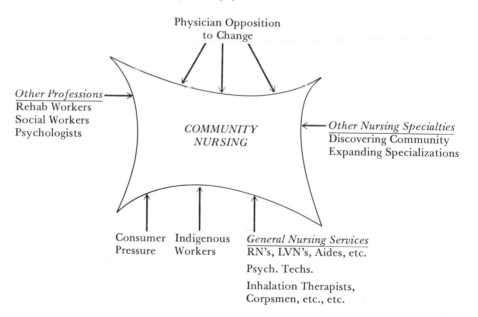

to negotiate their rights to help decide nursing staffing patterns in specialized areas of hospitals.

Certain kinds of client needs, long left to community health because others could not manage them, have suddenly attracted new categories of workers. For instance, drug abuse and alcoholism have become well-funded program areas and, consequently, battlegrounds for conflicting ideologies and professionals: lay, law-enforcement, religious workers, reformed users, or various mental and somatic health professionals. With substance abuse increasingly defined as mental problems rather than physical ones, the whole array of psychiatric practitioners have moved in with their claims of special expertise and the territorial battles escalate. Community nurses continue to participate but less noticeably. (When Ruth first volunteered at the Haight-Ashbury Free Clinic in 1967, its director could not figure what use a nonpsychiatric nurse could be.)

REACTIVE PROCESS IN COMMUNITY NURSING

Like any group movement community nursing has always had three sets of directions: the innovative leap forward, the reactive attempt to return to the past, and the holding operation that consolidates and institutionalizes change. The pressures defined above have been mounting in the last decade and community health nursing has found itself retreating from what had long been an advanced specialization. For many years, public health nursing was the only recognized, certified, high-salaried clinical specialty, thanks to early day activists in our field. All other advances in nursing had to be away from client service into teaching, supervision, or administration. Many sectors of nursing education maintained that only by narrower, in-depth specialization could nurses deliver expert nursing care. Thus, medical nurses moved into dialysis, cardiopulmonary disease, cancer care, diabetes, or other diagnostic specialties. Pediatric nursing specialties could focus at almost any stage of the age range, from newborns through adolescents, as well as in any of the major disease categories that apply to children. Maternity nurses could become experts in family planning or genetic counseling as well as prenatal and postpartum care.

The push in other areas of nursing for a client-centered specialization seemed of no particular concern to public health or community health nursing. However, as other specialties began to advance their own territorial limits into the community, the fact became clear that threats were being made on two fronts. Other specializations were not only invading our territory, they were also asserting that their expertise so outweighed ours in the various diagnostic categories they covered that they were justified in usurping our caseloads; we weren't needed anymore.

The first reaction was to shrink back before the certainty of the newcomers.

Community health nursing could envision a collective absolescence, even as individual nurses were moving into highly innovative areas of practice. Nurses learned in the Peace Corps, Model Cities, OEO projects, as well as in the experience of being the single nurse in a rural county, how much could be done when the needs were so great that health care professionals did not try to protect their own territorial rights. Attempts to create an overriding rationale to match those being publicized by the other specialized areas of practice bogged down in the complexities of the work community health nurses were actually doing. Community nursing groups from national to local levels have attempted to hammer out standards of practice that could apply across the board and have been baffled whenever these must be made operational. Some community health nurses tried to adopt the clinical specialist model of the late sixties. Now the catchphrase is nurse-practitioner, and community health nurses, like those in other areas of nursing, are trying to evolve yet another role to solve the dilemma.

COMMUNITY HEALTH NURSING PRACTITIONERS

Because there seemed to be a great deal of confusion about the definition of nurse-practitioner in community health, in 1973 we began a study of nurses who were so identified and we looked at the various formal and informal ways nurses are being prepared for such a role (Archer and Fleshman 1974; Archer 1976). The returns from several rounds of questionnaires make clear that nurses who label themselves as community health nurse-practitioners (CHNP) deal with the broadest possible range of activities. It also is clear that this broad range could be one of their characteristics: CHNP is a generalist and, if pushed, can operate with some degree of competence in nearly any area of care. Some respondents claimed in-depth knowledge about one or more specialized areas; others focused on primary care services (another watchword of the time) to various categories of clients. Some considered themselves CHNP without any client contact since they were teaching or administering programs that incorporated health-focused aspects they felt important to such a role.

These findings brought us to despair, for they suggested that CHNP was that old bane of nursing: supernurse. However, we began to see commonalities in the various descriptions of primary focus in job content, and we soon became aware of differences in the ways the CHNP reported their activities. From these we set up a typology (Archer and Fleshman

1974) and began to differentiate the features that characterize the predominant activities of each type. A first form of the typology was then sent back to the respondents who were asked to list their own activities under any of the functional categories that applied; each was also asked to list activities that did not seem to fit. After this round of testing the typology, which we modified from five to six categories under which the given activities could be placed with others of like kind, we consider it possible to describe CHNP practice in terms of its balance of multiple functions in direct, semidirect, and/or indirect relation to the health services client (table 16.1). In each of the columns, designated as fundamental community nursing linked with the particular specialty focus, we have tried to give examples to differentiate the way each operates. Although there are many other work elements that could be analyzed, we chose to look at the following aspects of each functional category: *Primary Activity,* the major focus of service delivery in the category; *Focus,* what portion of the health care spectrum is the special concern of the category; *Decision Making,* the particular nursing process used in working with the clients; and *Sites,* the locations in which the activities are most commonly carried out.

The first four functional categories are grouped under the heading of *Direct Client Services.* Here the nurse's primary interaction involves a health care exchange of some kind with a health care client, whether individual, family, or some other group. The fifth category, middle management/teaching, is identified as in a semidirect relation to the health care client. Although still concerned with the delivery of health services, these nurses must prepare, organize, equip, and supervise those who are the actual direct deliverers of care, whether students or workers. Finally, the sixth, administration/systems maintenance, is in an indirect relation to the health client. This area is concerned with creating the system within which the other levels of workers may function in the preparation for and actual delivery of health services (see figure 2.1, page 35). These latter two categories create some problems for nurses who insist that only direct health care delivery is "really nursing." As long as these managers and administrators are focused on health care delivery, they are a part of the whole clinical system and as important as all the others to the end product of that system.

A source of concern to some of our past readers is that what is detailed here is our prescription for the future of nursing. Actually, the patterns laid out here were derived from the responses of various nurses nationwide who replied to our survey instruments. In fact, we believe the diverse patterns of practice revealed by self-described CHNP may indicate the potential breakup of the field of community health nursing, as these various specialists begin to relate more closely with those in the specialty

TABLE 16.1 *Typology of Community Nursing Practice by Characteristics and Client Subsystems*

Characteristics	Direct Client Services				Semidirect Client Services	Indirect Client Services
	Subsystems by Nature of Client Services					
Functional Category	Community nursing plus diagnostic-disease-medical specialty.	Community nursing plus primary care.	Community nursing plus population group.	Community nursing plus place or spatial unit.	Community nursing plus middle management and teaching.	Administration and system maintenance.
Primary Activity	In-depth services to diagnostic category, usually but not always tied to illnesses.	Physical and psycho-social assessment; followup on deviations from norm and health promotion.	Wide-range service to designated group: positive health, overt illness, preventive actions.	Concern with widely defined health issues: delivery of comprehensive care to all in geographic area.	Management of personnel and material resources to facilitate delivery of direct client services.	Administration, research planning, system development, maintenance and repair, public relations, lobbying.
Clientele	Individuals or group members who fit disease category; their family members.	Individual-centered. Occasionally mother-child; some total family.	Group and/or members identified by shared characteristics.	All those within the spatial unit; communities, especially geographic; institutions.	Health workers on all levels, students on all levels.	System: Institution, agency, professional organization, funding agency.
Focus	Problem-centered on and related to organizing and delivering care to those in disease category.	Treatment and continuity of care for deviations from norm. Health promotion and maintenance.	Range of problems in client group, especially those particularly related to group membership.	Part of health care team serving geographic group; widest range of practice: primary, secondary, and tertiary perventive services.	Teaching, facilitating, and supervising others who deliver direct client services.	Administering, planning and evaluating direct and semidirect client services, resource development and allocation, research.

TABLE 16.1 (*Continued*)

Characteristics	Subsystems by Nature of Client Services					
	Direct Client Services				Semidirect Client Services	Indirect Client Services
Decision Making	Problem-solving processes, client management and teaching.	Sorting at entry point into care system: treat, consult, refer, follow.	Problem identification; matching resources to needs; transmission of information; advocacy.	Assessment, client-finding, counseling, teaching, referral. Epidemiological investigations and data gathering.	Teaching, consulting, allocating resources, evaluating those who give direct client services.	Planning, evaluating, controlling, allocating, forming policy for direct and semidirect client services.
Sites	Health agencies, inpatient and outpatient specialty clinics, occasionally specialist M.D. offices.	HMOs, OPDs, clinics, M.D. offices, health centers, health departments, independent practice.	Nonhealth and multipurpose agencies geared to serve client group: urban health centers, senior center, church, school, social service agencies, outreach programs, OPDs.	Local comprehensive health care centers, health departments, legislative and executive offices in branches of government.	Health service agencies, educational institutions in middle management, faculty, discharge planner positions, and in-service education.	Top management positions in service and educational institutions, professional organizations, research groups, management consultant firms.

Source: Sarah Ellen Archer, "Community Nursing Practitioners: Another Assessment." Reproduced with permission from *Nursing Outlook*, August Vol. 24 No. 8, p. 500. Copyright ● 1976, American Journal of Nursing Company.

area rather than with the field as a whole. This report, however, deals with a research approach and what follows from it will depend on the uses made of it by nurses in all these fields of practice.

CHN LINKED WITH DISEASE/DIAGNOSTIC CATEGORIES

One direction in which specialization may be developed is concentration on various factors related to a specific disease or diagnostic category. In traditional community settings these nurses have worked with the tuberculosis control or venereal disease services. Family planning and abortion counseling have more recently been the focus of such specialization. Some parts of community mental health have also evolved into diagnostically linked services for such categories as alcoholism or crisis intervention. The practitioner skills nurses may develop in these areas may well be of greater depth for being kept within bounds of a diagnostic category. Although illness provides the point of principal contact, the client transactions are not limited to this focus. Concerns about sexuality may, for example, fall quite legitimately within the purview of a nurse working with family planning. Those specializing in diabetic management must concern themselves not only with medical procedures but with the household adaptations that must be made by both clients and their families so that they may attain their optimum level of functioning. The clients such a nurse serves will be drawn from any of those fitting the diagnostic restriction, either as individuals or as members of the group. Often clients' families must be included in the care transaction. The nursing interventions are focused on problems directly related to and stemming from the diagnosis that organizes the specialty. In this area, the principal operation mode is probably the use of the entire problem-solving process directed to the diagnostic focus. In addition, the range of decision making that is involved with disease management is another major portion. These nurses tend to operate in health agencies, in inpatient and ambulatory services, in specialty clinics, and occasionally in the offices of specialized physicians. A generalist approach to this specialization may be seen in the visiting nurse services providing skilled nursing care services that are generally limited to third-party reimbursable diagnoses.

One possible source of conflict in such a combination specialization is that the disease restriction imposes a categorical limit to the concerns that are legitimate for such nurses. Their community health nursing aspect would often tend to pull toward either more comprehensive or wider distribution of services. If the community health becomes more important as a viewpoint, we may find that the nurse is engaging in a large number of "invisible" nursing activities: advising neighbors of the prime client, aiding families with health problems not strictly within the diagnostic limitations, employing nondisease-focused knowledge to aid client and family with wider health concerns. Needless to say, those of us with strong allegiance to comprehensive or inclusive health care do not approve of the limitations imposed by categorical programs and find them expedient only as funding sources for services not otherwise available.

CHN LINKED WITH PRIMARY CARE

Primary care practitioner is a new label for an old form of nursing activity that is gaining in stature as its various branches move toward special certification. Pressures on nursing in general have led some to move into a more independent role. Although the activities of many primary care practitioners are modeled on general practice medicine, the position of nurse-practitioners is firmly within a health care institution. The basis for their actions, categorized in the table as decision making, follows a triage or sorting process (see chapter 2). Here the decision to be made is to treat, to consult in order to treat, or to refer on. In practice, the conditions community nurses are permitted to treat are generally clearly circumscribed by the agency for which they work, as are the problems for which they must seek consultation or refer to more specialized practitioners, usually physicians. To some extent, these patterns change as individual practitioners prove their merit within the particular system. Until certification is generally established, the scope of practice is liable to be highly variable and more dependent on nurses' demonstrable abilities, the extent of trust in their skills, their own internal sense of strengths and limitations, and the agency's specific policies.

Although there is an awareness of the family and community bases from which their clients come, most primary care practitioners deal with individuals. Depending on the specialty, they may also see mother-child units or, less often, family groups. But the overwhelming majority of clients are individuals. Most transactions are illness-motivated, although some nurses are involved in the physical examination portion of multiphasic health screenings. Although these usually end up being generalized examinations of all the body systems revealing greater degrees of normality than abnormality, the examinations are still focused on the detection of pathology and decisions about the subsequent disposition for treatment. These nurse-practitioners are most often found working in ambulatory settings, such as outpatient departments, clinics, health maintenance organizations, physicians' group offices, or neighborhood health centers. In isolated areas or those areas with notably less than their fair share of health services, nurses have always had to deliver primary care. Many long-time office nurses have also developed the expertise to be entrusted more or less regularly with such responsibilities. Clients for this form of nursing may be drawn from those who presently seek care from similar medical general practitioners. There is little emphasis on case finding except insofar as publicity about the primary care practitioner makes health care more accessible or acceptable to people who had not made use of previously available services.

CHN LINKED WITH POPULATION CATEGORIES

Although all clients share an essential humanity, there are clearly identified commonalities within various groupings of people that make a focus on population groups a legitimate form of specialization. These people can be members of an ethnic or racial group, an age grade, (such as infants, school-age children, young adults, elderly), gender, (such as the clients of various women's self-help units), or even lifestyles (alternative, gay, or religious). The nurse will be concerned with the entire range of health-related services pertaining to the group's needs: for positive advancement of well-being, to cure overt or incipient illnesses, or prevent those to which they are most liable. Such a nurse tends to focus most on the health concerns usually encountered by group members, especially those connected in some way with their characteristics as members of the group. Sickle cell anemia, for example, is not limited to black populations but its presence in their genetic pool makes it a most apt concern for a nurse focusing on that group. Sexually active members of a gay community might well have need for venereal disease services but tend to have lower than usual interest in contraceptive advice. Chronic disease is not absent among young adults but it is not as frequent as such problems as allergy or suicide. Counseling in sexuality might well have far different content when directed to an elderly population than to other age groups. Because nurses with such a specialization begin from a more holistic stance, their expertise is more likely to be in establishing the parameters of typical health concerns and their practice of the decision-making process more likely to be in identifying problems, matching problems to the resources available to deal with them, and informing the client about possible actions to be taken. Such nurses are most likely to become advocates for the group or its members. In this capacity they may act to translate its characteristics to professionals or others involved in health services. They may also work to modify or create services that are more suitable to the group clients. The demand for bilingual health workers in areas with heavy concentrations of foreign-born people may be one that such a nurse can effectively champion. As advocates, nurses may also mobilize the client group to pursue its own special interest action by suggesting ways to exert leverage on decision-making bodies.

Such nurses might work in nonhealth or multipurpose agencies such as schools, jails, churches, and social service or outreach facilities. There may be employment in outpatient services and clinics as well as health centers in urban areas where population density would justify such specialization.

CHN LINKED WITH PLACE

In most areas of nursing the client is an individual or, at most, a group of individuals. The shift that occurs in this fourth category is a hard one to absorb. For nurses with this form of specialization, the client is the entire population that is present in some place or community of the types discussed in chapter 2. The place may be a community with a geopolitical base, ranging from a neighborhood to a nation. Some of the other types of communities can be organizations or institutions that comprise a total system or subsystem. In all the forms, the characteristic that is crucial to nursing practice is the involvement with the total population of the given community. Even if they are not actual clients, in this type of specialization everyone on site is equally at risk of being served.

Community health nursing has long had a relationship with various geopolitical communities, but few present health agencies actually serve the total population of their territories. In spite of the title and ostensible goals, public or community health agencies do not serve the entire public. Instead there is often a division between official agencies' clients and those who can afford to buy their medical care, as well as that portion of the population that is totally outside the medical care system. This latter group would include those who are not ill, for instance, or those whose notions of health and illness or the proper ways of dealing with problems are in conflict with the orthodox medical model.

For all the varieties of community nursing practice within this category, the primary focus is working with and through others to improve or provide health care services to the total membership of some location. The focus may be direct or semidirect (see chapter 1), again depending on the particulars. In a direct relation, the nurses would be part of the health team serving some total population. If semidirect, they would be planning with agencies or communities (and preferably both) about aspects of health care delivery. Direct service, with institutions as clients, would be provided by industrial nurses, those who work in summer camps, and those military nurses concerned with preventive and safety measures. Even though schools and jails also comprise institutional subsystems, their nurses' primary responsibility is for the students or inmates, not the teachers or guards; thus these nurses are placed under the population-linked type of specialization. Nurses who do work with the entire membership of an institution, however, would fit the present category. Community nurses may eventually find the Health Maintenance Organization (HMO) structure best suited to direct care to some entire geopolitical unit.

In dealing with total populations of any geographic unit much above a neighborhood, nurses will probably be involved in semidirect services. They may be found as staff members of a state health department bureau attempting to place contract health services in sparsely populated or impoverished rural areas that cannot maintain health department budgets of their own. World Health Organization nurses may well be involved at top decision-making levels in planning for care delivery for entire nations or multination regions. Participating with other community members to organize for action to produce their own health services is another instance of semidirect participation.

CHN LINKED WITH MIDDLE MANAGEMENT AND TEACHING

Insofar as some nurses practice primarily in this category, they have limited direct contact with consumers of health care. Instead, their "clients" are either the personnel actually engaged in delivering that care or the students being prepared for such service. We have defined this relation as semidirect since the ultimate concern is still focused on delivery of health services although these nurses are not in a position to do it themselves. (Of course, many nurses in these roles also maintain some form of clinical practice to keep in touch with that aspect of professional activities, but it is seldom a job requirement.)

Nurses working in this category can be found in the entire range of health services agencies and in the various educational institutions that prepare health care workers. Their titles may vary but they are located at the middle management level as supervisors, in-serve educators, discharge planners, care coordinators, or, in schools, as faculty members. These latter are often hard to see as middle management, but in the academic field, faculty members have a responsibility for the curriculum and the evaluation of their students that is more or less parallel to service supervisors' responsibility for program and personnel evaluation.

They utilize the range of skills from other fields that go into the techniques of teaching and supervising this other layer of health workers, either in the work arena or in their preparation. Supervisorial and in-service nursing staff, for example, use many of the same teaching skills employed by faculty in schools of nursing. Similarly, nursing teachers must often supervise and evaluate student performance. For this reason these job categories can be viewed as more similar than is assumed. In addition, incumbents of these positions get from their particular system somewhat more power and responsibility than those they supervise or teach.

CHN LINKED WITH ADMINISTRATION AND SYSTEM MAINTENANCE

Another step removed from direct contact with the health care consumer are those nurses whose "client" is some system, such as an institution, agency, or professional organization. They engage in diverse activities involved in administration, research, planning, public relations, or lobbying. They are responsible for some aspect of system development, maintenance, or repair. Thus such a nurse may be a member of a multi-disciplinary team planning a new health maintenance organization, or a dean of a university school of nursing charged with its total day-by-day operation, or even an administrator specifically recruited to introduce up-to-date practices in an agency stagnating after years of inept leadership.

It has occasionally been hard for nurses in this functional area to remain identified as nurses, since they tend to associate with people from other fields who also administer or otherwise work in systems operations. The unique contribution of a health care background may be seen, how-ever, in the kinds of decisions made by such nurses as opposed to ad-ministrators whose background is business and whose major criteria follow from a cost-accounting perspective. We can often see far different outcomes in decisions made by nurse-administrators because they remain significantly committed to the goals of community health. Otherwise, the nurse and non-nurse administrator are both concerned with generating funds and allocating them among the various departments, with plan-ning, overseeing, and evaluating both direct and semidirect client ser-vices, utilizing or engaging in research, or any of the other tasks involved at the top management levels. A health background, however, contributes an added dimension that we feel is crucial to retain in this category of community health nursing (see chapter 22 for more on administration).

Practitioner Preparation

The routes by which nurses become prepared for these roles are widely varied. Whether we start from a base of community health nursing and move toward the specialty or begin from the more usual form of that specialty and add a new consciousness of community health is not always an important distinction. Thus those of us who evolved from generalized community health can welcome colleagues who move out of traditional psychiatric institutional settings to community mental health. In chapter 14 we mentioned that Helen had been a community health nurse and her associate, Suzanne, a medical-surgical specialist. Their joint work with the Pomo health clinic gradually merged their special areas of knowledge until both became some blend of community health workers. Taking a family nurse-practitioner program added primary care skills to their roster of talents.

Community/primary care practice has generally developed out of an apprenticeship relation with some physician or, more rarely, with another practitioner already functioning in the role. Recently, formal educational programs in nursing have begun to emphasize the acquisition of primary practitioner skills.

The community/disease specialization tends to be derived from on the job evolution, motivated either by special client needs or the demands of the hiring agency. Special continuing education courses or in-service workshops contribute to this kind of expertise. Our own generalist-specialty, community health, is the only recognized one included in basic programs. Other specialization in nursing tends to develop at the post-baccalaureate level since basic nursing programs continue to teach all things to all students. Although some graduate programs may enable nurses to enter into a specialty, most require a prior base of study or experience.

There has been a great deal of ferment in the third category of community health nursing: community/population linkage . This area of specialization is an old division in nursing: Specialization with nursing of children has derived directly from motherhood, and school nursing has been a recognized nursing specialty from the start of this century. Geriatric specialization is more recent and the formalization of ethnic health care is also new. Further group identification as the basis for health service continues to evolve at an ever accelerating rate. The routes to preparation in this category may be formal programs, as with the earlier specialties, by *ad hoc* combinations of continuing education opportunities, or by the newest method: being a member of the population group itself. There seems to be a stage through which special populations have recently been going that insists that only a member of the population can adequately understand the circumstances to deliver health care stylistically suited to the group's particular needs. This has happened with certain portions of the free clinic movement, with some of the ethnic groups, women's self-help or special needs clinics, and services geared to other lifestyles.

The fourth model, community/place practice, features a wide variety of directions for preparation. Almost all of them reflect an individualized pulling together of diverse components: personal experience, professional preparation, formal and informal education, and self-directed learning. Until recently, the community-as-client model was an alternative nurse-practitioners derived on their own.

When our study began there was one exception to the do-it-yourself approach to role development: the Community Nurse-Practitioner Project at the School of Public Health, University of Texas, Houston. This ten-month program, leading to a master of public health degree, focused on entire communities with emphasis on community organization, planning, and epidemiology. The project was especially concerned with community self-help and the focusing upon the health of the total community as one's caresphere; a major part of the role is to discover with the community what its health priorities are, what resources are available, and what would be an effective and acceptable manner to approach the problem (Skrovan et al. 1974: 849). Although this project ended, the concept was adopted by nursing faculty at the University of Illinois and, at last report, was alive and well there.

The acquisition of skills used in the fifth category of our typology can cover the entire range of possibilities. Many nurses advance into middle management solely on the basis of longevity; in some places head nurses are simply those who have been there longer than the staff nurses. Some reveal special management skills in their daily work activities and are recognized for promotion. There are increasing numbers of in-service and continuing education workshops to provide skills in personnel and resource management. Formal teaching positions require higher education, which may be restricted to clinical or academic content and contribute little toward the development of teaching methods. Similarly, although many nurses enter graduate programs in preparation for middle management positions, they find few curricula designed to provide these functional skills.

It is perhaps paradoxical that although many top management jobs require a higher degree, programs in nursing contain little academic content devoted to the skills of, for example, deaning. These must be learned almost entirely by association with people already in such jobs or, if good role models are absent, by trial and error on the job. Of course, many of the same methods are used in middle management positions and it is generally from these ranks that nurses advance to the indirect service roles. It is often necessary to turn to fields outside nursing to acquire the needed methods, and many nurses are found taking courses in law, business, and public administration for these upper echelons. There is a growing tendency to look to these fields for candidates to fill administrative jobs and nurses are becoming concerned that decision making about nursing will be usurped by those who do not share a nursing perspective.

NURSES IN INDEPENDENT PRACTICE

Since the completion of the practitioner study, a new trend has become more noticeable that may add a new factor to the areas of direct client services. Until recently we could safely say that nurses were to be found as employees of various agencies and institutions. This situation has recently begun to change as more of us become impatient with the bureaucratic restrictions that keep us from using our entire repertoire of skills and talents. Besides, some of us notice the salary differentials between the independent professional and the hired hand. Thus a growing number of nurses have established themselves in independent practice. To some extent, such practices are a logical outgrowth of the movement toward higher degrees of professionalism. In addition, many nurses see some of the newer Nurse Practice Acts as requiring them to use their knowledge more fully than most agencies will permit. Independent practice is seen as a way to do so and be rewarded directly by clients and/or third-party payers. At the time we carried out the foregoing study of community nurse-practitioners, only two respondents identified themselves as independents. Gathering figures on the present numbers is still not possible, but many more nurses are so engaged and many others are highly interested in this challenging trend (Jacox and Norris 1977).

The idea of independent practice raises a great many issues that range from philosophical questions of the fee-for-service approach, of the propriety of yet another professional role, of team versus solo practice, down to the real life problems of how to learn all the crucial aspects of setting up practice. The general focus of discussion among present and potential independent practitioners is generally on the latter with much sharing of fee schedules, client recruitment, and public relations activities. Whether independent practice will become a major element in professional nursing probably hinges on attempts to include nurses as those reimbursed by third-party payers, both private and public (Archer and Fleshman 1978).

SUMMARY

Nurse-practitioner is one of the very new watchwords in nursing literature, but its meaning for community health is unclear. Our study of nurses who considered themselves such workers suggests that their functions may be subdivided into a logical set of types that we describe as community health nursing linked with varying emphases: (1) diagnostic/disease/specialty, (2) primary care, (3) population, (4) place, (5) middle management/teaching, and (6) administration/systems operation.

Community health has long been a generalist practice, but this approach has become hard to defend in the face of increasing specialization in the rest of nursing. The pressures from other social sectors upon community health have added to the need for some nurses to redefine their practice in specialist terms. How they have done so in the past often reflects the concurrent trends.

Like any logic, our constructs are derived from inductive research and, as the study goes on, may be revised to fit new data, collegial critiquing, or changes in the situation. The typology is not intended to determine practice or methods of preparing for specialization but reflects our analysis of what seems to be going on in nursing practice as of the time we completed that phase of our study. It appears to have been useful to other community nurses in seeing more clearly the multiple forms already emerging from nursing practice and may help to complicate our thinking processes to the greater benefit of nursing.

REFERENCES

ARCHER, SARAH ELLEN. "Community Nurse-Practitioners: Another Assessment." *Nursing Outlook* 24 (1976): 499–503.

ARCHER, SARAH ELLEN, and FLESHMAN, RUTH P. "Community Health Nursing: A Typology of Practice." *Nursing Outlook* 23 (1975): 358–64.

ARCHER, SARAH ELLEN, and FLESHMAN, RUTH P. "Doing Our Thing: Community Nursing in Independent Practice." *Journal of Nursing Administration* VIII (November 1978): 44–51.

COMMUNITY NURSE-PRACTITIONER STAFF. "Community Nurse Practitioner Project: Second Annual Progress Report." Mimeo. School of Public Health, Community Nurse-Practitioner Program, University of Texas at Houston, September 30, 1973.

JACOX, ADA K., and NORRIS, CATHERINE M. *Organizing for Independent Nursing Practice.* New York: Appleton-Century-Crofts, 1977.

KINLEIN, LUCILLE. "Independent Nurse-Practitioner." *Nursing Outlook* 20 (1972): 22.

LEWIS, M. D. "Health Care for Denver's Poor." *American Journal of Nursing* 69 (1969): 1469–71.

MILIO, NANCY. *9226 Kercheval: The Storefront That Did Not Burn.* Ann Arbor: University of Michigan Press, 1970.

PAYNICH, MARY L. et al. "Is There a Role for the Nurse Clinician in Public Health?" *Nursing Outlook* 17 (1969): 32–36.

SKROVAN, CLARENCE, ANDERSON, ELIZABETH T., and GOTTSCHALK, JANET. "Community Nurse Practitioner." *American Journal of Public Health* 64 (1974): 847–52.

17. Community Health Nurses and Community Mental Health

Carol Edgerton Mitchell

INTRODUCTION

Why are we talking about community mental health (CMH) in a book about community health nursing? For that matter, who is a community mental health nurse (CMHN). Are CMHNs nurse-psychotherapists moved out of the state mental hospital into community mental health centers? Are they community health nurses who like psych? Or are they some entirely distinctive type of nurse specialists or maybe a kind of supernurses? CMHNs have their own notions of what sets them apart from other nursing specialists, but as a group CMHNs have trouble agreeing as to just what those distinctions are, since all of the above definitions have been suggested by those involved in the preparation of nurses for such positions.

Five CMHNs were gathered; they dissected role complexities, discarded tired old cliches, and pinpointed commonalities. The discussion was lively; within the loosely woven fabric of mental health practice, individual philosophy, work style, and locus varied hugely. Ivy-covered institutions with authoritarian hierarchies (and imaginative crusaders), funky little clinics with uncomfortable traditionalists (and dedicated volunteers); health maintenance organizations with interdisciplinary combinations of all of these above are each a piece of the elusive whole. All have a role in services to clients and CMHNs operate in each. But, who are the CMHNs and what is their purpose? Representing some of the settings and styles of CMH nursing, the small group believed truisms of purpose and process could surface from an analysis of "those things we are really about . . . ."

Examples of CMH Nursing

One of the five nurses, through her own initiative and enthusiasm, had created "Obesity Groups" in a fast-paced, tightly organized, ambulatory care clinic. Members, coming from the wider clinic population, were patients for whom obesity was "only" secondary to a medical diagnosis. Identifying an unvoiced and professionally unattended client need—and recognizing it as an opportunity for appropriate role expansion—this nurse negotiated a tentative program with clinic staff, consultants, and clients and then designed a meeting format complete with goals, approaches, and methods of evaluation. There were soon four groups of young people and older adults gathered for weekly meetings. Centered on solving the hassles of daily living, the groups also provided peer support for the anxiety, discouragement, and general discontent of their members. The clinic staff watched the progress of these groups with considerable interest and suggested to the nurse that such a group approach be generalized. Groups could be established for adolescent diabetics or for elderly clients complaining of isolation; possibilities were limited only by resources and vision.

Across town, in three small rooms, there was a somewhat different approach to an emerging need. After negotiating her entry through a fiery women's action group, another of the five nurses had established a self-esteem counseling service for older women who were hesitantly approaching employment for the first time. Ebbing confidence was bolstered by supportive discussion of personal strengths and experiential assets; role playing difficult interpersonal scenes gave poise, deepened understanding, and promoted success. Postemployment followup allowed members to ease emerging role conflicts and to share success stories with newer clients awaiting that initial job interview.

A few city blocks away, a third nurse was involved in a collegial team effort with social workers and psychiatrists working at a psychiatric hospital's outpatient department and in the surrounding neighborhood. Using home visits for assessment of family strengths and dynamics, she worked with a caseload of "multiproblem" families of hospitalized and day-treatment psychiatric patients. Functioning both within the institution and in her clients' homes, she sharpened her awareness of the significance of language and place in interaction. The subtleties of ice cream socialization in a kitchen, professional discussion in the office, and philosophical variations at the team conference table were woven into here nursing practice.

Far removed from her colleagues in location and style, but harmonious in purpose, the fourth nurse was immersed in the judiciary system. Working in conjunction with a concerned parole officer who had facilitated her entry, she promoted peer support and problem solving through rap groups for parolees and honor farm inmates. Recognizing the fragility of her innovative approach, she was determined that the fledgling groups would progress and that their progress be demonstrated. Evaluation techniques were designed and woven into her program. Initial questionnaires and observations provided baseline data for ongoing measurement; frequency, content, and direction of intragroup interactions would become the guidelines for further action. Correlation of these early data with final evaluations were designed to help establish the value of her program. The uniqueness inherent in all pilot projects provided her with both flexibility of operation and uncharted areas of ambiguity.

The last of the gathered CMH nurses was consultant with a storefront neighborhood center for adolescents hassled by problems with school, parents, or the law; she was also a volunteer member of a family dropin center and referral service for situations related to alcohol abuse. At both centers, the groups—eclectic gatherings of concerned citizens and involved professionals—represented community response to institutionally ignored problems. Unlike some grassroots organizations, these two centers had been thoughtfully preplanned, thereby permitting their successful emergence from the "first-year frailty" that wreaks havoc with many new programs. Working relationships were now stabilized and goals more sharply defined; the heady feel of success was translated into great enthusiasm. Only recently, after value was demonstrated through their own efforts, had the groups been able to enlist official interest and budgetary support. Again, both internal and external evaluation were key elements of these programs and had been instrumental in "selling" the centers. But, selling requires a buyer: Community acceptance and involvement were promoted through frequent public relations campaigns and carefully publicized recruitment of volunteers for the programs' emergency telephone hotlines, dropin facilities, and numerous referral activities. Outreach for prevention and education was included through open house discussions at the centers and the provision of volunteer speakers at school, church, and work institutions.

The variety of what these five nurses were doing was evident. The range of activities could become mind-boggling by including colleagues engaged in: convalescent home consultation, stress-reduction programs in occupational health nursing, holistic health education at every level within school systems, discharge planning for mental hospital patients and consultation/implementation of their resocialization programs within their communities. Some work with police departments to assist victims of rape and wife beating; others work with the American Red Cross during disasters. Still others collaborate with innumerable private and public agencies to educate, assess, intervene and evaluate all manner of self-destructive behaviors and painful personal predicaments. Whether a situation of drug abuse, separation by divorce, depression and withdrawal of retirement, or family disruption attendant upon a suddenly handicapped child, a CMHN may be present.

The commonality linking this whole array of professional activities centers upon a shared definition of community mental health as holistic, people-in-their-environment-effort to promote peoples' abilities to function optimally. Health, itself, reflects a focus upon inherent strengths and possibilities, rather than a preoccupation with malady or weakness. Weaving the purpose and process of their colleagues in community health with the theory and skills of those in mental health, the ensuing blend operationalized the philosophy that there can be no "health" without mental health and no "reality" without inclusion of the ecosystem. Only in the interactions of body and mind and of person and environment does health become evident. The significance of this relationship, fundamental in ancient Eastern philosophies and acknowledged in the classical Latin exhortation *mens sana in corpore sano* (a sound mind in a sound body), is currently being explored through a mushrooming of mental health approaches to self-actualization. Crisis group, encounter, sensitivity training, psychodrama, primal therapy, transactional analysis, and many, many more make up a varied enough smorgasbord to offer some appropriate kind of growth experience for almost everyone.

BASIC CONCEPTS IN CMH

The philosophy of community mental health represents a holistic approach common to the efforts of all five nurses. Incorporating the community health model of primary prevention, health promotion, maintenance, and rehabilitation, it emphasizes comprehensive and continuous care, planned for and delivered within the clients' own community (National Commission on Community Health Services 1966: ch. 12). The dynamics of adaptation and the implications of stress are core concepts and the subtleties of community—or system—entry, facilitate their application.

ADAPTATION

Through the dynamics of adaptation an individual moves toward illness or health. Adaptation represents growth, a continuous process of mutual demand-response cycles rather than a static state of attainment.

From origin to final dissolution, an entity must constantly interact with its milieu, or ecosystem; this is as true for the newly formed rap group as it is for the middle-aged, and currently unemployed, woman. Since these reciprocal demands generate compromise responses, each demand permits further progression in adaptation. The reciprocity inherent in a rap group is readily recognized, but there is a similar interactional relationship between the group as a totality and its sheltering environment. If the group fails to meet its responsibilities, expenses, maintenance, shelter will be withdrawn; should the shelter prove inhospitable, depressing, uncomfortable, the group will move on. There is a similar adaptive reciprocity between CMHNs' perceptions of their purpose and their organizations' expectations of their functions—as well as in the comfort of each others' philosophy. Seldom, however, are the processes' mutuality in balance. When institutional and individual philosophies are in conflict, morale declines; and when a social environment demands youthful beauty, verve, and economic productivity, the "over-forty" female may withdraw. As adaptation suggests optimal, bilateral response to mutual demands, so maladaptation indicates an unbalanced response that unduly favors one party of the interaction at the expense of the other.

Additional dimensions are given these interactions by continual—and opposing—demands for both change and stability. While the fact of maturation assures the inevitability of change, there is also present a counter tendency for stability, an inclination to organize experience into patterns and to rely on these "easy" repetitious responses for smoother operations. Mrs. A. M., forty-nine years old, recently widowed, and now looking for first-time employment, is tugged onward by her yearning for betterment while simultaneously she hesitates, fearful to leave the security of her old ways. Adolescents, beckoned by physiological and social maturation, attack the same authority systems that give them the comforting stability that enables them to attack.

STRESS

As adaptation is the dynamic process of growth, so stress is the instigator. Described variously as strain, pressure, intensity of force, it seems to have acquired a somewhat negative connotation in common usage. Advertising suggests that stress requires pills for the head, powders for the stomach, and salves for those portions between. In truth, stress is essential for our very structure; for only in the intricate balance of stress and counter stress do even our individual cells maintain their integrity. Both the physics of muscle action and the mental health concern for the interrelationships of people and their ecosystem are grounded in the study of stress. Levi provides a comprehensive working definition of the stress reaction as ". . . the nonspecific response of the body to any demand made upon it" (1972:11), and Hans Selye, father of stress-adaptation research, succinctly identifies the stressor as any external agent initiating the stress response (1956:261). Central to these considerations is the absence of a positive or negative value of stressors. Stress or distress, agent of greatest joy or deepest sorrow, stressors all invoke change.

Scientific interest in stress is relatively new. Selye began his pioneer laboratory studies of measurable physiological and behavioral changes associated with the General Adaptation Syndrome (stress reaction) in 1936. His first book on the subject, in 1950, reported observations and measurement of laboratory rats and guinea pigs subjected to a variety of stressors such as lowered temperature, injury, and overcrowding. Human subjects have also been monitored for cardiovascular, sympathoad-renomedullary, and renal reactions to experimental and life stress. Some of the sophisticated findings have been translated into popular measures by which we may calculate and assess the desirability—or possible lethality—of our present life stress quotient. Lethality of stress sounds ominous. Even as life stress is an integral element in human maintenance and growth, there is a finite capacity for adapting to stressors. Selye's rats, coping valiantly, developed maximum adaptability and then, as stress continued, lost the adaptability and died (1956:88–89). Levi analyzed reactions of invoice clerks pressured to improve their performance. Work output did increase, and so did excretions of adrenaline, noradrenaline, and creatinine along with significant complaints of fatigue and physical discomfort (Levi 1972:ch. 6). But negative stressors are not the only ones to evoke distress. Working within a carefully screened laboratory setting, Levi studied another group of human subjects in their reactions to various stimuli. Bland films of natural scenery provided baseline reaction data against which subject response to violent, frightening, and humorous films were contrasted. Adrenaline excretion was significantly elevated during the pleasant as well as the unpleasant films. There was no appreciable difference in arousal (Levi 1972:ch. 3).

The feeling of "let down," so common after achievement, is typified in the new mother's "baby blues" and the graduate's "postcommencement droop." Both may be linked to the ability of adrenaline to trigger excitement or euphoria that may be followed by depression. Helping people to anticipate this and other common and very normal occurrences can help them deal more effectively with the results of these and other "passages" (Sheehy 1976). This kind of anticipatory guidance is an essential part of community health nurses' roles just as it is of community mental health nurses' roles.

Periods of life complicated by exceptional or snowballing demands for adaptation may be marked by emotional distress, physical illness, and even death. Overstimulation of adaptive potential, as summarized in studies of World War II guerrilla forces, is first indicated by fatigue, then confusion and increasing irritability, and, eventually, the listless surrender of emotional exhaustion (Toffler 1970:345). Transcultural studies of relationships between stressors indicate that the high cost of adaptation is common to the human situation (Holmes and Masuda 1972:71). We are beginning to recognize the major role of stress on physical conditions such as hypertension, heart conditions, and even the onset of cancer. Change events can even be ranked in the order of their impact on the stress-adaptation systems: death—or loss—of a spouse, followed closely by divorce and marital separation, have primary weight; marriage is midway on the value scale, with retirement and marital reconciliation coming fast behind. These stressors seem to transcend cultural variation as do many other life events. Some other stressors, however, may be culturally defined, and the significance of all are further determined by individual perception. Progression from street to jail to court to probation might signify a number of things: disgrace, chagrin, fury, or pride. Illegitimate birth may indicate shame or distinction.

The measure of stress factors, thoughtfully correlated with the signs and symptoms of adaptive and/or maladaptive response, becomes our mental health indicator. Audy suggests this indicator may qualitatively and quantitatively be measured in our ability to rally, or bounce back, from the insults, or stressors, we encounter (Audy 1971:145). Through increased self-awareness, we can monitor our stress status and consciously provide for increased sensory stimulation when the environment is dull or we can build in peaceful respites when our circuits suffer from overload. Such prescriptive use of stress is appropriate for CMHNs working with lonely clients isolated through long institutionalization or recently impaired function from cultural stimulation; they can also use it as their problem-solving approach with other clients bewildered by the overlapping demands imposed by a fast-shifting social milieu. Interventions aimed at facilitating the adaptive use of stress provide common linkage for a myriad of roles.

Community Entry

Treatment of psychiatric illness, the forerunner of community mental health care, traditionally was administered within institutions designed for that specific purpose. The very architecture of these fortress-like buildings spoke of fear and its containment. Moreover, the usual institutional location—an out-of-sight-out-of-mind distance from town—enabled community denial of mental illness and further encouraged the chance passerby to appreciate this restrictive approach to "public safety." It fit the times, for the early 1900s, both treatment and architectural styles were congruent with the state of the art in psychiatric care and understanding. Now, when mental health difficulties are conceptualized as adaptation problems as much as psychiatric illness, the locus of intervention can no longer be confined to stoutly walled institutions. Since adaptation is concerned with social interaction, the interventions of mental health are aimed at facilitating interpersonal living, preferably in the natural environment of the home or community. Yet, generations of separation and concealment have left a legacy of stigma, of awkwardness and suspicion overlaying most concepts of the psyche. These vestiges hamper both the effectiveness of health worker and the receptivity of consumer. The problem is magnified as traditional professional styles—appropriate to authoritative control—are discovered to be inappropriate in the newly desirable community open systems, and the traditional practitioners—fearing or actually sensing this ineptitude—may withdraw from outreach efforts necessary for realistic community interaction. They choose, instead, to wait in their new community center offices for the appearance of "properly motivated patients" who are responsive to their efforts. Locus of intervention may shift from the mahogany desk of the psychiatric hospital to the color-coordinated desk of the mental health center; the therapeutic style, however, may be unchanged.

Community members, interpreting the professionals' apparent withdrawal as lack of commitment, may scorn available services. Only a little self-persuasion is needed for many long-suffering persons to convince themselves that (a) there is no mental health problem, (b) if there were, it would be someone else's, and (c) the "head shrinkers" are too out of touch with reality to be of much use anyway. Without a full-blown emergency, consumers tend to avoid traditional mental health agencies. This statement is true both of the services offered, since only a tiny segment of the community may become socialized into mainstay patients, and of the service location, since fearful complaints of possible traffic problems, fire hazard, and crime potential accompany proposals for almost every community location of mental health services.

Not only, then, is effective community entry by mental health professionals essential to allow a meaningful and effective fit between mental health agency and community, but it requires great sensitivity and fastidious attention to detail to overcome the traditional separatism that can maintain or increase the gap. Certainly, community assessment is a first step of the process since the characteristic profile of the particular neighborhood, town, or county needs early delineation. "Basic doorbell ringing," as it wryly has been called, pretty much describes the methodology. This entry assessment does far more than gather information, it is also a "soft sell" of both health professional and potential health service. Too, it attempts to contact consumers' reality, to acknowledge interest, and to encourage involvement even while it introduces consumers to the philosophy and personnel of the mental health agency. Effectiveness of entry is evaluated through use of agency services and through their continued responsiveness to community needs.

The Alcohol Information Committee (AIC) in one county demonstrates this entry process. The seven to eight committee members included a school health nurse, a community health nurse, and a CMHN. All were taxpayers and established community members, but were still bound by the necessity of another entry, one that would permit their meaningful activity within an area of specialized interest. Potential working relationships within the community emerged during the committee's subsequent entry assessment as newspaper reporters, elementary and junior high principals and teachers, traffic judges, police officials, and civic leaders were contacted. All defined alcohol abuse as a major community problem, even though they unanimously echoed the difficulty of intervention. Secondary and tertiary prevention programs, focused upon help for the acute and chronic stages of alcoholism, carried stigma with them. A community attitude of denial that any problem existed was pervasive. The hidden costs of absenteeism, health deterioration, accidents, residential fires, motor vehicle fatalities, and family disruption remained uncounted. The implications of four to five "significant others" assumed to be painfully linked with each alcohol abuser were also being ignored. The potential for primary prevention of alcohol abuse was huge. The AIC wanted to use the momentum generated through its entry assessment for greatest possible effectiveness. Because its resources were limited, it had to focus upon the particular portion of the alcohol abuse problem most accessible to change. Choosing a limited target goal that has a high probability of success, can go a long way toward building an organization's public credibility and generating additional resources.

Because of their concern for their young people, county residents were greatly distressed at the prevalence of pre- and early-teen problem drinking. For this reason, the AIC believed that energy to alter the present picture of alcohol abuse by young people could be organized. Active intervention was most important to the people whose concern was much more focused on the overt symptoms of alcohol abuse by young people than on the possible causes for this behavior. The community assessment had delineated both specific problem areas and persons interested in challenging them. A talent assessment of committee members revealed abilities and interests specific for the purpose. The committee's successful community entry, facilitated by this organizational–situational match, was soon evident in well attended classrooms, PTA meetings, and county workshops exploring youthful *and* parental alcohol abuse. The nurses on the AIC further incorporated alcohol counseling and consultation into their practice: with students worried about self, family or friend; with teachers wondering how they might better approach the problem within their own classrooms; and with persons concerned about self, spouse, or child. Friendly contact with the local press translated into positive publicity, and the committee was gratified to see its efforts acknowledged county-wide and rewarded by public response and budgetary support.

EPIDEMIOLOGY

Not limited to the pursuit of Typhoid Mary nor the discovery of brucellosis, epidemiology is essential in mental health. When the focus shifts from treatment of manifest psychosis, obesity, or child abuse to one including a concern for prevention, much of the population at risk may be obscure and the interventions may be ill-defined. Evaluation of statistics gathered from incidence reports, treatment programs, and neighborhood surveys can reveal multicausal relationships. These serve as foundational hypotheses for new approaches and further evaluation. With an understanding of the background complexity of child abuse, the CMHNs put on the "epidemiologist hat" and use data to estimate tendencies and plan interventions. Parents who were themselves abused tend to repeat their own damaging experiences with their children. Their anxiety and guilt may prevent them from reaching out for help. Patterned bruises, fractures, or malnutrition can indicate that a child has been abused. CMHNs become educator, case finder, child advocate, and resource for parents. The community information programs they plan or implement may break the vicious cycle in some situations: Their consultation with individual and groups of troubled parents may lessen the infliction of injury while their participation in detection programs facilitates early care and treatment. Followup questionnaires assess the value of these interventions and provide information for new approaches. Epidemiology is a thread of continuity running through all phases of CMH nursing activities.

SYSTEMS ASSESSMENT

Systems assessment is essential in the practice of community mental health. Resources available in the interacting systems represented by client, staff, clinic, community, family, and CMHNs must be recognized and enlisted. A key in this assessment is the determination of strength, or power, within the resource network and consideration of the methods by which this strength may most effectively be marshalled. Probable consequences of alternative actions need to be weighed, for the ripple effect of an event extends a dozenfold.

For example, Laura, a timid, overweight adolescent, diffidently stated her determination to shed pounds, hopeful of gaining peer group acceptance. Faithful in "Obesity Group" attendance, but still showing no shrinkage, she later reported bountiful meals over which mother persided, urging, "Clean up your plate, I've spent the whole afternoon cooking!" The situation required a reassessment of purpose and power, a selection from alternative nursing actions that would align meaningful parts of Laura's home environment with that of the clinic's.

During a problem-solving session she had designed for both Laura and her mother, the nurse encouraged a more open communication style that in turn enabled Laura to ask for her mother's help. Pleased with the role of coplanner, Mrs. E. was soon enthusiastically discussing special low calorie menus she would prepare. Mother, in joining the CMH subsystem, lent strength rather than sabotage, and Laura's pounds were soon disappearing. We are, as John Muir said, all hitched to everything else; the interwoven network of each person's support system includes subsystems that interfere with positive change as well as those that facilitate it. Consideration of the real—and potential—value or threat of these systems is essential for a meaningful assessment.

RECIPROCITY

The last, but equally important, part of the CMH approach is reciprocity of involvement. Nowhere is assuring clients' genuine participation more essential than in activities centered around their own well-being. There are few captive audiences in the community; instead there are persons and groups imbedded in their own support systems in the community. They watch with varying degrees of eagerness or rejection while still another "helpful stranger" approaches. Studies indicate the futility of "do for" programs planned for client needs as perceived by professionals and disavowed by clients (Brown 1971:331–45 and 393–409). And health centers resound with their staffs' disillusioned complaints of clients who never follow directions, keep appointments, or even seem interested. Only a merging of professional and client goals can lead to mutual and meaningful efforts.

"Contract setting" for services and support may be helpful (see chapter 6). With this approach, the health worker and client discuss objectives and the methods by which they may be achieved. Done early enough in the interaction—and reconfirmed as needed—this arrangement encourages mutuality. Problems can arise when discussion reveals no mutual fit between CMHN and client goals. If reality is distorted on either side, further exploration may clarify issues and permit teamwork. While compromise sometimes may be necessary—and there are occasional stalemates—such a respectful effort to elicit a client's perception of needs is conducive to reciprocity. The health worker, then, becomes an advocate for the client's health and must sell the idea of reciprocal involvement.

For example, Anna, fifteen years old and a high school sophomore, was reported to be falling far behind in her special education classes. Any discussion of this problem, though, collapsed under her dull monosyllabic replies. Finally, Anna sighed, paused, and then defiantly stated that pregnancy was her real worry. Once her real concern surfaced, mutual involvement was possible and problem solving proceeded briskly. While the initial focus centered on Anna's primary concern, by agreement it smoothly spread to other areas, including school.

CMH NURSING IN PRACTICE

SITES OF PRACTICE

With such a holistic man-environment view, and a process that includes epidemiology, systems assessment, and reciprocal involvement, community mental health is practiced in all kinds of places. Bower, a consultant for the National Institute of Mental Health, divides the practice area into three categories: (1) primary institutions such as family, schools, health institutions, churches, governmental agencies, and occupational areas; (2) transitional institutions such as courts, hospitals, and social agencies; and (3) correctional institutions, such as prisons and mental hospitals (Bower 1967:18). Such an expansive territory allows traditional facilities and approaches to coexist with storefront clinics and innovative treatment modalities. The present emphasis upon provision of comprehensive and continuous care within the client's own community has encouraged attention to physical and emotional accessibility of services: entranceways that can be negotiated by the handicapped, transportation systems available to the elderly, and services comprehensible to the non–English-speaking client. Decentralized neighborhood units augment regional centers and a continuity-of-care spectrum is developing that can permit concentration on a client's mental health needs through halfway houses, dropin clinics, crisis intervention centers, and other services.

LEVELS OF PREVENTION

To be "comprehensive," mental health services must include provisions for the three levels of prevention: primary, secondary, and tertiary. Primary prevention and health promotion include education and consultation. Secondary prevention, or early treatment, includes twenty-four-hour emergency service with provision for diagnosis, evaluation, care, and treatment. Tertiary services may include the above activities as well as a range of pre- and posthospitalization services (Caplan 1964:16–17). These are designed to help clients establish, restore, and maintain their optimum level of functioning while minimizing their disability and preventing further complications. Surely, secondary prevention is the intervention level that captures the lion's share of interest and resources. There's nothing like an acute health problem to galvanize action and there's no level of intervention that more dramatically yields results. Our successes with secondary prevention have generated the need for more effective tertiary efforts and, of late, increasing emphasis has been given to the rehabilitation of the survivors of acute episodes (see chapter 9).

Primary prevention tends to be given lowest priority. With skyrocketing costs of illness, it seems wonderously simple that an ounce of prevention is worth several pounds of cure. Nevertheless, primary prevention is both our present challenge and our present frustration. It is a remarkably complex level of mental health intervention to implement and evaluate. Ethical issues such as "manipulation," "big brotherism," and "freedom to choose" need to be addressed—and resolved—prior to the planning of preventive programs of counseling and consultation with identified high-risk groups. Also, economics is often problematic, for "squeaking wheels get the greasing" and crisis situations are far noisier and better attended than are the quietly consistent efforts to facilitate positive mental health. The desirability and continuity of primary prevention programs remain tentative, at best, without energetic and excellent advocacy. Perhaps the surest way CMHNs can encourage the inclusion of primary level services into their budgeted activities is to pinpoint—as did the Alcohol Information Committee discussed earlier—a "workable" concern, illustrate and publicize the problem, design a response, gather a wide base of support, collect evaluative data, and then use both the support and the data to negotiate for budgetary support.

While theoretically separate, the three prevention levels and their approaches often overlap considerably in a single interaction. An example arises from interactions in the family dropin center, which, like most services oriented towards an abrupt, crisis-like situation, takes an approach of secondary prevention. Let's look at the multiple levels of prevention incorporated into care given Mr. and Mrs. R.

Case Study

Mr. and Mrs. R. came into the center early one Sunday night. After brief introductions and explanations of the center's purpose and procedures, they sat at the small round table, drinking coffee with two staff members. Mrs. R. spoke bitterly of her husband's "constant drinking" and the impossible demands it placed on their budget and family life. Mr. R., red-eyed and somber, admitted his drinking had become a problem with his job; the foreman had warned him about missed Fridays. One staff member, a volunteer and former alcoholic, listened supportively. Then he introduced the R's to the wider services his group had available: education of other family members regarding alcohol, group support for the problem drinker, and emergency service for acute situations. The other staff member, a CMHN, helped the R's assess their own situation and identify some of the stressors that seemed to lock them into repeating patterns of futility.

While he drank moderately throughout the week, Mr. R. celebrated "weekends" by stopping—on Thursdays—at a favorite bar to "unwind" from the week and to brace himself for the weekend. Mrs. R. met these actions with heated accusations and smouldering withdrawal; their downward spiral was perpetuated as Mr. R. countered with additional drinking so that he usually reached oblivion by late Saturday. Communication was such that the two would sometimes talk *at,* occasionally talk *to,* but never talk *with* each other. Referral services were available for carefully supervised detoxification, and Mr. R., after a lengthy round-table discussion of alternatives, decided that referral was his best option. Mrs. R. stated that she would try the center's community meetings and that when her husband was feeling better, they would perhaps go to a nearby couples' mental health group focused on effective open communication. Three hours after the R's came into the center, they were on their way. Followup evaluation would be done via postcard checklists given to the R's just before their departure and by telephone contact with the detoxification unit.

In various combinations, most of the elements of CMH activities are present in this interaction with Mr. and Mrs. R. By encouraging the couple to assess themselves and to identify their own stressors, the CMHN incorporated the three prevention levels into her intervention: primary prevention in the avoidance of specific problem areas; secondary prevention for early intervention arising from the couple's enhanced ability to handle emerging crises; and tertiary prevention in the return to and maintenance of the family's optimal level of functioning. The couples' communication group referral was another triple-phased approach, as was the introduction of specialized alcoholic services.

Reciprocity is evidenced here in the initial "contract setting" when the R's entered the center through the mutual discussion of alternatives and finally in the process of evaluation. Systems analysis occurred when the CMHN assessed indications of strength and motivation, as well as weakness and potential danger within the R's relationship. She considered the values assigned to the employment system by Mr. and Mrs. R. and the pressures these values might exert on the R's adaptive efforts. Subsystem linkages between the center and the R's were consciously strengthened in the hope they would increase accessibility to other helping systems such as the detox unit and the alcoholic and the couples' groups. Earlier assessment had suggested the appropriateness of these varied systems as referrals. Epidemiology had already provided information on incidence and spread, indicated probable high-risk populations, and named some of the variables the CMHN could expect would influence outcomes in cases like the R's. These data provided guidelines for expectations and interactions.

Similar multilevel CMH approaches are carried out in traditional secondary level prevention as well. In meetings with families of adolescents hospitalized for mental illness, efforts were, for example, directed at maintenance of wellness in those family members exposed to the additional stress accompanying the stigma of hospitalization. Realistic problem solving was encouraged and communication channels were opened to the family. In addition, mutual support was expressed and the CMHN provided anticipatory guidance—that is, advance planning related to areas of special risk. Interventions were built upon family strengths and were designed to minimize regression and provide long-term support through referral to a wide range of community rehabilitative groups.

Institutions chiefly concerned with rehabilitation—or tertiary prevention—also use the previous two levels of care. As in the adaptation cycle, each completed intervention becomes a springboard for the next. And so, interventions with the probationers' rap group represent rehabilitative work for past maladaption while looking toward the future via primary prevention. Joe's rap group gave him opportunity to test angry feelings at racism, to problem-solve present implications of smoking grass or cutting classes, and to plan specifics that could move him toward stated goals; in this example, all levels of prevention are represented.

Within these parameters of care, institutional philosophies modify role performance, establish priorities, and define goals. CMHNs will find their personal style and professional stance affected by the particular institutions within—or against—which they function. They will also have an impact on the institution. The institutional stylistic range is very wide and is based on many variables; these include community involvement, nursing responsibility and accountability, volunteers and lay workers, treatment modalities and underlying psychosocial theory, and many more. A continuum could be designed for each of these variables. A related continuum represents length and place of service offered, ranging from twenty-five minutes on a telephone hotline to a life of hospitalization. We would have difficulty in sketching a profile of a model mental health facility other than to identify it by its outer shell and by its core of one or more of the levels of mental health preventive care.

CMH NURSING ROLES

Within the variety of institutional forms, current CMH nursing roles have been identified as (1) therapist or counselor, (2) consultant—to staff and to others, (3) liaison for the client and/or community agencies, (4) team member with various obligations and responsibilities, (5) client and/or community advocate (DeYoung and Tower 1971:74), and increasingly (6) clinical researcher, and (7) manpower facilitator. Education preparation may be an indicator of role, with the therapist position often held by those CMHNs with advanced degrees. However, in some facilities demonstrated clinical expertise determines role assignment (DeYoung and Tower 1971:23). Hazy role boundaries may be a problem or an opportunity, depending on the situation. While the ambiguity of blurred expectations is sometimes stressful, especially when an innovative nursing approach elicits raised eyebrows rather than a clear yea or nay from associates, the accompanying freedom for creativity can be hugely rewarding. Especially in the new, "in-process-of-becoming" community organizations, collegial interdisciplinary team work is encouraged by the very absence of patterned pasts. In such places, learning through mutual discovery seems to be the norm.

The main challenge here is the query, "But what do nurses *do* outside hospitals?" A formal internship or an unacknowledged wait-and-see period may be needed before one's demonstrated CMH nursing abilities answer the question and open the doors. All three nurses in the opening example who worked in small community settings encountered this initial skepticism, wary testing, and final acceptance in their role negotiations (see chapter 18).

Institutions, emergent and stabilized, undergo the same kind of adaptation cycle that moves us all toward maturation. Environmental demands for change and growth foster role adaptation everywhere; imaginative foresight allows the nurse to capitalize upon the opportunity. CMHNs may expand their role by organizing and providing therapy through swimming lessons for hospitalized psychiatric patients or by negotiating with a straight-laced hierarchy for adolescent "rap" groups on birth control and sexual values. Through these role negotiations dynamic forces of change are being incorporated into expanded CMH nursing practice.

An increasing number of CMHNs are filling the role of manpower facilitator. Arising from the emphasis on mutuality of involvement, nonprofessional neighborhood workers and volunteers are increasingly being incorporated into health center teams. Approaches used to incorporate them will vary. Professional language can quickly become a barrier to real communication, as can any other jargon. Total staff involvement in orientation programs, in-service education, and evaluation often makes the difference between success and fragmentation. McGee identifies three types of reaction to nonprofessionals among professional consultants in his study of community crisis intervention centers. The first reaction is facilitating, which is marked by efforts to decrease anxiety, offer support, and encourage independence. The second approach is that of uneasy supervision, which is cautious and critical, while the third style is perfunctory—that is, showing indifference and apathy (McGee 1974:106). An effective use of self, as in the role of facilitating consultant, enhances harmony and helps provide a climate where real mutuality can flourish.

Roles, then, are also responsive to environmental stressors and shape themselves in various ways. Roles emerging from situations are inductive and thus designed to answer specific need. Home visits made for assessment and family counseling exemplify inductive roles when an expansion of recognized skills is formalized to meet present demands. In home visiting, on-the-site experiences can indicate a need for new approaches, and the success of these modifications will illustrate their underlying theory base. Other roles are deductive—that is, designed by principle and then operationalized. In the examples presented earlier, the obesity and the probationer rap groups were both rather abstractly founded in theories of support systems and then applied to appropriate new populations for evaluation. Many other roles of the CMHN are complex combinations of both inductive and deductive roles. The dropin family clinic is an example, as are both the counseling group for older women and the sexual values discussion with adolescents. However, all are focused on promotion of mental health, and all seek to consider clients within their unique, interacting, and ever-shifting environment.

RESEARCH AND EVALUATION

Running through the fabric of community mental health is a bright strand of research and evaluation. A repeated criticism leveled at community mental health is that its research and evaluation have been inadequate and, therefore, must be strengthened. CMHNs have vital contributions to make in developing, perfecting, and utilizing research and evaluation techniques that will provide essential data on the process and client outcomes derived from many kinds of mental health interventions. We must all become increasingly involved in clinical research from both qualitative and quantitative frames of reference (Hargraves, Attkisson, and Sorensen 1977).

Only through critical evaluation can approaches be improved, discarded, or redesigned. Measurable objectives, incorporated into programs from the beginning, provide the yardstick for determining success. If data gathering for evaluation is interspersed throughout the program, trends can be detected early enough to be used effectively. The probationer rap group, for example, centered upon such a design while the family dropin center used a terminal evaluation plan for each client. The Alcohol Information Committee, focusing upon primary prevention, used audience response evaluation forms following all of its workshops and an attitude and knowledge questionnaire administered both before and after its classroom programs. Effectiveness of individual counseling/consultation was evaluated through the clients' own reports of progression and through the CMHN's assessment of situation improvement. Large agencies can effectively use a random selection evaluation program: one that gives every third or fourth client an evaluation form to complete anonymously and return.

Clinically based hunches, formalized through annotated observations, may also reveal clues or perhaps disintegrate and reshape the evaluation into new patterns that yield different answers. Who uses the dropin center? At what hours, and what seems to be the most common precipitator for the visits? How did clients hear of the services? What is the most effective advertising medium for which neighborhood? The questions almost ask themselves; the answers require probing. As cost consciousness becomes a major factor, evaluation becomes essential. When the funding body is considering a budget cut, evaluation data will be needed to support the value of the services given. We want to be sure essential figures are available.

SUMMARY

Community mental health nursing is a vigorous and evolving field. Under the umbrella of preventive care and ecosystem considerations, individual and institutional philosophies blend the components of CMH nursing into an intricate variety of health services. CMH nursing deals with clients' needs in the clients' setting, which can be home, school, business, or any other locale. Activities in CMH nursing focus around the three levels of prevention. Primary prevention and health promotion focus on education and consultation. Secondary prevention is mainly concerned with early diagnosis and treatment. Tertiary prevention includes both of the other two levels and concentrates on pre- and posthospitalization services with the objective of helping clients establish, restore, and maintain their optimum level of functioning.

Key concepts discussed in the chapter include stress-adaptation patterns and their implications in physical as well as mental functioning. Epidemiology forms the basis for gathering data about communities' mental health needs; these data guide CMHNs in developing their many roles to fit with community needs. Systems analysis or assessment also plays a part in this process. Client involvement is stressed as essential in developing CMH programs; this principle of reciprocity is receiving increased attention in program planning and evaluation, although more is still needed.

Case examples illustrate many of the CMH nursing roles, which include therapist or counselor, consultant, liaison, team member, client advocate, clinical researcher, and manpower facilitator. These roles may evolve inductively—that is, from observations in specific situations so that skills are applied in order to meet present needs. Roles may also be deductive—that is, predesigned on principles and then operationalized to meet the situation at hand. More often than not, the inductive and deductive methods are combined in working with clients.

Research and program evaluation are essential components of any program, CMH or otherwise. Much criticism has been levelled at CMH programs because they have not been able to quantify the results of their activities as well as other sectors of the health/care system can. At this juncture, community mental health services join the other community health services in the dilemma of documenting the effectiveness and efficiency of preventive programs—that is, proving that something did *not* occur and that had the event occurred, the cost of treating it would have been far greater than was the cost of the preventive program. Consciousness throughout the health care system regarding the need for research and evaluation is providing new and sounder techniques to begin to answer questions of program effectiveness and efficiency. Participation in the development and implementation of these tools and the evaluation of their results is a facet of the community mental health nurse's role.

REFERENCES

AUDY, J. RALPH. "Measurement and Diagnosis of Health." In P. Shepard and D. McKinley, eds., *Environ/Mental. Essays on the Planet as a Home*. Boston: Houghton Mifflin, 1971.

BEISSER, ARNOLD R., and GREEN, ROSE. *Mental Health Consultation and Education.* Palo Alto, Calif.: National Press Books, 1972.

BLOOM, BERNARD L., and BUCK, DOROTHY P., eds. *Preventive Services in Mental Health Programs.* Boulder, Colo.: University East Campus, 1967.

BOWER, ELI M. "Preventive Services for Children." In *Preventive Services in Mental Health Programs,* Proceedings of a Mental Health Institute held at Salt Lake City, Utah, May 31 to June 2, 1967. Boulder, Colo.: Western Inter-State Commission on Higher Education, 1967.

BROWN, ESTHER LUCILLE. *Nursing Reconsidered: A Study of Change, Part 2.* Philadelphia: J. B. Lippincott, 1971.

BROWNING, CHARLES H. "Suicide, Firearms, and Public Health." *American Journal of Public Health* 64 (1974):313-17.

CAPLAN, GERALD. *Concepts of Mental Health and Consultation, Their Application in Public Health Social Work.* Washington, D.C.: U.S. Department of Health, Education and Welfare, 1959.

————. *Principles of Preventive Psychiatry.* New York: Basic Books, 1964.

DeYOUNG, CAROL D., and TOWER, MARGENE. *Out of Uniform and Into Trouble; The Nurse's Role in Community Mental Health Centers.* St. Louis: C. V. Mosby Co., 1971.

GLASSER, WILLIAM. *Reality Therapy, A New Approach to Psychiatry.* New York: Harper & Row, 1965.

GOLDSTONE, STEPHEN E. "An Overview of Primary Prevention Programming." Paper presented at the Pilot Conference on Primary Prevention, April 2-4, 1976, Temple University Conference Center, Philadelphia.

HARGRAVES, W.A., ATTKISSON, C.C., and SORENSEN, J.E., eds. *Resource Materials for Community Mental Health Program Evaluation,* 2nd ed. Rockville, Md.: National Institutes of Mental Health, 1977.

HOLMES, THOMAS H., and MASUDA, MINORU. "Psychosomatic Syndrome (Life Crisis-Illness)." *Psychology Today* (April 1972):71-72.

JAHODA, MARIE. *Current Concepts of Positive Mental Health.* New York: Basic Books, 1958.

KLEIN, DONALD C. *Community Dynamics and Mental Health.* New York: John Wiley & Sons, 1968.

KRAMER, MORTON. "Some Perspectives on the Role of Biostatistics and Epidemiology in the Prevention and Control of Mental Disorders." Presentation at Rema Lapouse Mental Health Epidemiology Memorial Award Session, November 8, 1973, San Francisco.

LEVI, LENNART. *Stress and Distress in Response to Psychosocial Stimuli.* New York: Pergamon Press, 1972.

LIEBERMAN, E. JAMES, ed. *Mental Health: The Public Health Challenge.* Washington, D.C.: APHA, Interdisciplinary Books, Pamphlets & Periodicals, 1975.

McGEE, RICHARD. *Crisis Intervention in the Community.* Baltimore Md.: University Park Press, 1974.

McLEAN, ALAN, ed. *Mental Health and Work Organizations.* Chicago: Rand McNally & Co., 1970.

MORGAN, ARTHUR, and MORENO, JUDITH. *The Practice of Mental Health Nursing: A Community Approach.* Philadelphia: J. B. Lippincott, 1973.

NATIONAL COMMISSION ON COMMUNITY HEALTH SERVICES. *Health Is a Community Affair.* Cambridge, Mass.: Harvard University Press, 1966.

PALMER, JAMES O., and GOLDSTEIN, MICHAEL J., eds. *Perspectives in Psycho-pathology.* New York: University Press, 1966.

PANZETTA, ANTHONY F. *Community Mental Health: Myth and Reality*. Philadelphia: Lea & Febiger, 1971.

PARAD, HOWARD J., ed. *Crisis Intervention: Selected Readings*. New York: Family Service Association of America, 1970.

PASNAU, ROBERT O. *Consultation-Liaison Psychiatry*. New York: Grune & Stratton, 1975.

REINHARDT, ADINA M., and QUINN, MILDRED. *Family-Centered Community Nursing. A Sociocultural Framework*. St. Louis: C. V. Mosby, 1973.

ROSENBAUM, C. PETER, and BEEBE, JOHN E., III. *Psychiatric Treatment: Crisis/Clinic/Consultation*. New York: McGraw-Hill Book Co., 1975.

SELYE, HANS. *The Stress of Life*. New York: McGraw-Hill Paperbacks, 1956.

SHEEHY, GAIL. *Passages: Predictable Crises of Adult Life*. New York: E. P. Dutton & Co., 1976.

SINGH, R. K. J. *Community Mental Health Consultation and Crisis Intervention*. Palo Alto, Calif.: National Press Books, 1971.

STENGEL, ERWIN. *Suicide and Attempted Suicide*. Baltimore: Penguin Books, 1969.

SUCHMAN, EDWARD A. *Sociology and the Field of Public Health*. New York: Russell Sage Foundation, 1963.

SZASZ, THOMAS. "Illness and Indignity." *Journal of American Medical Association* 227, no. 5 (February 1974).

TOFFLER, ALVIN. *Future Shock*. New York: Bantam Books, Random House, 1970.

TYHURST, JAMES S. "The Role of Transition States—Including Disaster—On Mental Illness." Symposium on Preventive and Social Psychiatry, Walter Reed Army Institute of Research, Washington, D.C., 1957.

ZIMBARDO, PHILIP G. "Social Psychology: Tool for Improving the Human Condition." In Julius Segal, ed., *Mental Health Program Reports—6*. Rockville, Md.: National Institute of Mental Health, 1973.

18. Community Nursing in Schools: Developing a Specialized Role

Dorothy S. Oda

INTRODUCTION

If you are a nurse yourself and have the audacity to ask a group of nurses to define *nursing*, you will probably get reactions of astonishment, disbelief, discomfort, annoyance, anger, or all of the preceding—usually in that order. Seemingly, we who have gone through the rigors of nursing education are expected to just "naturally" know what nursing is. Most nurses are affronted when asked to define nursing, especially by another nurse. We usually go through the "you know" syndrome of verbal shorthand in assuming that one knows what the other is talking about. For example, currently every nurse is expected to understand instantly what primary care, expanded nursing role, nurse-practitioner, and school nursing are—you know.

In the same manner, nurses in a school setting are assumed to know clearly what a school nurse role is; otherwise why are they working there? Furthermore, school nurses are expected to naturally communicate this information to the pupils, teachers, parents, principal, school psychologist, and others in the school and community with whom they work. Why then are there so many reports and studies regarding the conflicting perceptions of the school nurse role (Eidens 1963; Forbes 1967; Fricke 1967; Regan 1976)? Clearly, the school nurse role is largely one about which there is a notable lack of agreement. Is a school nurse a first aid expert? a

495

health educator? a mental health counselor? a mother-surrogate? a health consultant? an attendance checker? or official lice detector?

The fact that school nurses have had role problems is really not surprising when we consider some factors involved in developing such a specialized nursing role. In many ways, school nurses have long been involved in a role-defining process that was "ahead of its time." To explain, specialist roles in nursing are just now coming into their own—that is, being recognized by nursing itself as well as by other disciplines. For example, employment advertisements are currently filled with positions for clinical nurse specialists in a variety of settings and nurse-practitioners for various client groups.

These newer nursing roles have much in common with the school nurse role. Clinical nurse specialists and nurse-practitioners are often one-of-a-kind in a work setting as is the school nurse. The specialized services of a clinical nurse specialist or nurse-practitioner can be open to option—that is, the staff can choose whether to utilize their expertise (or to assist them in their roles) to a full or a minimal extent. In the same way, health service in a school setting is a supportive one and is also subject to elective use by students and staff. In such situations, nurses have to motivate others to appropriately use their services.

Current literature verifies that specialized nurses are experiencing many problems related to role development (Vaughn 1973; Moore 1974). When roles are new or unclear and services are not mandatory and open to optional use, the role definer must know how to handle and promote the specialist role itself. What is needed for the effective development of any specialized nursing role is a systematic process such as the one discussed later in the chapter.

There is remarkable consensus in the literature that the role of the school nurse is not yet well understood, even though statistics and history reveal that school nursing has endured and grown since 1902 when Lillian Wald placed the first school nurse in a New York school. In an effort to understand and explain what the seemingly enigmatic school nurse role is about, in this chapter we ask (and try to answer) the following questions: What is school nursing? What are school nursing services? What are some issues and concerns in school nursing? What are some current practices influencing school nursing? The answers are then placed within a framework for developing a specialized school nurse role.

SOME PERCEPTIONS OF SCHOOL NURSES

Elementary school pupil: I'm sure glad you're here today, you can tell the teacher I don't feel good so I better not go back to class for awhile.

High school student: You mean you can't even give me an aspirin for a headache? I thought you were a real nurse.

Parent: I feel much better knowing that a trained nurse is at school in case there's a serious accident.

Teacher: You know more about health and things, could you give a class on diet and nutrition?

Secretary: It's certainly nice when you're here and can take care of all the cuts and bruises.

Principal: Thank you for the detailed accident report. It makes it clear that the student disobeyed the rules and broke his arm as a result.

WHAT IS SCHOOL NURSING?

The American Nurses' Association (ANA) in 1966 stated as a "philosophy" of school nursing: "School nursing is a highly specialized service contributing to the process of education . . . . It must be diligently pursued through health and educational avenues . . . ." Under functions, the ANA further stated: "The basic reason for a nurse being a member of the school's professional staff is that the art and science of nursing, properly applied, aid the school in accomplishing its task of facilitating the learning of its student" (ANA 1966).

A more recent publication from the American School Health Association begins the introduction as follows:

> School nursing as a professional entity is now in its eighth decade. School nurses have repeatedly attempted to define their role in the school and their responsibilities within the school health program. The primary focus of school nursing is enhancing the child's or youth's individual ability to utilize his intellectual potential and to make worthwhile decisions affecting present and future physical, social, and emotional health [ASHA 1974:1].

Bryan, writing about the dimensions of school nursing, is of the opinion that "School nursing is as versatile as the nurse practicing it, as full of variety as there are differing school community needs, and as creative and innovative as the individual nurse" (1973:1).

We might guess that every school nurse will understand and agree with all of the foregoing statements regarding school nursing. The problem of understanding and defining school nursing lies not with those who practice it, but with others who come in contact with it. Would parents understand what school nurses do after reading these same statements? Probably not, except in very general terms. Therein is another example of nursing's verbal shorthand syndrome. However industriously school nurses work, there remains the need to *clarify and communicate the nature of their professional services to others.*

A number of factors are involved in school nurses' trouble in role clarification and communication. There is a gap between educational preparation and practice settings; there are work setting differences; there is a wide age range of client populations; and there is the necessary variable in the school nursing role that results from the unique interactions of each school nurse and the specific school setting.

Nursing education traditionally prepares nurses for positions in health care service. Whether their practice is in a private physician's office, an acute hospital, long-term care facility, or community health agency, the primary purpose is health care delivery. In a school setting, the main purpose is the education of students. Health service in schools is a supportive one along with such services as guidance, counseling, psychological testing, and social welfare. Health and health topics tend to have lower priority than basic classroom subjects such as reading and mathematics. Therefore, health education is open to optional selection and emphasis by both teachers and students. Yet, the simple fact that students are unable to learn well when they cannot see or hear clearly or when their physical or emotional condition impedes their ability is well established. The school nurse, therefore, must skillfully and persistently promote health-related subjects such as veneral disease or substance abuse and specific preventive activities such as vision and hearing screening.

The variability of the school nurse role has been mentioned as being related to individual nurse ability and inclination. An additional reason is a form of dual role assumed by nurse-teachers in some areas of the nation. These nurses combine a nursing background with teaching preparation. Many nurses without this specific preparation in teaching do a great deal of direct classroom teaching while others act only as resources to the teachers. Some states require school nurses to have the equivalent (though not the same) academic background as teachers do for certification. These school nurses are employed on the same salary basis as are teachers. State certification varies across the nation, with twenty-three of the states having school nursing certification mandatory. However, these requirements vary widely from registered nurse licensure to postbaccalaureate work and advanced degrees for certificate renewal (American School Health Association 1976).

The nurse who is new to school nursing usually suffers from a form of culture shock induced by characteristics of the work setting. There is no head nurse, no other staff nurse in the same school, no physician on the premises (ordinarily), and no other familiar persons associated with health care services. No nursing care plans or definite assignment of patients or clients guide activities for the day. Most school nurse interns doing fieldwork plaintively ask, "What am I supposed to be *doing*?" The second most frequently asked question is, "Who is the school nurse responsible to?"

These are some of the unique and challenging aspects of school nursing. School nurses themselves must determine what health services are needed, desired, apppropriate, acceptable, and feasible. Aside from a few mandated services, they literally create their own health service programs. The accountability lines are to the school site administrator, usually the principal, and to a central administrative office nursing supervisor, if available, or to the director of special educational services.

School nurses work with an essentially well and ambulatory client population whose ages and grade levels range from preschool to adulthood. Therefore, school nurses must have knowledge of growth and development throughout the life span with particular emphasis in the phases in which the majority of their clients are. They must understand age-related health concerns such as family dynamics and the preschool child, adolescent pregnancy, and the developmental crises through which members of their client group or their families may be going. School nurses must be familiar with community resources and be able to match these appropriately to the individual student's and their families' needs in initiating referrals or suggesting that clients avail themselves of sources of assistance.

The main focus in school nursing regardless of the age, grade, or other characteristics of the client population is on what can be called *educational health*—that is, those aspects of health that influence the individual student's or the group's learning ability. The client is always viewed as a unit of the family, school, and community, rather than as an isolated individual. Figure 18.1 illustrates the ecosystem factors that impinge on the student and his or her learning ability.

WHAT ARE SCHOOL NURSING SERVICES?

School health programs have traditionally been divided into three parts: school health education, healthful school living, and school health services (Wilson 1964; Nemir and Schaller 1975).

School health education is the process of providing learning experiences that favorably influence understanding, attitudes, and conduct relating to individual and community health. This aspect is sometimes called school health and safety instruction and includes general hygiene and accident prevention. Learning experiences can be by direct instruction, integrating health topics into other school subjects, special projects, or activities and individual health guidance whenever opportune (Bryan 1973: 12).

The concept of *healthful school living* includes the physical and social environment of the school and its effect on pupil health. *School health services* are concerned with the health condition of the schoolchild and can in-

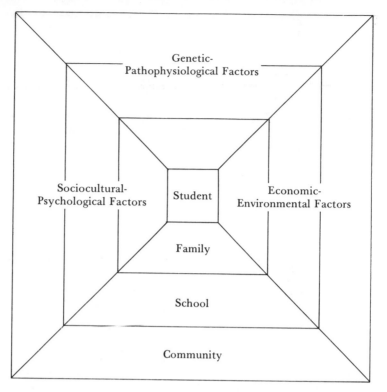

18.1   *Comprehensive Educational Health Components*

clude observation, appraisal, screening tests, followup for referral and care, communicable disease control, and emergency care.

While school nursing services encompass all of the above-mentioned *school health programs,* the definition of *school nursing services* is perhaps better clarified by a framework that identifies three intertwining and overlapping components: health supervision, health counseling, and health education, (see figure 18.2).

Health supervision includes such activities as health assessments, vision and hearing screening, emergency care, and health deficit identification. *Health counseling* involves providing interpretation of health information, guidance and counseling regarding health behavior, and recommendations regarding individual and group health conditions. *Health education* refers to planning, promoting, and implementing health instruction as well as providing consultation services in health-related matters.

These three components of school nursing service are not distinct in actual practice and can move in the directional flow shown in figure 18.3. For example, emergency care often results in the school nurse doing followup and referral not only to deal with the emergency at hand but also for the purpose of teaching the student how to prevent future

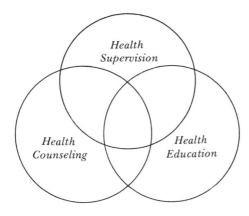

18.2   *School Nursing Services*

emergency situations. However, certain aspects can be dealt with individually as well. For another example, preventive health education about venereal disease does not necessarily require either health supervision or health counseling activities. Not all counseling necessarily originates from the nurse's identification of a problem. Students with personal or family problems may refer themselves to the school nurse for assistance.

The three major nursing service categories are broad responsibility areas. Daily tasks such as recordkeeping, communications, overall health program planning, as well as minor ministrations and major emergency care differ from school system to school system and therefore are not specifically detailed here.

Another way to view figure 18.3—School Nursing Service Flow Chart—is as a representation of *levels of service*. Again a strict division is neither possible nor intended. Professional school nurses have been hard

18.3   *School Nursing Service Flow*

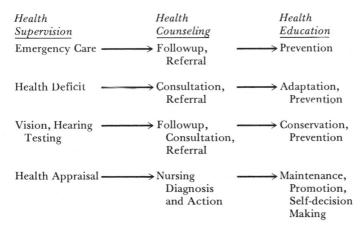

put to prove qualitatively, if not quantitatively, that what they are capable of doing can be differentiated from what nonprofessional personnel such as health aides can do. The flow chart identifies components and processes of problem solving and case management techniques used by school nurses.

Health supervision, the first level, can be carried out by paraprofessional persons such as assistants or volunteers with school nurse supervision. Health counseling, the second level, can be done to some extent by persons with health service preparation, such as licensed vocational nurses, but it is primarily in the domain of the professional nurse because of the extent of the expertise required. Health education, the third level, is most often the responsibility of the professional or certified school nurse. What is important to note here is that greater expertise is needed to manage student situations at levels two and three than is necessary at level one. For example, a paraprofessional may be able to do vision and hearing screening tests. Followup counseling and initiation of appropriate referrals for care require skills paraprofessionals do not ordinarily have such as interpersonal relations and knowledge of community resources. The health education necessary to help the student to prevent subsequent sensory loss and to maintain his or her level of function is definitely the responsibility of the professional school nurse. The process of increasingly complex problem solving from level one to level three is illustrative of the qualitative difference between paraprofessional and professional school nursing practice.

WHAT ARE SOME CURRENT PRACTICES INFLUENCING SCHOOL NURSING?

The Family Educational Rights and Privacy Act (H.R. 69, P.L. 93-380, 1974) mandates accessibility of public school records, including cumulative health records, and thus affects recording methods. Under this Act clients have the right to see all kinds of records kept on them by public and private agencies. Thus, great care must be taken to include in records only information that is highly pertinent to the individual client. Many school nurses and other health care professionals are developing a recording style that describes behaviors and situations rather than resorting to the verbal shorthand syndrome. For example, instead of recording that a child is hyperactive, a more pertinent recording of the child's behavior is ". . . Teacher reports that Tommy cannot remain seated for longer than five minutes. Even during this interval, he is noted to move about in his seat, motion to other children, and kick his feet." To facilitate this kind of recording, the Problem-Oriented Record adapted from Weed's (1969) Problem-Oriented Medical Record has been adapted for school use (Boone 1974; Oda and Quick 1977).

A few school districts have begun to computerize student records including health records. This practice is undoubtedly a trend of the future and makes the development of increased standardization of recording necessary. Computerized records are a great boon to highly mobile segments of the population such as the children of migrant farm workers since the process makes centralized information and retrieval services for these children's school scholastic and health records more feasible (Stennett et al. 1971).

Health screening in schools has usually included vision, hearing, and dental areas but has recently expanded to scoliosis, hypertension, sickle cell, cardiac high risk, and other conditions to keep up with medical and technologic advances. Much of the impetus for these increased screening procedures has evolved from epidemiological studies of school-age children and their risk factors for the development of chronic illnesses. Because of the realization of lifestyle influences on people's health and abilities to function, greater emphasis must be placed upon positive health education and health promotion in the school-age population with the objective of assisting them to develop lifestyles that are conducive to their improving and maintaining their own abilities to function. As noted these kinds of teaching activities are solidly within the purview of the professional school nurse. Increasing attention must be focused on helping young people to avoid tobacco, alcohol, and other drug abuse; obesity; sedentary lifestyles; and risk taking that results in accidents. In the prevention of all of these hazards, the school nurse's role as both a health educator and role model can be of critical importance.

Practitioner preparation in school nursing is now a reality, and nurses with additional health assessment, maintenance, and management skills can provide a broad range of direct primary health care services to school children (Silver, Igoe, and McAtee 1976). Since 1970 when the prototype Denver, Colorado, program began operation, comparative studies have been made on traditional and school nurse role effectiveness (Hilmar and McAtee 1973; McAtee 1974).

There is little doubt that school nurse-practitioners with their special skills can add to the quality, availability, and continuity of health care for children. However, as Silver et al. note:

> Since most school nurses cannot assume the duties of a school nurse-practitioner unless relieved of clerical and other routine tasks, school health aides (adults or high school students with a special interest in health) assist with office activities and minor first aid [Silver et al. 1971:581].

The writers make clear that for school nurse-practitioners to be able to use their particular expertise appropriately and effectively, auxiliary help of some kind is essential.

WHAT ARE SOME CURRENT ISSUES AND CONCERNS IN SCHOOL NURSING?

The preparation necessary for entry into school nursing is still open to controversy. The present range is from a two-year associate degree or three-year diploma school registered nurse license to a baccalaureate degree (not necessarily in nursing) with the registered nurse licensure. The trend appears to be toward a minimum of a baccalaureate degree in nursing as indicated by recent publications (Bryan 1973:17; American School Health Association 1974). School nursing as a specialty is thought by the American Association for Health, Physical Education, and Recreation (1972: 22) to require graduate level preparation.

The type and level of school nurse education cannot be separated from the issue of state certification for school nurses. There is considerable difference among the states regarding certification for school nurses. The most recent figures available show that twenty-three states have mandatory school nursing certification requirements. Four states are currently developing certification requirements and fourteen states indicate no plans are being developed for certification (American School Health Association 1976). A further complicating factor is the lack of uniformity of requirements for certification for school nurses even among the states that have mandatory or permissive certification.

Nurses working in school settings can have a variety of titles. Some school nurses feel that the term "health" denotes the more positive aspect of their work and incorporate it in their titles; for example, health counselor, student health counselor, and health consultant. Other titles used include nurse-teacher, school nurse-teacher, health teacher, school community nurse, school public health nurse, as well as the original designation of school nurse. The newer expanded roles in school nursing are usually identified by such titles as school nurse-practitioner, school nurse specialist, nurse specialist in school health, and clinical specialist in school community health. By whatever name nurses choose to call themselves, the nurse image will remain in the perception of others in the school. Therefore, astute and enterprising nurses can use the caring, positive image of the nurse to advantage in the school setting. They must, however, set limits to the pathology-oriented, "emergency care and band-aiding only" image.

The trend toward expanded roles in school nursing will eventually have an influence on school nursing in general. First, school nurse-practitioners can provide primary care in those areas in the nation where such services are not otherwise available and so are necessary and appropriate for provision in schools. Secondly, clinical specialists in school health prepared at the master's level can provide high-level clinical competence and expertise in areas such as college health, mental health, and work with exceptional children and special education. For example, the School of Nursing, University of California, San Francisco, continued has a federally funded project for a trilevel preparation program for school nursing that includes a master's level, Nurse Specialist in School Health. Finally, any additional skills acquired by school nurses now operating in traditional or expanded roles will improve their capabilities in health counseling, health assessment, and health maintenance. Stated differently, skills that are presently considered expanded role skills will, in all probability, become basic or standard skills over a period of time.

As mentioned earlier, school nurse-practitioners need assistance with clerical and routine duties in order to use their expanded skills apppropriately. While there are pros and cons regarding the use of paraprofessional personnel in school health services, we must point out that many reports deal with paid assistants (not volunteers or work-experience students) who are additional school staff usually supervised by school nurses. Generally, the proponents indicate a wider and improved nursing coverage of schools and the release of the school nurse from time-consuming routine tasks to attend to more serious health problems and needs in the school (Dunphy 1966; Bryan 1973). The opposing view warns of the misuse of assistants by replacing school nurses and possibly diminishing the level of health service (Tipple 1964). As a matter of fact, when school district budgets must be trimmed, one of the first items cut is usually that for school nurses' salaries, which has been the case since the passage of Proposition 13 in California in 1978. The school nurse is often replaced with someone whose expertise is limited to carrying out health supervision activities. Thus the essential services of the school nurse in health counseling and health education are sacrificed.

Some school districts allow and encourage the use of parent and student volunteers in the nursing or health office while others forbid or discourage it. The question of the protection of student health record confidentiality has been raised with the use of community or student volunteers in the health office. These volunteers must be taught that records are confidential and must not be discussed with anyone. When feasible, the use of volunteer assistants can add or improve health services while adding no additional costs to the school budget.

The supervision of school nursing services presently follows one of two patterns. Under ideal conditions, a school nurse supervisor or coordinator of health services is located in the central administrative offices. This arrangement provides support and direction of nursing services by a nurse manager. A more common situation exists where school nursing services are a part of special educational services or pupil personnel (support) services and the director has a teaching or counseling background. Some school districts have a senior school nurse who carries some supervisory responsibilities along with a school nursing assignment. Other districts have a self-appointed or a rotating spokesperson selected from the school nursing staff. There are school districts with such a small enrollment that there may be only one nurse who is responsible for all the district's schools and is accountable directly to the superintendent.

There are a number of variations to the sponsorship of school nursing services. The predominant employment source is the local school district. Some school districts contract for school nursing service from the county public health nurses. A few have a combined service where services are jointly sponsored, and we must add, there are some school districts that have no school nurses at all.

Developing a Specialized Role

The school nurse role, as with other specialized roles, is most effectively developed when it is approached in a systematic manner. Being expertly prepared—theoretically and clinically—is not enough, nor is it simply a matter of commitment to quality care with dedication to hard work. A nurse specialist does not work in a social vacuum, and role study does not deal with isolated nurses (Sarbin and Allen 1968). Role implementation is an interactional process involving nurses and others with whom they work.

The essence of developing a specialized nursing role consists of (1) clearly identifying the role purpose and function for oneself and others; (2) implementing the role through goal-directed interactions; and (3) achieving positive recognition and support of the role. These are the three phases of role development and are operational elaborations of the concepts of clarification and communication (Oda 1977). Figure 18.4 represents a summary model of the three-phase role implementation process using clarification and communication concepts, which are further developed into operational phases.

PHASE I

Role Identification means that the role purpose must be clarified and articulated based on a philosophy of practice. Nurses may have to gain entry to a system, negotiate their role, know *what* they will do as well as what they will not do, *why* they will do it, and *when* they will expect to

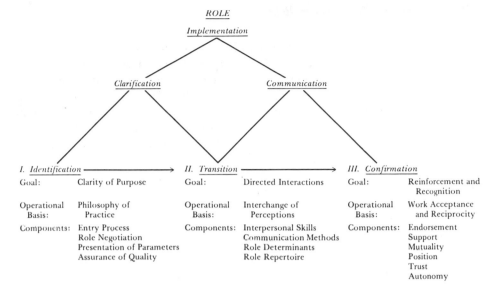

ROLE

Implementation

Clarification   *Communication*

I. *Identification* ————————⟶	II. *Transition* ————————⟶	III. *Confirmation*	
Goal:	Clarity of Purpose	Goal:	Directed Interactions	Goal:	Reinforcement and Recognition
Operational Basis:	Philosophy of Practice	Operational Basis:	Interchange of Perceptions	Operational Basis:	Work Acceptance and Reciprocity
Components:	Entry Process Role Negotiation Presentation of Parameters Assurance of Quality	Components:	Interpersonal Skills Communication Methods Role Determinants Role Repertoire	Components:	Endorsement Support Mutuality Position Trust Autonomy

18.4   *Role Development Process in Nursing Specialization*

achieve their goals to a certain degree. These are parameters of practice and give assurance of nurses' competence as specialists with a particular service to offer.

PHASE II

Role Transition involves interactions that are guided by "goal direction" or movement toward the objectives of the nurse-defined role. The interchange of perceptions must be a mutual process. Nurses, as role definers, take the initiative and monitor the direction, but are also willing receivers of the perception of others. Interpersonal skills and communication methods are important components of this phase as determinants of the role are discovered and modifications in the role are made as necessary over a period of time. The ultimate goal is to create a role fit between what the role definer or specialized nurse feels is appropriate and what others in the work setting view as appropriate.

PHASE III

Role Confirmation is achieved when nurses receive recognition and support for their defined role and are permitted a high degree of autonomy. Evidence of role confirmation is when coworkers and superiors accept the role and include the nurses in work activities that make optional use of their expertise. This cooperation and collaboration component has definable levels of work acceptance and reciprocity. The first or lowest level is simple *endorsement* such as the positive mention of the nurse's work without action to back it up. The *support* level indicates some activity in response to nurse requests. Then, when work is initiated and carried out actively together, a level of *mutuality* prevails. The continuation of mutual experiences provides a recognized *position* or status achieved through proven competence. Next, a certain level of *trust* is gained, built on a bank of successful and productive interactions. Finally, when a role is fully accepted, increased *autonomy* is granted with less dependence on others for decision making and role performance.

Using the role development process, the school nurses as providers of specialized nursing service, can operationalize their role in the following manner:

Role Identification: Determine which services are essential or have high priority, which are to be maintained at a lesser priority, and which are nonessential or inappropriate; articulate some role limits so that nursing service does not become overextended and diluted into an ineffectual, nonvisible, and highly dispensable service to schools.

Role Transition: Utilize a variety of formal and informal communication methods such as newsletters, memos, reports, and bulletin board displays, as well as conferences over coffee and lunch, classroom presentations, and participation at meetings to increase visibility and interactions; continuously articulate the role and define and redefine the role parameters by emphasizing areas that are relevant health matters and reordering other demands (but not ignoring them); according to students, staff, and parent input, modify priorities and shift role boundaries if appropriate. Responsiveness and flexibility are critical components as rigidity, particularly at the outset, in role development is counterproductive to effective interpersonal relationships.

Role Confirmation: Gain positive support and recognition in the form of integration and inclusion in school activities as a faculty member; constantly solicit and receive referrals and requests for consultation for health matters and resource material; achieve significant independence in determining role functions and acceptance by others of role limits with increased personal accountability.

SUMMARY

This chapter presents several dimensions of school nursing: the variations in school nurse role perceptions, new developments and issues in school nursing, and a discussion of specialized role development. What is not done here is identifying a universal school nurse role. This role identification problem in school nursing is no simple matter and has prompted at least one writer to question whether such a role even exists (Hawkins 1971). As we have seen, no one, universal definition is realistic in this form of nursing practice. The essential nature of nursing in schools consists of a constant nurse identity and a variable role according to the educational health needs of the students, school, and community (Oda 1973). School nurses practice nursing in a school setting but adapt their activities in health supervision, health counseling, and health education *individually* to the pupil, the school, and the community in which they function. This variability is a role requirement in school nursing. Nurses can differentially interpret this tailoring of activities to the given situation as a restriction to functioning or a challenge to creativity. It can truly be said that, "school nursing is what you make it."

School nursing practice will continue to be diverse according to regional, economic, and legal variations in requirements for school health services. In one or two areas of the nation, there are (or being planned) school nurse-practitioner–run clinics in the school setting. At the other extreme, a few school districts are replacing school nurses with health aides in the interest of "economy."

The overwhelming majority of school nurses are highly committed persons who work conscientiously and industriously for the health maintenance and promotion of school populations of all ages. They have been highly successful in upgrading school nursing as a recognized speciality in the nursing profession. The area in need of further efforts is the improvement of the image of school nursing. For example, the restrictive, historical band-aider image needs to be overcome while keeping the positive, caring aspect. The nuisance disease-checker-only image needs to be changed while keeping the community health concern aspect. The health counselor, consultant, educator, and resource person attributes of the role need emphasis and promotion.

The flexibility, independence, and inventiveness necessary for effective school nursing practice should be integrated into the preparation of school nurses. For school nursing to increase in importance and recognition, *role clarification and communication* are absolutely essential as an interactional skill basic to this form of nursing service, which is open to optionality and is located in a non–health care delivery setting. Other nurses who work in non–health care agencies or so-called nontraditional health care settings such as independent nursing practices and holistic healing centers need to go through the process of developing a specialized role. Because this process is the same regardless of the setting, the general discussion of role development should be of use to nurses in a variety of settings.

Nurses with a firm philosophy of practice and a commitment to optimal student health for learning will find school nursing an exciting speciality. School nursing demands of its practitioners statesmanship abilities, a wide role repertoire of nursing behaviors, and the capability to be persistently persuasive.

REFERENCES

AMERICAN ASSOCIATION FOR HEALTH, PHYSICAL EDUCATION, AND RECREATION. *School Nursing for the 70's.* Washington, D.C.: The Association, 1972.

AMERICAN NURSES' ASSOCIATION. *School Nursing.* New York: ANA, 1966.

AMERICAN SCHOOL HEALTH ASSOCIATION. *Guidelines for the School Nurse in the School Health Program.* Kent, Ohio: ASHA, 1974.

———. *School Health in America: A Survey of State School Health Programs.* Kent, Ohio: ASHA, 1976.

BOONE, SHIRLEY F. "A New Approach to School Health Records." *Journal of School Health* 44 (1974):156–58.

BRYAN, DORIS S. *School Nursing in Transition.* St. Louis: C. V. Mosby, 1973.

DUNPHY, BARBARA. "In Defense of School Nurses' Aides." *American Journal of Nursing* 66 (1966):1338–41.

EIDENS, C. O. "Work of the Secondary School Nurse-Teacher as Perceived by Selected School Staff Personnel." *Journal of School Health* 33 (1963):187–88.

FORBES, ORCILIA. "The Role and Function of the School Nurse as Perceived by 115 Public School Teachers from Three Selected Counties." *Journal of School Health* 37 (1967):101–06.

FRICKE, IRMA B. "The Illinois Study of School Nurse Practice." *Journal of School Health* 37 (1967):24–28.

HAWKINS, NORMAN G. "Is There a School Nurse Role?" *American Journal of Nursing* 71(1971) :744–51.

HILMAR, NORMAN A., and McATEE, PATRICIA A. "The School Nurse-Practitioner and her Practice: A Study of Traditional and Expanded Health Care Responsibilities for Nurses in Elementary Schools." *Journal of School Health* 43 (1973):431–41.

MOORE, ANN C. "Nurse-Practitioner: Reflections on the Role." *Nursing Outlook* 22 (1974):124–27.

McATEE, PATRICIA A. "Nurse-Practitioners in Our Public Schools? An Assessment of Their Expanded Role as Compared with School Nurses." *Clinical Pediatrics* 13 (1974):360–62.

NEMIR, ALMA, and SCHALLER, WARREN E. *The School Health Program.* Philadelphia: W. B. Saunders Co., 1975.

ODA, DOROTHY S. "The Nature of Nursing in Schools: A Study of a Coordinate Work Role." Unpublished doctoral dissertation, University of California, San Francisco, 1973.

———. "Specialized Role Development: A Three-Phase Process." *Nursing Outlook* 25 (1977):374–77.

———. *The Preparation of School Nurses: A Multilevel Curriculum.* A training grant (5 DIO NUO 1565–02) funded by the Division of Nursing, Health Resources Administration, U.S. Department of Health, Education and Welfare, Washington, D.C., 1975–1978.

————, and QUICK, MARY JANE. "School Health Records and the New Accessibility Law." *Journal of School Health* 47 (1977):212–16.

REGAN, PATRICIA A. "A Historical Study of the School Nurse Role." *Journal of School Health* 46 (1976):518–21.

SARBIN, THEODORE R., and ALLEN, VERNON, L. "Role Theory." In Gardner Lindzey and Elliot Aronsen, eds., *The Handbook of Social Psychology*, Vol. I, 2nd ed. Reading, Mass: Addison-Wesley Publishing Co., 1968, pp. 488–567.

SILVER, HENRY K., IGOE, JUDITH BELLAIRE, and McATEE, PATRICIA ROONEY. "The School Nurse-Practitioner: Providing Improved Health Care to Children." *Pediatrics* 58 (1976):580–84.

STENNETT, R.G., CRAM, D.M., GIBSON, DOROTHY, and DUKACZ, KATHRYN. "Exploring the Possibilities of Computerized Student Health Records." *Journal of School Health* 2 (1971):59–64.

TIPPLE, DOROTHY C. "Misuse of Assistants in School Health." *American Journal of Nursing* 64 (1964):99–101.

VAUGHN, MARGARET. "Difficult Tasks: Defining the Role of the Clinical Specialist." In J. P. Riehl and J. W. McVay, eds., *The Clinical Nurse Specialist: Interpretations*. New York: Appleton-Century-Crofts, 1973, pp. 200–01.

WEED, LAWRENCE L. *Medical Records, Medical Education and Patient Evaluation*. Cleveland: Press of Case Western University, 1969.

WILSON, CHARLES C. *School Health Services,* 2nd ed. Washington, D.C.: National Education Association and The American Medical Association, (Chicago) 1964.

19. Community Health Nurses as Discharge Planners

Suzanne Brodnax

INTRODUCTION

Discharge planning is a critical, and all-too-often missing, link between discrete elements of the health care delivery system: the hospital and community agencies. Through thoughtful planning that ideally starts before the clients enter the hospital or at least as early as the first contact with them while in the hospital, the nurse anticipates clients' needs for care and support after they leave the hospital and begins to develop plans of care to meet these needs. The nurse uses a holistic approach to assist the client and family ". . . to regain as normal and productive a role as possible; providing for efficient, compassionate, and economical methods for the delivery of health services (Bristow et al. 1974:4). Thus the discharge planner is instrumental in helping clients to return to their optimal level of functioning.

The discharge planner confers on an ongoing basis with the client, family, physician, and members of the home care agency and hospital staffs to coordinate services and maintain clear channels of communication. Health professionals in the hospital and in community agencies function as teams. As a member of each of these teams, the discharge planner is the liaison between the two and ensures that their efforts on the client's behalf are complimentary and coordinated. The client, aided by the discharge planner, travels smoothly from one team to the other,

512

thereby benefiting from the best of both. The "Patient's Bill of Rights" includes the right of the client to expect this continuity of care (Quinn and Somers 1974).

For example, public health nurses hired by a hospital, work full time to coordinate services for clients with their continuing health needs (LaMontagne 1975). These discharge planners develop an intimate knowledge of their clients' needs and community resources. They often consult with hospital nurses who detect long-term care needs, such as medication and vital sign monitoring for a person with cardiac disease, in order to develop teaching plans that can then be smoothly continued by the home care staff or caretaker. Discharge planners also advise community nurses on hospital policy and practices; for example, how to help a client get an appointment in a special clinic to facilitate the client's care. Discharge nurses act as liaisons by locating and coordinating the many services a client may require and thereby avoiding fragmentation and costly duplication.

In some settings, discharge planners work with a specific population and provide some additional services. For example, one community health nurse works half time in the emergency room of a large medical center. As part of her job, she refers clients to a variety of community services and also assists other staff to learn to make these referrals. The other half of her time is spent working in the home setting with selected clients who had been seen in the emergency room. This arrangement of her time gives her and the rest of the emergency room staff an excellent opportunity to see the impact of their nursing care on the client as well as to insure that clients are able to receive the additional services they need. Providing for this kind of continuity is especially important since an increasing number of clients are using the emergency room as their sole source of medical care. Having a nurse with whom the client is familiar do a followup often increases the probability that clients will follow through on the suggestions that are made, including information on where to find other health care resources. The hospital staff feels comfortable referring clients for evaluation and followup of their care management in the home because they, too, know the nurse who will do the followup. As we might anticipate, staff, client, and community health nurse satisfaction is high.

In maternity nursing, hospital- or clinic-based nurses are also providing direct and indirect home care followup services. Postpartum hospital nurses make phone calls to newly discharged mothers to assess the situation and to reinforce teaching or make indicated referrals. Some of these hospital nurses are making home visits to mothers and babies who are discharged within a few hours of delivery. These visits are to assess their condition as well as to teach self-care and infant care. Again, client-staff satisfaction is high. Continuing care needs are assessed and met while nurses receive valuable feedback. This feedback is invaluable in helping the hospital nurses to modify their teaching and care as needed and to take pride in a job well done.

In other maternity settings, hospital nurses who do not make home visits on newly delivered and discharged mothers and babies keep in close touch with nurses in community agencies who make these visits. Another instance where this kind of followup after discharge is essential is with premature infants, especially in light of the relatively high incidence of child abuse of which these youngsters are often victims. Whatever pattern for this followup is used, the end results are that the new mother and baby receive care and teaching in their home. These services reduce the number of serious complications and greatly assist in the development of sound parenting. Feedback to the hospital nurses assists them to give quality nursing care to all of their clients.

Some institutions such as Montefiore and Kaiser hospitals have their own home care services that provide clients with needed followup, teaching, and care in their homes. People who have been treated in the hospital for such conditions as diabetes, heart disease, and cancer involving surgery, such as colostomy and mastectomy, are automatically candidates for these services. Care and nurturing of this kind also reduce the incidence of complications and prevent costly readmissions. The same results are obtained by other hospitals' use of discharge planners to work closely with visiting nurses' associations, combined health departments, and other home care services to see that people who are discharged with continuing needs for teaching and care have these needs met.

Often the ideal situations such as those just described are far from the real circumstances in which community health nurses engaged in discharge planning have to work. Many clients leave the hospital with continuing needs for care that are, and often will remain, unmet, even though resources to help them exist in their communities (Wensley 1963; Sister Ambrose 1974; Zeigler 1974). Many reasons contribute to this discrepancy between the ideal and the real. A few of these include:

1. Failure of many providers within the hospital to realize that most clients are far from cured and ready to resume their normal activities of daily living at the time of discharge—even after a "simple" procedure much less a complex one. Therefore, the job of discharge planner is complicated by the constant need to remind nurses to teach patients and their caretakers how to deal with their needs and doctors to refer the patients to community agencies who can offer supportive services.

2. Territorial jealousies and boundary protection (see chapter 11) that affect how the discharge planner is viewed. If discharge planners

are placed in the hospital from a community agency, often the hospital nurses see them as intruders. If discharge planners are hospital based, community agency nurses tend to view them as hospital nurses who may not understand community nursing. Only with time, through patient work, and tireless communication can discharge planners develop a track record that gives them credibility with their colleagues in nursing inside the hospital and in the community. Many nurses do not have the patience to see this process through, but the rewards to those who do and the benefits to the clients and their caretakers are worth all the effort.

3. Very personalized credibility and development of the role of discharge planner. For example, when a nurse who has painstakingly developed the linkages between acute care and community agencies leaves the position of discharge planner, the whole network may fall apart. The new nurse must thus start from scratch and rebuild the relationships that are essential for discharge planning to work. Administrative support is essential at all times, but particularly so at times of personnel transitions.

CASE STUDY

My experience as a discharge planner occurred as a result of an enormous number of mistakes that could and should have been avoided. In spite of all of these mistakes, the outcome was relatively successful. One of the greatest challenges we face is to turn really negative situations into what we ruefully call valuable learning experiences. There is much we can learn from these experiences, and so I share some of the negative as well as some of the positive aspects of my discharge planning experience with you here. As always, the shining experiences are those that occur with people.

THE SETTING

I was employed as a public health nurse in the home care unit buried deeply within the labyrinth of a metropolitan health department's bureaucracy. The home care unit came under the jurisdiction of public health administration, not public health nursing administration. Not only did this organizational placement wreak havoc with our own identity, it caused tremendous communication problems between the unit and other public health nurses. Public health administration did not understand our problems, and public health nursing had no authority to help us.

Our unit did not deliver direct client services but functioned as a watchdog to be sure that clients for whom any kind of home care had been authorized actually received it. We also initiated referrals, screened referrals from other parts of the agency for their appropriateness, made sure forms were filled out with the necessary working, reviewed billings to be sure services billed for had actually been provided, and spoke on request to community groups about home care services. I was responsible for authorizing payment of county funds to private service providers to supplement Medicaid allotments or to pay the full cost of home care services for clients who had no insurance and could not otherwise pay for their care. In the particular county in which I worked, home health care is purchased from private home care agencies and public health nursing is done by the health department, although in some counties, the health department provides both home care and public health nursing services through a combined agency. An additional facet of my job was to maintain close communication ties with the "liaison" public health nurses located in the county's hospitals. I was to encourage and assist these nurses to identify clients who needed home care services and to initiate appropriate referrals and followup.

Liaison nurses or discharge planners—or whatever the job title for nurses who are charged with the responsibility of insuring that clients receive needed followup care—have long been common personnel classifications. Studies have shown that 70 percent of the clients who spend five or more days in the hospital have at least one continuing need for nursing care; the average number of continuing nursing care needs at the time of discharge is 4.7 (Los Angeles County 1966). Smith (1963) indicates that the need for home care followup after discharge is higher in ethnic population groups of color especially for those living in urban ghettos. Our experience at Hightower, the county hospital serving many of the county's nonwhite urban people, was that almost 85 percent of this clientele would have benefited from continuing care at home.

Hightower, the county hospital where our home care unit was located, and its clinics were often the only source of medical care for our clientele. Even so, people came to Hightower as a last resort, and often by the time they finally sought care, they had to be admitted to the acute care facility at Hightower. By this time their physical conditions were, in general, very poor—diabetic coma, advanced pneumonia, cancer with widespread metastases, and far advanced, active tuberculosis—and their medical and nursing care needs were complex. A study done by the administration at Hightower documented the fact that because the client population was so seriously ill, usually accepted nurse-patient ratios were too low to permit sound nursing care. Many of the patients on the surgical floors—mainly trauma victims—and those on the gynecological and obstetrical units were in the best overall physical condition and could anticipate full recovery.

Some clients were discharged from Hightower to the long-term care county facilities and others were transferred to nursing homes, but the vast majority went back into the community—into the downtown's deteriorating hotels, Salvation Army, housing projects of varying repute and repair, and some even into the streets. Because of the wide variation in living situations, considering the client's "home" was imperative in any discharge plan. There was little sense in planning for the mother of several small children and no outside help to spend most of her first week at home after surgery resting and avoiding lifting. An elderly person living alone in a hotel room without running water, much less a private bathroom, would have difficulty taking a sitz bath four times a day.

The first discharge planner at Hightower was a nurse placed there under a grant from Regional Medical Programs. Unfortunately she stayed just long enough to alienate most of the people with whom she and subsequent discharge planners had to work. With no funds available to replace her, discharge planning activities were distributed among a number of public health nurses. Because these nurses were not located within the hospital structure and were not part of the hospital staff, none became identified as *the* discharge planner. This lack of a focal point for both responsibility and accountability for discharge planning activities caused a great deal of frustration for the public health nurses, confused the hospital staff, and resulted in considerable turnover. I was the sixth discharge planner, so called, in a period of five years.

Several years of political squabbling within the department culminated in the removal of the prior public health nurse from Hightower by the health department. This public health nurse had performed the following functions:

1. Assisting hospital staff, especially doctors, to refer patients for public health nursing services or home care;
2. Assisting public health nurses to obtain such information as medication dosages, return appointments, or data from patients' charts;
3. Assisting public health nurses to communicate with the patient's doctor about changes in the patient's condition or changes needed in medications due to drug reactions.

These functions laid the groundwork for the power struggle between the health department administration, who felt that the public health nurse—discharge planner—was serving the hospital's clientele, and the hospital administration, who felt that she was serving the health department's clientele. Each administration felt that the other should pay the public health nurse's salary, but both wanted to have her continue to function as described above. This situation typifies the many instances where everyone says a service is needed and valuable as long as someone else pays the bills.

What both administrations lost sight of was that the clients both served were the same people. The difference was that the settings in which the services were given changed as the clients moved from hospital to community. Such power struggles and shortsightedness are brought about by factors such as the necessity to justify budget expenditures in terms of the numbers of clients served or the units of service given. The public health nurse's position as what is all-too-often the missing link between hospital and community agencies made this cost accounting very difficult for both. Each lacked understanding of the situation, and both were unwilling to compromise for the good of the clients the public health nurse served in both of their settings. As a result, the health department removed the public health nurse from her liaison role and reassigned her. Thus hospital staff and clients in the hospital lost her services as did the clients in the community and community agencies staff.

My own reaction to the vacancy was a mix of anger, frustration, and despair. I had seen too many people discharged from Hightower in need of home care service. I feared that they would not receive the services they needed without a public health nurse to act as liaison and discharge planner. I wanted to work with hospital staff to cope in what I felt was an emergency situation. My supervisor advised me to stay out of the fracus for the time being. Hightower's administration claimed that they could manage without public health nurses in this role. They claimed that their head nurses could manage all the discharge planning that was needed and noted that many other hospitals survived very well without public health nurses' involvement as discharge planners. My thought was the hospital would indeed survive, but I had real doubts about the quality of survival that many of our clients would experience without help in managing when they went home.

THE PROBLEM

In fact, few patients received referrals after the liaison public health nurse left, and even these referrals did not usually go smoothly. In one such case, a young Chinese woman was diagnosed as having diabetes mellitus and was started on insulin in the outpatient clinic. Because the staff felt she was mentally retarded, her male companion was taught to give her insulin and a referral was made to the health department for nursing supervision. However, the referral suggested the possibility of the need for home care so the public health nursing supervisor referred the case on to a home health agency. Although the nurse visited on the day the agency received the referral, five days had already elapsed since the woman had been sent home with her insulin.

The nurse found that the woman was living alone—the male companion was only an occasional visitor—and that the woman was not retarded, but only spoke Mandarin and so was unable to understand English. She had been giving herself the insulin in her forearm, drawing up the wrong dose, and using the same glass syringe and needle each time without sterilization. In tribute to human hardiness, no irreversible harm had been done, but clearly the system was not working to the patient's benefit. The clinic nurse who made the referral had used an outdated nursing manual. She could have phoned the Visiting Nurses Association directly to make the referral and done the paperwork later. Bilingual interpreters were available to the clinic staff but had been unable to come at that particular time. Greater staffing flexibility to allow a translator to assist when needed would certainly have helped in this situation.

In another situation, one determined hospital head nurse detected the need for public health nursing—for medication supervision and patient teaching. The patient had been on the same medications before, but had had difficulty in taking them correctly apparently due to lack of either information or reinforcement. The head nurse filled out the referral form, found the correct nursing district, and phoned in the request for a nursing visit within a few days of the patient's discharge. When the patient was rehospitalized a few weeks later, the head nurse found out that no nurse had come. She called the district to learn that the referral was still on the desk of a nurse who had been on vacation during this time. The nurse covering the district could have at least sorted through the vacationing nurse's messages and referrals to be sure that those needing a fast response would get it and that no one would get lost in the shuffle. Failure to provide adequate district coverage in a nurse's absence can be costly in terms of the availability of patient care. In this case, the cost also included unnecessary loss of confidence in community health nurses by referring hospital staff. The head nurse was furious that the patient had not gotten care. The story was well circulated among the hospital nurses as a warning to those bold enough to consider dealing with the health department to think twice before doing so. As with many such situations, negative experiences are much more widely publicized than are successful ones.

One factor in the slow and painful acceptance of the need for discharge planning was lack of feedback. Feedback is critically important, as the systems discussion in chapters 3 and 11 emphasized, to ensure that the system continues to function responsively. Unfortunately even when hospital staff did make even sporadic referrals, their efforts were seldom reinforced by reports from community nurses on how their patients were doing. In instances where the head nurses had been concerned enough about a patient's welfare to initiate a referral, they believed that they were entitled to feedback from the community health nurses about what happened to the patient. When there is no such reporting back, hospital staff have difficulty justifying the time making referrals takes away from other duties and their enthusiasm for making referrals is dampened. Feedback helps hospital staff develop a sense of continuity of their patients' lives. Feedback about what is good and helpful, as well as what is missing in referrals, helps improve the whole process.

One way to generate feedback is to attach a feedback form to each referral that requests the data on the patient's status at home and other specific information the referring nurse desires. The completed feedback form can be routed to the head nurse who then shares the news with the staff and routes the slip to medical records for inclusion in the patient's chart. This information from the community can be of great value to hospital personnel on the next contact with the patient. Another source of feedback is to telephone the patient. In some areas, such as maternity, this approach works well. At Hightower, however, the expense of calls in time and money, the difficulty in contacting some patients by phone, and the lack of written data for later plans made telephoning an inefficient alternative. Calling the visiting nurse is another choice, but again at Hightower the same disadvantages applied, although phone calls could certainly have been used in specific cases or to supplement other information. Feedback, however gained, is invaluable, both to the staff and the patient, because of its effects on present and future care.

There were other less subtle barriers causing the head nurses' difficulties in performing the duties of discharge planner. They had been assigned the additional responsibility without any instruction, and they had not been given the released time from other duties to do it. In addition, the referral forms were confusing and very time consuming. The manual explaining their use was some twenty pages long. When the nurses did try to make referrals and could get through the forms, they were faced with a choice of two home care agencies and four district public health nursing offices. As in many places, the districts were geographically defined and one needed a census tract book to determine in which district a patient lived. Census tract books were rarely available on the units. Not surprisingly, therefore, referrals often were incorrectly routed, thereby causing delay in patients' being seen when they got home.

The fine line between home care and public health nursing, if indeed there is one, can be hard to understand. At Hightower we cynically described the difference in two ways: (a) if Medicare will pay for the care, it is home care; if not, it is public health nursing and (b) in general, public health nurses don't touch their patients; so if the care requires contact, it's probably home health care that is appropriate. Any referral to the Visiting Nurses Association (VNA) that was not appropriate was promptly referred to public health nursing.

The head nurses were understandably having a difficult time. Their orientation and experience were in the needs of hospitalized patients. Hospital care was so complex they didn't have time to look beyond their own four walls. The head nurses felt that a public health nurse should be appointed to serve as discharge planner in the hospital. Perhaps they felt that in their own best interests they ought not to do too well at making referrals themselves. A poor job would keep the need for a full-time discharge planner uppermost in everyone's minds and insure that the position would soon be filled. After a month of this half-hearted approach to discharge planning, during which patients were not having proper arrangements made for the continuity of care they needed, I asked Hightower's administration if our home care unit could be of any assistance on a regular basis. The answer was a quick "yes," and I was asked to make arrangements through the hospital's nursing administration staff.

GAINING ENTRY

The hospital's nursing administration staff suggested that I meet with the supervisors and head nurses to discuss the situation and see how we could work together to meet patients' needs for discharge planning and continuity of care. At the meetings, problems the hospital nurses discussed included lack of time for discharge planning, confusion with multiple agencies, difficulty in identifying patients needing referral, confusion and frustration with complicated forms, lack of feedback from community health nurses when referrals were made, and confusing procedures in the hospital's manual. When asked to identify areas in which we could be of most help to them, the head nurses agreed that they most needed assistance in deciding to what agency or agencies referrals for a given patient were appropriate. So I said that I would assume the responsibility for seeing that the referrals the head nurses made were routed to the proper place or places.

I also obtained permission from the nursing director during the first meeting to attend patient conferences that were held on the floors, make rounds as needed to assist with referrals, and be on call to help with any referral problems. I made rounds on all the floors, but concentrated on the medical units where the numbers of patients needing home care and/or public health nursing referral were high. On these units were many elderly people who were both poor and lived alone. People with chronic illnesses such as tuberculosis, diabetes, cancer, stroke, heart trouble, and crippling arthritis need a great deal of community-based care.

Under our new plan, each head nurse on the medical units kept a special folder into which personnel could put notes and questions if they missed me on my daily rounds. Gradually I became familiar with the doctors and began to get requests directly from them as well as from the nursing staff. I shared all these requests with the head nurse on the unit where they originated so that she or he was kept aware of what I was doing. Gradually the hospital's personnel got to know me and what I was doing, which thus enabled me to become increasingly effective in insuring that Hightower's patients would get followup care if they needed it.

INSIDE THE HOSPITAL

I was trying to create a discharge planning position through (1) pursuing administrative channels via phone calls, memos, and meetings with public health and hospital administration to keep them apprised of the situation, (2) facilitating communication and feedback between public health nurses and home care and hospital staff, (3) working with the hospital staff to improve their skills, and (4) in the meantime providing as much direct service as possible to patients needing discharge planning. The position was not a nine to five job, and running into the nursing administrator at seven at night on the units did give credibility to my statements that another body for discharge planning was needed—for what I didn't do, didn't get done. I enjoyed providing the service myself, but unless others became actively involved, I felt that when my energy fizzled, no one else was likely to carry on.

Just my presence on the units generated interest. When I worked on a referral, I did so by gathering information from such sources as Kardex and chart and by talking with the patient, and family when available, the nurses, the doctor, and the medical social worker. I tried to obtain a clear medical and psycho-socio-cultural understanding of the patient's situation. From such information, I could anticipate the basic nursing needs the patient might have after discharge and could develop and revise a care plan in collaboration with the doctor, patient, and others.

Patient interviews are highly desirable. They provide an opportunity to learn patients' perceptions of their needs and their expectations of care. Predischarge interviews should assess just how well prepared patients are to go home. Do they, for instance, know discharge is imminent? Do they share the hospital view of their readiness to go? Is there a home for them to go to, which is no idle question for many urban poor or elderly. Has the patient or a caretaker learned the necessary procedures that will be needed to get along until the nursing visit is likely to take place? One of the things I found unsettling was receiving a referral late Friday afternoon for a new diabetic or colostomy patient who had received no teaching in self-care during hospitalization. The unavailability of most services on weekends necessitates in such a case an immediate visit to conduct a crash course on the essentials of needed care to prevent complications that would result in readmission.

Patient interviews can also establish a feeling of continuity for clients, especially if they can be told when the home nurse will be visiting. Setting an exact date is not always easy to do when multiple agencies are involved, but the effort is worthwhile since clients feel less at sea or even panicky if they know for sure that a nurse has made an appointment for a home visit. I found clients were reassured, if at the very least, I verified their addresses and gave them my name and phone number so they could contact me should they need to change the appointment or should the nurse fail to arrive. Often folks go to stay with relatives or friends after discharge, and thus, verifying the address can get the nurse to the right place. Without a valid address, a nurse might arrive for a 7:00 AM insulin injection, find an empty house, and be unable to locate the patient, who then goes without the insulin. The information obtained from the Kardex and from nursing staff can be invaluable especially when continuity of a teaching program is desired.

The source of payment must always be considered, since it is often an unvoiced concern for the patient. For example, some patients refused desperately needed home care until they learned it was a Medicare-covered service. Few people want to admit that they can't afford what their doctor has ordered. Many providers balk at completing the lengthy forms required to insure that the patient gets reimbursed by some third-party payer for the expenses incurred. If these forms are not filled out and filled out properly, patients may be unable to get needed followup care at all or be saddled with gigantic bills which they cannot hope to pay. Thus, I cannot stress too strongly the necessity of nurses in discharge planning as well as all other direct client services being sure that insurance forms are properly completed (see chapter 12). If the patient or family expresses financial concerns or has inadequate insurance coverage, a referral should be made to social services for assistance *before* the day of discharge.

These aspects of discharge planning obviously take time. A referral can fail at any of the steps along the way so care must be taken to see that each procedure is carried out to insure that needed services are obtained. Getting the referral to the community agency is often the weakest link in the chain of events. The referral is usually phoned to the agency, since there is often too great a delay if the initial contact is by mail. Mail followup of the referral is then done. Again a request for feedback to the discharge planner should accompany the referral. The discharge planner can then share the feedback on the patient's transition from the hospital with the staff who initiated the referral. This positive reinforcement is essential, as already noted, to keep those referrals coming.

In practice I did much of this process on the hospital unit. At first I did so simply because it was too tedious to go all the way back to my office. Then I realized the nursing staff were observing what I did. One nurse commented: "I never knew what went into a referral—the other nurse just took some information and left. We never knew what she did with it." Clearly, most hospital personnel had little concept of patients' home care needs. Instead they observed what I did in my own process and then would request that activity. For example, the doctors and nurses noticed me interviewing a patient and would then ask, "Would you talk with Mr. Jones next." Only after I asked them why they felt I should do so did I finally learn they thought that Mr. Jones might need home followup of his diabetic teaching program. Possibly the hospital staff members viewed diabetic teaching as a discrete activity that could be prescribed as surely as any other therapeutic regimen. The staff would pick up clues that some home care would be needed, such as a patient being started on insulin, or going home with a pacemaker, or needing continuing IPPB treatments. Since they did not have time to pursue the patient's needs further, they would refer him or her to me instead. Their keen questioning about the patient's later progress indicated their lack of participation was due to other pressures, not to lack of interest.

In addition to staff suggestions, I did some case finding using the Kardex and weekly patient conference for leads. The kinds of things I was looking for are formalized in the Discharge Planning Questionnaire in table 19.1. The answers to these questions will provide excellent clues not only on whether to refer a patient but also to whom and for what. It is an example only. Specific formats need to be developed for individual settings.

A last-minute clue to the need for referral can come even as patients are being prepared for discharge. I asked myself these questions each time: What would I need to take care of this patient in a home setting? What am I using to care for the patient in the hospital and how does it translate to a home situation? If I used 15 med cards maybe the patient will need a medication schedule or other scheme, such as putting up a day's supply in a multicompartmented, labeled box. Does the patient know about the medication, its side effects, and so forth? Does the patient

TABLE 19.1 *Discharge Planning Questionnaire*

Medical/Physical—Reason for hospitalization? _____

How was patient getting care prior to hospitalization?   Self ____ Family ____

    Nurse ____ yes ____ no   Chore Service/Attendant ____ yes ____ no

Are new treatments being done for patient in hospital?   ____ yes ____ no

    Meds ____ Dressings ____ Diet ____ PT ____ Other treatments ____

Will patient probably be continuing these treatments at home?   ____ yes ____ no

Does patient require special equipment? ____ yes ____ no

    If yes, please specify: _____

Does patient need help with the equipment? ____ yes ____ no

    If yes, how? _____

Will patient probably need nursing care at home prior to next clinic visit?

    ____ yes ____ no

    Specify:

    Treatment supervision ____   Vital sign monitoring ____

    Activity monitoring ____   Medication supervision ____

    Special diet/med instruction ____

    Other (PT, OT, home health aide, chore service) _____

Psycho-Social-Cultural

Describe living situation prior to admission: _____

Any problems (social, financial, etc.)? _____

Will patient probably need out of home placement? ____ yes ____ no

    If yes, please explain. _____ ____

Did patient have difficulty following medical advice prior to admission?

    ____ yes ____ no   If yes, please explain. _____

Does patient have a new diagnosis? ____ yes ____ no

    If yes, what is it? _____

What has patient been taught about it? _____

Does patient need an interpreter? ____ yes ____ no

    If yes, what language? _____

Describe patient's behavior in coping with the current situation. _____

Does patient need assistance in understanding disease and treatment?

    ____ yes ____ no   If yes, please explain. _____

know what foods and liquids mix well or not at all with the medications? If half the Kardex is filled with the rotation schedule for treatments of various graft and donor sites, how will they be continued? Can the IPPB treatments and postural drainage and other physical therapies safely cease when the patient is discharged? If not, does the patient know how to do them and have the equipment? When there's no medication or treatment room to turn to, where will the syringes, bandages, clinitest, tablets, thermometers, blood pressure cuffs, scales, and so forth come from?

Another way of assessing a patient's needs is summed up by METHOD (Cucuzzo 1976), which means Medications, Economic, Treatments, Health Education, Outpatient Referral, and Diet. METHOD is a good starting point if we remember to add equipment and supplies, return appointments or source of followup care, and transportation. Can patients get to their homes, if indeed they have homes to go to, and can they get back for further care? Certainly the nurse caring for the patient is in the best position to plan for extending care past discharge when needed (Morcland and Schmitt 1974). After learning the continuing care needs, the art is to match them with a community resource or group of resources that will effectively meet them.

Eligibility for home services varies from state to state as well as among the various third-party payers involved in so much of our present health care. A variety of resources can be used to check eligibility in any community. Some of the following resources can provide information on who's eligible for what, when, and how often:

> Public health department, especially the nursing division,
> Visiting Nurses Associations or other home care agencies,
> Social services, especially if they have agency directories,
> Senior citizen organizations,
> Information and referral services,
> Homemaker services (try yellow pages),
> Public health department's communicable disease manual,
> Medicare information available from the local Social Security Office,
> Utilization review person of a major insurer, usually Blue Cross,
> Organizations like Heart Association and Cancer Society,
> Medicaid regulations,
> Other discharge planners.

The information so obtained should be fairly clear but there are always cases where the rules do not apply; for instance, if a doctor feels a service is medically necessary and Medicaid refuses to authorize it, the doctor can call the Medicaid authorizer and give medical justification for service; usually authorization will be given or a suitable compromise can be reached. Time is needed to learn the ins and outs and procedures often vary from month to month. Thus, alliances with other discharge planners are essential. The best approach I found was to do my homework first and to make myself known throughout the communication network so that I could be apprised of changes as they occurred.

Another nurse in my unit improved the direct client services we offered when she suggested that we do home assessments ourselves. These visits were made soon after patient discharge when the possibility that further services that could not be identified during hospital stay might be needed. If additional or different followup care was needed, the patient could be referred appropriately. The information gathered on these visits enabled us to provide needed feedback to hospital nurses about their patients in the community. This feedback added incentive for the staff to make referrals even when they were not certain whether one was needed. We were happy to advise them on the appropriateness of their referrals. Our home assessment visits could also be made prior to the patient's discharge when there were questions as to the suitability of the home environment. These questions could be physical ones concerning stairs or the bathroom or social ones about the availability of someone willing and able to learn the required nursing care.

Conferences involving patients and their families as well as the physicians and nurses can often prove unusually helpful. One of the home care unit's public health nurses set up a conference during which we suddenly learned that the patient had been swallowing prescribed tablets instead of placing them in his nebulizer and inhaling the mist. This explained his recent flurry of hospitalizations for asthma attacks despite what appeared to be an adequate medical regimen. With this practice corrected, I don't recall any further hospitalizations for the patient. It's amazing what can happen as an outcome of establishing clear communication.

There are several patients I remember well and would like to share with you as a way of illustrating different aspects of discharge planning. One "infamous" patient was a quadriplegic with multiple medical problems capped off by "terminal bed sores." His severe decubiti exposed tissue, tendon, and bone with no favoritism. He was well known to every home health agency as he required home care for catheter changes, dressing changes, range of motion exercises, and many other treatments. He was an expert manipulator and often played one agency against another. He had recently married a young woman who was suspected to be motivated more by the patient's reputation as a dope dealer than by true love. The daughter of a thrice relapsed TB carrier, she helped with his care from time to time. Attendants were found, care taught, attendants were fired, and the process was repeated.

During his most recent hospitalization at Hightower, his physician recommended a long-term rehabilitation program at one of the county's facilities. This plan was unacceptable to the man and he threatened to leave against medical advice. His doctor finally agreed—with the stipulation that there would be no home care either. Since this patient had at one time refused medically indicated hospitalization for months, I felt any effort to starve him, medically speaking, into a long-term program was not likely to be successful. I discussed this with the physician, who would have preferred to wash his hands of the whole matter, and I learned later that the patient and doctor had finally reached a compromise: The patient would go home with home care for two weeks and then be readmitted for extensive antibiotic therapy for his osteomyelitis and resistant urinary tract infection as well as a limited rehab program. Subsequently, the patient's condition improved. The doctor, instead of taking the simple course of dropping the patient, was making plans to continue his care. Discharging and forgetting a patient is far easier to do than planning for continuing care, but ask a patient if it's worth it.

In another situation I suggested daily nursing visits to a man who was newly diagnosed as having diabetes and who needed to be taught to give his own insulin. We discussed his gradually assuming responsibility for all his care. The nursing staff, however, said he had resisted all teaching efforts in the hospital and they felt he would do poorly at home. In addition, he had been taught injections using plastic syringes and would receive a glass syringe to take home. In hearing about the glass syringes and the process for sterilizing them, he volunteered haltingly that maybe there was something he could learn from that nurse after all. Only one problem remained: He usually didn't let anyone in his house but his wife. Finally he agreed that if he knew in advance when the nurse was coming and if she really was a nurse and if she could talk with his wife about his diet—well, maybe it would be all right after all. The referral was made. Later, reports indicated that he had let the nurse in and he had become quite adept at self-care. Seemingly, he had been in the early stages of grieving over his loss of health and had not been receptive to teaching during his hospitalization, but with the passage of time and some understanding, he was ultimately willing to learn.

As another example, the public health nurses also encouraged hospital staff to fill out morbidity reports on specific communicable diseases. Venereal diseases, once reported, received followup from the health department. Tuberculosis and other diseases also required followup, which could be extensive, as was the case when a man was admitted from the Salvation Army facility after being diagnosed as having active tuberculosis. A team of public health nurses did the contact screening and followup in that case. As discharge planner, I initiated a referral as soon as I learned of the case rather than waiting for his discharge weeks later.

A followup must be immediate in the case of a communicable disease in a transient population if efforts are to be of any use at all. In other instances referral is useful before a patient is discharged as well as after. Examples of these included the cases of a person with malaria and several varieties of worms who was admitted from a rural commune; another person with infectious hepatitis admitted from an urban collective; and a teenager with active tuberculosis who attended the local high school regularly and had a large group of close friends.

One case of tuberculosis was diagnosed on autopsy only and mentioned only in passing at a weekly conference, "Hey, does anyone remember old Mrs. B.? Would you believe she had miliary TB?" Apart from the screening necessary for hospital staff, the Visiting Nurses Association needed notification because the patient had had months of home care. I promptly notified the VNA so screening could be done and also made a referral to public health nursing for screening and followup of other close contacts. Without the intervention of the nurses in my unit, VNA would not have been notified for at least another month if the standard channels of communication had been followed.

At Hightower where patients were often hospitalized repeatedly, familiarity with the patients and carefully kept records were essential. Indeed, those records were very helpful in substantiating our comments on the need for a discharge planner. Our visibility also continued the pressure on the hospital administrators to provide this service for the hospital. My supervisor reminded them regularly that we were "on loan" for the crisis only. The hospital's nursing administrator admitted the head nurses were not able to do it. This statement, made at a county nursing directors' meeting, was seen by the public health nursing directors as a great change in position in hospital thinking. This admission plus the documentation of what our home care unit nurses had done, led the hospital administrator to designate a discharge planner position. Our colleagues in the health department felt that our efforts had been a real success. Discharge planning was finally recognized as a necessary and a full-time job. Now it would be up to the nurse appointed to fill the position to make the discharge planner position work.

REFLECTIONS

My experience was brief, intense, full of brilliant color: the man with the active TB admitted from Salvation Army housing, the young man with "terminal asthma," the quadriplegic dope dealer, the young mother with uncontrollable hypertension, the old gypsy woman dying of congestive heart failure with her ever-present tribe standing watch, and the woman afraid to move for fear her pacemaker would malfunction, which, ironically, did and required replacement. I am grateful they let me share a moment of their lives. I learned from them and I hope they benefited in some way from their contact with me.

The experience, as a whole, though fraught with many negative incidents, did have a major positive outcome. The hospital does now recognize discharge planning as a legitimate and necessary community health nursing activity. The discharge planner's position is full time, funded, and continuing. Communication and feedback on referrals from public health nursing remains poor and is likely to continue so until there are major changes in attitudes. However, feedback from the home care agencies remains excellent and has led to a majority of referrals for nursing care such as medication supervision and vital sign monitoring. These could go to either the VNA or the health department, which in turn sends them to the VNA. Public health nursing is cutting itself off at the knees in this area of care by failing to become actively involved in providing home care.

In the county where I worked, many well-trained, astute nurses have left the health department and have gone to home care agencies, clinics, hospitals, and other areas of employment. Seemingly, our difficulties with public health nursing were part of a much larger problem within the department. Public health nursing in neighboring counties functions far more satisfactorily. Thus, discharge planning can bring nurses into contact with the community agencies both excellent and disappointing.

SUMMARY

Discharge planning is a challenge to nursing for many reasons—not the least of which is the responsibility of coordinating two discrete parts of our health care system for the benefit of the patient. Without this bridge there often can be no delivery of home care. The patient contact and opportunity to be a patient advocate is satisfying and essential for those of us who are allergic to paper shuffling. The nursing and medical staff contact affords the opportunity for daily continuing education and professional growth. Discharge planning can satisfy an interest in being the "resident expert" in a special area of patient care. It challenges our ability to uncover community resources and sharpens our interviewing and teaching skills.

Community health nurses have a lot to offer in the role of discharge planner: Orientation and knowledge of the community are invaluable assets. For example, when a man is newly diagnosed as a diabetic requiring insulin, his eyesight is poor, and his address is a downtown hotel full of alcoholics, we can anticipate certain needs. Our knowledge of community resources also helps link clients with the programs they might be interested in and benefit from, such as social service, homemaker-chore service, or Meals on Wheels, as well as the visiting nurse or public health nursing service.

Can head nurses or medical social workers succeed at discharge planning? Certainly, if they have a basic knowledge of community resources, are able to anticipate the patient's needs for those services after discharge, and have the time and the interest in getting the patient and providers of service together. The hospital nurses in the case study lacked adequate time and knowledge of community resources and varied widely in their ability to project patient needs after discharge. A few home visits, support from nursing administration through making time available and presentations by community providers about their clientele and services might have made the difference between failure and success for the head nurses. But without positive feedback, the nurses' efforts would probably not have continued. Discharge planning needs to be done on a continuing basis if the patients are to gain access to those services developed to serve them.

REFERENCES

ALLEN, D. V., KUHNS, P. L., WERLEY, H. H., and PEABODY, S. R. "Agencies' Perceptions of Factors Affecting Home Care Referral." *Medical Care* 2 (1974):828–44.

AMBROSE, SISTER ANNE. "Discharge Plans—The Weakest Link." *Hospital Progress* 54 (March 1973):58–60.

BRISTOW, O., and STICKNEY, G. *Discharge Planning for Continuity of Care.* Richmond: Virginia Regional Medical Program, 1974.

DAVID, JANIS, et al. *Guidelines for Discharge Planning.* Thorofare, N. J.: Charles B. Slack, 1973.

ELCONIN, A. F., EGEBERG, R. O., and DUNN, O. J. "An Organized Hospital-Based Home Care Program." *American Journal of Public Health* 54 (1964):1106–17.

GREENLICK, M. R., HURTADO, A. V., and SAWARD, E. W. "The Objective Measurement of the Post-Hospital Needs of a Known Population." *American Journal of Public Health* 56 (1966):1193–98.

ISLER, E. "Helping Hospital Patients Out." *RN Magazine* 38 (1975):43–46.

LAMONTAGNE, MARGARET E., and MCKEEHAN, KATHLEEN M. "Profile of a Continuing Care Program Emphasizing Discharge Planning." *Journal of Nursing Administration* 5 (October 1975):22–33.

LAVOR, J., and CALLENDER, M. "Home Health Care Effectiveness: What Are We Measuring?" *Medical Care* 14 (1976):866–72.

LOS ANGELES COUNTY, CALIFORNIA, BUREAU OF PUBLIC HEALTH NURSING. *Continuity of Nursing Care From Hospital to Home—A Study in a Voluntary General Hospital.* New York: National League for Nursing, 1966.

MORELAND, HELEN J., and SCHMITT, VIRGINIA. "Making Referrals Is Everybody's Business." *American Journal of Nursing* 74 (January 1974):96–97.

NASH, D. T. "Making Use of Home Care Services." *Geriatrics* 29 (1974):140–45.

NIKKILA, M. "Securing Early Referrals for Home Care." *American Journal of Nursing* 62 (1962):59–60.

PEABODY, S. R. "The Home Care Program of the Detroit Visiting Nurse Association." *American Journal of Public Health* 51 (1961):1681–87.

QUINN, N., and SOMERS, A. "The Patient's Bill of Rights." *Nursing Outlook* 22 (April 1974):240–44.

SARGENT, E. G. "Evolution of a Home Care Plan." *The American Journal of Nursing* 61 (1961):88–91.

SMITH, L. C. *Factors Influencing Continuity of Nursing Service.* New York: National League for Nursing, 1962.

U. S. SENATE SPECIAL COMMITTEE ON AGING. *Alternatives to Nursing Home Care: A Proposal.* Washington, D.C.: U.S. Government Printing Office, 1972.

WENSLEY, E. *Nursing Service without Walls: A Call to Action Coast to Coast.* New York: National League for Nursing, 1963.

ZEIGLER, D., et al. *Patient Discharge and Referral Planning—Whose Responsibility?* New York: National League for Nursing, 1974.

20. Community Health Nurses in Ethnic Communities of Color

Teresa A. Bello
Ruth Ann Terry

INTRODUCTION

Historically, public health nurses have worked most frequently with people who are economically, socially, and culturally outside of the so-called mainstream of society in the United States. The majority of public health practitioners have been and continue to be white and members of the middle class and thus are separated economically, socially, and culturally from many of the clients they serve. Although community health nursing is broadening its focus so that people from all walks of life throughout the community are served, many of the clients and too few of the providers are ethnic people of color. To be able to work effectively in helping ethnic people of color attain and maintain their optimal level of functioning, community health nurses must understand more about the cultural and social values and aspirations of ethnic people, as well as the conditions under which many live in our society. To these ends we have written this chapter.

A generally accepted fact is that some form of oppression exists in most societies. However, the basis for one group's dominance over another may vary. For example, oppression may be based on belief in the supposed superiority of male over female. When a given society embraces such an idea and authenticates it through its social system and practices, the result is oppression of females. The oppressor is male; the oppressed,

533

female. Since the ideology is rooted in sexual beliefs of superiority and inferiority, this form of oppression can be called sexual oppression, or sexism. When an ideology of innate superiority based on skin color exists (for example, white versus nonwhite) and this ideology permeates the entire society by granting the preferred group social privilege or status, then oppression takes the form of racial oppression or racism. Both the oppressor (white) and the oppressed (nonwhite) are profoundly affected by this belief system of racial superiority. That has been the experience here in the United States.

This chapter attempts to explain, from a nonwhite perspective, ways in which racism influences and often determines the behavior and practice of nurses working in nonwhite communities. Racial or ethnic minority groups may vary in constitution in various parts of the country. At times we may mention a particular one but, for general purposes, a reference to any particular minority is intended to be extrapolated to ethnic people of color.

Institutional racism refers to the

> . . . operating policies, priorities, and functions of an ongoing system of normative patterns which serve to subjugate, oppress, and force dependence of individuals or groups by (1) establishing and sanctioning unequal goals, objectives, and priorities for blacks and whites, and (2) sanctioning inequality in status as well as in access to goods and services [Stafford and Hadner 1969:70].

Individual racism distinguished from *institutional racism* refers to those offensive acts and behavior committed by individuals or groups based on a personal sense of racial superiority. Differentiating institutional racism from individual racism is often difficult since the two go hand in hand as oppression is maintained over time.

Generally, institutional racism provides the structure for individual racist acts—that is, in order for individual people to practice personal racism, they must have a framework or structure that allows and/or sanctions such behavior. For example, newspapers recently reported that sterilizations were performed on a number of black adolescents without the knowing consent of their parents. Numbers of health professionals, including community nurses, were involved in carrying out this agency policy. Such actions could not have been carried through in the absence of certain shared social values, racist in nature, which superseded professional values and good judgement. No action, especially one with such long-term and irreversible consequences, should ever be undertaken without both parent and adolescent being actively involved in the decision-making process and signing that informed consent has been given. In the cases in point, individual and institutional racism even resulted in ignoring state and federal laws under which these violations were prosecuted. Personal racism in this example is demonstrated by the health practitioners' decision that sterilization was the only viable solution to the problems faced by these adolescents. Such single-mindedness by the health practitioner reinforces the insidious nature of personal racism: That only one solution is possible for a devalued ethnic group in society despite what is known about contraceptives. Ryan calls this ideology a brilliant one for justifying a perverse form of social action, designed to change not society, but, rather, society's victim (Ryan 1971:7).

Freire further illuminates the operation of racism by describing in detail certain aspects of oppression. One is that oppression dehumanizes the oppressed. This dehumanization occurs through the imposition of the oppressor's values onto the oppressed, thus transforming the oppresseds' consciousness to reflect the oppressors'. Thus, to be considered human, one must conform to the image conveyed by those with the power to prescribe such humanness (Freire 1971:2, 3). We often call this syndrome laying your trip on someone else. Most of us deal with this kind of phenomenon on a daily basis. However, those of us with sufficient individuality and ego strength are able to distinguish between what we think is right for us and what is being imposed on us by others. Ethnic people of color have continuous and pervasive trips laid on them by members of the majority society. Ethnic people of color are discounted by whites who believe they know what is best for nonwhites, even to the point that institutional norms are created which encourage and sanction discriminatory behavior.

When protected by the larger society and its norms that sanction and reward individual racist behavior, people may engage in prejudicial behavior both consciously and unconsciously—that is, some people act like racists even though they have never been in contact with ethnic people of color and consciously disclaim negative feelings about ethnic people of color. One may engage in racist behavior solely by passively accepting racist practices as the status quo. Community health nurses may be a case in point, as we shall discuss.

"Blaming-the-Victim" Syndrome

Many community health nurses find working in ethnic communities of color difficult and, for some, initially frightening. When questioned about their fears or feelings, one finds that the fears or feelings are based upon stereotypes, misconceptions, and a lack of adequate information about the culture of the people with whom they are working. Rather than perceiving the community's culture as only *different* from their own, these differences are viewed as being *a deficit*, seen from a *"less-than"* orientation.

The authors are often confronted with statements such as "these people will not keep their appointments" or *"they* just aren't interested so why bother with preventive health teaching." What may result is what Ryan calls "blaming the victim" (1971). This attitude in itself is hampering and maladaptive. It encourages the nurse to focus on the alleged deficits or perceived shortcomings in the client rather than to step back and look for other causes for such behavior. A familiar example is the scheduling of all morning clinic appointments for 8 AM. As a result, many clients are kept waiting two hours or more. If clients are fortunate, a health professional may spend at least ten minutes with them, learn something about their health status, and try to help them. When clients begin to arrive at 10 or 11 AM, instead of asking "what is wrong with clients who do not keep appointments?" maybe we should be asking, "what is wrong with our delivery of health care?" or "how continuous or coordinated is the health care system?" Obviously the clients have already diagnosed the problem. According to Ryan, to "make up" for the noncompliant behavior of client, we develop new programs aimed toward correcting the deficiencies of the clients' behavior while ignoring and leaving unchanged the obvious inadequacies of our health care delivery (1971:8).

Blaming the victim is defined as an ideological process, which is to say that it is a set of ideas and concepts deriving from systematically motivated, but *unintended,* distortion of reality. It is based on a belief system that maintains the status quo in the interest of a specific group (Ryan 1971:10). This blaming-the-victim process begins benignly enough as follows:

First,   identify a disadvantaged group; for example, ethnic people of color who tend to have higher mortality and morbidity rates for hypertension.

Second, fund a few hypertension studies in the black community to study the people and discover that their diet is high in cholesterol, simple carbohydrates, and salt, that they smoke heavily, and that there is much obesity.

Third,   identify these behavioral symptoms as the causes of the people's hypertension and prescribe treatments. Do not look for the underlying causes of these behaviors, such as stress brought about by deprivation and injustice or for the intrinsic rewards these behaviors bring with them.

Fourth, blame the people for not following sound medical advice and for not taking better care of themselves when they do not change their behavior.

Throughout this entire process, the real cause of peoples' hypertension is never looked for, much less uncovered. The focus is on the victim and the solution is to change the victim, rather than to deal with the larger societal factors that are making the victim sick—that is, deprivation and injustice. As long as this process continues, racial oppression will exist.

COMMUNITY HEALTH NURSING AND OPPRESSED GROUPS

The process of community health nursing, as for nursing in general, prescribes that community nurses assess a given situation, identify a problem, explore possible alternative plans and actions, institute the best plan of action, and evaluate the effectiveness of the plan. The process in itself, however, can function as an oppressive act if nurses undertake it unilaterally without clients' participation. We must begin by asking whether the data and the interpretation of the data are valid to identify the problems? Then we must ask questions like: Are these problems in each of our *client's* assessment, or is the interpretation based on our own conviction of what the situation should be? Is the plan of action derived from our own experiences, the client's problem-solving framework, or some combination of the two? Do we evaluate our plans for each client based on what we did, or is there some shared assessment with each client regarding the value of the intervention? The following illustration is a case in point.

A community health nurse made an initial visit to a Filipino family for the purpose of well child supervision. When the community health nurse arrived, the husband was home alone with the young children. Inspecting the home, the community health nurse began questioning the husband about sleeping arrangements as there was only one bedroom. The husband explained that their two preschool children slept in the bedroom with their parents. The community health nurse, raising her eyebrows, immediately launched into the "privacy" and "sexual" reasons why the children should sleep in a separate room. The husband explained that there was one bedroom, no space in the living room or the kitchen to place the children's beds, and that the family was too poor to move into a larger house. Besides, the house was owned by his nephew who had invited him and his family to live there. The nephew slept on the sofa in the living room. This explanation did not deter the nurse, who continued her sermon while the husband, suffering from acute embarrassment, tried to distract the children from hearing what she was saying.

To begin with, the purpose of the visit was well child supervision. Launching into a discussion about sleeping arrangements is a precipitous entree on any first visit. A strange woman discussing such an intimate topic with the husband is taboo to many families, Filipino and otherwise. Her being a nurse did not change her stranger status. The family's sleeping arrangements were practical for the circumstances. The extended family nature of this arrangement is common among most Filipino families, in which there is an overriding desire to provide for and share with kin. Filipino parents are just as constrained as white and other parents about displaying the sexual act in front of anyone, even young children. The discussion of sex in front of children is another taboo. Placing the children in the living room with the nephew would cause embarrassment as it would seem that the parents were infringing upon the nephew's privacy. While this example represents an oversimplification of the cultural traits of Filipino families, it serves to illustrate the husband's perspective that the nurse ignored. The nurse's immediately prescribing a change of behavior is an example of an oppressive act. The thought did not occur to her that her behavior was an infringement upon the family's right to be as they were rather than as she wanted them to be.

Some readers may consider this community health nurse's behavior as gross and rare and have immediately recognized the need for change. Others may be thinking that the nurse simply did not understand the family's cultural and economic realities. In fact, the nurse's behavior disregards the need for accurate data collection and interpretation, reciprocity in the nurse-client relationship, and common courtesy. The nurse's behavior was not out of ignorance but out of racism. She laid her trip on the family, which is oppression. The fact that the nurse felt she had a mandate to prescribe behavior change on the basis of her own standards is the subtle message of oppression we so seldom recognize.

This example also illustrates the mechanism of cultural domination as a means of social control over people of color that minimizes, distorts, and/or negates the contributions of a particular group's culture. The goal of such dominance is to remove or reduce the influence of the group's culture as a mobilizing and sustaining force. The oppressed deny their own group culture and buy into the culture of the "superior" group. Assimilation is a logical outcome of cultural dominance. According to the melting pot theory: the more you are forced to imitate us and our behavior, the closer you will come to being one of us and enter the mainstream of our society. Such was the experience of each successive wave of European ethnics who immigrated to the United States.

Koshi points out that the myth of a monolithic American culture acts as a barrier to the recognition of ethnic/cultural pluralism in our society. Once our society begins to legitimize this pluralism, all people, ethnic people of color and white ethnics, will be able to choose their own cultural identity rather than be forced into the dominant one (1976). The rub comes when ethnic people of color are confronted by another social control device: limited social mobility by the prescription of "place" for them. There are certain jobs, certain neighborhoods, and certain behaviors that are deemed to be appropriate for people of color (Blauner 1972).

OFFENSIVE MECHANISMS

While Blauner describes the larger societal process, Pierce, a black psychiatrist, describes an effective way in which oppression is maintained at the person-to-person level through the process of offensive mechanisms (1970). Nurses are familiar with the idea of defense mechanisms and the important role they play in maintaining the personal integrity and functioning of the individual in the presence of high levels of anxiety. The literature abounds with contextual definitions and descriptions of these kinds of behaviors so that the practitioner understands what they are and how they function for a variety of individuals. With these insights, the practitioners can determine whether or not a given person's defense mechanisms ought to be strengthened or weakened in order to optimize his or her level of functioning. Most often defense mechanisms are appropriately labeled reactive phenomena.

Pierce advances the concept of offensive mechanisms and how they function in race relations in America. These behaviors are not reactive but are small, "continuous bombardments of micro-aggression by whites to minorities" (Pierce 1970:280). The cumulative effect of this micro-aggression is reinforced racism. In order for racism to be effective, offensive mechanisms in interaction between white and nonwhite must be explicit. Pierce identifies the relationship between individual racism and offensive techniques:

> Racism is a mental health and public health disease characterized by perceptual distortion, contagion, and fatality. The vehicle for these characteristics is the cumulative effect of offensive mechanisms, individually exhibited but collectively approved and promoted by the white sector of society [Pierce 1970:282].

Three commonly used offensive mechanisms are: "We love you minorities to death"; "You minorities are sick"; and "We whites are right" (Pierce 1970). We believe seeing how Pierce's elaboration of offensive maneuvers is sometimes employed in the everyday work of community health nurses can be beneficial. Thus descriptions of each of the offensive mechanism and examples from the authors' experience that illustrate each are presented in the following sections.

"We love you minorities to death." At the end of this interplay, the minority person feels that the white person has said, "You people are unappreciative of whatever we try to do to show you that we love you to death."

One of us was a consultant to a nursing school whose white faculty members were struggling with ways to introduce content about the care of people of color to their students. What prompted the call for consultation was a crisis in the classroom. After attending a workshop designed to increase nursing faculty awareness about the lack of curriculum concerned with the health problems of people of color, one of the faculty members, although not convinced of the need for it and against the skeptical attitude of other faculty members, had decided to present information about the health care of black patients. In class, she began her discussion on the hair care of black patients by describing the physical differences of blacks and how important it was to know these differences. Using one article written about hair care of blacks, she tentatively ventured into the subject. At that point, the only black student, obviously shaken, angrily stated that there was no difference between whites and blacks. The student's point was that both racial groups were human beings and that the faculty member was using black differences for the purpose of suggesting a deficit. The teacher was shocked at the student's response as this black student was perceived as one who did not consider herself as "minority" and seemed unconcerned about the health problems of ethnic people of color; furthermore, the teacher felt that the student did not appreciate the time and effort she had gone to in preparing this material. The least the teacher expected was a positive response from the black student; however, rather than explore the black student's objections, the faculty person apologized profusely, to the point of tears.

The consultant asked the faculty member why hair care was not discussed routinely under bed-bathing and care of the skin in the following manner: It is a fact that in certain parts of the body, the skin produces hair follicles, and these are numerous on the scalp. Sebaceous glands surround the hair follicles to prevent the hair from drying. A particularly oily scalp needs frequent washing to prevent dandruff. If the patient already has dandruff, failure to wash the hair results in a bad odor and thinning or loss of hair. If the patient's scalp is particularly dry, washing should be less frequent. In either case, appropriate washing for the hair promotes a healthy scalp. The type of hair follicle present varies with racial groups and hereditary characteristics. If a person has fine hair such as is the case in white persons, the scalp is easy to clean. If the hair is very curly or kinky as is usual in black persons, washing the hair and scalp is most easily accomplished by a preliminary combing and massage. The consultant further suggested the use of community resources to assist the teacher with the preparation and presentation of material that was new to her.

The faculty person acknowledged that she had never considered the importance of integrating the subject of hair care of blacks under basic nursing content. Apparently, her ambivalence about presenting the topic, her feelings about black people's differences, and her lack of information overrode her objective presentation of the material. These attitudes became paramount during her lecture and precipitated the black student's response. The teacher's discomfort with the material as well as her feelings about black people came through and caused the black student's response. As a consequence, the whole context took on a negative aura for the white students as well as the black student. Because of the teacher's inability to deal directly with the black student's response, she lost an opportunity to explain her perspective and create a constructive learning situation. Instead, the white students picked up that an open discussion about hair care of black patients can be traumatic.

One positive aspect of this crisis was that the black student spontaneously spoke up for the first time. The student could not allow the teacher's offense to go unchallenged. She was compelled to counter it rather than participate in behavior that condoned or reinforced the "rightness" of the presentation. Content about ethnic people of color in nursing curricula is usually presented within a "differences"—which really means "deficit"—context. That such content be presented is crucial, to insure that all clients receive a high standard of nursing care. However, the manner in which the presentation is made must not degrade, dehumanize, or appear as an afterthought.

"You minorities are sick."   At the end of this offensive maneuver minorities feel that whites have communicated, "You are sick, and we must do all that is in our power to protect you from yourselves."

For example, a common practice for many Chicano women is to sponge bathe rather than shower or immerse in a tub bath during menstruation. A community health nurse visiting a Chicano home was told about this practice by an adolescent female and interpreted it as unhygienic. She began to lecture the mother about the merits of bathing. In defense the mother explained that bathing would "stop the period." Not hearing or understanding, the community health nurse continued her teaching plan and stressed such different behavior as unhealthy. Had the nurse been less concerned with deviance and pathology and more concerned with cultural practices and their meanings, she might have listened, weighed the relative "danger" of sponge baths, and intervened in a different way. If sponge baths are truly violations of some principle of hygiene, then the bed baths we nurses give in the home and hospitals ought to be reexamined.

"We whites are right."   This interplay is probably the most basic of offensive mechanisms stemming from feelings of racial superiority. The minority perceives the white's message to be, "My way is what is right and

how things ought to be—any other way is wrong or is merely for my amusement, edification or some other form of exploitation."

Consider the following example. A workshop for nurses took place on an Indian reservation. The Indian tribe owned and operated the restaurant and hotel where the participants were lodged. The program included walks through the nearby town and homes, after which the participants were to discuss their observations. Many complained that there were no "real" Indians around to talk with and whose homes they could visit. Even when they were reminded that they were on a reservation and that every person not a workshop participant was an Indian, they continued to demand a meeting with "real" Indians, replete with ceremonial dress and tepees. The Indians listening to the discussion left in disgust; the project participants "knew" what "real" Indians looked like.

Had the Indians present responded by seeking out Indians who fit the white nurses' stereotypes of "real Indians," they would have assumed a pro-racist position by validating the behavior of the white nurses and negating the feelings and behavior of their own group. In all likelihood, some of the white nurses left the workshop feeling deprived because they had not had the entertainment they expected from Indians who fit their stereotype.

Toward a Responsive Practice of Nursing

Nursing's stated philosophy is to deliver quality nursing care to all people. Yet, most community nursing is done in economically impoverished areas and in minority communities that are sociologically and culturally different from those of the majority of community health nurses. This discrepancy often sets up a conflict between the nursing ideology and what nurses actually see, which can be endured only as long as fictions are devised and practiced by the nurses. Most practicing community health nurses are white and middle class, and these attributes place them in sharp contrast to many clients. Some of these nurses are painfully aware of the numerous social and cultural differences between themselves and their clients and of their inadequate knowledge on which to base and formulate appropriate interventions. Some, however, compensate by becoming excessively authoritarian, as we have shown, or by fostering their clients' complete dependence. It is incumbent on white community health nurses then to understand the numerous offensive maneuvers they employ, whether intentional or not, that can minimize and degrade clients and can, in turn, transform the nurses into insensitive practitioners. Unless all nurses have this understanding and act accordingly, client-centered care will remain as yet another phrase whose sound is magical to the ear and not become an actual part of nursing practice.

Reciprocity and risk taking are concepts that can decrease nurse behaviors that are oppressive to others. Reciprocity is the process of give and take in a nurse-client relationship. The nurse avoids prescribing behavior and strives toward sharing decisions. Risk taking denotes a flexible attitude that permits the nurse to be creative with interventions and to tailor them to the individual client situation. When clients are encouraged to participate as equals in decision making, the risks potential in innovations are shared. Through this process, care becomes more client centered than procedure oriented.

Several patient-care benefits can be derived through the recruitment of potential nurses from communities of color. Such nurses (who are also victims) are concerned about the dehumanization of health care in institutions and among providers and can identify the oppressive nature of certain behaviors and practices. Also, being a victim sensitizes one to the subtleties of oppressive acts and often instills a reluctance to act oppressively toward others. The following case illustrates this point as well as the use of the concepts of reciprocity and risk taking.

A client was described in the nursing record as slow and possibly retarded. She was thought to be difficult to teach since she could not repeat the information given to her by the regular community health nurse. The client was also described as having mothering problems because she seldom spoke to her ten-month-old son.

A black nursing student was assigned to this client. After the first home visit, the student went to her brown instructor and related that the young woman was unresponsive, but did not seem retarded. The nursing student said that she felt uncomfortable doing all the talking and asked whether the instructor could help her identify what she was doing, because she recognized her behavior could be a factor in the case. The instructor asked the student to review the home visit in detail, particularly her own behavior and the client's response. The student's description made clear that she was asking "yes" and "no" questions, and that as her frustration level increased, she asked questions that already contained the answers; for instance, "you don't have any trouble with the baby, do you?" After pointing these facts out to the student, the nursing instructor said to her: "I notice you are a quiet person yourself. You hardly ever speak in clinical conferences except to answer a direct question and never volunteer more information than what is asked." "That's true" the student replied. The dialogue that ensued follows:

Instructor:　Well, how do you feel when you think you're expected to respond to every question.
Student:　Uncomfortable.
Instructor:　What do you do?

Student: I just sit and look and wait, wishing the pressure to talk would go away.

Instructor: You mean the person who is expecting you to talk?

Student: Yes.

Instructor: How do you think Mrs. J. feels, since she is a quiet person, too?

Student: The same; I never thought about it that way!

Instructor: Why don't you try a different approach?

Student: You mean just sit there in silence and try not to expect an answer?

Instructor: Yes, you could do it that way. How do you handle silence?

Student: I do all right if I don't feel I have to break it.

Instructor: Well, since this is a new situation for you, why don't you try telling Mrs. J. that you notice she is a quiet person just like you are, that you don't want to make her feel the pressure of talking to you and telling you everything? Why don't you also ask what she expects from you as the nurse and how you can ask her for information about improving the relationship?

Student: I'll try it. I know how she probably feels about my visit. I hope she doesn't tell me never to come back!

The instructor asked the student to personalize her approach, admit to imperfections, and to take the risk that the client would react negatively.

The student returned from her second visit elated and smilingly described what had happened on the visit. At first, the client was taken aback. She never thought about expecting anything from the community health nurse. She assumed we come because we are sent. Since she was asked, she said she wanted to know about good health care for her family and herself. She also explained to the student that the reason she was so quiet was that when she was a child, she was tongue-tied and lisped. Her family and other children had made fun of her. She had to go to a speech therapist regularly. The other nurse who visited reacted to her speech by responding in baby talk. The client interpreted this behavior as demeaning, but was afraid to confront the nurse who would think she was rude. She was afraid to talk to her ten-month-old son for fear he would imitate her poor speech. The astute and sensitive student looked into the baby's mouth and discovered that his frenulum linguae *was* short. The student described to the mother the kind of care indicated so as to prevent a similar situation in her son. The mother worked through her fears by sharing them with the student and from then on could not be kept from talking! The student also became more verbal in clinical conferences.

In this example, the student began by going to her instructor to tell her of her frustration and to admit an inability to communicate. Because she cared about her client, she took the risk of being told she was doing something wrong. Although the previous nurse set the stage for the student to blame the client for unresponsive behavior by what was recorded in the nursing notes, the student chose to investigate her own behavior as a possible deterrent to the establishment of the relationship. Reciprocity occurred between the student and the instructor and between the student and the client in the process of exchanging information and attempting to uncover the reason for the communication problem.

To be a risk taker, each community health nurse must care about the well-being of each client and be willing to entertain the hazardous idea that the nurse's own attitudes and behavior may be stifling to client progress and inappropriate for the circumstances. Oppression is perpetuated by community health nurses who do not take such risks because they cannot accept client differences as valid or conceive that their own behavior is so involved and instead try to impose their standards of behavior onto the clients.

SUMMARY

If nurses and nursing are serious about improving the care delivered to all clients, we must become aware of the different realities ethnic people of color confront in this society. We must develop some awareness and understanding of racism and the many ways in which it is manifested in contemporary society. Toward this end, nurses must know that two models of racism exist in our society—institutional and individual—even though making clear distinctions between them is difficult at times. When white nurses can understand that there are two forms of racism, they are in a better position to analyze their attitudes and interventions. Did they act in a certain way because of personal attitudes of superiority, or did they act in a certain way because structural expectations precipitated these actions? Nurses then can thus become more aware of the determinants of their performance and more able to change these behavior patterns. Ethnic nurses of color must also become more assertive in identifying ways their colleagues minimize people of color. To do less is to engage in and foster pro-racist behavior.

Learning new techniques that will help us to take more seriously the perceptions of people of color and to value their interpretations of situations and behaviors is essential for all community health nurses. We must also examine the system and its constraints on clients' behaviors. Examples of ways to avoid the "blaming-the-victim" syndrome are to deal with special care needs of ethnic peoples of color and to develop reciprocity and risk taking in client *and* nurse for truly client-centered quality community health nursing for all peoples.

REFERENCES

"Asian Americans: The Neglected Minority." *Personnel Guidance Journal* 51 (1973):385–416.

BECKER, HOWARD. *The Outsiders.* New York: Free Press, 1963.

"Becoming Aware of Cultural Differences in Nursing." Speeches presented during the 1972 American Nurses Association Convention. Kansas City, Mo.: American Nurses Association, 1973.

BELLO, TERESA A. "Cultural Sensitivity in Nursing Practice." *Imprint* 23, no. 1 (February 1976).

BLAUNER, ROBERT. *Racial Oppression in America.* New York: Harper & Row, 1972.

BOZOF, RICHARD R. "Some Navajo Attitudes Toward Available Medical Care." *American Journal of Public Health* 62 (1972).

BRANCH, MARIE, and PAXTON, PHYLLIS. *Providing Safe Nursing Care for Ethnic People of Color.* New York: Appleton-Century-Crofts 1976.

BRINTON, DIANA. "Value Differences Between Nurses and Low-Income Families." *Nursing Research* 1 (January–February 1972).

BROWN, TURNER. *Black Is.* New York: Grove Press, 1969.

CLEAVER, ELDRIDGE. *Soul on Ice.* New York: McGraw-Hill Book Co., 1968.

COMER, JAMES P. "White Racism: Its Fact, Form, and Function." In Reginald Jones, ed., *Black Psychology.* New York: Harper & Row, 1970.

DELORIA, VINE. *Custer Died for Your Sins.* New York: Avon Books, 1969.

DRYER, WILLIAM G. "Working with Groups." In Adina M. Reinhardt and Mildred D. Quinn, eds., *Family Centered Community Nursing: A Sociological Framework.* St. Louis: C. V. Mosby Co., 1973.

EVERY, DALE VAN. *Disinherited: The Lost Birthright of the American Indian.* New York: Avon Books, 1966.

FREIRE, PAULO. *Pedogogy of the Oppressed.* New York: Herden Company, 1971.

GOSSACK, MARTIN M., ed. *Mental Health and Segregation.* New York: Springer Publishing Co., 1963.

HESS, GERTRUDE, and STROUD, FLORENCE. "Racial Tensions: Barriers in Delivery of Nursing Care." *Journal of Nursing Administration* (May–June 1972).

HILL, ROBERT. *The Strengths of Black Families.* New York: Emerson Hall Publishers, 1972.

JONES, RHETT S. "Proving Blacks Inferior: The Sociology of Knowledge." In Joyce A. Ladner, ed., *The Death of White Sociology.* New York: Vintage Books, 1973.

KOSHI, PETER. "Cultural Diversity in Nursing Curricula." *Journal of Nursing Education* 15, no. 2 (1976).

"Mexican? American?" *Civil Rights Digest* 3 (Winter 1970).

NORMAN, JOHN C., ed. *Medicine in the Ghetto.* New York: Appleton-Century-Crofts, 1969.

OSOFSKY, GILBERT. *The Burden of Race.* New York: Harper & Row, 1967.

PADILLA, AMADO, and RUIZ, RENE. *Latino Mental Health: A Review of Literature.* Washington, D.C.: U.S. Government Printing Office, 1974.

PIERCE, CHESTER. "Offensive Mechanisms." In Floyd Barbour, ed., *The Black Seventies.* Boston: Porter Sargent Publishers, 1970.

Race Relations Reporter. Race Relations Information Center, P.O. Box 12156, Nashville, TN 37212.

ROACH, LORA B. "Color Changes in Dark Skins." *Nursing '72* (November 1972).

ROMANO-V., OCTABIO L. "The Anthropology and Sociology of Mexican-American History." *El Grito* 2 (1968):13–26.

RYAN, WILLIAM. *Blaming the Victim.* New York: Vintage Books, 1971.

SELLERS, RUDOLPH. "The Black Health Workers and the Black Health Consumer: New Roles for Both." *American Journal of Public Health* 60 (1970): 2154–70.

SOLIS, FAUSTINA. "Current Problems in Mental and Public Health Services as Related to Mexican-American." *Cabinet Committee Hearings on Mexican-American Affairs*, El Paso, Texas. Interagency on Mexican-American Beliefs, 1800 G Street N.W., Washington, D.C. 20506.

STAFFORD, WALTER W., and HADNER, JOYCE. "Comprehensive Planning and Racism." *Journal of the American Institute of Planners* 35 (1969):68–74.

STAPLES, ROBERT. *The Black Family: Essays and Studies.* Belmont, Calif.: Wadsworth Publishing Co., 1971.

STORLIE, FRANCES. *Nursing and the Social Conscience.* New York: Appleton-Century-Crofts, 1970.

TERRY, RUTH ANN. "The Responsibility and Role of UCSF, School of Nursing As Perceived from a Minority Viewpoint." *School of Nursing,* February 6 and 7, 1974.

U.S. DEPARTMENT OF HEALTH, EDUCATION AND WELFARE. *Perspectives on Human Deprivation: Biological, Psychological, and Sociological.* Washington, D.C.: U.S. Government Printing Office, 1968.

VALENTINE, CHARLES. *Culture and Poverty.* Chicago: University of Chicago Press, 1968.

VASQUEZ, RICHARD. *Chicano.* New York: Avon Books, 1971.

WAGNER, NATHANIEL N., and HANG, MARSHA J., eds. *Chicanos: Social and Psychological Perspectives.* St. Louis: C.V. Mosby Co., 1971.

WILCOX, PRESTON. *White Is.* New York: Grove Press, 1970.

21. Community Health Nurses in Administration

Carol Dana Brancich
Patricia Porter

INTRODUCTION

Why do they do that? This question probably sounds familiar since it is frequently heard wherever two or more staff nurses congregate. The "they" are, of course, nursing administrators. Knee-deep in day-to-day details of direct client services and often lacking frequent face-to-face contact with management staff, community health nurses often do not have the knowledge or understanding of the management staff's contribution to the nursing organization. Reasons for this lack of understanding vary from institution to institution

Certainly there are nurse-administrators who believe that staff have no need to understand the whys of administration, and consequently they make no attempt to communicate the rationale for their decisions and actions to the staff. We believe that nurse-administrators and staff share a common goal: the provision of high-quality health services to clients. This sharing of a common goal mandates cooperation between staff and administration for its attainment, precisely because each level of staff addresses a different aspect of the system for delivery of health care services. Thus appropriate distribution of functions to various levels of staff is essential for the efficient provision of sound client services. A communication network that facilitates the sharing of information and rationale for decisions made at all levels is the glue that holds the system together.

548

In this chapter we discuss some of the functions that are most often the responsibility of staff designated as "management" or "administration." These functions can be organized into a variety of categories. We have chosen to use the following categories for our discussion: planning, organizing, directing, and controlling. Our intent is to provide you with some insight into the *whys* and *wherefores* of nursing administration.

RESPONSIBILITIES OF NURSE-ADMINISTRATORS

PLANNING

Nurse-managers, in community health have traditionally been more interested and often more involved in program planning than have their counterparts in hospitals. Programming in acute care centers has generally been in response to medical services' needs. These needs have been identified by physicians and hospital administrators, and nursing service directors have responded with the necessary number of nursing personnel to support medical services. Nursing directors in community health agencies, on the other hand, have been in positions that allowed for assessment of community needs and some flexibility in programming to meet identified needs.

ASSESSMENT OF COMMUNITY NEEDS

An essential step in planning for the development of programs to meet community needs is the process of community assessment. For a community health nurse, doing community assessments is as essential an activity as is doing individual and family assessments. When nursing management staff are aware of community needs, they can then make plans for addressing these needs.

The responsibility for planning decisions ultimately rests with the nursing director. To make these kinds of decisions she must gather information from many sources. For example, a nursing director may be a member of a number of commissions and boards in the community that have both consumer and provider input regarding needs for health services. One example might be a children's commission responsible to the county's governing body. In this capacity, the nursing director is constantly exposed to community groups requesting health services for children. To respond appropriately to these requests, the director must learn about the kinds and quality of resources available in the community to meet these needs in addition to those her agency can provide. This information can then be augmented by data from staff nurses' assessments of families and segments of the community. Together this information enables the director to decide how and where to allocate the agency's resources to complement or augment existing services or to create new ones to meet community needs. If any of the data are missing, then the decision may not be in the community's best interest.

CONSIDERATION OF FUNDING SOURCES AND MANDATED SERVICES

Needs assessments are only part of program planning. While it would be marvelous to be able to plan realistically and to implement programs for all identified needs, such a utopian situation does not exist for there is always the factor of limited resources. As is pointed out in chapter 11, the entire health care system is becoming increasingly acutely aware of the limitations on resources available to it and the necessity to make very hard choices accordingly. Most often resources are controlled by funding sources outside of the agency in which the nurse-administrator functions. For community health programs these funding sources usually include federal, state, and local governments. A further consideration is that many community health services are legislatively mandated. In most states these include communicable disease services—for example, tuberculosis control and treatment of venereal infections—and maternal-child health services such as Early and Periodic Screening, Diagnosis, and Treatment (EPSDT). Political, social, and economic climate changes often occur, thereby necessitating new directions and the refocusing of service delivery.

For example, in our state in the past few years, we have seen state health department funding expand priorities from maternal–child health programs to include programs for the aged. While we can applaud the state's insight and action regarding the needs of the aged and support this shift, our agency has highly developed and utilized programs in maternal–child health that are at risk due to reductions in funding. Because of the shift, our agency's nursing staff now spend more direct service time on programs for the aged and less time on maternal–child health programs. This change has caused an outcry among staff and consumers, with both groups identifying the need for maternal–child health services and believing in their value. We encountered some interesting situations when in response to reduced funding we changed our criteria for the admission of children to our well child clinics. The new criteria excluded many middle-income families who could afford private care but who preferred the well child services that they received from the public health nurse. These politically aware consumers called their elected officials to protest; they in turn called the director of nursing. Thrilled as we were with this overwhelming endorsement for our quality services, we had to acknowledge that we could no longer afford to provide them to all comers. This particular situation has led us to explore a sliding-scale fee system for reimbursement for well child services since such an arrangement would allow us to meet a community need and assist us with meeting operating expenses.

Given current funding problems, a reasonable approach to programming must involve the setting of priorities. These priorities are best supported with hard data that identify community's needs. When funding is reduced even for very popular programs, revised and deminished priorities must be set within the program; for example, outreach to large numbers of teenagers in a family planning program may have to take precedence over expensive fertility workups for a limited number of clients. As Bailey and Claus have stated so well in their discussion on budgeting, ". . . the budget is a means of expressing the philosophy, goals, and objectives of the decisionmaker" (1975:97). The possession of information pertaining to mandated services and funding sources is essential for staff; otherwise, they may feel that their direct participation in any given program area is at the whim of nursing management decisionmakers. Having provided nursing management with their assessment of community health needs, the staff has a right to expect to receive nursing administration's rationale for program decisions.

POLICY AND PROTOCOL FORMULATION

Another part of nursing management's planning process involves the formulation of policies and procedures (protocols) for the various program areas. Contrary to popular belief, policies and procedures are designed to assist staff in providing direct services. How? First of all, we will make the assumption that the policies that direct the staff reflect an acceptable standard of nursing care in the community. The standards may be adapted from those advocated by a variety of sources, such as the Joint Commission on Accreditation of Hospitals, National League for Nursing and American Public Health Association Accreditation Standards for Community Health Agencies, and the American Nurses' Association. Adherence to policies, then, assures that acceptable care is *consistently* delivered by each staff member. Policies are also designed to allow service delivery to occur as *efficiently* as possible, according to the limited resources. Nurse-administrators formulating policies are often more aware of the nature of those limitations than are staff nurses.

An example of this administrative perspective is a situation we encountered in our agency at different times during the past few years. We provide family planning services to clients in our county with money from federal, state, and local governments. Our policy stipulates that only residents from our county may receive services in the clinics. Rationale for the policy involved two issues. First, services are partially funded by local tax monies and are designated for citizens of the county; and secondly, followup of clients in another county by district nurses is impossible, thus precluding a major component of our family planning services. Although staff members are aware of the rationale for the policy, they have had difficulty in saying "no" to out-of-county clients and in assisting them to find another source of care. However, nursing administrators have enforced the policy and have had to assume the role of "bad guy" in an attempt to provide family planning services of a high-quality to consumers in our county. We feel that this role is an appropriate one for administrators.

Consistency and efficiency are clearly factors supporting the need for policies in an agency. In this age of accountability it behooves health care delivery systems to attend to issues such as cost-effectiveness and predictable outcomes resulting from acceptable care delivered consistently. Policies are also a way of dealing with these issues.

Procedures have a place in planning a health care delivery scheme as well. They provide direction for how specific tasks are to be performed. We are all familiar with the voluminous amount of materials present in procedure manuals maintained in most agencies. The amount of detail varies with the philosophy of nursing management and more recently is being dictated by nursing licensure laws as described in chapter 13. As Stevens (1975:112–13) has described, using quotes from Perrow, there are many staff views of policies and procedures. Some staff members view them strictly as limitations on their decision-making power, while others interpret them more positively as guidelines and delineations of what they *can* do.

We prefer to view procedures and protocols as positive components of the system. However, they require mutual input and support from nursing management and staff. Individually and collectively, staff members are best able to assess their level of functioning and to provide nursing management with suggestions as to the areas in which they need more or less detailed procedures. We have found that overemphasis on procedures and protocols has resulted in staff members' requesting endless lists of specific behaviors. For example, the protocol for family planning directs the nurse to do a medical history to determine client eligibility in a clinic designed for well persons seeking contraceptive services. Serious medical conditions, such as cardiac disease or a history of cancer, contraindicate provision of services in our clinics. Other conditions may require nursing judgment as to the severity of the condition or the medical management required. It is unwise if not impossible to attempt to list all the behaviors community health nurses should carry out. At some point nurses must rely on their professional judgment. Writing procedures and protocols in a situation in which a nursing service is composed of entry level community health nurses as well as those with advanced preparation and extensive community health nursing experience requires that a fine line be drawn between what is defined in procedures and protocols and what is left to the nurses' professional judgment. Constant assessment by staff and management of the tasks to be performed and the functioning level of the staff to perform them is essential. Procedures and protocols, if appropriate to a setting, a program, and a functional level of staff, increase the likelihood of maintaining established standards for quality of the care provided to consumers.

ORGANIZING

The effective and efficient organization of nursing staff is an essential ingredient in a successful health delivery system. Needless to say, staff organization is also complex. Many factors must be considered as the nursing organizational framework is designed (or redesigned as the case may be) in order to implement program decisions and achieve program goals. Basically, the framework must allow for the performance of a variety of tasks by varying levels of personnel. Our contention is that a well-defined system of labor distribution is one key. We believe that nurse-administrators are responsible for the establishment and maintenance of the labor distribution system. We also believe that in fact if staff organization is not focused appropriately, the delivery system malfunctions.

DIVISION OF LABOR

To illustrate our beliefs, we have chosen to use Archer's and Brancich's (forthcoming) division of labor according to client service focus as shown in figure 21.1. This model categorizes the community nursing service system into direct client services, semidirect client services, and indirect client services, as described in chapter 1. The activities within each of these categories are assigned to various levels of staff and managerial personnel according to the amount of time each group spends on the activities within the category. There are a few overlapping or shared areas of responsibilities. However, areas of primary responsibility are also clearly defined. The areas of primary responsibility are specific to different levels of personnel.

Direct Client Services. Staff functions are highest in direct client services and top, administrative functions are most numerous in indirect client or system's services—and in our view should so remain. As we previously stated, nurse-administrators have the responsibility to keep the staff's activities focused appropriately. A classic example of this focusing is that of assigning staff public health nurses to represent the agency officially at community meetings. The personal satisfaction derived by the assigned

21.1 Division of Labor Between Levels of Personnel: Community Health Nursing Service Settings

COMMUNITY HEALTH NURSING SERVICE SETTINGS

SUBSYSTEM	Direct Client Service Focus	Semidirect Client Service Focus	Indirect Client Service Focus
Responsibilities	Direct Client Service Responsibilities: Client teaching Client care Client rehabilitation	Day-to-day Staff Development Responsibilities: Day-to-day staff supervision responsibilities Peer supervision and review responsibilities	Facilitating Attainment of Client-Centered Goals: Program planning, control, and evaluation Liaison with other agencies	Organizational Survival and Development Responsibilities: Resource procurement, allocation, and accounting Intra and extra-organization relations Research and program development and evaluation

Time Commitment of Levels of Personnel

100%
75%
50%
25%
10%

Legend:
☐ Directors and Assistant Directors of Nursing
▨ Supervisory and Staff Development Personnel
■ General Staff

Source: Sarah Ellen Archer and Carol Dana Brancich, *Nursing Management: Theories and*

nurse will undoubtedly be great. However, the loss of direct client service time is irreplaceable. The situation reverses itself when the director of nursing spends time on individual client case management conferences and is thereby losing time that could be better spent in such activities as budget revision meetings. There is no question that participation in case management provides personal and professional satisfaction for the director. However, the void that is created by the director's absence from administrative activities results in decisions being made *for* the director, and *for* nursing, and not *by* the director of nursing. In time, the entire organizational system will malfunction, as will the nursing service subsystem. The lack of understanding of this dynamic balance of functions is common among general nursing staff and often leads to misunderstanding between staff and administration.

Figure 21.1 not only clarifies the role and activity distinctions between staff and management but also reinforces the often not-so-obvious differentiation between the management roles of supervisors who provide semidirect client services and administrators who provide indirect client services.

Semidirect Client Service Activities. The level of personnel who spend the majority of their time in semidirect client service activities includes supervisors and staff development people, as shown in figure 21.1. Their semidirect client service activities are aimed at the development of the staff who provide direct client services. This task is coupled with the review of staff performance according to defined client care standards. Success in these activities dictates success in attaining program goals. The successful first line supervisor has a personal working relationship with each and every staff member in the supervisory unit. The magic formula of course is to encourage and to coordinate staffs' abilities so that clients' needs are met.

As part of their role for ensuring that staff are able to meet client needs, supervisors spend a great deal of time evaluating employees. Creating a climate that is conducive to the expression of employee performance by both supervisors and supervisees is ideal. When a safe environment for such interactions is created, the stage is set for constructive, dynamic exchange. This interchange is most important when evaluating health care professionals regardless of rank. Each supervisor is called upon to use her talents in assessing employees' performance and in eliciting employees' self-directed comments. The evaluation process is simplified when looked at in the context of measuring employees' ability to perform according to the agency's established client care criteria. How well employees perform the tasks outlined in the procedures is the subject matter of evaluation conferences. Both supervisors and employees will then be evaluating the latter's level of performance by using a clearly defined and common set of behaviors and expectations.

For example, let us assume that Sue Jones, newly hired staff public health nurse, is receiving her first two-month postemployment evaluation. Part of Sue's assignment in these two months has been interviewing new family planning clinic clients, to obtain a brief social profile and a medical history. These tasks are defined within the family planning protocols that delineate what questions are to be asked and how to approach problems brought to light through the questioning (see chapter 13). Sue knows what is expected of her and the supervisor knows what to expect of Sue. They can then compare how each perceives Sue's actual interviewing and so "evaluate" her performance on the basis of specific criteria.

Again, we reinforce the importance of creating a safe environment within which this interchange occurs. Evaluation should be a positive growth experience for both the employee and for the supervisor. An honest appraisal of what one does well and setting of objectives for employee growth should be the outcome. Hostility and fear have no place within the evaluation process.

Continuing education, like employee evaluation, is an essential component of semidirect client services activities. Staff development includes formal educational experiences (lectures, seminars, supervised practice) and informal educational experiences (employee evaluations, periodic consultation, anecdotal teaching). Structuring the formal experiences is a matter of establishing training priorities and then carrying them out. Available time, financial, and human resources of course need to be carefully considered. These often dictate how training is indeed done. Supervisors must be constantly alert for informal educational experiences.

Shifts in priorities do occur such as from tuberculosis teaching to family planning counseling to ambulatory care practitioner training. These shifts normally occur due to the changes in health care needs within the community served or as a result of the development of specially funded programs. However, staff changes also produce alterations in training priorities thus requiring a continuity and flexibility in staff development programming. Our experience has been that long-term priority setting or programming for staff development is best accomplished with direct staff input. A vehicle for such communication might well be a representative committee elected by the staff to meet regularly with the staff development person. Staff development is a two-way street and open communication between the involved parties is a major key to its success.

Indirect Client Service Activities.   The nursing administrator's or director's role includes developing and fostering a system in and through which client services are provided. We call this array of functions the indirect client service or system focus. More simply stated, administration tends to the environment—that is, setting goals and priorities; assuring adequate space, the appropriate kinds of positions and supplies, and adequate budget; and through these functions, providing leadership and direction. Maintenance of the environment has both an internal and external focus. Nursing administration must develop and nurture relationships with other departments within the parent system as well as outside it. The personnel department is an example of the former and a Visiting Nurses Association and the American Cancer Society are examples of the latter. Internal environmental maintenance includes perpetuating a climate conducive to the expression of individual needs and concerns, one that encourages participation of staff in many program and operational issues.

For example, in our experience staff members working together in committees have been able to identify problems and to propose and negotiate solutions with nursing administration. The negotiations have often led to a better mutual understanding of the staff's needs and the administration's limitations. There is definitely power in a group—constructive power—that plays an essential role in negotiations. Most often the negotiations end in a compromise; neither side wins or loses. After having experienced a number of these situations, we have sensed a change in the approach of staff in presenting their needs to us in nursing administration and we have changed our posture as we respond. Of significance was the development of a formalized system for communication flow between nursing administration and staff. In this system, the Professional Performance Committee sends a member of its steering committee to the weekly nursing administration group meetings. This representative has the responsibility for disseminating information to staff and gathering input from them to bring to future meetings. The administrative group has gained much respect and admiration for staff members who have brought input from staff that is often directly opposed to administration's positions. On occasion, the staff representatives have come away from the discussions at the meetings with a different understanding of the situation and a position that differs considerably from the one with which they came. On sharing this information, these staff members are often able to sway staff opinion. That takes courage and commitment. Both administrators and staff have grown considerably as a result of our negotiations over issues. Our repeated experience upon reaching a compromise has been to find that we are all at the same place. We in nursing administration have worked very hard to develop a climate in which staff trusts us and we trust them. We have been honest about the limitations under which we have to work. Naturally, as with any system, there are problems, but we have been able to work them out usually to everyone's satisfaction. All in all, we have developed a workable system.

In sum, the division of labor in a health care delivery system is as follows: the administrator's primary role is to devise, revise, and maintain the system; the supervisor's and staff development person's primary role is to ensure a well-functioning staff; and the staff's primary role is to deliver high-quality direct client services. No one of these levels can carry out its role without the other two. Thus they are both interrelated and interdependent. Pulling together, they produce an efficient and effective nursing service. Delegation of tasks within this framework promotes utilization of each person's skills and knowledge. Research studies of employee motivation and job satisfaction indicate that employees gain job satisfaction from assignments that utilize their expertise, allow for development of new skills, and provide opportunity for job advancement (Herzberg 1968; Szilagy, Sims, and Terrill 1977).

DIRECTING

Certainly we are all familiar with the baton-wielding conductor directing the members of a symphony orchestra. We attribute the overall success or failure of the musicians' efforts to the brilliant or lackluster direction provided by the conductor. In fact, symphony aficionados have been heard to mutter critically that the orchestra itself was quite capable yet failed to achieve harmonious excellence due to ineffective conducting. We have also heard critical muttering that nursing staffs, although quite capable, fail to "click" due to ineffective direction from their leaders. We have discussed the importance of a well-balanced labor distribution system. Let us now take a closer look at the responsibilities ascribed by the Archer-Brancich Division of Labor model to those who direct.

The role of the nurse-administrator, as we have seen, is that of attending to the system—to its development and to its survival. Systems, be they symphony orchestras or nursing departments, require a structure through which decision making and decision implementation are accomplished. According to Katz and Kahn (1966) the development of an organizational structure is dependent upon five things:

Specialization of tasks;
Standardization of role performance;
Centralization of decision making;

Unification of practice;

Avoidance of duplication of function.

Certainly all five items are operant in the vast majority of organizations.

We experience little difficulty in observing how a symphony conductor attends to all five points. As the conductor directs the various orchestra sections in playing the written score, we clearly see the orchestra moving as an integrated system toward achieving its goal. The same clarity is not necessarily true in observing nursing organizations and their administrations. Perhaps the difficulty lies in that ease of observation is dependent upon nonparticipation and involvement. Whatever the difficulty, too often the staff question "Why do they (administrators) do that?" reflects the lack of clarity with which nursing-administration's role is seen.

Let us carry our analogy between symphony orchestras and nursing departments one step further and attempt to clarify the director's role somewhat. Each system has its own unique set of goals and objectives: the orchestra to produce beautiful music and the nursing department to produce excellent nursing services. The symphony has a written musical score that delineates each section's part, (horns, violins, and so forth) and each member's part within each section (1st horn, 2nd violin, and so forth). The linking processes of communication and balance produce a harmonious relationship. The conductor creates the environment by directing the component parts to insure harmony. The nursing staff has a set of written nursing policies and procedures that delineates each section's role (outpatient clinic, public health nursing, and so forth) and each staff member's part within each section (supervising public health nurse, R.N., and so forth). The nursing director tends to the environment by directing the component parts to assure coordination and efficiency. How marvelous it would be to be able to set a nursing department upon a stage and to listen to and watch its live performance as a whole. Undoubtedly, most of us would experience both delight and stage fright in such a situation.

Styles of directing are as diverse as there are persons directing. And it is here that perhaps critical disclaim abounds. Idiosyncratic symphony conductors are often the most successful. The success of these individuals rests with common organizational goals and values shared by the organizational members, namely, the musicians. Agreement as to purpose and goals allows for individuation of behavior. Too often we totally negate what is being done because we are turned off by how it is done. Nursing directors are often the most vulnerable to this criticism. Frequent and dynamic communication between staff and nursing director assists in correcting any dissonance. The old adage "Practice makes perfect" applies to communicating and repeatedly using one's administrative style. Certainly as a symphony orchestra practices over and over, they respond more and more quickly and easily to the conductor's cues. The same pattern would seem to work as well for nursing staffs and their administrators.

The foregoing analogy has dealt with the intraorganizational relations shown in figure 21.1. We have emphasized and elaborated upon this point since it is in all probability the very point that concerns staff nurses most. However, we do not wish to underemphasize other nursing administration responsibilities within the organization. Resource procurement, allocation, and accounting will be dealt with in the next section on controlling. Suffice it to say at this time that all directors, administrators or symphony conductors would and should involve themselves totally in the fiscal affairs of their organizations.

Other activities in figure 21.1 that are attributable to persons responsible for the system include extra-organizational relations. In community health nursing the dualistic nature of this responsibility is pronounced. Community health nursing administrators must attend to extra-nursing organization relations (i.e., the personnel division, the accounting division, the statistical/data division) and extra-agency organization relations (i.e., the school nurses, the local heart association, the local department of social welfare). The mutual dependence of numerous groups, people, and programs in the provision of community health services demands the involvement of top nursing administrators with other top administrators within the community's pool of resources. Linking all these various systems together at top management level facilitates the staffs' working together to the benefit of mutual clients.

The last points in figure 21.1 of research and programming deserve more time and space than can be allotted here. We have touched on program planning and development in the earlier sections entitled "Planning" and "Organizing." The subject of program evaluation and research (clinical, of course) are areas that nursing administrators often find little time to do. Yet, the continual survival of any organization or system is dependent upon its ability to prove its effectiveness, quantitatively and qualitatively. If it cannot or does not, then its purpose for being is indeed questionable and in time will be challenged. Unfortunately, community health nursing has had little experience and therefore little success in documenting service outcomes. Health attitude and/or behavior changes are difficult to measure. How parenting skills have increased is not as readily measured as is the admission, surgery, and discharge of a cholecystectomy patient. Community health nursing badly needs and deserves more attention in this area. Our parting comment on the subject is a fervent plea to encourage more direct efforts in community health nursing. Chapter 8 provides some guidelines on where to begin.

CONTROLLING

To provide high-quality services at a reasonable cost is the order of the day (in fact of *every* day) for the community health nurse administrator. Spiralling costs for health care have focused a great deal of attention on cost control. Nursing administrators as administrators must respond to the pressures being exerted to contain costs. As nurses they must also respond to ever-increasing demands for services while ensuring that high-quality and quantity of nursing services are being provided. A double (or is it a triple) bind, you say? Indeed so!

FISCAL ACCOUNTABILITY

An essential factor that all nursing staff members must be aware of and share in is that the cost of providing care is everyone's concern. Fiscal accountability is not just the responsibility of the accounting staff and/or of "administration." Today's health delivery system is delicately balanced by the amount and types of funding received, which then allows for (and even dictates) the provision of certain services. Not only do nursing staff members share in the responsibility to contain unnecessary expenses, they are called upon to generate revenue. Nursing staff are the implementors of services and of late have become the instruments for reimbursement for services rendered.

Community health agencies heretofore have required fiscal subsidies. In official agencies this subsidy has usually taken the form of local tax monies mixed or matched with state and federal monies. Voluntary agencies have been subsidized through private and public contributions, client-fee collections, and occasional public tax monies. However, within the past few years both types of agencies have begun to collect monies from the government (Medicaid and Medicare) and insurance companies for what is called fee-for-services rendered. Needless to say, it behooves staff nurses to acquaint themselves with the realities of their agency's funding and to follow the policies and procedures set forth regarding client eligibility and fees. Chapter 12 will help you to do this.

FISCAL PROCUREMENT

Let us move on to the administrative process called fiscal procurement and its direct relationship to the types and degree of controls ultimately placed upon nursing services. An example of the type of control fiscal procurement can place upon nursing services is beautifully portrayed in public family planning programs. State and federally established financial criteria must be met by the client before "no charge to the client" contraceptive services can be provided. If the client does not meet the financial criteria, a private (self-pay) payment system must be used. Clients meeting the financial criteria have their services paid for by state and federal monies. However, these monies pay for very clearly defined procedures, in some instances dictate how often the procedures can be performed, and always dictate how much money will be reimbursed per procedure per client. A computerized system monitors how often clients are seen and what types of services are being performed. The service agency submits its bills for services rendered and is reimbursed accordingly. The computer is used as a check-and-balance system to validate that the regulations set forth are being met, so payment can be made. The process of procuring family planning funds carries with it program regulations and limitations. It not only regulates who will be seen but how often they will be seen, what services are allowable, and how much money will be paid to the provider-agency.

FISCAL ALLOCATION

Let us now move on to fiscal allocation. As funds (through services provided) are being generated, instant and continuous monitoring must occur. As these public family planning funds are being audited, so are the number and types of clients served and services given. Quantitative and qualitative factors can be documented equally. The evaluation of these factors provide a data base for decision-making process through which the appropriate allocation of funds occurs. Expanding services or increasing staff are substantiated through actual growth data. Amounts and types of supplies may be purchased after evaluation of documented usage and needs. Again the provision of services and purchasing of supplies must be balanced by the amount of monies being generated.

In actuality the process is cyclical: Funds are initially sought; monitored as to their increase, equalization, or decrease; and then allocated (or recycled) accordingly. This delicately balanced funding–service cycle exists in all kinds of agencies. The cycle's continuing growth is dependent upon the further involvement of the government and other payment sources in the funding of services provided (commonly referred to as fee-for-service third-party payment mechanisms).

As previously stated, the nursing administrator must be equally concerned with cost control and with quality control. The trick seems to be in direct and simultaneous involvement in budget, program, and service. Much of what we have previously described in the sections on planning, organizing, and directing must be brought to bear directly on fiscal control. Knowledge of community needs, staff abilities, and current funding mechanisms need to be smoothly orchestrated. We feel strongly that in today's cost-effective health world that the top nursing administrators must be prepared to do just that. They must be as available and prepared to be involved in fiscal procurement, allocation, and monitoring as they are in more traditional nursing services issues. Only when this involvement occurs can fiscal considerations be seen in perspective with other facets of nursing administrators' responsibilities.

Nursing administrators, especially the directors, must be recognized as full members of their agency's decision-making bodies in control of funds. Noninvolvement or less than full membership results in services decisions being made for the nursing service department and not with it. Invariably quality of care becomes the issue. Nursing needs a full voice whenever fiscal matters are being decided. As the largest provider of direct personal services, nursing has a great deal of investment in any decision affecting its providership. The Archer-Brancich model clearly sets the responsibility for this role with the top nursing administrators. Nursing staff members often need to be educated to the significance of their administrators' role in fiscal matters. That role must be supported from within the nursing service department as well as from the agency's administrative unit. The nursing organization's survival and development is dependent upon the demonstrated success of its administrative staff.

SUMMARY

In this chapter we have presented some major functions of nurse administrators: planning, organizing, directing, and controlling. As with all tasks, a division of labor is essential to a smooth running and efficient organization. This division of labor is illustrated in figure 21.1, which also delineates functional areas of primary responsibility for staff, supervisory, and administrative personnel. These are direct client services, semidirect client services, and indirect client or system-focused services, respectively. As the figure shows, these functions are complementary and overlapping, rather than being mutually exclusive.

Throughout the chapter we have emphasized the role of staff nurses in providing input to nursing administration to improve the quality of services clients receive. Fiscal accountability is a fact of life for all agencies, and we have given some guidelines for all levels of personnel working together to maintain an efficient and cost-effective community health nursing service.

REFERENCES

ARCHER, SARAH ELLEN, and BRANCICH, CAROL DANA. *Nursing Management: Theories and Processes or So You Want to Be a Nurse-Manager?* North Scituate, Mass.: Duxbury Press, forthcoming.

ARGYRIS, CHRIS. *Personality and Organization.* New York: Harper, 1957.

ARNDT, CLARA, and HUCKABAY, LOUCINE M. *Nursing Administration: Theory for Practice with a System Approach.* St. Louis: C.V. Mosby Co., 1975.

ARNOLD, MARY F., BLANKENSHIP, L. VAUGHN, and HESS, JOHN M., eds. *Administering Health Systems: Issues and Perspectives.* Chicago: Aldine-Atherton, 1971.

AYDELOTTE, M. "Administration and Directors of Nursing." *Hospital, Journal of the American Hospital Association* 48 (1975):61–63.

BAILEY, JUNE T., and CLAUS, KAREN. *Decision-Making in Nursing: Tools for Change.* St. Louis: C.V. Mosby Co., 1975.

————. *Power and Influence in Health Care.* St. Louis: C.V. Mosby Co., 1977.

BARNARD, CHESTER I. *Functions of an Executive.* Cambridge, Mass.: Harvard University Press, 1938.

BLAIR, E.M. "Needed: Nursing Administration Leaders." *Nursing Outlook* 24 (1976):550–55.

BLUM, HENRIK L., and LEONARD, ALVIN R. *Public Administration: A Public Health Viewpoint.* New York: Macmillan Company, 1963.

COLTON, M. "Nursing's Leadership Vacuum." *Supervisor Nurse* 7, no. 10 (1975):29–38.

DOUGLASS, L., and BEVIS, E.O. *Nursing Leadership in Action.* St. Louis: C.V. Mosby Co., 1974.

ETZIONI, A. *The Semi-Professionals and Their Organization.* New York: The Free Press, 1969.

FREEMAN, RUTH B. "Nursing Practitioners in the Community Health Agency." *Journal of Nursing Administration* 4, no. 6 (1974):21–24.

GANONG, J.M., and GANONG, W.L. *Nursing Management.* Germantown, Md.: Aspen Systems Corp. 1976.

GRAVES, H. "Survival in the System." *Journal of Nursing Administration* 3, no. 4 (1973):26–32.

HERZBERG, FREDERICK. "One More Time: How Do You Motivate Employees?" *Harvard Business Review* 46 (1968):53–62.

KATZ, D., and KAHN, D.L. *The Social Psychology of Organizations.* New York: J. Wiley and Sons, 1966.

KERR, D. "Administrative Styles: 10 Routes to Survival." *Modern Hospital* (1973): 65–70.

LAMBERTON, E. "A Greater Voice for Nursing Service Administrators." *Hospital, Journal of the American Hospital Association* 46, no. 4 (1972):101–08.

LASSEY, W.R., and FERNANDEZ, R.R., eds. *Leadership and Social Change.* La Jolla, Calif.: University Associates, 1976.

LAWSON, J.B., GRIFFIN, L.J., and DONAT, F.D. *Leadership Is Everybody's Business: A Practical Guide for Volunteer Membership Groups.* San Luis Obispo, Calif.: Impact Publishers, 1976.

LEININGER, M. "The Leadership Crisis in Nursing: A Critical Problem and Challenge." *Journal of Nursing Administration* 4, no. 2 (1974):28–35.

LEVINSON, HARRY. *Organizational Diagnosis.* Cambridge, Mass.: Harvard University Press, 1972.

LONGEST, B.B. *Management Practices for the Health Professional.* Reston, Va.: Reston Publishing Co., 1976.

MILLER, DORIS. "How Should We Prepare Our Nurse Administrators?" *Hospital, Journal of the American Hospital Association* 46, no. 7 (1972): 120–26.

NOURI, C. "Supervisor Development for Nursing Leaders." *Journal of Nursing Administration* 2, no. 2 (1972): 52–60.

SANZOTTA, DONALD. *Motivational Theories and Applications for Managers.* New York: AMACON, A Division of American Management Association, 1977.

SCHAEFER, J. "The Satisfied Clinician: Administrative Support Makes the Difference." *Journal of Nursing Administration* 3, no. 4 (1973):17–21.

STEVENS, BARBARA. *The Nurse as Executive.* Wakefield, Mass.: Contemporary Publishing, 1975.

SZILAGY, A.D., SIMS, H.P., and TERRILL, R.C. "The Relationship of Leadership Style to Employee Job Satisfaction." *Hospital and Health Service Administration* 22 (1977):8–21.

WARSTLER, M.E. "Some Management Techniques for Nursing Service Administrators." *Journal of Nursing Administration* 2, no. 6 (1972):25–34.

22. Community Health Nurses' Involvement in Legislative Processes

Jean Moorhead

INTRODUCTION

Much of the determination of what shall be done in health care in the United States is the result of federal, state, and local legislation. These laws and the regulations developed for their implementation, often define what services are to be given, to whom these services are to be made available, which providers will be paid for delivering these services, and how much this reimbursement will be. As noted in chapter 12, whatever kind of national health care plan this country has, government involvement in health care is bound to increase. Another fact of legislative life is that lawmakers are influenced by what they hear and from whom they hear it. Thus vested interest groups, such as those mentioned in chapter 11, have real power because they can effectively lobby elected officials to address problems and devise solutions that are compatible with the groups' interests.

Nursing is a vested interest group. We have concerns for nursing, for our clients, and for the quality of health care available—or unavailable—to us all. We are finally beginning to utilize our power, individually and collectively, as the largest group of health care providers in the nation. Gone are the days when nurses—or anyone else, for that matter—can sit back and refuse to become involved in legislative processes. We *are* involved. The only question is whether our involvement will be active or passive. As a registered lobbyist and legislative representative for my state's nurses' association, I am an active participant on behalf of nurses and nursing in the lawmaking and regulatory process in our state. I cannot do my job effectively, nor can other states' or ANA's legislative representatives, without active involvement by nurses from all kinds of practice and in all manner of specialties.

This chapter is a call for us all to become more active in shaping the legislation that so vitally affects health care in this country. To be effective participants, we must have confidence that our involvement will make a difference and that we know what we are doing. I address both of these needs. I know that individual nurses can influence health care legislation. As proof, I give an example of a bill I authored and persuaded two legislators to carry through the state legislature to amend the penal code to permit minors to get medical treatment and counseling for substance and alcohol abuse without parental consent. I think this example is particularly appropriate for us as community health nurses. The problem addressed is a consumer problem and thus is especially illustrative of our potential as community health nurses to initiate change. I acted as an individual community health nurse, not in my position of legislative representative for the nurses' association. Thus, I know from personal experience that as an individual nurse, I can and have made a difference. You can, too. To help you learn how, I have included in this chapter general discussions of legislative processes at the state and federal levels. Although the state-level procedure is for my state, the steps are generalizable, in principle, to all states

CASE STUDY: FROM PROBLEM STATEMENT TO LAW

BACKGROUND AND ENTRY

As a practicing community health nurse and faculty member, I had long been aware of the inability of minors twelve years and older to get— or health care providers to give—needed medical treatment and counseling for alcohol or other substance abuse without consent from their parents. Obviously, parental consent is desirable *if* a parent is present and will give permission for needed treatment. These ideal circumstances do not always exist, and withholding needed treatment because of lack of parental consent can endanger the young person's life. I finally decided that someone had to introduce the problem into the legislature and get the penal code changed to permit needed care to be given to minors twelve years and older even without parental consent.

I prepared a one-page, typed problem statement based on my study of the problem and its effects on the young people involved and went off to meet with the aide to the legislator whom I hoped to interest in carrying the idea through to law. I saw the problem as a health problem and so went to a member of the Health Committee for entry into the system. The legislative aide advised me that the problem was probably within the jurisdiction of the Assembly Health Committee. However, before she completely agreed to have her legislator make a commitment to me, she did some further checking. She called several substance abuse clinics in the large urban area of the capitol and asked about their treatment of minors. She telephoned an advocate for the Childrens' Lobby. From both telephone calls, the aide received reassurance that my concerns were legitimate and my legislative proposal sound. At this point the aide arranged for her legislator to author or sponsor my piece of legislation.

WRITING THE BILL

Now that an author was excited about the proposed legislation, my next step was to get my idea from the one-page statement into correct "bill language." This transition is accomplished by the author's office with the technical assistance of the Legislative Counsel. The Legislative Counsel is comprised, in my state, of about sixty attorneys who know exactly what part of the law you are adding to or changing and who will put your ideas into the correct language. In my case, the author allowed me to take my proposal to the Legislative Counsel and to work with an attorney on the first draft of the bill. Several options were left up to the author. For example, she could stipulate the age of the minor that she wished to have covered by the bill. We all agreed upon age twelve, based on previous family planning legislation and the political reality that an eight- or ten-year-old seeking drug abuse help would not make a palatable bill.

After three sessions with legislative counsel, the author's copy of the bill was ready. The bill was forwarded in this form then to the author for her final concurrence.

FIRST READING AND COMMITTEE ASSIGNMENT

Because my author was an assemblywoman, the bill was introduced into the Assembly. The clerk read the short synopsis of the bill and it was given the next number in chronological order. The speaker of the Assembly then made the assignment of the bill to a policy committee. Much to my dismay, the bill was assigned to the Judiciary Committee and *not* to the Health Committee. The bill was then sent out to be printed, and thirty-one days had to pass before it could be heard in the committee.

REASSIGNMENT TO HEALTH COMMITTEE AND HEARING

The author's office was instrumental in getting the bill changed from the Judiciary Committee to the Health Committee. First the staff researched similar changes in the penal code dealing with minors. In the case of minors obtaining abortions, they found the precedent for having a penal code change heard in the Health Committee. This information was then hand carried to both the Judiciary Committee consultant and to the Health Committee consultant. In both cases these consultants each lobbied their bosses, the assemblymen who chaired the respective committees. With grave doubts, both chairmen reluctantly agreed to the change.

Finally, the bill came up for hearing before the Assembly Health Committee. We needed to have a variety of people testify in favor of the bill in an attempt both to inform and to persuade the members of the committee that the bill should be approved. We arranged for a pharmacologist from a well-known drug abuse clinic, a senior citizen who is a lobbyist for the rights of minors, and two young counselors from drug clinics. The bill was heard along with a similar bill that was introduced to change the same section of the penal code involving medical care, without parental consent, for minors twelve years of age or older who had been raped. The two bills had been scheduled for the same day and the chairman suggested that they both be heard simultaneously. I was dubious about this idea from the start. Both sponsoring legislators presented their bills, and the Health Committee immediately passed the rape bill.

I had thought the timing was good for a bill regarding minors. I reasoned that minors had been controversial a few years earlier, but by now the public, as reflected by the legislature, would have accepted that minors should be given medical rights. We had the support of all health and education groups, even the state Parent-Teacher's Association. In fact, there was no opposing testimony except for the legislators themselves. One legislator even said "I have no minors in my district who take drugs." I knew he came from an affluent area of some high substance abuse. When a legislator is locked in like that, however, there is not a lot that you can do to lobby someone whose mind is so firmly shut. There is no way that I could say, "You have got to be kidding." So, we just forgot that one vote.

The substance abuse bill, unlike the one on rape, was deliberated at great length. The concern stemmed from the standpoint that parents have rights too. The committee members wondered whether we, in society, have not gone too far by permitting minors to get abortions, obtain family planning, and get V.D. treatments without parental consent. It appeared to some legislators that the time had come to stop all of this permissiveness. Obviously, with that attitude, the bill was not going to get out of the committee unless some acceptable amendments were offered and accepted. One of the committee members said, "I don't want any of those hippies who counsel in those clinics deciding that parents don't need to be notified. I will only vote for this if it stipulates that a professional will be contacted to decide whether to involve the parents." Other amendments were offered and accepted, but the debate took about two hours. That is a very long time to watch your ideas being tossed, turned, and changed around. However, after all of this, the bill finally passed the Assembly Health Committee by one more than the minimum number of votes needed. The author and I knew that we had a long road yet ahead of us before the bill could become law.

PASSAGE BY THE ASSEMBLY

Because there were no appropriations required under the bill, it skipped hearings before the Finance Committee, which is ordinarily the next step in the legislative process, and went straight to the Assembly floor. The second reading in the full Assembly was uneventful. However, on the third reading, the same types of questions that had been raised in the Assembly Health Committee were again asked. It was obvious at the end of the discussion that there were not enough votes to pass the bill. To prevent its failure, the author asked that the roll call be left open, so that other members could vote when they came into the session. She then made her way through the capitol until she found enough colleagues who supported the bill and brought them in to vote. The bill passed the Assembly by one vote.

SENATE PROCESS AND PASSAGE

Following the bill's passage by the Assembly, the press heralded it as the "controversial bill for minors." With this kind of publicity, it was with fear and trepidation on our part, that the bill was introduced into the Senate. We said, "Well, we got it assigned to the *Assembly Health* Committee, so obviously now it will automatically go to the *Senate Health* Committee." Well, as you might assume, it went to the *Senate Judiciary* Committee. I was ready to give up on the bill even though it had been my idea originally. I was that pessimistic about its Senate passage.

The day that the bill was due to be heard in the Senate Judiciary Committee, the author was in her own home district because her daughter had entered an animal in a 4-H show and this legislator/mother felt that, as a mother, it was important to be with her daughter. Although a legislator can authorize a staff member to present a bill, whenever this is done, other members interpret that the author places a low priority on the piece of legislation. The author had promised me that she would get back for the hearing if she possibly could, and so did not ask a staff member to be on call. The Judiciary Committee hearing wore on. As 4:30 came, the chairman announced that the committee would adjourn in ten more minutes and called the substance abuse bill for hearing. My heart sank: "There goes the bill," I thought. At that moment, in walked the author from her district two hundred miles away.

As she and the same witnesses we had used at the Assembly Health Committee took their places at the podium to testify on the bill, the committee's chairman asked her how the 4-H competition had gone. He then went on to compliment her on what he called "an admirable piece of legislation." I thought, "Aha, the chairman is making a strong statement; he is saying to the committee that he likes the bill!" A gentlemen in the audience jumped up and said, "Wait a minute, the city I represent has some very important concerns regarding this bill." The author said, "Mr. Chairman, I can add that we have taken some amendments and I think we can straighten out the bill." Another Senator then said, "Move the bill," and the bill passed out of the committee—7 to 0.

The whole process went by so fast I wasn't sure what had happened. Afterwards I realized that, with only ten minutes allotted before adjournment, no one on the committee wanted to waste time on hearing testimony pro or con! The chairman was well within his rights to simply refuse to recognize the concerned gentleman from the audience as well as my faithful string of witnesses. Although we were all a bit crestfallen by the speed of the event, the moral to this episode is that you never know nor can you anticipate what might happen in any committee. Judiciary Committee passage was a big victory, but the process was not finished.

From the Judiciary Committee the bill went to the Senate floor for its second and third readings. As had been the case in the Assembly, the final roll call had to be held open—in this instance three times—to get enough supporters of the bill to get it passed by one vote. We had made yet another hurdle.

CONCURRENCE

Since the Senate had added some amendments that did not appear in the Assembly-passed version, the next step was for the bill to be sent back to the Assembly for its concurrence on the Senate-added amendments. I was concerned before about parental-rights legislators having another chance to kill the bill even though it had gotten this far. The author shared my concerns, so we did some homework before the revote was scheduled.

We went back over the voting records of all of the Assembly members and compared their performance on the bill that gave minors the right to have medical treatment in the case of rape without parental consent and our bill. We found that a number of members had voted for minors' rights in the case of rape but against minors' rights in the case of substance abuse, our bill. Thus they were not voting consistently on the principle of minors' rights. The author took this information on their voting records and showed it to each of her colleagues who had voted against our bill but for the rape bill. As a result, when our bill was voted on in the full Assembly for concurrence with the Senate version, it passed overwhelmingly and without debate.

ON TO THE GOVERNOR

The governor in my state has twelve calendar days either to sign a bill into law, to veto it, or to allow it to become law without his signature. His legislative staff prepares a report on each bill received. This report centers around the analysis of the bill undertaken by the various appropriate departments of the executive branch. In this case, the staff of the Department of Health had taken a "support-if" position, which, translated, meant that *if* they could ascertain the fiscal impact of such a bill, and *if* that impact were not monumental, then they would be in support. However, since the bill was not asking for an appropriation, it had not gone to the fiscal committees, and therefore, the Finance Department had not studied it. The governor's office reflected the concern of the Health Department by calling the author for reassurance that millions of minors would not suddenly appear at clinics for "free" treatment without parental consent. The author's office called several meetings among those of us working on the bill and the governor's office to explain how small we believed the impact would be. We explained that many clinics treated the minors illegally now and that this bill would only technically remedy existing practice. We also pointed out that the bill was permissive—that is, a clinic would still be able to refuse a minor if he couldn't pay or the clinic was filled.

On the tenth calendar day the author called me at home on a weekend and requested that I call the governor's office myself. She gave me the name of the governor's aide and suggested I talk with him as I was the sponsor of the bill. I called, feeling nervous and scared. Fifteen minutes later, I hung up feeling fairly assured that the bill would pass. I spoke honestly and confidently about the bill. I answered questions about this bill's priority in relation to health care needs in the state. I gave it my all—and it felt good. On the twelfth night the governor signed the bill. It became law on January 1, 1978.

DISCUSSION OF THE LEGISLATIVE PROCESS

Once again I must stress that if I can influence this kind of legislative change, you can too. Words cannot describe the sinking feeling when you think your bill is about to be killed or the ecstacy when you see it finally signed into law. The legislative process is full of surprises and uncertainties. I think you need to bear that in mind when you look at any legislative flow chart such as the one in figure 22.1, the chart looks all

22.1   *How a Bill Becomes Law*

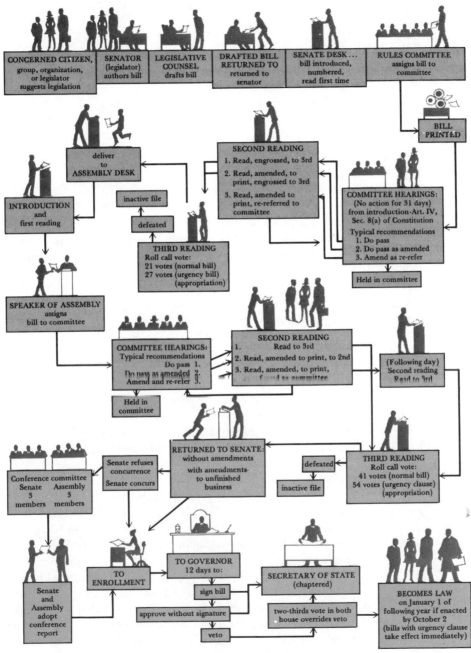

(A simplified chart showing the route a bill takes through the California Legislature)

Reprinted with permission from California State Senator Peter Behr.

neat and tidy. But remember, legislators are people just like you and me. On a good day they can be kind and supportive; on a bad day they can be miserable and vindictive. There are some specific techniques and ground rules that may not enable you to make the lawmakers' days good ones, but at least if you know about them, you may not inadvertently make their days bad.

THE STATE LEGISLATIVE PROCESS

APPROACHING YOUR LEGISLATOR

One of the first myths to be dispelled is that legislators sit in their of-fices dreaming up legislation. That rarely happens. Each legislator has a staff of aides who do much of the work for the elected official. These staff people are hired because they are experts in areas in which the legislator is interested—or in which his or her constituents are interested. Legisla-tion gets drafted because people like you and me define problems that can be dealt with legislatively. This definitional process involves the kind of homework I did in preparing the information needed to draft the sub-stance abuse bill. When you go to a legislator, you need to have at least a one-page, typed problem statement that you can leave with the legislative aide. Also before you go, be sure that the problem you want addressed deals with statutes that the legislator can change and not regulations. For example, in the case of the substance abuse bill, I knew that the law prevented minors from receiving needed treatment for alcohol and other substance abuse without parental consent. This then, was a legislative problem since the statute had to be changed. If, on the other hand, the problem had been that clinics and emergency rooms were not giving minors the needed treatment regardless of parental consent, then I would have had to deal with the regulatory body, in this case the Health Depart-ment, to get the problem solved.

If you approach a legislator as an individual, you will probably begin with your own locally elected representative. He or she will indicate whether the problem you address is in his or her area of interest. If it is, then the legislator may agree to work with you. If it is not in his or her scope of interest, you will be referred to another representative who is on one of the committees that deals with the area in which your problem lies. In the case study example, I defined the problem as a health one although the legislature initially defined it as a judicial one. Eventually the author and I worked through the system and got the bill into what we thought was the proper committee, at least in the Assembly. Don't be discouraged if you are referred on to other members of the legislature. Lawmakers, like all of the rest of us, are increasingly specialized.

When you arrive at the appropriate legislator's office, the legislative aide will begin working with you on the problem. The legislative aide must have enough information about the problem to take to the legislator so that the latter can decide whether he or she will carry the bill. Legislative aides *can* put you off, but I think if you are going to be put off, now is the best time to have it happen. If you believe that the staff is evasive, it is best at that point to say, "O.K., who do you think that I should see?" or "Are you telling me that I have an idea that does not have any merit and that I should forget it?"

Often a more effective way to get attention focused on a particular problem is to go through an organized group within whose interests the problem lies. Many groups, such as professional organizations, unions, voluntary organizations, universities, and others have mechanisms for promoting legislation that affects them. A number have lobbyists whose job it is to promote legislation in which their organization is interested. Experienced lobbyists also know which legislators might be appropriate to carry a specific piece of legislation. I shall talk more about lobbyists later.

Prior to the opening of the legislative session, most legislators have some sort of a staff meeting in which they just deal with what they are interested in introducing. So, if you have met with that legislative aide and your one-page problem statement is already in the works, you are making progress towards a bill. Once a legislator and his staff make a commitment to you to carry or sponsor your idea in bill form, this commitment extends through the entire legislative process; you need to realize that when you persuade the lawmaker to introduce your idea, you too are making a commitment for the whole process.

WRITING THE BILL

Once you have found a legislator who says, "Yes, that idea has merit and we will follow through with it," you personally do not have to possess the expertise to write your idea into "bill" language. Two methods are used to put your idea into the appropriate legislative language: The legislative staff can do it, or they can authorize you to go to legislative counsel. The attorneys in our Legislative Counsel are specialists in writing legislation and know exactly what part of the law it is that you are adding to or changing. They will put your proposal in the correct language. Your idea then goes back to the author in correct bill form. This version is called an author's copy of a bill. At that point your bill is ready for introduction.

In the case of my bill, I was permitted to go to the Legislative Counsel by the author, in order to work on the bill language. The attorney writing the bill had no personal knowledge of the subject matter. So, as the attorney asked me questions about the problem of minors and substance abuse, she was relating the discussion to concise bill language. At the conclusion, she had learned the subject matter (substance abuse/minors), and I had learned how to draft a bill from a one-page problem statement.

INTRODUCTION AND COMMITTEE ASSIGNMENT

A legislator waits for what he or she decides is the best time to introduce a bill. If they have a lot of ideas ready at one time, they don't introduce a series of ten or twelve bills all in one day. They try to space them because in our state there must be thirty-one days between the time the bill is introduced and when it is heard in the first committee. Once a member introduces a bill, the speaker of that house of the legislature assigns it a number and designates the committee that will consider it. Then the bill is sent to be printed.

The committee assignment is crucial. If, for example, you have a health issue and the bill does not go to a health committee, you may be in trouble because the kind of interest and expertise on committees differ. To me, the substance abuse bill was clearly a health issue. When it was instead assigned to the Judiciary Committee, I was sure we were done since most of the members are attorneys. My concern was that they would not be as sympathetic to a health-related idea.

It is much harder to get a bill changed from one committee to another than it is to get it to the appropriate committee the first time around. When a bill is assigned, it becomes the property of the chairman of that committee and therein lies the problem. A chairman who feels very protective about his assignment may not want to give any bills up. So, you try to get your bill to the right committee on the first assignment.

ORGANIZATIONAL REVIEW AND LOBBYING

After the first reading and assignment to a committee, the bill is sent out to be printed. There is a required period of time before the committee can hear the bill. It is during this waiting period that the public is supposed to find out that the bill has been introduced. Newspapers and professional organizations that monitor legislation receive copies of the bill and ask their readers and members for review and comment. Lobbyists for organizations whose interests are directly affected by the proposed legislation begin their work in favor of or in opposition to the bill. There are over six hundred registered lobbyists in our state. Thus a lot of lobbyists are monitoring every bill that is introduced and are providing a lot of input into the system.

An example of this process is what takes place in our state nurses' association's legislative office. We automatically receive a copy of every bill that is introduced into the state legislature. Our legislative analyst scans each bill and decides whether it has any impact on nursing. When she decides that indeed the bill does have implications for nursing, we must then determine what the organization's position is on the bill, before I can begin to lobby for or against it. In our state the waiting period between assignment and hearing is thirty-one days. That's plenty of time to develop an organizational position on the proposed law if we already have a policy that addresses the issue. If there is no policy, then we must obtain input from as many of the 18,000 nurses who make up our organization as possible. To do so, we send the bill out to the regional offices, and they send it to their legislative committees. The results of the committees' discussions are tabulated and our organizational position is formulated on this basis. The thirty-one-day waiting period can thus put us on a very tight time schedule.

Hopefully, by the time the committee to which the bill has been assigned meets, our organization is ready to take a position on the bill. Timing is important. If our position is to support the bill, then we notify the bill's author that the nurses' association is supportive of his or her bill and why we favor it. This information is sent by letter in order that the author may use such support letters to try to get his or her colleagues to vote for the legislation (you may let the legislator's office know verbally also). I usually call and say that we are in support and that our letter will follow. Then it is pretty much up to the author and staff to decide how they want to "work" that bill.

An author's response to our support varies. Sometimes the reply is "thank you" and there is nothing more implied. Sometimes we are told, "We really need your help, would you be willing to lobby that committee and would you be willing to have someone testify?" When this request occurs, we ask our regional nurses' association offices to get involved. If our membership at the grass roots level is known to the district office staff of a legislator on the committee, then these members can be most effective at the lawmaker's district office. Once again our impact is not on the legislator per se, but on the legislative aide or the staff. Sometimes, and we are always delighted when it happens, someone from the legislator's district office will call one of our nursing regional offices and say "We have a vote up on a bill and we do not thoroughly understand it; will you come over and give us some kind of input?"

When our organizational position is to oppose a bill, etiquette demands that we inform the legislator's office that we are in opposition to the bill and why. It does not do any good to write a letter and just say, "We are absolutely opposed, period." The intent of the legislator is to produce the best piece of legislation possible, and that is most often done through compromise. So, in such letters state specifically why you are opposed: "We are opposed for the following reasons . . ." or "We believe that if the bill were amended in this way or that, we might then be able to support it." Let the legislator know what it would take to put you, or your organization, in a support position.

So, let us say that you have let the author's office know that you are opposed. The author's staff may accept your letter and say, "Well, we will see what we can do," or they may say, "We cannot do anything about it." If so, then you reply, "We will be there to oppose." I think more times than not what happens is that the author will facilitate a meeting between you and the bill's sponsors hopefully to find a compromise. Getting together and trying to hammer out the differences of a bill is very exciting and very time consuming! If either side does have opposition, at least each knows where it is coming from and can honestly lay out the differences. Obviously, if you are in an opposed position, the author's staff is not going to call you and ask you to please appear for the hearing. If no compromise can be reached, they very much hope you will go away forever. You must monitor the hearings carefully, therefore.

With a *position* thus developed on a given issue, the nursing association staff can work in concert with the membership to best present nursing's viewpoint to the legislature or other administrative agencies. I cannot stress enough, *to each of you,* that your interest, input, and help is essential to regional interest groups, state interregional groups, and national organizations. When positions are developed from lively group discussions and thorough deliberations, they are good positions for nursing

A word of caution, however: Credibility so carefully obtained can be destroyed by unilateral action purporting to be "official." Obviously outright misinformation or bad guesses destroy us. More subtly destructive, though equally damaging, is advocating a position as though it were an official position when in actuality it is personal and unofficial. Sending communication, either written or verbal, that implies official endorsement only confuses the receiver, particularly when other communications follow—all claiming to be the "true" position. By the time several of these communiques are received, the same comment is usually forthcoming: "You nurses can't get together on anything." Hence, down goes our credibility and our impact as the largest group of health care providers.

COMMITTEE HEARINGS

The committee hearing occurs after the waiting period. At this hearing the author presents the witnesses he or she has gathered to testify in support of the bill. The way in which these witnesses are set up is crucial to the bill's progress. A broad spectrum of people is usually more effective than having several people testifying, each of whom is a carbon copy of the last. In the case of the substance abuse bill, we had a pharmacologist, a senior citizen, and two drug counselors testify at the committee hearing. Each of the two counselors took a different approach to the bill so that their testimony was not redundant. In most instances, if the bill deals with health, the author's staff will want consumers as well as providers to appear so that the committee does not get the idea that the providers are merely looking after their own interests. Obviously supporters of the bill want it to pass, and so supporters need to cooperate with the author's staff to help the process along.

Sometimes people ask, "Should you bring busloads of people to a hearing?" Legislators hate busloads of people for exactly the reason that busloads of people are brought—people produce pressure. If you really feel very strongly pro or con, it is at the committee hearings that your group can absolutely fill the room. That pressure definitely will be felt. The smart thing to do is not to have everybody in your group think they are going to testify. Have one spokesperson do it for the group and let that person point out, "I have all these people with me and this is what we want to say."

Organizing the opposition to a bill is often more difficult than getting people together to support it. As I noted, the author's staff is not going to keep you informed about when the bill will be heard by the committee. You'll have to do that yourself. The way I do this monitoring is by reading what in our state is called the Daily File. A Daily File is put out every morning for both our Assembly and our Senate. Thus, whenever I go into the capitol, I stop by our bill room and get a copy of the Daily Files so that I know what is happening that day in both houses. Each state has a daily publication similar to our Daily File for everyone's information.

A notification that a bill is scheduled to be heard must be printed for three days in the Daily File. Many times what happens—and causes people to get frustrated with the process—is that a bill appears in the file and you appear to hear that bill before the committee, but it is not heard because it has been pulled from the calendar. If the author's staff realizes they do not have enough votes to pass the bill, they will pull the bill off the committee's calendar for that day. A bill can be scheduled three times before it must be heard by the committee. The author therefore has two opportunities to take the bill off the calendar and can do so even while walking into the committee room. So you may arrive ready with your opposition testimony, only to find out that the bill has just been removed. Naturally your first response is to get annoyed. But this action by the author may mean that you are making progress and that other legislators are not willing to vote favorably on that measure. Pulling a bill off calendar is also a way to dissipate the opposition. For example, you get lots of members of your organization to come to the capitol all revved up about something and the bill is not heard. The next time you ask them: "Don't you want to come back?" "Aren't we still as upset as we were last week?" The answer is usually not as enthusiastic. Stalling is an effective technique, and the best thing you can do is to check with the author's office before making a trip to the capitol.

During a committee hearing, one of the first questions to be asked of you when you testify for the opposition is whether or not you notified the author of your position. Protocol demands that you extend this courtesy to the author, and if you did not, the committee is less interested in what you have to say. Now, if you come in late and for some reason you have not found out about this bill and it is a terrible piece of legislation and you need to testify, notify the author in person at that point. In other words, don't pull surprises. It does *not* improve your credibility! Also, if you arrive late at a committee hearing and you don't know whether something has been pulled or not, ask the sergeant at arms in the committee room and he can tell you exactly what bills have been heard and which bills have been pulled off the calendar.

Share the reasons for your opposition to the bill with other people and groups, because many times if your concerns are really legitimate and other people have voiced the same concerns, the author will start amending the bill. The committee can accept those amendments as author's amendments. So you see it is important that the legislator and other groups know where you are coming from, because those changes don't have to take place after the fact. Those changes can go on right there during the testimony. That means you have to be flexible yourself and able to accept or reject changes that take place during the committee hearing. I am allowed enough leeway in testifying so that if the amendment that my organization wants is accepted, I can then say "Yes, we will now support the bill." Or I can say, "We now withdraw our opposition," if I don't want to go as far as saying that we support it. That is why you have to remain flexible.

This description then is an outline of the way a committee hearing proceeds. The bill is next voted on and it passes or fails at that point. When there are not enough votes to get a bill out, the committee can decide to meet as a subcommittee. When enough members are in the room, they can vote as a full committee. Another voting tactic is "holding the roll call open," which means that if some members are not present when the bill is voted on, they can cast their votes when they arrive. It used to be that the roll call could be held open indefinitely, and you never knew after the committee hearing was over whether or not your bill got out or if it were dead. Now, at the conclusion of each committee, the roll call is closed. This arrangement sometimes gets very frustrating for a lobbyist—if you are one vote short, you find yourself literally running around the capitol trying to get that last legislator there to vote. Legislators cannot vote by proxy. Finally, there is the "suspense file." An author, knowing he or she does not have enough votes to pass the bill and having used up the two options to pull the bill off the calendar, can have the bill heard and then ask that it be held in the suspense file without a vote being taken. The issue is just about dead when this technique is used, although the option is open for a later vote.

If the bill passes the committee, it is then on its way to becoming law. If the bill fails in committee, it is dead for that session. The author may rewrite it and introduce it at a later session.

PROCESS THROUGH THE HOUSE

After a bill is passed by the committee, unless there is no appropriation of money involved, it goes to the Finance Committee for review. In the Finance Committee, only the author and fiscal experts usually testify. If the bill passes the Finance Committee, it proceeds to the floor of the legislature for a second reading. This is a formality in our state. The third reading is when the clerk does read the bill, the author discusses it, and there is debate from members of the legislature as they see fit. This third reading is by no means a rubber stamp of committee action as my example shows. The final vote is then taken.

All bills must go through both houses in states that have bicameral legislatures. The bill may be introduced simultaneously in both houses or may go through one before being introduced into the other. The process in both houses is basically the same as the one outlined here. Both houses must pass it before it continues on to the governor. In cases, such as my substance abuse bill, where the two versions of the bill differ, the differences must be reconciled into a final amended version. If concurrence cannot be reached in both houses, the bill is sent to a conference committee. This committee, comprised of two or three legislators from each house, works out the final compromise. If the committee's amendments are not accepted by both houses, the bill is dead. Because my bill passed the Assembly on concurrence of Senate amendments, it did not need to go to a conference committee.

THE GOVERNOR

My state requires positive action for the governor to veto a bill; otherwise it becomes law with or without his signature. He has twelve calendar days to decide whether to veto. If a bill becomes law, it next goes to the secretary of state to be chaptered—that is, entered into the appropriate place in the state's legal codes. The secretary of state's office has the chaptering information in the morning when the governor has done his signing by midnight. Once a bill is chaptered, it becomes known by its chapter number because at the beginning of the next legislative session, the numbering of bills begins all over again.

KEEPING UP WITH THE STATE LEGISLATURE

In addition to the Daily Files that I have already discussed, there are three other documents you need to know about. One is the Daily History. The Senate and Assembly each produce what is called a Daily History that shows actions taken on Assembly and Senate measures to and including that day. I do not use this document too often because the bill room also produces a weekly history both for the Senate and the Assembly. The Weekly History brings you up to date on everything that occurred that week. It gives a short synopsis of the history of a bill, when it was read the first time, what committee it was referred to, when the waiting period was over, when it was heard and in what committee, and whether it passed or failed. In other words you get a summary of exactly what has happened to a bill. There is also a Legislative Index that lists everything: the bills, the constitutional amendments, the concurrent resolutions, and other legislative documents. The Legislative Index is produced several times during the session.

You may, as citizens, view the floor session of either house. It is interesting to watch the legislative process: Debate goes on, and the legislators vote by electronic means. There is a big board up on the wall, and as the legislators turn on the switches on their desks, a light beside each legislator's name lights up—green to indicate a yes vote and red to show a no vote. When the roll call is closed, the votes are tallied, and the totals come out as a computer printout that is available to the author. Sitting in the gallery for the first time is an exciting and interesting experience. The more you know about the behind-the-scenes processes, where the real work is done, the better you will be able to understand what is happening before you.

THE FEDERAL LEGISLATIVE PROCESS

As you can see from figure 22.2, much of what I have said about the legislative processes at the state level is also true for these processes at the federal level. There are a few significant differences, however.

1.   There are no specific deadlines. The bill, therefore, can move as fast or as slowly as needed, which thus makes keeping track of bills more difficult at the federal than at the state level.

2.   There are no automatic processes a bill must follow from introduc-

22.2   *Federal Legislation Process*

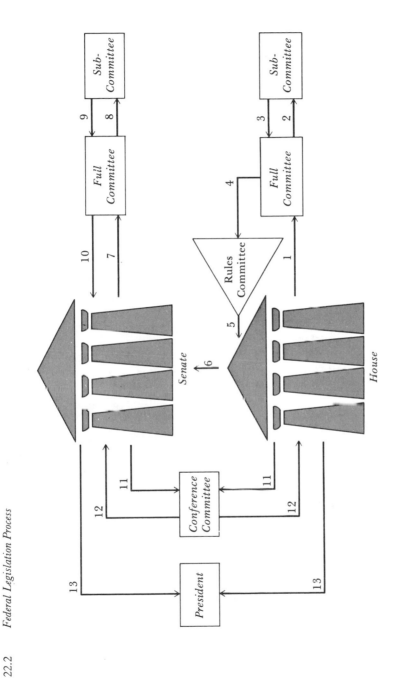

Source: Charles J. Zinn, *How Our Laws Are Made* (Washington, D.C.: U.S. Government Printing Office, 1976).

tion to passage or defeat. A bill does not automatically get a hearing in each related committee. It may be heard in several committees simultaneously, if needed.

3.   There may be no hearings on the bill. A bill introduced in either the Senate or House of Representatives is assigned to a committee and then becomes the property of that committee chairman. He may schedule a hearing or not depending on his interest in the bill, or upon the pressure he gets to hold hearings. In many cases, no hearing is ever held and the bill is then dead at the end of the session. However, when a committee or subcommittee *decides* to act on a legislative proposal, hearings are generally conducted. Depending upon the nature of a bill, hearings may be conducted for a few hours or last for several days or weeks. Sometimes, but not often, the chairman of a committee or subcommittee will limit the type and number of individuals and organizations that may testify. The purpose is either to expedite the committee's deliberations or to create an environment of one particular attitude or conclusion of the hearing. In addition to legislative functions, committees and subcommittees also have the power to conduct "oversight hearings." The purpose of an oversight hearing is to analyze, appraise, and evaluate both the execution and effectiveness of laws administered by the executive branch and to determine whether there are areas in which additional legislation is necessary or desirable. Usually, however, when the executive branch and Congress are controlled by the same party, there is less interest in oversight hearings.

4.   There are differences in the way bills are numbered, depending on how many co-authors an author can persuade to add their names to the bill. If more than twenty-five legislators sign on as co-authors of a bill, the bill is then given a new number and introduced under that new number also. The name of the primary author remains the same but the twenty-four additional names differ. The additional bills are not necessarily numbered in consecutive order. In other words, HR 2156, 3116, 4102 may all be the same bill, but representing seventy-five different co-authors.

5.   There are differences in the way amendments are handled. At the state level, amendments are written into the original bill and the number that was assigned to the bill originally stays with it throughout the process. At the federal level, amending takes place in a "mark-up" session. The bill is worked on and amended by a committee. Instead of then being reprinted in the amended form, the bill is printed in its "clean" form and reintroduced with a *new* number.

FLOOR ACTION

When the committees have completed their deliberations, the bill is ready for a vote by the Senate or House. However, there are several procedural items that precede the actual vote.

1.   In the House, the completed committee bill is sent to the House Rules Committee (see figure 24.2). The committee has the power to establish the length of time for debate and to determine whether floor amendments will be allowed. Except for the House Rules Committee review, procedures are the same for the House and Senate.

2.   The bill is placed on a calendar and given a calendar number. In the Senate there is only one calendar, while in the House there are three: the House Union Calendar, which is utilized for revenue raising or appropriations of funds; the House Calendar, which is used most often for public bills and resolutions; and the House Private Calendar, which is for bills of a private nature, such as claims against the government. Bills placed on a calendar are voted upon in order of numerical sequence, although both Houses have established rules to bypass this sequence for quick consideration of a particular measure.

3.   A bill may be amended further during floor debate. Again, because of the need to rely upon committee conclusions and expertise, amendments on the floor need considerable support for favorable passage.

4.   When a bill has been passed in one house, it is sent to the other house for action and the entire legislative process is repeated. Often, both the Senate and the House will be considering bills of a similar nature. It is unlikely that both will pass identical bills; for example, in the case of the reimbursement for nurse practitioners' bill in the 95th Congress, the Senate version preceded passage of the House version by several months. If the bills do not pass each house in identical form, then a conference committee is arranged.

ON TO THE PRESIDENT

The president has four options when a bill is sent to him. First, he can sign the bill. It immediately becomes law and is sent to the General Services Administration for publication. Second, he may veto the bill within ten days (not counting Sundays) and return it to Congress. If this action is taken, the Constitution requires him to submit a statement describing his objections. Third, the president may allow the bill to become law without his signature by taking no action for ten days when Congress is in session. Fourth, his last option is the "pocket veto"—that is, if Congress adjourns before ten days have elapsed after the passage of a bill, thus preventing the president from returning the bill, the bill is "dead" or "pocket vetoed." A two-thirds majority vote in each house is required to override a veto.

KEEPING UP WITH CONGRESS

Just as it is important for the Congress to have access to information and resources during its deliberations, it is equally important for those participating in the legislative process to know the information resources available from the federal government and when Congress acts or plans to act. The following sections provide an overview of what is available and how it may be obtained.

DAILY CONGRESSIONAL ACTIVITY

Floor Debate, Scheduling, and Voting.   In order to determine when a bill is scheduled for floor debate, contact the Majority Whip's Office by telephone (Senate Majority Whip, 202-224-2158; House Majority Whip, 202-225-5606).

For recorded messages that are revised throughout the day on floor debate, scheduling, and voting, the Democratic and Republican Cloakrooms may be contacted (Senate Democratic Cloakroom, 202-224-8541; Senate Republican Cloakroom, 202-224-8601; House Democratic Cloakroom, 202-225-7400; House Republican Cloakroom, 202-225-7430).

Bill Status.   There are three ways to determine the status of a bill by telephone. First, the Bill Status Office (202-225-1772) can give you an update on any Senate or House bill, including date of introduction, sponsors and co-sponsors, date of committee hearings, and current status of the bill in the legislative process. Information is current (within the preceding twenty-four hours) and requests should be made by bill number. Second, the committee or subcommittee having jurisdiction over the bill also can provide current information. Third, if the bill has been referred to the floor for action, the Majority Whip can provide current information on when it will be scheduled for a vote (Senate Majority Whip, 202-224-2158; House Majority Whip, 202-225-5606).

FUTURE CONGRESSIONAL ACTIVITY

Committee Hearings and Schedule.   In addition to reading the listing of the committee schedules in the *Congressional Record,* you can make inquiries directly to the committee or subcommittee staff. Some health committees distribute periodic press releases on committee schedules or hearings. (See the Daily Hearings section below.)

Week's Floor Schedule.   The week's floor schedule in both the Senate and the House is determined by their respective Majority Whips. Contact their offices for specific information (Senate Majority Whip, 202-224-2158; House Majority Whip, 202-225-5606).

Additionally, both Whip offices distribute weekly press releases on the upcoming week's schedule. To be placed on the mailing list, write: Senate Majority Whip, S–148, Capitol, Washington, DC 20510; House Majority Whip, H–107, Capitol, Washington, DC 20515.

Presidential Signature.   To determine whether the President of the United States has signed a bill that has passed the Congress, contact either the White House Records Office (202-456-2226) or the Archives (202-523-5237) and refer to the bill by number.

Vacations, Adjournments, and Recesses.   For vacations, adjournments and recesses, contact the Whip's office for information.

Daily Hearings.   To determine what hearings are to be conducted for a given day, the following will be helpful: *Washington Post,* "Today's Activities in the Senate and House"; United Press International, "Datebook"; and Associated Press, "Datebook." The *Congressional Record* lists hearings for the next day, while the week's last edition lists publicly announced hearings for the following week (see ordering information below in the Publications section).

The House Interstate and Foreign Commerce Subcommittee on Health and the Environment places interested parties on a mailing list for press releases that announce public hearings in advance. Similarly, the House Ways and Means Committee distributes announcements.

Rules Covering Debate.   For information on rules covering current debate, contact the Senate or House Parliamentarian, respectively (Senate Parliamentarian, 202-224-6128; House Parliamentarian, 202-225-7373).

PUBLICATIONS

Congressional Record.   The *Congressional Record* is a verbatim transcript of the proceedings of the Senate and House. It includes a "Daily Digest" summarizing floor action, committee activities, and committee meetings scheduled for the next day. The last edition of the week (usually Thursday or Friday) lists hearings scheduled for the coming week. Single copies may be purchased by sending twenty-five cents to the *Congressional Record* Office, H–112, Capitol, Washington, DC 20515 and specifying the date of the issue requested. An annual subscription for forty-five dollars may be ordered from the Superintendent of Documents, Government Printing Office, Washington, DC 20401.

Digest of Public General Bills.   This digest lists all bills, in numerical order, as introduced in Congress. Enacted bills are also listed showing subject and author. Published five or more times each session of Congress with supplements, it is available from the Superintendent of Documents, Government Printing Office, Washington, DC 20401.

Bills, Committee Reports, Conference Reports, Public Laws.   To obtain one free copy of a bill, send a self-addressed label to the Senate Document Room (for Senate items) S–325, Capitol, Washington, DC 20510, or House Document Room (for House items) H–226, Capitol, Washington, DC 20515. Make requests by bill number, committee report number, and so forth. Materials may also be picked up in person at the same location.

Committee Prints and Hearing Records.   To obtain a free copy of a committee print or hearing record, send a self-addressed label to the Publications Clerk of the committee from which the document was issued. Hearing records are generally available two months after the close of hearings.

General Accounting Office (GAO).   GAO publishes a free monthly listing of reports. To be placed on the mailing list, write: General Accounting Office, 441 G Street N.W., Washington, DC 20548. Nonprofit organizations may obtain free copies of GAO publications by writing to the above address, Attention: Distribution Section, Room 4522. State the publication requested and indicate that the request is on behalf of a nonprofit organization. Others should remit a check for the specific amount to the same address.

Legislative History.   One can trace the reverse chronology of a law by obtaining a copy of the law from the Senate or House Document Room or from the Government Printing Office. At the end of each law is a summary list of actions taken on the statute prior to enactment, including dates of passage.

Washington Health Newsletters.   Congressmen and their staffs in the health field also make use of newsletters that periodically distribute summaries and analyses of what is happening in Congress and elsewhere in Washington. Many of these newsletters are available to the general public and are excellent sources of information and advice. They are produced by both commercial firms and nonprofit organizations. A compilation of these newsletters, listing ordering information, is available from: Health Policy Center, The Graduate School, Georgetown University, Washington, DC 20057 (202-624-3092). Ask for the "Catalogue of Washington Health Newsletters." (See also National Health Council 1976.)

LOBBYING AT THE FEDERAL LEVEL

All of the previous discussion regarding the "How To's" and "How Not To's" of lobbying on the state and local level are equally applicable at the federal level. The American Nurses' Association maintains an office in Washington, D.C. (202-296-8010) and has three full-time nurse lobbyists. These lobbyists need the back-up, grass roots kind of input and support that only each of us individually and collectively can provide from our individual states. Communication with each other is key to coordinated nursing effort.

The American Public Health Association (202-467-5000) and the National League for Nursing (212-582-1022) are two other organizations where legislative activity is generated by nurses at the state level. With a policy position on a given subject, determined by a consensus of the membership, the best lobbying and testifying is done by individual members with expertise in that area of health.

CONCLUSION

In either state or federal process, the important ingredient is *you*, the individual nurse. Because one by one, we, as nurses, add up to a total that represents the largest number of health care providers. As the largest number, we need to assume a *larger* voice in the direction of health care in America!

Effectiveness and thus success in the legislative arena depend upon *credibility*. Credibility is built, like friendship, slowly and upon mutual trust. It is nurtured by being honest and straightforward plus providing the legislator and his/her staff with accurate, up-to-date information within the procedures and protocols of the legislative process. Nursing will continue to have credibility as long as members use our various organizations' internal structure for the purpose of expressing, debating, and eventually deciding on issues of concern to us.

Many people believe that nurses have had little "clout" legislatively because of the fragmentation caused when each group works independent of the process provided for within our organizations. Our potential is fantastic, but we must learn to "play by the rules." Working through the process does not preclude dissenting personal opinion, if it is so labeled.

I urge all of you to become involved in issues of importance to you—but get involved in the most *productive* manner!

SUMMARY

The legislative process is examined in this chapter from the viewpoint of a community health nurse interested in the future of nursing. First, she discusses her legislative triumph in her state whereby she took a problem—minors needing substance abuse treatment but unable to get it without parental consent—and found a state legislator to author the bill. Her bill is followed to its signing by the governor. Second, a general state legislative process is examined, step by step. Techniques of lobbying are explained and discussed. Finally, the federal legislative process is examined as it differs from the state process. And, the Conclusion section emphasizes that the final ingredient, *you* the individual nurse, cannot be underrated. Until you become active and aware politically, our collective nursing voice will not reach its ultimate potential!

REFERENCES

ALFORD, ROBERT R. *Health Care Politics: Ideological and Interest Group Barriers to Reform*. Chicago: University of Chicago Press, 1975.

ANDERSON, JAMES E. *Public Policy-Making*. New York: Praeger Publishers, 1975.

BARKLAY, ROBERT. *Washington Newsletter*. Washington, D.C.: American Public Health Association, monthly publication.

BENNIS, W., BENNE, C., CHIN, R., and COREY, K. *The Planning of Change*, 3rd. ed. New York: Holt, Rinehart, Winston, 1976.

CALIFORNIA CENTER FOR RESEARCH AND EDUCATION IN GOVERNMENT. *Legislative Process*. Sacramento: California Center for Research and Education in Government, 1977.

CATANSES, ANTHONY J. *Planners and Local Politicians: Impossible Dreams*. Beverly Hills, Calif.: Sage Publications (Sage Library of Social Research), 1974.

DELOUGHERY, GRACE L., and GEBBIE, KRISTINE M. *Political Dynamics: Impact on Nurses and Nursing*. St. Louis: C. V. Mosby, 1975.

GREEN, MARK J., FALLOWS, J., and ZWICK, DAVID R. *Who Runs Congress?* New York: Grossman Publishers, 1972.

COUNCIL OF HOME HEALTH AGENCIES AND COMMUNITY HEALTH SERVICES. *Guidelines for Meeting with Legislators*. Government Relations Pamphlet No. 1, Publication No. 21-1640, 10-76. New York: National League for Nursing.

———. *Guidelines for Presenting Testimony on Legislation*. Government Relations Pamplet No. 2, Publication No. 21-1642, 10-76. New York: National League for Nursing.

———. *Guidelines for Writing Your Congressman*. Government Relations Pamphlet

No. 2, Publication No. 21–1641, 10–76. New York: National League for Nursing.

Health Law Newsletter. (Available from National Health Law Program, 2401 Main Street, Santa Monica, CA 90405.)

Health Policy Making in Action: The Passage and Implementation of the National Health Planning and Resources Development Act of 1974. New York: National League for Nursing, 1975.

HOTT, JACQUELINE R. "Nursing and Politics: The Struggles Inside Nursing's Body Politic." *Nursing Forum* 15 (Fall 1976):325–40.

KALISH, B.J., and KALISH, P.A. "A Discourse on the Politics of Nursing." *Journal of Nursing Administration* 6 no. 2 (1976):29–31.

LAWRENCE, JOHN C. "Confronting Nurses' Political Apathy." *Nursing Forum* 15 (Fall 1976):363–71.

McKINLAY, JOHN B., ed. *Politics and Law in Health Care Policy.* New York: Prodist, 1973. (A Milbank Memorial Fund Resource Book.)

MICHAEL, JAMES R., ed. *Working the System: A Comprehensive Manual for Citizen Access to Federal Agencies.* New York: Basic Books, Inc., 1974.

MONSEN, JOSEPH R., JR., and CANNON, MARK W. *The Makers of Public Policy: American Power Groups and Their Ideologies.* New York: McGraw-Hill Book Co., 1964.

MOYNIHAN, DANIEL P. *Maximum Feasible Misunderstanding: Community Action in the War on Poverty.* New York: The Free Press, A Division of the Macmillan Company, 1969.

"N–Cap, Handbook for Political Action," 1st ed. (mimeo). Kansas City, Mo.: American Nurses' Association, 1975.

NATIONAL HEALTH COUNCIL, INC. *Congress and Health: An Introduction to the Legislative Process and Its Key Participants.* New York: National Health Council, Inc., Government Relations Handbook Series, February 1976.

PERLMAN, JANIS. "Grassrooting the System." *Social Policy* 7 (1976):4–20.

POWELL, DIANE J. "Nursing and Politics: The Struggles Outside Nursing's Body Politic." *Nursing Forum* 15 (Fall 1976):341–62.

REDMAN, ERIC. *The Dance of Legislation.* New York: Simon and Schuster, 1973.

ROSS, DONALD K. *A Public Citizen's Action Manual.* New York: Grossman Publishers, 1973.

ROUCK, FRANCIS E. *Bureaucracy, Politics, and Public Policy.* Boston: Little, Brown and Co., 1969.

SILVERMAN, MILTON P., and LEE, PHILIP R. *Pills, Profits, and Politics.* Berkeley and Los Angeles: University of California Press, 1974.

SOMERS, ANNE R., ed. *Promoting Health: Consumer Education and National Policy.* Germantown, Md.: Aspen Systems Corp., 1976.

STRICKLAND, STEPHEN P. *Politics, Science, and Dread Disease: A Short History of United States Medical Research Policy.* Cambridge, Mass.: Harvard University Press, 1972.

ZINN, CHARLES J. *How Our Laws Are Made.* Washington, D.C.: U.S. Government Printing Office, 1976.

23. Community Health Nurses and Community Organization

Teresa A. Bello

INTRODUCTION

By its very nature community nursing provides a unique opportunity for establishing diverse nurse–client relationships. The skills of community health nurses include bedside nursing techniques; assessing client, family, and community strengths, needs, and resources; and planning and evaluating nursing actions. Through home visiting, community health nurses see clients' normal environments and become aware of client/family/community dynamics that influence behavior. Through skilled interviewing, community health nurses gather information about clients and their families. Through utilization of technical skills, psycho-social and physiological knowledge, and information collected from families, community health nurses effect close relationships with clients and their families. The opportunity to establish a nurse–community relationship whereby nurses become involved with community residents not as clients, but as colleagues, all working together toward common goals, is often missed or considered tangential to community health nurses' roles.

In community organizing, as community health nurses, we work with residents, but decisions are made by the community people as to what should be done and how. The process is not easy and requires concerted effort on our part to rid ourselves of the tendency to jump into action and make decisions for the people involved and instead to take the time and effort needed to actively involve the people affected by the plans and decisions in their development (see chapter 2).

The need for community health nurses to involve ourselves in community organization is very pressing but is often missed. In many areas of our country the community's health status is below par and health care delivery is inadequate. The usual response is to build more facilities, but that action does not really address the real problems, which so often are access to health care facilities, the need for health education, and the lack of a health care model that focuses on health promotion and primary prevention rather than upon disease.

What community health nurse does not know the frustration of policies that prevent us from delivering needed nursing care and health teaching because the clients are not eligible for care under one of the third-party payment plans and cannot afford to pay for the services themselves? Or policies that prohibit us from transporting clients when public transport is not available and clients' physical conditions preclude their standing, waiting, and maneuvering onto a bus or even driving their own cars? If community health nurses include in our practice a community organizer role, perhaps we could anticipate more accurately the needs of the community we serve and thereby direct our efforts and theirs toward developing more meaningful services.

However, in our present system, we lack power. Power for nurses to say what is good nursing care and be flexible in our practice. Power for the community residents to be heard as they relate their needs for and perceptions of good health services. One way to achieve power is through participation in community organization practice. Many nurses participate in community organization in a limited way, such as by arranging mothers' groups to discuss special concerns. What is proposed in this chapter is participation by community nurses in community organization practice on a large scale. Such participation pays off for all concerned, particularly nurses, and community organization may be the one area of practice where our efforts are appreciated by all because in working with clients toward common goals, the results of those efforts will be longer lasting. The following case study is an example of what is meant by community organization as an integral part of community health nurses' practice. I know it can be done and that it works, because I did it myself.

CASE STUDY: COMMUNITY ORGANIZATION IN ACTION

East Los Angeles (ELA) encompasses an area of approximately forty-four square miles. The predominantly Spanish-speaking/Spanish-surnamed population numbered about 400,000 in 1970. The proximity of the Mexican border leads to a constant influx of Mexican nationals and retention of the mother country's cultural values. It is a low-income, high-density area with all the attendant health problems.

At the time of my involvement in ELA, the area had no grassroots community-based organizations concerned with health. Recognizing this lack, a group of four community residents and a state health consultant from Comprehensive Health Planning wrote a proposal that would establish such an organization. The organization would be called the ELA Health Task Force.

When the proposal was funded, flyers were posted and calls were made to announce a community meeting to be held in a local church hall for the election of a board of directors. That particular setting was chosen for the elections to increase the likelihood of community residents' attending and being elected. Holding such a meeting in an official agency would have reduced this likelihood.

The purpose of the task force was to make the community's perception of health needs known to official agencies and to develop a health care delivery system with community involvement in planning and implementation. The goals were that the task force would (1) be a model for future community-based health task forces; (2) be the coordinating agency for all health-related programs in ELA; and (3) be the administrative agency for these health programs.

Before the total board was elected, the four grassroots residents who wrote the proposal hired a small staff to take care of the clerical work, to disseminate information about the task force, and to solicit broader community support. The persons hired were community residents with clerical skills, community organizing skills, and a need for a job. They primarily functioned independently. The four residents declared themselves board members and managed the budget. They moved quickly to avoid the loss of federal monies and yet hesitated to rush into an election until as many as possible community residents were informed of the pending election.

The board that was finally elected consisted of both grassroots and professional persons. While the terms *professional* and *grassroots* suggest numerous meanings, in this context *professional* meant individuals employed by an official agency and *grassroots* described community residents who were not employed by an official agency. One could be a community resident and still be considered a professional. The grassroots residents recognized that the locus of loyalty could be influenced by an income. For example, they were aware of instances where a community resident would be critical of an official agency because of poor service and insufficient input from the community. The official agency would then offer a community worker position to the critical resident who in a few weeks would not understand why other community residents were still critical!

The only noticeable change instituted by the official agency in such a case would be the hiring of the resident. The resident, who would feel elevated in personal status because of the job and a paycheck, would in turn direct his or her energies toward conserving his or her position and ignoring the previous injustices. While some residents would openly reject the employed resident, others would understand the necessity and dignity of a job. This divide-and-conquer tactic of the agencies taught the residents to be suspicious of the official agencies' motives and of the residents employed by those agencies.

With the exception of the state health consultant (hereafter simply called the consultant), all board members were amateurs at management, administration, and parliamentary procedure. Initially, the consultant suggested that the board needed such skills and attempted to arrange training in these topics for board members. The majority, feeling important and honored by their community election, rejected the suggestion. Their thinking was that dedication and hard work alone would get the job done. Also, they rejected the bureaucratic procedures that seemed to cement the official agencies into inactivity. Surely, the board could function adequately and swiftly without the rules and regulations that they perceived would only impede progress and preclude reciprocity with the community residents. The fear was that the board would become as insensitive and inflexible as the "establishment."

Consequently, the first few board meetings were spent feeling each other out and trying to define tasks. Were the professionals' interests in serving the community or in serving the official agency? Were the grassroots persons' interests in serving the community or in becoming politically powerful? What was the purpose of a board of directors? Whom did the board direct? How did the board direct?

The grassroots members were experienced in organizing and attending special interest community meetings where they had voiced their concerns. They were also proficient in arranging for and attending meetings with county supervisors, directors of hospitals, and state and federal officials. However, program development and management were unfamiliar strategies in their practice of community organization. Much meeting time was spent recalling the various experiences the board members had in the past when they confronted the "establishment." Horror stories of the poor quality of medical and nursing care were also recounted time and again.

PRESSURES ON THE BOARD

The community residents, hearing that the task force was to be a champion of their rights, began calling the task force staff to relate incidents of poor health care delivery and ask for help in alleviating the situation and developing more accessible, acceptable, and appropriate services. The staff, in turn, began asking for direction from the board. Many board members began realizing there was a repetition of topics from one meeting to the next. Then and not until then did the board recognize the necessity for training. Community pressure increased movement in this direction, and a motion to request and fund a training course was approved.

As the training sessions progressed, the tasks and the methods for their accomplishment became clearer: Fiscal decisions were to be made on sound data rather than "gut feeling" since the total board would be legally liable. Minutes of the meetings were required and considered legal documents. Freedom to indiscriminately absent oneself from a board meeting was not possible; a quorum was required to be present for a vote. The board learned they were responsible for the staff's actions. The task force bylaws were to be heeded rather than ignored, which meant establishing the specified committees. Even as the board was trying to establish itself as a formal, legitimate group, the members insisted that community meetings be held weekly to inform their constituents of what the board was doing and to hear feedback from them.

Some of the board members began to write a project proposal for the recruitment and retention of Mexican-American nurses who would be under the aegis of the task force and a local college. The report of this action to the community residents generated so much interest that an invitation was extended to the soon-to-be-retired leader of the local school's nursing department to speak about her nursing program and her thoughts about the project proposal. The community residents also wanted to give her their input. Unfortunately, during her visit a hubcap was lost from her very expensive sportscar. Infuriated, she called the sheriff and shouted to the attending residents: "You people are responsible for this. I came to you in good faith. I'm only trying to help you poor people!" Fortunately for the task force and the community, she retired shortly thereafter.

The project for recruiting and retaining Mexican-American nurses was instituted after much heated negotiation with the local college fiscal administrator. The project was to be contracted out to the the task force; however, the fiscal administrator insisted that no monies could be spent by the task force without approval from two nursing faculty members who were to be designated as project director and codirector. This requirement was a change from previous discussions with representatives from the local college and the federal funding agency. The fact was that the project was ultimately approved and funded because of community support and the local college's promise to work closely with the task force, and when the compromise was finally reached, it was viewed by the community as a dramatic victory for the task force and the board. The local official agencies began to reassess their thinking about the task force. No longer could the task force's legitimacy be questioned by anyone.

As the board began to function smoothly and with confidence, a leadership conflict arose between the consultant and a grassroots board member. The consultant was accused of making decisions and forcing them on the board and acting independently from the board and trying to use the community as a stepping stone to power. The consultant was shocked and his only defense was that he was trying to get things off the ground in the best and fastest way possible. His only interest, he maintained, was in seeing the organization become really viable. The board was split among the "grateful for the help" members, the "we would rather do it ourselves" members, and the "what are you talking about" members. The conflict was resolved by the consultant's resigning and dropping out of sight. Despite the feeling of guilt among the few "grateful for the help" members, the board pulled itself together by focusing upon its goals. Concurrently, requests from other grassroots communities for help in establishing task forces and writing project proposals inundated the staff. A request from the staff came to the board for more personnel. It was approved and the task force was on its way to establishing itself as an activist community-based organization.

MY PERSONAL INVOLVEMENT

I was one of two community nurses elected to the board and would like to focus on my experiences as a member of it. I am both Spanish speaking and Spanish surnamed and came to ELA to work in a federally funded project.

My presence at the meeting where the elections took place was due to the insistence of my boss and my own curiosity about the organization. I had heard rampant rumors that this organization was militant and wanted to check it out myself. A few of my coworkers were at the meeting, and when I was nominated by one of my friends, I nominated her. What fun! Then, to my surprise, I was elected. Oh, no, I thought. That meant meeting in the evening after work.

I was regarded as both professional and grassroots. Being of the ethnic group, my casual style of operation, and my ignorance of what I was involved in worked in my favor. I did not relate my experience and participation on the board of directors to anything as broad as community organization practice. Rather my activities were in fulfillment of the contract for being elected. The other board members regarded as incidental the fact that there was a nurse among them. Only as questions arose about a disease or medical treatment was I consulted.

Struggling with the new role of being a director on a board, I searched my mind for applicable associations or experiences. The association conjured up images of General Motors and Rockefeller Foundation. Obviously, that would not do. My experience in leadership was being the treasurer in my high school Thespian Club. That would not do either. I decided I must be a novice.

I then directed my energies toward trying to decide how board activity was related to health and nursing. I went to the library. No help. The word "health" conjured only the association of physical well-being. I began to think about my experience as a nursing student. I was called upon to translate for every Spanish-speaking patient on the ward to which I was assigned. I remembered the delight of the patients to see a nurse with whom they could relate. I also remembered my pangs of anger during clinical conferences where the discussion of Spanish-speaking patients assumed a denigrating theme. I relived my own family's deplorable experiences with the health care delivery system. Slowly, "health" began to take on a different meaning: Health is personal involvement of a nurse to speak out against poor health care, and it is active participation in community efforts to alter the situation.

Although my ethnic background was similar to that of the community residents, I was unfamiliar with most of them and the community dynamics. Following this realization, the obvious next step was to gather more information about the community—the residents, the formal and informal leaders, the network of support systems and how to hook into them, and community politics. I had to learn about the behavior patterns of an urban group that seemed more assertive and outspoken than the more familiar migrant rural group. The only way to proceed was to listen attentively to the discussions before, during, and after the board meetings, to listen to coworkers' comments about the community, to listen to the merchants, to attend other community meetings, to read the local newspapers, and to keep an eye open for what was really going on. During home visits, my clients' comments about other residents and the surrounding environment were viewed as just as important as their comments about illness.

As I mentioned earlier, gathering this information was done more out of a natural inclination than as a formula for successful community involvement. Essentially, careful preparation for meaningful community involvement was occurring by my development of an awareness of the community context in which I was to operate. This information increased my sensitivity to the nuances in this particular urban community and decreased my fear of having to function in a vacuum. In informal conversations, I was able to use this information in explaining why ELA needed such an organization as the task force and why the residents should join. I discussed community politics with factual information rather than stretching rumors to sound like facts. "Community wants and needs" took on a human perspective. Those words were no longer rhetoric, but reality.

These realizations and activities increased my desire to get the board moving. Uncomfortable with the lack of direction evidenced in the initial board meetings, I used this tactic: I mentally labeled each member of the board as aggressor, blocker, facilitator, or gatekeeper and then pointed out these behavior patterns to them as charmingly as possible. Functioning in a low-key manner decreased the possibility of becoming a threat to the male leadership. Charm, knowledge, and skill were effective mixers.

As the board's task became clearer, I asserted myself by increasingly active participation in board activities, such as rewriting bylaws, functioning in the communications committee, writing and editing proposals and letters, recruiting new members, social protest picketing, and negotiating with the local colleges or administrators. My crowning glory occurred during that fateful community meeting attended by the leader of the local school's nursing department. Angered by the woman's tirade and remarks, I stood up and responded eloquently. Amazed by my sudden courage, I barely heard the thundering ovation in the meeting hall. The only thought that ran through my head was that this must be "health" because it felt so invigorating!

Another result of my activities in the community was the reevaluation of my goals and commitment to the official agency for which I worked. As a new community nurse I had initially been excited about working in a setting that served my ethnic group; I believed an impact could be made to change the health care delivery system. Because of my idealism and inexperience with the resistant-to-change forces of bureaucracy and inflexible colleagues, I was unprepared to handle my frustration. For example, often clients could not keep well-baby, physical, or recheck appointments because of lack of transportation, but policy precluded our transporting clients and/or administering immunizations in the home. So children were unimmunized and preventive health care was spotty. I was also bothered by an insensitive Anglo nurse employed at the clinic who treated clients disrespectfully and without concern for their cultural practices—extreme modesty of the children being one. It didn't make sense to me. We health professionals were supposed to raise the standard of health in ELA but could not even deliver it. We talked about this discrepancy at staff meetings, but the focus would be shifted to the numbers of home visits that were made, the numbers of new clients registered, the numbers of dollars spent, and so on. Apparently, to justify the existence of our project, the quantity of this and that became priority. Seemingly, for every suggestion made to improve nursing services, there was a policy to prevent its implementation. Not knowing how to be a change agent and fearful of being considered militant, my enthusiasm waned. I complained all the time to my supervisor who assured me she understood.

Then, I was elected to the board. After the task of the board became more clearly defined and my role emerged, my sense of commitment increasingly transferred to the board. Repeated successes with the board in attempts to effect change enlarged my scope. As my experiences on the board helped solidify my role as a community organizer, I became able to see ways in which changes could be made in the agency. My growing identity with the community and acceptance of the community organizer role as part of being a community health nurse made salient the fact that I worked in an agency that was insensitive to the basic needs of its clients and that was technically part of the problem. My commitment to the agency's activities revived in an altered and more exuberant form.

My observation and data gathering processes were put into effect at the agency. I discussed the situation with other staff members who I knew were fed up. We discussed strategy and the limits of our commitment— for instance, resigning or risk of being fired. Together with other nursing staff, I met with the administrators of our project. With the feeling of fear and intimidation balled-up in my gut, I took on the project medical director. The results of the meeting were that the insensitive nurse was not rehired; the policies on transporting clients and administering immunizations were changed; and the administrators began to work with the community to get bus service to the clinic. The nursing staff agreed that this must be "health" because it felt good.

Discussion

Community organization, like most fields, has a body of knowledge that has been developed both from practical experience and abstract projections to explain what goes on in situations like the ELA example. Although, with the exception of the ouside consultant, all of us on the ELA Health Task Force board flew by the seat of our pants, we demonstrated the applicability of many community organization theories even though we were totally unaware of them at the time. Our experience on the board is typical of many life experiences, where we become deeply involved in a situation before learning about a theoretical framework and where, as a result, there is often no linear progression from theory to practice. Indeed, involvement often motivates a search for more knowledge about the subject and a desire to study the process. Not until several years after my experience on the ELA board did I finally encounter the literature on community development and community organization. Only then did I get a theoretical perspective on the events I had lived through. The rest of this chapter is devoted to passing along some of the information I have acquired about community organization. This information will help you to understand the ELA example better as well as enable you to get new perspectives on situations in which you are, have been, or will be involved.

FINDING A FOCUS

Until a community becomes focused on some mutual concern, individual members have a tendency to complain about local problems and frequently to propose conflicting solutions to them. Without organization, they lack the power to expect, demand, or force change. If a defeatist attitude about the likelihood of change also exists, little progress can be made. If the latter is reversed, however, the mere idea that change may be possible creates a self-fulfilling prophecy and induces behavior that effects change. The ELA Health Task Force board's experiences certainly exemplify these realities. Before members of an organization can acquire the ability to predict and control their social environment, they must acquire the political clout to make change. The labor union movement has shown well that the larger the population base, the greater the impact the organization's spokespersons have on the political processes that affect the population.

Behavior in meetings, viewed from outside the context of the members' perspective, often seems unsophisticated and unproductive. However, transformation of consumers from a social or complaint orientation to readiness for action cannot be shortened too much without losing some of the assets the community members already have. Telling war stories is often a necessary prelude to girding for further action: "We did it before and we can do it again." Community organizers should recognize this inevitable part of the process and allow enough time for it to be completed.

In addition to a sense of impatience, professional community organizers often have preconceived ideas of the behavior and value system of the community. Biddle cautions that attitudes that a worker with people has toward those people will either enhance or negate development (Biddle 1974:245). What you expect is what you will get.

Looking at the case study example, we see the grassroots board members' concept of community organization practice: arranging community meetings to discuss issues or a crisis situation, confronting agency administrators about those issues and crises, acting as interpreters for those who needed services, and making themselves known to community residents as advocates and to the established agencies as articulate spokespersons. This process is similar to that involved in organizing a labor union or a special interest group, and it makes some sense.

BOARD TRAINING

Before the board of an organization, whether lay or professional, can develop and use its inner resources, it must learn to function as a board. The ELA board in the case study made what is a very common mistake and one that we see happening on Health Systems Agency and other community boards. The ELA board elected not to have any formal board training. As noted in the case study, the members felt that hard work and dedication would suffice for them to attain their goals. They, as members of most other boards find out sooner or later, found that certain rules and procedures were necessary to get anything done, to account for monies received, to deal with other organizations and agencies, and even to manage their own meetings. The challenge to the community organizer who wants to help community boards move toward their goals is to persuade them of the necessity of learning needed procedures, gathering sufficient background information on which to base decisions, establishing and maintaining lines of accountability and communication, and proceeding in an orderly manner through meetings. The community organizer must know how to do these things himself or herself and be able to teach them to the board members in an acceptable way.

In the ELA experience, the grassroots board members bickered and spent much meeting time discussing their past victories, thus making it difficult to move as quickly as the consultant desired. This behavior pattern was usually interpreted as an example of a phenomenon Altshuler describes: poorly educated laymen with irreparable handicaps as decisionmakers—concerned with only themselves and the immediate, fearing anything unfamiliar, deliberating endlessly (1970:45). But uneducated laymen are not the only ones who behave so; labor negotiation sessions or university faculty meetings often show the same patterns. Thus it does not seem too farfetched to suggest that all groups need some training in processes of meeting and communicating so that they can move effectively toward meeting their objectives (Bradford 1976; Pfeiffer and Jones 1978; Schindler-Rainman and Lippett 1975).

COMMUNITY ORGANIZER MODELS

In most theories on community organization practice, the focus is on the *external agent* who has skills and certain qualities and who moves in and builds up the disorganized community. While there may be use for this perspective, the disregard of the skills communities possess to sustain their existence is an injustice to the integrity and abilities of community residents. Viewing success from the perspective of the professional community organizer precludes recognizing the community's past and present strengths that may also facilitate movement toward the organizer's goal.

The ELA consultant could be described as an external agent. He was the expert from outside the community proper, an Anglo who tried to implant a program in the form of an organization—the task force. He was a problem area specialist who clearly practiced ethical absolutism in that his actions often suggested he knew better than the community about its wants and needs. In our experience the creation of the task force as a community need was not at issue; the issue was more a question of loyalties. Only when one of the board members began to feel the board was being manipulated did he begin to ask questions about the consultant's motives. This situation is common in many community situations: The leadership figure is gradually suspected of self-aggrandizement in activities that were previously thought done entirely for the betterment of the population.

If success is measured by the degree to which an external agent implants programs, the ELA consultant was successful; however, his behavior resulted in a crisis in leadership. Unlike the catalyst-teacher model of organizer (Biddle 1953:78), he had not fostered the development of decision-making skills in the previously unskilled board members. Only later did the board members realize he had been remiss by constantly giving all the solutions readymade and failing to expand on their own abilities. This approach is common among persons educated and defined as professionals; their knowledge is presupposed to solve all problems and their actions are passively accepted. The consultant's resignation was a growth-producing experience: The board members were able to assert their confidence and independence as thinkers and problem solvers.

Another community organization model involves the optimal use of inner resources. Here the organizer encourages community members to identify their needs and to work cooperatively in meeting them. The central objective is to get people working on their own problems. Disadvantages include a slow, unsophisticated action process and the action taken is less likely to be under the control of the professional. As we saw in chapter 2, the inner resources method enables people to learn how to work together on problems they perceive to be important and by so doing the projects the community undertakes will have meaning and permanence that imposed projects do not.

The ELA board's method of problem solving using inner resources is illustrated by the following example. A membership drive was needed for the task force to qualify for more program monies. Initially, trying to be sophisticated, the board members haggled over the best method to approach this complex problem. A grassroots board member, tiring over the failure to agree, mentioned that he knew a community resident who helped organize union membership and was now unemployed because of a disability. He could be trusted to do a good job or his esteem would suffer in the eyes of the community. Everyone agreed that the idea was a good one. The man was hired and he set up a systematic membership drive complete with a timetable. The community resident was able to use his skill and increase his self-esteem and financial gain, and one more community problem was solved.

Even the inner resources approach that encourages communities to identify their own wants and needs and work cooperatively in satisfying them can still smack of the paternalistic approach if care is not taken to avoid conveying an attitude of "let's help the poor community to move."

In the ELA case the board's recounting of past victories at meetings was an affirmation of its ability to confront the establishment. The members felt they were the warriors in the "war on poverty." While the larger society often places a negative value on such tactics of demanding to be heard the board's community compatriots knew the courage that was required to confront an authority figure who did not have the nerve or did not see the need to face the community residents and listen to them.

COMMUNITY NURSING AND COMMUNITY ORGANIZING

Community health nurses, as a result of our education, often fall into the trap of thinking that we know what is good for clients. This perspective handicaps nurses or, for that matter, any other professional group involved in community organization practice, for our preconceived ideas about the community can stifle our ability to listen critically and see the community process and thus recognize its strengths as well as its needs. Again, we need to know "what's really going on" (see chapter 8).

Community involvement can also have an impact on a nurse's relationships in the community and in much larger arenas. The reciprocal effects of my own involvement in the ELA Health Task Force board are diagrammed in figure 23.1 as an example. My first contact with the task force board was my half-frivolous nomination and surprising election to the board (1A). At that time my identity as a community nurse was as a member of the agency that employed me (1B). I was ready to do what I perceived the agency and its stated goals required; my role concept there was clear. I saw no need for the agency to be changed let alone that I might be the one to do it. As I became involved with the board, I began to revise my own goals and roles as a community member (2A). However, the experience there spilled over into my perception of the agency for which I worked, and for the first time I began to see its policies and actions in a new light and to question its goals. Reflecting a growing alienation, the diagram (2B) shows me moving away from identification with my agency. Having committed myself to learning my role as a board member, I became wholly immersed in the community perspective (3A).

23.1   *Reciprocal Effects of Involvement in Community Organization Practice*

Task Force Board of Directors Involvement

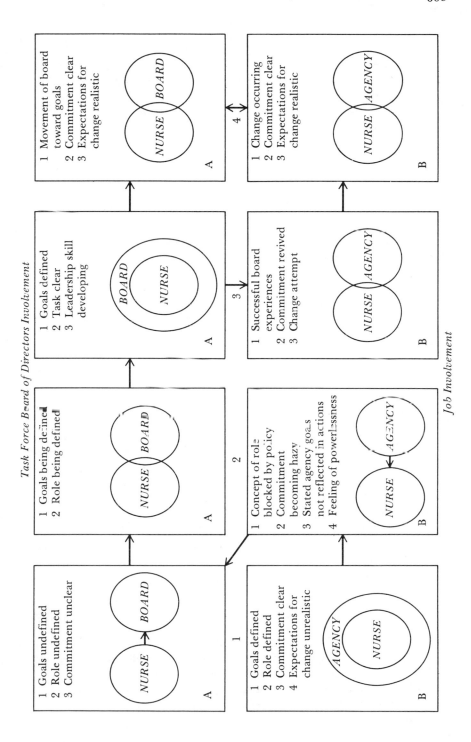

Job Involvement

Being able to have some successes on the board, I turned my interests back to my agency. Since I continued in my nurse role, I began to consider how and whether I could carry this out by making changes in the agency's actions (3B). Time and experience with the board helped me clarify points of difference that were not overwhelming obstacles and gave me a more realistic view of my dual position as both professional and grassroots (4A). Success in making changes with the aid of colleagues in my health agency also gave me a new relationship with my work role— neither totally alienated nor blindly accepting as before (4B). At this point I am at the same level of involvement in both agency and board. I am now equipped with interpersonal skills in dealing with change and better understand my roles in both systems. (Although my experiences are presented in seemingly logical sequence, you need to understand that such processes do not always occur that way. Nor was my understanding of its logic acquired until a good deal of time and learning had passed!)

As outsiders, community health nurses come with concepts and theories learned external to the community context. Some of us may be convinced that textbook knowledge is sufficient or that the well-meaning feeling alone causes enlightenment. Textbook knowledge alone lacks a reality base and must be tested before it is applied. If nurses hope to become a part of the community action, we must be able to set aside those concepts and theories and become students ready to learn from the real community. That stripping process removes the sense of security from community health nurses who are convinced they know what is best before they ever get there.

What is often forgotten is that the community residents do their homework by learning about any unknown persons who present themselves. Our behavior as nurses is scrutinized and our comments are interpreted. While at the outset community health nurses may seem to be given much attention, the astute community residents are assessing us simply by listening and observing. The community residents too have ideas and theories learned from experiences in the larger society and in their community. The residents have preconceived ideas about nurses. Our responsibility as community nurses is to learn this fact and to dispel those ideas that interfere with our ability to function.

A Guide for the Community Health Nurse Community Organizer

This section presents a guide for community health nurses to use in community organization practice. It has been developed from the experiences some of us have had in such practice, and it runs a close parallel to the planning process discussed in chapter 3. There are numerous definitions of and approaches to community organization (Alinsky 1971;

Altshuler 1970; Biddle and Biddle 1965; Cox 1973; Ross 1967), but all have the common thread that community organization is a process. Like all processes, this one looks deceiving on paper since it is neat and orderly, while in practice the steps are not necessarily followed in the order outlined here. Realistically, community health nurses may become involved at any of the steps along the way.

Community also has numerous definitions depending on the perspective of the people asked to define it. The different conceptualizations of community, as noted in chapter 2, include a specific geographic area or a particular interest, social, or ethnic group. Most often, community health nurses become involved in community organization with a group of clients who are residents of a given geographic area. While the focus of this guide is a community group in a specific area, as noted in the ELA case study, the community organization process can be just as effective in the work setting.

STEP 1: YOU—THE POTENTIAL COMMUNITY ORGANIZER

Questions to ask:

What are your personal objectives and goals as they relate to the community?
What are your motives for community involvement?
What is your style of working in the community?
Are you willing to modify your style based on feedback from the community?
Will you be able to receive and objectively evaluate negative criticism?
What is your time commitment?
In what "community" do you want to get involved?
With whom in the community can you work?

As a community health nurse involving yourself in community organization, you should begin with a thorough examination of your motives for this activity. If you believe it is an integral part of nursing, you should be able to talk about goals related to nursing. You should also know yourself as a person and be able to recognize your own strong characteristics and your weaknesses. Community organization is a process that effects changes in all of the principals involved. Change may be rewarding or painful depending upon one's ability to "know thyself." At the grassroots level, community nurses must be prepared for constant questioning, directly and obliquely. Without being unduly cynical or suspicious, community members may well question why yet another outsider comes in to "do good for the folk."

According to the *Organizer's Manual* (O.M. Collective 1971), this step is very important. Involvment in community organizing removes you from your safe and secure bureaucratic work environment where you have a title and some status. You may find yourself with a group of persons who do not place a value in your title or status and may even be suspicious of you because of your title or status. If you become involved with the group because, unconsciously, you wanted to increase your status or exhibit your leadership skills, you are in store for much emotional trauma (see also Lassey and Fernandez 1976).

You can be assured that someone in the group will notice your behavior that reflects your status consciousness or your desire to lead and may well call it to your attention, often abruptly. If you are unaware of your own motives, when confronted you may become defensive, feel uncomfortable, and lose your desire to be involved. In this kind of a situation, no one wins.

Since there are many ways to work in a community, you should be aware of your own style. Whatever that style is, you should be comfortable with it since copying another's style often is like wearing another's clothing—the fit is not good. You should think carefully about your own style and be aware that you will need to learn how to be flexible and adaptable since feedback from the community may make clear that unless you modify your approach you will not get very far.

As community organizers, we should be able to receive and give feedback about our performance and the performance of others constructively so that a climate of trust and mutual respect can be developed within the group. Since community health nurses are very often outsiders, how we convey our reasons for involvement, emotional tone, and responses to community input will greatly influence whether a trusting relationship can develop. Trust takes time to evolve. Unless you have sufficient time and are willing to commit it to work as a community organizer, then don't even start. Community organization is far more than a 9 A.M. to 5 P.M. undertaking.

STEP 2: IDENTIFICATION OF THE PROBLEM, CONCERN, OR ISSUE

Questions to ask:

Who identified the problem, concern, or issue and brought it to the fore?

Is the problem real or perceived as potential?

Do you understand the problem from the community's perspective?

Do you have the background—education, life experience, empathy, and so forth—to deal with the problem?

Can the problem be defined in terms that are easily understood by all concerned, especially the "target" community or group?

Is it a chronic problem or is it new?

Is the identification of the problem politically inspired?

Is the problem already a priority for any agency or community group? What are they doing about it? What have they done in the past?

Is the problem influenced by faulty communications between agency and community?

Is the problem a problem or a dilemma?

This step and the questions that you need to ask are particularly important since the problem that is brought to the community health nurse's attention is often not the real problem but merely a symptom or outcome of the problem. After all, community problems are multidimensional and highly complex.

For example, a group of community health nurses became concerned about the low immunizations level in a low-income community. They managed to get agency permission to increase the number of immunization clinics held in one week; they advertised on the radio and in community newspapers and told their clients to tell other clients. However, few people attended the immunization clinics. Discouraged, some of the nurses criticized the community residents; however, one undaunted nurse decided to find out why the clinics were sparsely attended. She questioned her clients who identified that the single most frustrating barrier was the lack of adequate transportation to the clinics. Although there was a bus system, schedules were unreliable and often people were kept waiting on the street for an hour or more. The mothers were unwilling to gather up their several young children, wait for an unknown length of time for a bus to get to the immunization clinic, wait there to be seen, and then have to stand around again waiting for a bus to take them home. In the meantime the children would be tired, hungry, in need of diaper changes, and fussy because of the immunizations. The mothers also indicated that they considered their time too valuable to waste on all this waiting. The time that the immunization clinics were held was also identified by the mothers as a barrier. The mothers preferred that the clinics be held after 5 P.M. so that they could leave those children who did not need immunizing at home and also have access to the family automobile.

All of this information served to define the problem in a very different light than had been originally perceived by the community health nurses. The methods of dealing with the problem also took on new dimensions. Obviously having more immunization clinics between the hours of 9 A.M. and 5 P.M. was not the answer. Unless community pressure could be organized and brought to bear on the bus company to improve the reliability of its services, the day-time transportation problem would continue. Unless community pressure could be organized and brought to bear on the agency to have evening and Saturday clinics, the time barrier problem would continue.

When the community health nurse reported her findings to her colleagues, a couple of them voiced disgust that the mothers would not use the bus in spite of the waiting problems—after all, they reasoned, the bus system was "better than nothing." Many of the nurses were unwilling to work during the dinner hour and evenings because they wanted to be home with their families. Saturday clinics met with the same negative response. For those nurses who really wanted to help the community address its problems, there seemed little choice but to encourage the community to organize to change either the bus company's or the agency's policies.

A word or two about dilemmas is appropriate here. A dilemma, unlike a problem, has no real solution. Often when dealing with a dilemma we find that all of the possible alternatives for dealing with it are undesirable. In other instances no matter what alternative is selected, its outcomes are negative or undesirable in terms of others' points of view. The kinds of complex social issues with which community health nurses often have to deal are increasingly assuming the dimensions of dilemmas. Inadequate or unsafe housing is an example. Often people live in substandard housing either because they cannot afford other housing or because none is available to them. If their present housing is condemned, they have to move, but there is no place for them to move. If their present housing is renovated, they may well not be able to afford to live in it any more and there still will be no alternative housing available for them. These are the kinds of knotty dilemmas community health nurses face all the time, if we permit ourselves to become really involved in our communities' needs. Finding ways to deal with these dilemmas as well as problems and other concerns is what leads many of us into community organization. In most instances, it is only through concerted community-wide effort that these kinds of situations can be effectively addressed.

STEP 3: ASSESSMENT OF THE PHYSICAL COMMUNITY

Before undertaking community organization practice, you must base yourself in the community and develop a "sense of community." One way to begin is by a *personal assessment approach*. Using a map, you pick out an area within the community. With notebook in hand, you park your car and proceed to walk street by street conscientiously observing anything and everything.

Questions to ask:

Is there air pollution or noise pollution?
What do the houses in the area look like? Are they freshly painted? In

what condition are they? Are they single- or two-story houses? What colors are they painted? Are there fences around them? Are there "Beware of Dog," "No Solicitors," or "Do not Disturb" signs?

Are there trees in the area? Are there flowers or lawns?

Are there apartment buildings in the area? How do they look? Are there fences and where are they located?

Are there cars parked in the area? What year and condition are they?

Are there people walking on the streets in the area? Are they younger or older? Are there children? What is the ethnic composition of the residents seen? How are they dressed?

How heavy is the traffic? Are there street signs? Are there highways, freeways, bridges, railroads, or canals? Are there buses or bus stop signs? Are there benches for sitting and waiting?

You should then draw a map of your own that indicates the above characteristics of the community. You should also talk to the community residents you see and ask some additional questions: Are they friendly? Have they noticed a physical or people change in their neighborhood? To what do they attribute the change? Do they know the local politics and what is their viewpoint? How long have they lived there? Do they know the history of the area? You should also listen astutely for key value words or phrases such as, "Those guys ruined this place," "The politicians are all crooks," "Who cares about us," "Don't walk the streets at night," "All the young people left." These phrases can set an emotional tone for the data and alert you to sensitive topic areas.

This descriptive process approach is familiar to community health nurses since it is the basic format we use for data collection on clients, families, and their home environment. The process is merely extended to the entire community setting. Again, we are asking our basic question, "What's really going on?" As is the case in reporting any descriptive data, care must be taken to avoid interpretation of what is seen or heard before all data are collected.

For example, a community walk by nurses was undertaken in a settlement situated on an Indian reservation. The nurses met to report the data they had gathered. One woman began by saying the Indians she spoke to were unfriendly and hostile to her because she was Anglo. Another woman reported the indigenous Anglos were hostile and unfriendly to her because she was an Anglo from another state. Both of these women spoke out with their reports. Their experiences were similar except that the out-of-state woman became curious rather than fearful. Thinking that a business person would be likely to answer questions, she walked into a real estate agent's office and struck up a conversation. She learned that recently oil was discovered on the reservation. That discovery brought in

Anglos from other states who were exploiting the local community in their quest for riches. They camped their trailers anywhere without consideration of ownership, sanitation facilities, or environmental impact. The local residents regarded their behavior as uncivilized and selfish. Consequently, they were hostile and suspicious toward any unknown Anglo. This nurse's findings exemplify the necessity to exercise caution in translating your experience into action on the basis of partial data only.

The approach by which you ask questions of a community resident is important. Kent favors the "native" question approach whereby the resident is initially asked for directions to a particular street or where a place to eat is located. From that beginning other questions about the neighborhood may be asked (Kent videotape). If you begin by identifying yourself, your occupation, and your place of employment you put yourself outside the residents' informal communication process. While you may be impressed with your credentials, the community resident may be placed on guard by them. That is not to imply that you lie to the residents or refuse to tell them who you are.

You may find that any approach tried will be unsuccessful. That in itself is indicative of "something going on" in the community. Before continuing to approach residents, try other avenues such as the local newspaper or local radio station, read the posters or leaflets appearing in the neighborhood, read bulletin boards in laundromats, talk to the priest or pastor of the church(s). Try talking to children or adolescents. They provide information from yet another perspective.

Along with the personal assessment approach, nurses contemplating community organization practice need *data collected from official agencies,* such as local and state health departments, census bureaus, bureaus of vital statistics, and schools. Boyle lists several essential factors that should be examined including geographic and environmental factors, demographic and socioeconomic data, objectives of the official agencies that deliver health care, levels of education, the economic situation, and the distribution of power (1973:176–79) (see also health indicators in chapter 2).

With the personal and official data collected, you can formulate a meaningful picture of the total community and an understanding of the residents' wants and needs. However, you need continual assistance to interpret the data and feedback about your actions as you try to implement change. This assistance could come from an understanding community resident or a professional person whose ethnic background is the same as the community or a professional person who lives in the community.

Community health nursing is enlarging its knowledge and awareness of the client's immediate environment to include social, economic, psychological, and cultural factors. Knowledge and awareness of the total community environment must broaden as health care moves away from established agencies. Community nurses must take responsibility for improving the inadequate health care that is delivered by our agencies because of unrealistic policies. We must no longer regard our clients as "those people" if we wish to remain in the community. Such an attitude places a clear distance between us and our clients that cannot help but interfere with our attempts to establish working relationships with them.

STEP 4: ASSESSMENT OF COMMUNITY STRENGTHS, RESOURCES, AND INTERESTS

Questions to ask:

What are the community's skills and limitations?
What is the base of information about the problem or issue?
What are the community's goals, objectives, and priorities?
Do they conflict with yours?
Is there enough interest to sustain the effort needed to deal with the problem?
What are the mechanisms for sharing information?
Is there an identifiable work group? Is it formal or informal? Are there other community groups that will join in?
Is there effective leadership within the community?

In this step the community health nurse-organizer assesses the community's level of sophistication regarding its own leadership, dynamics, parlimentary procedure, objectives, goal development, and management in general. As noted in the ELA case study, training for most groups and boards is essential if they are to function effectively and efficiently. Your first step in developing a plan for board training is to learn where the board is in terms of its members' skills. As a wise community organizer, you will need to find a leader or group of leaders from within the community through whom and with whom you can work. The most skillful community organization is one that everyone believes evolved from within the group itself, without outside help or interventions.

Community organizers need all of their group process skills to help community groups define their goals and priorities, leadership, communication mechanisms, bases of support, and the level of interest to sustain the effort needed to deal with the problem. One of the most effective roles community health nurses can play in this kind of situation is to facilitate the group's progress toward what it wants rather than trying to lay our trip on the group. This process often requires tremendous patience. Needless to say, in most instances the process would be much quicker if the community group would just take our advice and get on with it. The drawback is that the accomplishments, if there are any, are not the community group's own, but rather are another instance of their compliance to an outside force. If community organization is to meet its short-term objective, which is to deal with the situation at hand, as well as its long-term goal, which is to develop the capability within the community to deal effectively with later problems, then we must take the time to help the community learn and do for itself. We cannot help the community meet its own goals if we do not agree with those goals. Thus there must be considerable congruence between the community's goals and objectives and our own. If there isn't, then we had better let someone who is in sympathy with the goals work with the community.

STEP 5: ASSESSMENT OF POLITICAL INFLUENCES IN THE COMMUNITY

Questions to ask:

Who are the identified leaders, both formal and informal, and whom do they represent?
Is their representation broad or limited?
Can they effect changes at higher levels?
What is their financial base?
What are the hidden issues?
Who benefits or loses if the problem or issue is solved? Who benefits and who loses if the problem or issue is unsolved?
Who are the protagonists: grassroots versus professionals? staff versus management? insiders versus outsiders? young versus old?
Which side controls what part of the media?

As community organizer, the community health nurse must attempt to determine what the power base is in the community and how that power base may be shifted. Naturally, you cannot discover all that there is to know in a brief period of time and without the help of others. However, you should know that even as the problem or issue becomes clarified, political influences may continue to be difficult to pin down. You should also know that political influences may prevent the problem or issue from being clarified. As mentioned earlier, community problems are complex, and the reality we face as community organizers is that someone benefits if a problem remains unsolved. Simplistically speaking, the one with the most power usually prevails. Therefore, the more informed we community health nurses are regarding a community's power base and political influences, the less time we will waste looking for support where none is to be had.

STEP 6: EVALUATING ALTERNATIVE COURSES OF ACTION

Questions to ask:

What are the alternatives for dealing with the problem?

What are the pros and cons of each of these alternatives in such areas as probable outcomes, acceptability to the community, probable long- and short-term effects on the community, and cost in all kinds of resources?

Because there is almost always more than one way to address a problem, this step is necessary to enable the community group to study the alternatives from a variety of perspectives. As many possible alternatives as can be thought of should be considered in this step. All-too-often communities jump at what appears to be a likely alternative without taking the time to look more closely for other, possibly better, alternatives. Since by this step in the process community people are often impatient to do something, your help as community organizer is really essential in stressing the need to consider alternatives carefully.

The conclusion of this step is the selection of the best alternative for dealing with the problem on the basis of the kinds of criteria listed under the questions to ask in each step of this guide. A matrix for decision making such as discussed in chapter 11 can be of great assistance in insuring that all possible alternatives are carefully and systematically considered. Once the best alternative is selected, criteria for evaluation of the process and outcomes of its implementation must be developed from the community's goals, objectives, and priorities. The more specific and measurable these evaluation criteria are, the better the evaluation of the group's actions will be.

STEP 7: REDEFINITION OF OBJECTIVES, PRIORITIES, AND THE COMMUNITY HEALTH NURSE'S GOALS

Questions to ask:

Are the objectives and priorities actually what they seemed to be in steps 2 and 4? Are you and the community group still in agreement?

Now that the community assessment is completed, can the goals, objectives, and priorities realistically be met? If not, how should they be restated or revised?

Has the community assessment process uncovered other, and perhaps more important, problems?

Are you too tired or overextended to actively continue in the community organization process? Can your role be turned over to others?

Are other major actors too tired or overextended to carry on?

This step is a stock-taking phase similar to step 7 in the planning process discussed in chapter 3. Here the community health nurse-organizer needs to take the time to see where the process actually is and to validate with the community that the direction in which they are going is the one they want. All-too-often by this step both the community organizer and the community is very close to being burned-out by the effort expended so far. Pausing here for a reevaluation of the situation oftentimes enables everyone concerned to catch his or her breath. It is also an excellent opportunity for everyone to reassess and regroup. Many will be discouraged by this step in the process since much time and energy will have been spent for what appears to be naught. Looking at what has been done as well as what lies ahead is an opportunity to overcome some of these feelings.

This step and step 6 are often undertaken simultaneously and the selection of the best alternative upon which to formulate a plan of action provides a rallying point for flagging energies. This step is also an opportune time to see whether you can take a less obvious role by encouraging the community people to assert more leadership.

STEP 8: DEVELOPING A PLAN OF ACTION

Questions to ask:

What are the best strategies to implement the selected alternative?
Can you buy it?
Can you sell it to those whom it affects?
Does it fit with your style and that of the community?
Can it be realistically carried out?
What groups, agencies, and so forth should be actively involved in the implementation and how?

This step is the nitty-gritty of deciding how the alternative the community group has chosen to deal with the problem will be implemented. The group has already considered time, cost, feasibility, and other criteria in selecting the alternative in step 6. Now it makes the actual, specific plan for doing what it is the members have decided to do.

STEP 9: IMPLEMENT THE PLAN

This step is the action portion of all that has gone before. Here the community group and the organizer implement the plan that has been developed.

STEP 10: EVALUATION OF THE OUTCOME OF THE PLANNED ACTION

Questions to ask:

How many goals and objectives did the plan meet?
Why were we successful (if the plan worked)?
Why were we unsuccessful (if the plan failed)?
What have we learned from the process that will help us next time?
Where do we go from here?

Even if the outcome, as evaluated by the criteria defined in step 6, is not a total success, often some progress has been made. As organizer, you may have to spend a great deal of energy helping community people see that some progress, however small it may be, has been made. Community people, and we too, want everything to come out just as it was planned, which is rarely the case due to the kinds of political processes that almost invariably take place (see chapter 11). What the community members must be helped to see, unless the plan is a real success, is that they have learned a great deal that can be utilized in subsequent efforts. Thus the evaluation process becomes not only assessing what has been accomplished and why, but also looking at what is to be done next.

SUMMARY

Community organization is another skill and another important role for community nurses interested in community autonomy. The case study of my own election to the board of a community action group describes a transformation process that changed both my expectations and my actions in relation to that community and to my own health agency. The experience also gave me a base for identifying strengths and weaknesses in many of the theories of community organizing that affect how this skill is often practiced. As a community member I observed how grassroots board members could be prevented from developing innate strengths for action as well as ways these could be maximized to the ultimate benefit of the entire enterprise.

The crucial influence of the community organizer is considered at length, and the discussion stresses the importance of resisting the professional's urge for efficiency by doing for people things they need to learn to do for themselves even if that does take longer. Patiently permitting the necessary stages to progress from a social to an action stance is one way a community organizer can multiply the effectiveness of involved community members. A guide to help community health nurses become actively involved in community organization is presented in the final section.

REFERENCES

ABRAMS, HERBERT E. "A Community Perspective on Health Care." *Nursing Outlook* 19 (1971): 92–94.

ACKERMAN, N., and BLAISDEL, S. "An Internship in Community Health Nursing." *Nursing Outlook* 23 (1975): 374–77.

ALFORD, R.R. *Health Care Politics: Ideological and Interest Group Barriers to Reform.* Chicago: University of Chicago Press, 1975.

ALINSKY, SAUL D. *Rules for Radicals: A Pragmatic Primer for Realistic Radicals.* New York: Vintage Books, A Division of Random House, 1971.

ALTSHULER, ALAN A. *Community Control.* New York: Pegasus, 1970.

BARKER, R.G., and SCHAGGEN, P. *Qualities of Community Life.* San Francisco: Jossey-Bass, 1973.

BOYLE, JOYCEEN S. "Community Assessment." In A. Reinhardt and M. Quinn, eds., *Family Centered Community Nursing.* St. Louis: C.V. Mosby, 1973.

BRADFORD, LELAND P. *Making Meetings Work: A Guide for Leaders and Group Members.* La Jolla, Calif.: University Associates, 1976.

BRADSHAW, BARBARA R., and MAPP, C. BERMELL. "Consumer Participation in a Family Planning Program." *American Journal of Public Health* 62 (1972): 1336–39.

BRILL, NAOMI I. *Working with People: The Helping Process.* Philadelphia: J.B. Lippincott Co., 1973.

COX, FRED, et al. *Strategies of Community Organization.* Itasca, Ill.: F.E. Peacock Publishers, 1974.

DILLICK, SIDNEY. *Community Organization for Neighborhood Development, Past and Present.* New York: Wm. Morrow and Co., 1953.

ETZIONI, AMITAI. *A Comparative Analysis of Complex Organizations.* New York: Free Press, 1961.

GLASER, BARNEY, and STRAUSS, ANSELM L. *The Discovery of Grounded Theory.* Chicago: Aldine-Atherton, 1967.

GOLDSMITH, H.F., et al. *Typological Approach to Doing Social Area Analysis,* DHEW Publication No. (ADM) 76–262. Washington, D.C.: Superintendent of Documents, U.S. Government Printing Office, 1975.

GROSNER, CHARLES F. "Community Development Programs Serving the Urban Poor." *Social Work* (1965): 15–21.

HAWLEY, WILLIS D., and WIRT, FREDERICK M. *The Search for Community Power,* 2nd ed. Englewood Cliffs, N.J.: Prentice-Hall, 1974.

HENRY, PAUL. "Pimps, Prostitutes, and Policemen: Education of Consumers for Participating in Health Planning." *American Journal of Public Health* 60 (1970): 2171–74.

HOLLAND, T.P. "The Community: Organism or Arena." *Social Work* 19 (January 1974): 78–80.

HUNTER, FLOYD. *Community Power Structure.* Chapel Hill: University of North Carolina Press, 1953.

———, et al. *Community Organization: Action and Inaction.* Chapel Hill: University of North Carolina Press, 1956.

KAHN, SI. *How People Get Power: Organizing Oppressed Communities for Action.* San Francisco: McGraw-Hill Book Co., 1970.

KENT, JAMES. *Descriptive Approach to Community Organization* (Videotape). Denver: Foundation for Urban and Neighborhood Development, 1972.

———. *A Death of Colonialism in Health Programs for the Urban Poor.* Denver: Foundation for Urban and Neighborhood Development, 1972.

———, and SMITH, HARVEY. "Involving the Urban Poor in Health Services through Accommodation—The Employment of Neighborhood Representatives." *American Journal of Public Health* 57 (1967): 977–1003.

KORNHAUSER, WILLIAM. "Power Elite or Veto Groups." In Seymour Martin Lipset and Leo Lowenthal, eds., *Culture and Social Character.* New York: Free Press, 1961.

KRAMER, RALPH M., and SPECHT, HARRY, eds. *Readings in Community Organization Practice.* Englewood Cliffs, N.J.: Prentice-Hall, 1975.

LASSEY, WILLIAM R., and FERNANDEZ, RICHARD R., eds. *Leadership and Social Change,* 2nd ed. La Jolla, Calif.: University Associates, 1976.

LUTHER, THELMA, and BREWER, WILMA D. "Stimulating Community Action in Health." *Nursing Outlook* 18 (1970): 41.

MILIO, NANCY. *9226 Kercheval: The Storefront that Did Not Burn.* Ann Arbor: University of Michigan Press, 1970.

———. *The Care of Health in Communities.* New York: Macmillan Publishing Co., 1975.

NATIONAL COMMISSION ON COMMUNITY HEALTH SERVICES. *Health Is a Community Affair.* Cambridge Mass.: Harvard University Press, 1967.

O.M. COLLECTIVE. *The Organizer's Manual.* New York: Bantam Books, 1971.

OZARIN, LUCY D., and THOMAS, CLAUDEWELL S. "Advocacy in Community Mental Health Programs." *American Journal of Public Health* 62 (1972): 557–59.

PARKER, ALBERTA W. "The Consumer as Policy-Maker—Issues of Training." *American Journal of Public Health* 60 (1970): 2139–53.

PFEIFFER, J. WILLIAM, and JONES, JOHN E. *The 1978 Annual Handbook for Group Facilitators.* La Jolla, Calif.: University Associates, 1978.

REINHARDT, ADINA, and QUINN, MILDRED D. *Family-Centered Community Nursing: A Socio-Cultural Framework.* St. Louis: C.V. Mosby, 1973.

ROSE, ARNOLD M. *The Power Structure: Political Processes in American Society.* New York: Oxford University Press, 1967.

ROSS, MURRAY G. *Community Organization Theory: Principles and Practice,* 2nd ed. New York: Harper & Row, 1967.

RUYBAL, S.E., BAUWENS, E., and FALSA, M.J. "Community Assessment: An Epidemiological Approach." *Nursing Outlook* 23 (1975): 365–68.

SCHATZMAN, LEONARD, and STRAUSS, ANSELM L. *Field Research: Strategies for a Natural Sociology.* Englewood Cliffs, N.J.: Prentice-Hall, 1973.

SCHINDLER-RAINMAN, EVA, and LIPPETT, RONALD. Talking Your Meetings Out of the Doldrums. La Jolla, Calif.: University Associates, 1975.

SELLER, RUDOLPH V. "The Black Health Worker and the Black Consumer—New Roles for Both." *American Journal of Public Health* 60 (1970):2154–70.

SUTTLES, GERALD D. *The Social Construction of Communities.* Chicago: University of Chicago Press, 1972.

TURNER, JOHN B., ed. *Neighborhood Organization for Community Action*. New York: National Association for Social Workers, 1968.

WARREN, DONALD I., and WARREN, RACHELLE B. "Six Kinds of Neighborhoods." *Psychology Today* 9 (June 1975): 74–80.

WARREN, ROLAND. *The Community in America*, 2nd ed. Chicago: Rand McNally and Co., 1972.

PART V

Postscripts and Cautionary Tales

Ruth P. Fleshman
Sarah Ellen Archer

To cover the whole area of community health nursing and not end up with a lot of loose ends, stray ideas, pressing concerns, and a lot of dilemmas is impossible. It would be tidier to quit without bringing up these extra bits. But then we'd have failed to share that other aspect we feel so strongly—not only are we unsure whether there are really right answers in this field, we're not sure we know the really important questions. For that reason we have included this last chapter as a miscellany of thoughts and notions that are not always easy to fit into any logical framework or theoretical structure. We think they're important to wrestle with, so here are some of them.

IS PRIMARY PREVENTION AN ENDANGERED SPECIES?

Recently we have noted a trend for official public health agencies to become increasingly involved in the diagnosis and treatment of disease. Our colleagues in public health administration assure us that this trend disturbs them too. However, they explain that health departments can be reimbursed only for these diagnostic and treatment procedures. Home nursing visits for health promotion are decreasing since only visits for skilled nursing care, as defined by third-party payers, can be billed for. Community health nursing time, they tell us, is much more economically used by having clients come to the clinic to see the nurse. Many community nurses have been prepared to do physical assessments and are being used in clinic settings in place of more expensive physicians. The pressure to follow the medical or disease-focused model results in a loss of health-, OLOF-, and client-centered services. Many of our colleagues who have done generalized public health nursing before and now find themselves in such clinic settings tell us they are not allowed time to work with clients on primary prevention beyond routine immunizations.

There never has been much money available to pay for primary prevention. If there had been, the task of carrying out this mandated activity wouldn't have been left to official health agencies. Health departments, until recently, concentrated most of their resources on primary prevention and some secondary prevention in the area of communicable diseases. But, as we say in chapter 9, now the noninfectious diseases and conditions are the ones for which primary preventive measures must be developed and promulgated. Since the private sector of the health care industry has always concentrated on the treatment of disease, they can never be expected to raise their heads above the flood of demand for just that product. Of course, a few HMOs are beginning to try to do just that since they see how undiminished disease incidence will inevitably erode the economic bases of their enterprise. However, unless the public sector takes back its responsibility for the *public's health,* significant primary prevention will never be done.

The appropriate role of health departments in this case is to educate taxpayers and their elected representatives to appropriate sufficient funds for primary prevention of major noninfectious conditions. With infectious diseases, we could pray another not-too-bad epidemic to persuade the money-holders. Our present major killers in the other category are still largely beyond individual control. Community nurses, especially public health nurses, have a tremendous potential to work in concert with other public health workers in educating the public about what we know and what we still need to know about primary prevention for these diseases. Such government service should continue to be a supported public obligation and primary prevention should be adequately funded. If public health doesn't do it, no one else will, and we shall all be the losers.

DILEMMAS OF CLIENT-CENTERED CARE

A client comes to an emergency service, a doctor's office, or a neighborhood health center. He has clearly been using drugs, is high, has drugs on his person. He asks for services unrelated to his drugged state and makes no unseemly moves. But there is no question that he is violating the laws regarding possession and use of illegal substances. The health workers are faced with a dilemma: to ignore his law-breaking behavior and treat him, or notify law enforcement officials and demand his arrest.

I know from experience how I would deal with the problem, but I cannot expect that every nurse would share my decision. The nature of a dilemma is that neither choice is easy. But I might guess that a large percentage would assess the immediate and long-range hazards of both choices and come down on the side of saying nothing and going about giving care.

Now, let's change one of the conditions: The client asks for treatment of a needle abscess on his ankle. Shooting up in one of his few remaining veins has induced an inflammatory reaction that is grossly infected, painful, and in need of immediate attention.

Although we have many ethical standards that advise us against moralizing about clients' illnesses, it is hard for some of us not to regard certain illnesses as the client's own fault and somehow deserved for violating social norms. Health workers are often abrupt, preachy, and physically hostile toward clients with socially disapproved illnesses; VD is only one example. It is a small bit easier, in these circumstances, to use an illness or its treatment as just punishment.

Let us now add a client who not only fulfills all of the above but, in addition, is argumentative and impolite and refuses to follow requests or directions. He uses obscene language and seems determined to insult everyone in sight.

It does become difficult indeed for us to maintain an even temper in the face of insults. It may help to consider how painful that abscess may be—perhaps his withdrawal symptoms are also sneaking up on him—and we could be a bit sympathetic at his impatience with all those forms we have to fill out. But clients need to realize that we too are human!

As the doctor finally gets started on treating the abscess, he cuts a little before the anesthetic is fully effective and the client takes a swing at him. He misses, but . . . .

Health workers have an obligation to deliver services to clients who may not always be proper or even polite. As health care actually does become a right and not a privilege, we will not be able to expect gratitude or subservience; after all, we don't thank the registrar of voters for letting us exercise our constitutional right to cast our ballots. On the other hand, work conditions are not supposed to be a threat to safety—unless we get hazard pay too. When client actions go beyond simple impoliteness and pass over to the threatening or even dangerous depends as much on our perceptions as on the reality of the behavior. What we do not understand often frightens us. There are also some of us who are foolhardy in our unwillingness to admit danger exists. Like other hard choices, the definition in this situation often depends on the individuals and the circumstances in very specific interactions.

There are also dilemmas in the relation to certain legal issues. Community nurses are especially liable to encounter clients who are violating one or more laws: drug users, illegal immigrants, moonshiners (in many states even homemade beer is illegal). Any of these force us to make decisions only by juggling a number of equal contradictions. There are, of course, the legal constraints that the client has violated, and concealing or condoning them may put the nurse in a law-breaking position too. We must balance a set of loyalties: to the client, for whom we are supposed to have some special obligation; to the system that employs us and pays us to do that job (Is there a stated policy? Are there informal understandings about what is actually to be done?); to ourselves as individuals (Does this situation violate a deep personal belief? Are there special circumstances that make this situation especially sensitive?). In addition, we all carry a professional perspective that commits us to health care delivery, not to maintenance of the legal or judicial systems around us. There are many times when decisions cannot be a clear-cut victory of right over wrong. It may sometimes require balancing a number of poor choices and picking the one with the lowest risk. The violent client, if unarmed, may well be dealt with either by persuasion, by the staff ganging up on him, or by calling the police. The presence of weapons changes the whole scene, whether one or both sides hold them. Being an innocent bystander is not one of our favorite roles!

PRAGMATIC APPROACHES TO THERAPIES

Sometimes we have difficulty in sorting out fads from new trends and even early good results from hysteria and quackery. In our neighborhood right now, for example, everyone is talking about holistic health, which seems to include all the good things anyone has ever heard of. The point is that we can no longer automatically dismiss alternative approaches simply because orthodox Western science does not recognize the underlying philosophy or training methods. We must realize that specialized education within one frame of reference should not deter us from trying to understand a discipline that starts from thoroughly different premises. Some of us are becoming aware of the many ways of managing health problems that have remained resistant to orthodox medicine. Individual testimonies do not suffice to prove or disprove any therapy, but too many clients report aid, relief, help, cure, or whatever from treatments that do not match the logic of conventional anatomy and physiology for us to ignore them. Examples include chiropractic, acupuncture and acupressure, homeopathy, herbalism, massage and other forms of body work, meditation, and yoga. These are often the more conservative therapies used. Many nurses are already involved with some of these practices, either as clients or as practitioners. Although some nurses try to adopt the whole fabric of these modalities, rejecting all the critical skills of Western scientific method seems wasteful.

While providing services that comfort clients in distress is one of the more rewarding aspects of any therapeutic occupation, a better approach in the long run would seem to call for systematically gathering sufficient data that such new-old therapies could move out of the realm of exotica into more general acceptance. Many practitioners and clients are turned off by some of the more mystic trappings to some of the treatments, but we have found it possible to teach relaxation to very straight, elderly clients who would have been instantly alienated by reference to yoga or even meditation. In spite of the conflict between philosophy and therapy, many such techniques have proved useful in many clinical practices and are being tested for their general usefulness in some diseases with strong psychosomatic components.

POWER STRUGGLES

If any one thing should be clear by now, it's that there's no reason to expect a happy ending. Battles are being fought now that will only lead directly into new challenges, defenses, conflicts, and more battles. One that's ongoing right now is the altered position of physicians in the hierarchy of the health care team. Tradition has always vested all the decision making in their hands, and other job categories were created simply to carry out the tasks they could not (or would not) do themselves. Physicians have been divesting themselves of functions and responsibilities without making a major shift in their image. Those of us in the one-down relation have chafed under the necessity of paying lip service to an authority we do not always accept. But, except in a few instances, we have been unable to devise a system that can dethrone the ruler without armed rebellion. We can look at the countries that exist well with constitutional monarchs. These monarchs have many symbols of power and a great deal of influence but a clearly defined job description and a handsome salary.

As group practices have developed, many physicians have left solo practice in seeking the comfortable support of peers. Some major groups have taken the step of employing other physicians, not as equal partners, but as workers under their direction. The expansion of HMOs may make the salaried position for physicians more commonplace. When control of the income passes from physicians to clinic administration, much of their power to demand performance passes too. Although we may find it necessary to continue awhile to defer to the image, it may not be too long before physicians realize that their specialty is not the whole of the health care package.

MALDISTRIBUTION

Governmental support has been provided for professional education in the hope of increasing the number of workers available to rural and other underserved areas in the present scheme of things. More workers are indeed graduated but tend to flock in the same proportions to the same overserved areas. In fact, our impression is that some rural areas are even more depleted than before as the old-time "docs" die off and new ones don't move in to replace them. Many nursing programs generally promise that extended-role nurses will, of course, fill just that gap. But they don't! Such nurses often want high salaries to justify all that education and status, and almost the only place where nurses with added skills can move into high salary positions is in major urban centers with huge clienteles available to cover their costs.

How can this situation be changed? The United States does not have any tradition of mandatory service—even the military draft has been suspended, and nurses were never subject to draft even in wartime, but instead always volunteered in numbers sufficient to meet military needs. Some other nations stipulate one year payback service for all recipients of educational support. Of course, some people manage to have their families buy their way out of that obligation but enough had to repay with service that some outlying areas got some aid. But after the designated time is up, they still flock back to the cities. Thus it is not surprising that our voluntary efforts have gotten little publicity and one might expect them to have had little impact as well. The Public Health Service has tried to provide medical teams for unserved areas, but there are hardly enough teams to go around for all the communities who have no professionals at all.

INDEPENDENCE, SHARED POWER, AND COLLABORATION

A useful point to remember is that there are reciprocals—the other side of the coin—and consequences to any course of action. Nurses moving toward independent practice may not consider the full impact of the loss of the support system they had when within an institution. When restrictions become unbearable, the notion of independence has great allure, but carries whole new problems: managing the income tax without automatic withholding; arranging health and disability insurance as well as malpractice coverage commensurate with the risks. It may well be a relief no longer to have to take orders within the hierarchy, but it also means having no one else to take the responsibility (or blame) when things don't go well. Having the authority to make decisions requires taking the responsibility for the consequences. The traditional medical model has vested both power and responsibility entirely in physicians who often act as though they are one step just below divinity. This relationship is changing. High time! For those of us who do not aspire to full independence, another approach may be possible. Nurse-practitioners who do not hesitate to share decision making with their clients find them not only much more cooperative with the resulting treatment plans but also more willing to accept whatever outcomes arise.

Legal advisors have tried to help practitioners prevent malpractice suits by telling them to be certain to make no claims that have a high likelihood of not being fulfilled. Sharing the notion of differential risks, the odds involved in the various choices, the range of possible outcomes, and the relative uncertainties of practice makes the client more aware of the complexities of any care situation. Claiming omnipotence, accepting total responsibility, and withholding choices tend to maximize the likelihood of clients' bitterness at any degree of failure. For example, one of us listened in on the phone call made by the family of a terminally ill cancer victim to a quack treatment "clinic" and was impressed with the cagey tactics used on them. The manager did not promise a cure; he admitted things sounded grave and mentioned that his clinic had "had some success with this kind of cancer" but he could not tell how things would go for this man. By extending the promise of doing all he could to help when doctors had given up, he offered them a hope so that when the client finally died, they did not resent having spent all that money.

Collaboration within community health agencies provides still another alternative to traditional work roles. Entire volumes can be written about the development of interdisciplinary teams, but one major comment should be made here. The trend in professional preparation has been toward rarefied specialization and greater separation of the various groups, thereby removing any chance for students to practice cross-professional work. Interdisciplinary teams cannot be created from scratch and then expected to set right out about their primary tasks. Group process must take its toll as individuals sort out identities and professional stereotypes before making more realistic assessment for role realignment within the team.

The adjustments involved for everyone to work through to a true team relationship are painful and tedious, but many who go through them report the result more than justifies the trauma. A goal focused on client service rather than territorial or system maintenance may well keep the procedure more humane. Teams report that in the end the special skills and talents of team members receive greater emphasis than the role stereotypes would have allowed; for example, the aide may well be the most appropriate intake worker, the nurse may prove the best primary therapist, the social worker may be best at organizing parent discussion groups even when the topic is diet. As long as job descriptions order the work content the likelihood increases that client needs not only will go unmet when they don't fit but will go unrecognized when they don't match anyone's professional territory.

INVISIBLE PREPARATION

Until recently, identifiable content and practice in public health or community health nursing were required in all baccalaureate nursing programs accredited by the National League for Nursing. Thus we could be sure that graduates of NLN approved programs were prepared to take entry-level jobs as public health nurses, which is no longer the case. In chapter 16, we discussed how all of nursing has discovered the importance of community as a central concept. As a result nursing curricula claimed to integrate this concept throughout the program. However, such integrated curricula now have no identifiable community health nursing courses or field experience, and to all appearances, the community health nursing content is lost. Early analysis from a study of nursing agencies and schools of nursing seems to show that approximately one-third of the service respondents do not consider that students are prepared for public health nursing experience. The result is that many community health agencies require baccalaureate graduates to have at least one year's experience in nursing before they will hire them as community nurses. In addition, many nursing agencies find they must also set up costly in-service "orientation" programs to teach young graduates such basic tools as epidemiology, interviewing, and health teaching before they can carry out the daily activities of their jobs. We think we might have been more than a bit upset had we learned that our professional education had not prepared us to practice our profession. We wonder whether today's consumers of nursing education may be able to work for a better outcome for the practice of community health nursing.

GAIN–LOSS IN CHANGE

Change is exciting, stimulating, interesting, enlivening, everywhere. It is also hard, painful, unsettling, scarey, unpredictable. In spite of the best and most thorough planning, we can't ever anticipate all outcomes. Insofar as growth is change, every living thing must change. There comes a point, however, when change can become destructive. The fibrillating heart cannot do its job because the pulsing becomes too rapid and erratic. A program that is revised from week to week can never demonstrate its accomplishments at any one thing. How, then, can we look at the changes going on in our own field and those around us with total serenity? We need to look not only at the excitement but also at some of the reactions that can arise from change or the threat of change.

If, for instance, our clients become fully participating members of the health team, many of our own enjoyable roles will be taken from us. An advocate is needed only when the clients cannot represent themselves, and demystification of health care may eventually remove the need for such a function as they learn how to fend effectively for themselves. This same process may also diminish the one-up power of special knowledge, especially if we keep sharing it through an educative process. Of course, there will always be the legitimate stature that accompanies special expertise, but that kind of division of labor puts us in an equal status with our clients, many of whom happen to be specialists in their own fields: cooks, electricians, mothers, singers, historians.

These examples of zero-sum games show that when one player acquires functions, the other one's functions decrease. This same situation appears to be operating in the struggle between nurses and hospital administrators over the issue of shared decision making on staffing patterns. Nurses' acquisition of power in this area is clearly perceived as a diminution of the power of the administration, as if it were some fixed quantity. Some physicians also seem to perceive the demands of pushy nurses to take on certain skills as a threat. In such a view, if we do more, we are taking it away from someone else, which is true only as long as the focus is on the job description: X is permitted to do 1, 2, and 3. Y does 4, 5, and 6. If Z comes along and offers to take on 2 and 5, both X and Y get scared they pretty soon won't have any job at all. Reconsider, for example, the reaction of the Pomo health professionals described in chapter 14 to the new nurses coming into their community.

If jobs are directed to objectives, especially in human services, there will always be more to do, either quantitatively or qualitatively. But there is a constant change in the how. The kind of arguments that can arise from this sort of change are quite different from the defensive moves described above. People may be no less furious, but at least there might be less attack/defense when "opponents" are simply debating how best to go about accomplishing their collective business.

ROOM FOR ALL

In chapter 3, Archer laid out a scheme for deciding what were the most appropriate actions for community nurses—by sorting through a whole bunch of criteria. A variation on this theme comes up when we are faced by community problems that we are not prepared by education or experience to deal with, but that are not being addressed by anyone else. The history of public health and community health nursing is filled with women who would not conform to the expected behaviors and took the initiative to correct some health condition that no one else bothered with. Those early-day heroines have modern counterparts, but as always, there are the others who can't resist sniping at nonconformity. The progressive movement of any occupational group is a balance of the forward drive of innovators and the stabilizing influence of the conservators. What is important is that they be able to coexist in the same field. Many of the experimenters are more or less openly impatient with whichever nurses fail to endorse their directions or convert immediately to their cause. But there is an equal intolerance among those who feel they safeguard the true spirit of nursing against the barbarians. If nursing is to attract and retain creative and innovative people, there must be leeway for the pursuit of a wide variety of activities. Such a perspective not only safeguards the rights of the traditionalist but prevents the accusation being leveled against those who venture into new territories: "That's not nursing!" We can turn it around and demand to know: "Why not nursing?"

A field as large as nursing—we are, after all, the largest single category of health workers—has to contain widely diverse types of people, and we would be highly unrealistic to expect total agreement on anything, let alone a controversial topic. Perhaps this is one of the reasons philosophies of nursing are all so vague and platitudinous; if one got specific, there might well be only two nurses who could agreeably subscribe to it.

This section may seem peculiar unless you have experienced the discouragement of standing out on an innovative limb and discovering potshots are being fired at you by other nurses! Thus it is a warning not to assume that all our colleagues think just like we do; we need to watch out for other nurses. It is also a plea to each of us to remember that no one has a monopoly on the Right Way to do things. Just as I have a right to do my thing without having your trip laid on me, so too I have no right to demand that you give up what you are doing.

PAYING YOUR WAY

It's important for students, researchers, or anyone else who operates in the community as part of their occupation to consider the balance between what personal reward they get and what return they give for it. Researchers are becoming aware that subject cooperation cannot be assumed, and the old willingness to answer questions just because they're asked is less operative now than it used to be, especially around universities that spawn student-researchers bursting out on the world with their bright-eyed questionnaires. So too with people who live in various target areas: this season's favorite ghetto or deprived population; our town's redevelopment project; the occupational group of the year. A lot of people have found their time taken up by one after another inquirer who feels a divine right to ask questions and then vanish into the sunset. Students also feel their educational goals override all else, without thinking at what cost to other people with other fish to fry. Health workers and other community do-gooders also have a reputation for making promises of good things to come and then never being able to produce them when the budget priorities come up.

The point for students (and their faculty) to realize is that using other people for learning purposes puts you in their debt. The question here is, then, how do you repay that debt? Sometimes the payoff is in reciprocal service: using an educational experience to provide some needed health service to clients or, conversely, turning a routine service situation into a learning experience. With research (or studies or student projects), client contributions of time, effort, responses, or even desk space in an agency should be repaid with some return: a copy of the paper, a final report of the experience, at least a sincere "thank you." Some of the more innovative client-aid learning experiences have come directly from student concerns. For one example, Filipino men living in a run-down hotel received unexpected health service when some students set up a nursing clinic in their lobby. Small-scale projects can serve as pilots for bigger ones or even grant proposals aiming for the improvement of client care. Students find such projects far more stimulating than routine academic exercises, since they see reality at work in the complexities of a real community project.

CERTIFICATION, LICENSURE, AND ACCREDITATION

The continuation of community health nursing as a generalist field of nursing seems to be implied in the content to be tested in ANA's program of certification in that area of practice. The brochure, *Community Health Nursing Certification,* describes the procedure and states: "The examination is designed to identify content relevant to the provision of direct patient care in all areas of community health nursing" (ANA 1974:4). The areas of content to be covered in the test include the following:

> Process of change,
> Epidemiology,
> Disease prevention (primary, secondary, tertiary),
> Populations at risk,
> Rehabilitation,
> Ecological considerations,
> Economic, cultural considerations,
> Principles and theories of power structure (legislative, politics, decision making),
> Group process,
> Family and community dynamics,
> Coordination and continuity of care,
> Health and safety education,
> Health and social problems,
> Health care planning with patient/family/community,
> Health promotion and health maintenance (ANA 1974:4).

Additional documentation will be needed in case studies from the candidate's special area, a report to illustrate innovation and/or initiative for improving health care, and three evaluative references from others.

Both licensure and certification have, historically, been searches for public legitimation. Much of the impetus for uniform nurse licensing criteria around the turn of this century came from attempts to protect the public by establishing minimum standards. Presumably, possession of a state license or certificate gives assurance that the holder is able to practice that trade safely. There are many grounds for debating that assumption. For example, one of our colleagues arrived at work from a duly licensed beautician with green hair—maybe the fact that she still had hair made him safe? In more vital jobs, such as nursing, is safety the only quality control we would want to have guaranteed? In only a few areas—and so far not in nursing—is there any attempt to provide for reassessment of the continued maintenance of even that standard. In most states we require drivers to repeat their tests at intervals, and the elderly must often prove their ability to perform to some minimal standard because of their possible failings. But a nursing license can remain in force a lifetime without retesting, evidence of continuing education, or even relatively regular employment. In times of explosively changing knowledge, we have difficulty imagining a standardized exam that can test for currency of information. For example, one of us recently took a civil service test for nursing that still asked questions about the Salk vaccine for polio. Anyone who has recently taken state boards knows what we're talking about. Some states have begun to require evidence of continuing education from health professionals, including nurses. Interestingly, much opposition to this idea has come from the ranks of nursing with the claim that it insulted our professionalism by enforcing mandatory requirements. The cynics among us wondered why continuing education needed to be mandatory—if we were all so very professional as to do it without being forced to. In our state nonetheless a vast number of nursing courses are being developed now that we are all required to take some before relicensure.

Professional organizations attempt to establish advanced levels of certification to promote some particular vision of excellence. Presumably not everyone passes these exams so it is clear that such certification is intended as a gatekeeper—that is, to keep the practitioners within some reasonable number and above some qualitative minimum. However, what begins for protection of the public often ends up protecting the practitioner. Physician licensure, for example, has been interpreted as a way of excluding practitioners who do not conform to the single approach to training and practice endorsed by the medical establishment. Nursing educators have tended to insist that higher education must be the only route to advanced specialization; nursing service has been equally adamant in pushing practice as a prerequisite. The nature of compromise suggests that some blend of the two will end up as the final pattern. Perhaps we might complicate the thinking by suggesting that there could well be many routes to excellence, without having to blend the various components.

Another form of credentialing is the accreditation of schools by the state or by special professional organizations—in our case, the National League for Nursing. Specially designated teams descend, at regular intervals, on each nursing school and consider a wide range of factors that ostensibly measure the degree to which a school exceeds the minimum expectations for such institutions. How many faculty are available for how many students? What percentage of graduates pass the state examinations? How well does the program conform to its stated philosophy and objectives? Has it appropriate resources—library, classroom, and so on—to serve students? The items go on and on.

All three kinds of evaluation—licensure, certification, and accreditation—have objective criteria on which the final assessment is based. But in view of the length of time needed to create and standardize tests and other evaluative devices, it is hard to imagine one that can keep up with the changes in the field. Since both the League and ANA take innovation into account, we might well wonder just how it is measured. Individuals and programs have been denied approval because they were too innovative for the criteria used, but in view of the lead time necessary to create the evaluation tool, these innovators may be more in touch with current needs than are the evaluations.

Just as nursing education is confusing, so too are the various methods of credentialing nurses of all kinds. It may prove interesting to consult the findings of the ANA study group at the University of Wisconsin-Milwaukee whose two-year study, completed at the end of 1978, tried to look at all the present forms of granting credentials in order to propose a single system for all the various areas of nursing.

Before leaving the topic of licensure, there is one further development of which we all need to be aware. Although we have many questions about the values of individual licensure, it poses far fewer problems than the proposal for institutional licensure. This plan, endorsed by many institutional administrators, would eliminate all health licenses below physicians and give the training or hiring agency the responsibility for the functions of its workers. At least, with individual licensing your personal license goes with you when you move, and you received it for your performance on some competitive examination with evaluation proceeding from criteria developed within our own profession. Institutional licensure would end any nursing claim to participate autonomously in decision making and place us in a dependent relation to the institution where we work. Health workers would no longer be free to travel with their license as a passport. Hospital administrators may actually see this approach as a solution to their turnover problems with staff. We see institutional licensure as a clear danger to developing any professional independence and a return to the handmaiden role we've been working to live down. We doubt that this form of licensure will even protect the public from unsafe practices; we have no doubts that it will extinguish any glimmer of creativity and innovation in nursing.

COMMUNITY HEALTH NURSES' INVOLVEMENT ON PLANNING FOR COMMUNITIES' HEALTH

We are absolutely convinced that nurses' active, continuous, and informed participation in all kinds of community health planning activities is essential, not only for the value our input can have to community endeavors, but also for the benefits and knowledge we obtain and can share with our clients through our involvement. Health care planning, whether it is done by Health Systems Agencies, boards of health, mental health advisory boards, state legislatures, voluntary organizations—such as Heart, Cancer, and Lung Associations—or by groups targeting on specific populations—such as the aged, high-risk mothers and children, and the handicapped—is too important for us to permit it to take place without input from nurses, especially community health nurses. Because communities are our clients as much as are individuals and families, our involvement in planning for health care is part of our professional responsibilities whether or not this is explicitly stated in our job descriptions.

This responsibility to participate in community health planning activities may be a relatively new idea for some of you, so we want to explain a bit about why we believe it is so important for us as nurses. Helping clients, whether they are individuals, families, groups, or communities, to attain and maintain their optimal level of functioning is an integral part of all of our roles and requires that we come from a holistic perspective (see chapters 1, 2, and 3). Because of this perspective and because we see clients in their own environments, we can bring data to community health planning groups that few other providers will have. Because of our commitment to promoting clients' optimal level of functioning through primary prevention and health education (see chapters 9 and 10), community health nurses are less likely than are other providers to become caught up in disease care and complex medical technological issues. At many community health planning group meetings, for example, we have often found ourselves reminding colleagues that we must look at the needs of those who are healthy as well as of those who are ill. Because the needs of the ill are often more apparent than are the needs of the healthy—by far the larger group—the healthy peoples' needs are often overlooked in our rush to help the obviously needy. For example, a community planning group considering the needs of the aged community almost always reacts with surprise when reminded that less than 5 percent of this group is institutionalized at any one time and so we must address the provision of services for the 95 percent of the aged living outside of institutions.

Thus we often have an educative function with community health planning groups.

As we have often said in this book, consumers are frequently better able to talk with nurses than they are to other providers in community health planning groups, especially women consumers, for many reasons. Consumer involvement is essential if programs and agencies are to really address peoples' needs. People affected by the outcomes of planning groups' deliberations should be involved in those deliberations. Community health nurses are often in an excellent position to identify people who will be affected and to motivate them to participate. Finally, as nurses, we have much to gain professionally from active participation in community planning activities. We can learn a tremendous amount about the communities in which we work. This information can help us better understand needs and resources and so be more able to work with individuals and families. Although some community planning meetings are crashing bores, most are interesting and some are fun. They provide splendid opportunities to meet community influentials and to observe as well as practice a variety of styles of participation. In the long run they are well worth the time and effort spent.

NURSING PRACTICE MOVES TOWARD LIBERATION

The increasing move of community nurses into practitioner roles is a trend that will undoubtedly continue for quite a while. Greater numbers of nurses are feeling that basic nursing education alone is clearly inadequate to form the basis for a professional practice of any kind let alone one of high level skill. In the past, development of specialized nursing knowledge failed to win recognition from the medical elite. We have tried to hack out a variety of special areas to claim independent expertise. Our skill with psychological aspects of patient and family care was a bandwagon a few decades ago. Sociocultural contributions to health care issues occupied our attention in the last decade. Primary care is this season's watchword.

As long as advanced nursing specialization is carried out within institutions controlled by the present power structure, gaining legitimacy will depend far more on personal charisma than actual expertise for individual nurses. Almost every one of us is aware of how little of our full potential can be used.

Community activists have long urged nurses to look to clients for support, and some of us are beginning to see how it pays off. Practice in a community-centered setting can demonstrate consumer legitimation of the new nurse role in ways few physicians ever have. Acceptance has been shown by the fact that clients knowingly use nurses' services, pay for them, express satisfaction with the quality of care, and return to use their services again. Some in fact create problems by openly preferring nurse-practitioners to their physician preceptors.

As insurance companies begin to realize that nurses are capable of carrying out certain medical procedures, they will be fast to notice that nurses cost less than physicians. And the companies will begin to pay nurses' fees rather than physicians' higher ones. When physicians cease to be paid for a service, they will cease giving it. This cycle may seem just another simple-minded economic theory, but it is probably of greater influence than all the interdisciplinary task forces on practitioner legislation will ever be.

When nursing was one of only two respectable trades for women, our profession had a large number of aggressive and active members. After a period of relative quiescence, the conjunction of increased professional expertise with the rise of the women's movement has begun to restore some awareness of our own potential strength. Many active feminists have great scorn for nursing as a mousy women's job. Even some of our more militant nurses despair when the entire group does not rise up with one purpose. There is a growing consciousness that waiting for someone to recognize our virtue doesn't do it; that offering quiet and rational justifications for our value as a coworker in health care doesn't get heard. Like other organizing groups, some of us have begun demanding our right to participate in decision making that affects us and our clients. Even though we are not a totally female profession, the linkages between nursing and the women's movement are both timely and essential. Wilma Scott Heide, president of the National Organization of Women in 1974 and herself a nurse, addressed that year's ANA national convention with an apt exhortation for both women and nurses by saying we've got to "come out of the booth, in the corner, in the back, in the dark."

Index